W9-BRS-979

BY THE EDITORS OF

CONSUMER GUIDE®

AND HUNDREDS OF LEADING DOCTORS

THE
HOME
REMEDIES
HANDBOOK

CONSULTANT:
JOHN H. RENNER, M.D.

President and Medical Director of the Consumer Health
Information Research Institute and Member of the
Board of Directors of the National Council Against Health Fraud

PUBLICATIONS INTERNATIONAL, LTD.

The brand-name products mentioned in this publication are service marks or trademarks of their respective companies. Mention of these products in this publication does not constitute an endorsement by the respective proprietors of Publications International, Ltd., nor does it constitute an endorsement by any of these companies that their products should be used in the manner recommended by this publication.

Neither the Editors of Consumer Guide® and Publications International, Ltd., nor the consultant, authors, medical and technical advisors, or publisher take responsibility for any possible consequences from any treatment, procedure, action, or application of medication or preparation by any person reading or following the information in this book. This publication does not attempt to replace your physician, pharmacist, or other health-care provider. Before undertaking any course of treatment, the publisher, authors, medical and technical advisors, and consultant advise you to check with your doctor, pharmacist, or other health-care provider.

Copyright © 1993 Publications International, Ltd. All rights reserved. This book may not be reproduced or quoted in whole or in part by mimeograph or any other printed or electronic means, or for presentation on radio, television, videotape, or film without written permission from:

Louis Weber, C.E.O.
Publications International, Ltd.
7373 North Cicero Avenue
Lincolnwood, Illinois 60646

Permission is never granted for commercial purposes.

Manufactured in U.S.A.

8 7 6 5 4 3 2 1

ISBN 1-56173-747-X

CONSULTANT:

John H. Renner, M.D., is the president and medical director of the Consumer Health Information Research Institute (CHIRI), a nonprofit organization dedicated to providing reliable and accurate patient health education for preventive care, wellness, and self-help. Dr. Renner also serves as a member of the Board of Directors of the National Council Against Health Fraud; as clinical professor of family practice at the University of Missouri in Kansas City, Missouri; and as an adjunct professor of preventive medicine at the University of Kansas Medical School in Kansas City, Kansas.

CONTRIBUTING WRITERS:

Sue Berkman is a veteran science/health writer who writes for a variety of consumer and professional publications, including *Woman's Day, Good Housekeeping, Health,* and *Women's Health and Fitness News.* She has also coauthored two books on health.

Linda J. Brown is a freelance writer specializing in health and the environment. She writes an environmental column for *Good Housekeeping,* and her articles have appeared in *Self, Omni,* and other national magazines.

Jenny Hart Danowski researches and writes consumer articles for newsletters and magazines in the areas of health, fitness, and psychology. Her work has appeared in Whittle Communications' health and living publications, *Woman's Day,* and *Men's Health.*

Bobbie Hasselbring is the former editor of *Medical SelfCare* and has authored five books on health and psychology. She currently writes a column for the *Oregonian* and has become a nationally recognized health writer. The American Heart Association awarded her its 1991 Award for Media Excellence.

Susan G. Hauser is a freelance writer who works as a contributing writer to the *Wall Street Journal* and as a special correspondent to *People Magazine.*

Susan Nielsen writes regularly on health and consumer issues for such magazines as *Good Housekeeping* and *Family Circle Magazine.* She has been an associate health editor of *Redbook Magazine,* as well as a senior editor for "The Better Way" section of *Good Housekeeping.*

Brianna L. Politzer is a freelance writer specializing in health, medicine, and nutrition. She has worked as a newspaper reporter and an editor. She has contributed to many health publications, including *Medical Tribune News Service, American Health,* and *AIDS-Patient Care.*

Diana Reese is a medical writer who has written for such national publications as *American Health, Health, Longevity, HealthWatch,* and *Physician's Weekly.* She was previously senior editor on health publications at Whittle Communications.

COVER ILLUSTRATIONS:
Leonid Mysakov

INTERIOR ILLUSTRATIONS:
Lorie Robare

MEDICAL AND TECHNICAL ADVISORS

Sabiha Ali, M.D. Neurologist, Houston Headache Clinic, Houston, Texas **David Alpers, M.D.** Professor of Medicine and Chief of the Gastroenterology Division, Washington University School of Medicine, St. Louis, Missouri **Douglas Altchek, M.D.** Assistant Clinical Professor of Dermatology, Mount Sinai School of Medicine, New York, New York **Philip C. Anderson, M.D.** Chairman of Dermatology, University of Missouri–Columbia School of Medicine, Columbia, Missouri **William C. Andrews, M.D.** Executive Director, American Fertility Society; Professor of Obstetrics and Gynecology, Eastern Virginia Medical School, Norfolk, Virginia **Barbara J. Arnold, M.D.** Associate Clinical Professor, University of California Davis, Davis, California **David H. Avery, M.D.** Associate Professor of Psychiatry and Behavioral Sciences, University of Washington School of Medicine Harborview Medical Center, Seattle, Washington **Demetrius H. Bagley, M.D.** Professor of Neurology and Professor of Radiology, Jefferson Medical College, Thomas Jefferson University, Philadelphia, Pennsylvania **Covert Bailey** Fitness/Weight Expert; Author, *Fit or Fat* and *The New Fit or Fat* **Diane Baker, M.D.** Clinical Professor of Dermatology, Oregon Health Sciences University, Portland, Oregon; Advisor, National Psoriasis Foundation **Peter A. Banks, M.D.** Director, Clinical Gastroenterology Service, Brigham and Women's Hospital; Lecturer on Medicine, Harvard Medical School, Boston, Massachusetts **Joseph P. Bark, M.D.** Chairman of Dermatology, St. Joseph Hospital, Lexington, Kentucky; Author, *Retin-A and Other Youth Miracles* and *Skin Secrets* **Andrew Baron, D.D.S.** Clinical Associate Professor, Lenox Hill Hospital, New York, New York **Ronald G. Barr, M.D.C.M.** Associate Professor of Pediatrics and Psychiatry, McGill University; Director of the Child Development Program, Montreal Children's Hospital, Montreal, Quebec, Canada **Erwin Barrington, D.D.S.** Professor of Periodontics, University of Illinois in Chicago, Chicago, Illinois **Michael Baskin, M.D.** Assistant Clinical Professor, Department of Orthopedics, Oregon Health Sciences University, Portland, Oregon **Rodney Basler, M.D.** Chairman, Task Force on Sports Medicine, American Academy of Dermatology; Assistant Professor of Internal Medicine, University of Nebraska Medical Center, Omaha, Nebraska **Judy Basso** President, Chronic Fatigue Syndrome Association of Minnesota, Minneapolis, Minnesota **Evan T. Bell, M.D.** Specialist in Infectious Diseases, Lenox Hill Hospital, New York, New York **Loomis Bell, M.D.** Chief, Pulmonary–Critical Care Medicine, St. Luke's–Roosevelt Hospital Center; Clinical Professor of Medicine, Columbia University College of Physicians and Surgeons, New York, New York **Richard Bennett, M.D.** Assistant Professor of Medicine, Johns Hopkins School of Medicine, Baltimore, Maryland **Michael S. Benninger, M.D.** Chairman, Speech, Voice, and Swallowing Disorders Committee, American Academy of Otolaryngology–Head and Neck Surgery; Vice-Chairperson, Department of Otolaryngology, Henry Ford Hospital, Detroit, Michigan **Wilma Bergfeld, M.D., F.A.C.P.** Head, Clinical Research, Department of Dermatology, Cleveland Clinic Foundation, Cleveland, Ohio **Paul A. Bergh, M.D.** Assistant Professor of Obstetrics and Gynecology, Division of Reproductive Endocrinology, Mount Sinai Medical Center, New York, New York **Cheston M. Berlin, Jr., M.D.** Professor of Pediatrics and Professor of Pharmacology, Pennsylvania State University College of Medicine, Milton S. Hershey Medical Center, Hershey, Pennsylvania **Lawrence H. Bernstein, M.D.** Family Physician, Storrs, Connecticut **Robert A. Berselli, M.D.** Orthopedic Surgeon, Portland, Oregon **Henry J. Bienert, Jr., M.D.** Orthopedic Surgeon, Tulane University School of Medicine, New Orleans, Louisiana **Henry Blackburn, M.D.** Mayo Professor of Public Health and Professor of Medicine, University of Minnesota, Minneapolis, Minnesota **Zachary T. Bloomgarden, M.D.** Assistant Clinical Professor of Medicine, Mount Sinai School of Medicine, New York, New York **Janet Bohanon** Cofounder, National Chronic Fatigue Syndrome Association, Kansas City, Missouri **Larry Borish, M.D.** Staff Physician, National Jewish Center for Immunology and Respiratory Medicine, Denver, Colorado **Jon H. Bosland, M.D.** General Ophthalmologist, Bellevue, Washington **Dennis Bowman** Director, National Communications, Arthritis Foundation, Atlanta, Georgia **Charles Boylan, M.D.** Specialist in Pediatric Ophthalmology, A Children's Eye Clinic, Seattle, Washington **Richard C. Bozian,**

M.D. Director of Research, Monarch Foundation, Cincinnati, Ohio; Professor of Medicine, Assistant Professor of Biochemistry, Director, Division of Nutrition, University of Cincinnati, Cincinnati, Ohio **Earl J. Brewer, Jr., M.D.** Former Head, Rheumatology Division, Texas Children's Hospital, Houston, Texas; Former Clinical Professor, Former Head, Rheumatology Division, Department of Pediatrics, Baylor College of Medicine; Author, *Parenting a Child with Arthritis* **James E. Bridges, M.D.** Family Physician, Fremont, Nebraska **Lee J. Brooks, M.D.** Assistant Professor of Pediatrics, Case Western Reserve University; Director, Sleep Disorders Center, Rainbow Babies and Children's Hospital, University Hospitals of Cleveland, Cleveland, Ohio **Jeffrey L. Brown, M.D.** Clinical Associate Professor of Pediatrics, Department of Pediatrics, Department of Psychiatry, The New York Hospital–Cornell Medical College, New York, New York **Vera Brown** Skin-Care Expert; Author, *Vera Brown's Natural Beauty Book* **W. Virgil Brown, M.D.** Past President, American Heart Association; Professor of Medicine, Director, Division of Arteriosclerosis and Lipid Metabolism, Emory University School of Medicine, Atlanta, Georgia **Allan Burke, M.D.** Assistant Professor of Clinical Neurology, Northwestern University School of Medicine, Chicago, Illinois **John Buse, M.D., Ph.D.** Assistant Professor, Department of Medicine, Section of Endocrinology, University of Chicago; Director, Endocrinology Clinic, University of Chicago Medical Center, Chicago, Illinois **Jay E. Caldwell, M.D.** Director, Alaska Sports Medicine Clinic, Anchorage, Alaska **C. Wayne Callaway, M.D.** Member, 1989–1990 Dietary Guidelines Advisory Committee to the U.S. Department of Agriculture/Department of Health and Human Resources; Associate Clinical Professor of Medicine, George Washington University, Washington, D.C. **William B. Carey, M.D.** Clinical Professor of Pediatrics, University of Pennsylvania School of Medicine; Director, Behavioral Pediatrics, Division of General Pediatrics, Children's Hospital, Philadelphia, Pennsylvania **David B. Carmichael, M.D.** Medical Director, Cardiovascular Institute, Scripps Memorial Hospital, La Jolla, California **Bruce R. Carr, M.D.** Paul C. MacDonald Professor of Obstetrics and Gynecology, Director, Division of Reproductive Endocrinology, University of Texas Southwestern Medical Center, Dallas, Texas **William P. Castelli, M.D.** Director, Framingham Heart Study, Framingham, Massachusetts **Michael Castleman** Former Editor, *Medical SelfCare* magazine; Author, *Cold Cures* **Col. Ernest Charlesworth, M.D.** Assistant Chief of Allergy and Immunology, Wilford Hall U.S. Air Force Medical Center, San Antonio, Texas **Daniel S.J. Choy, M.D.** Assistant Clinical Professor of Medicine, Columbia University College of Physicians and Surgeons; Director, Laser Laboratory, St. Luke's–Roosevelt Hospital Center, New York, New York **Edward R. Christophersen, Ph.D.** Professor of Pediatrics, University of Missouri at Kansas City School of Medicine; Chief, Behavioral Pediatrics Section, Children's Mercy Hospital, Kansas City, Missouri **Sebastian G. Ciancio, D.D.S.** Past President, American Academy of Periodontology; Professor and Chairman, Department of Periodontology, Clinical Professor of Pharmacology, Director, Center for Clinical Dental Studies, School of Dental Medicine, State University of New York at Buffalo, Buffalo, New York **Alvin J. Ciccone, M.D., F.A.A.F.P.** Associate Professor, Department of Family Medicine, Eastern Virginia Medical School, Norfolk, Virginia **Amanda Clark, M.D.** Assistant Professor of Obstetrics and Gynecology, Oregon Health Sciences University, Portland, Oregon **Jack W. Clinton, D.M.D.** Associate Dean of Patient Services, Oregon Health Sciences University School of Dentistry, Portland, Oregon **Peter F. Cohn, M.D.** Chief of Cardiology, State University of New York at Stony Brook Health Sciences Center, Stony Brook, New York **Cheryl Coleman, R.N., B.S.N., I.C.C.E.** Director, Public Relations, International Childbirth Education Association; Childbirth Educator, Hillcrest Medical Center, Tulsa, Oklahoma **Edmond Confino, M.D.** Associate Professor, Director of Gynecology, Department of Obstetrics and Gynecology, Mount Sinai Hospital Medical Center, Chicago, Illinois **Sonja Connor, M.S., R.D.** Coauthor, *The New American Diet*; Research Associate Professor, School of Medicine, Oregon Health Sciences University, Portland, Oregon **Paul Contorer, M.D.** Chief of Dermatology, Kaiser Permanente; Clinical Professor of Dermatology, Oregon Health Sciences University, Portland, Oregon **James R. Couch, Jr., M.D., Ph.D.** Professor and Chairman, Department of Neurology, University of Oklahoma Health Sciences Center, Oklahoma City, Oklahoma **Joan Couch, M.S.A.T.C.** Assistant Professor and Athletic

Trainer, University of Delaware, Newark, Delaware **Donald R. Coustan, M.D.** Professor and Chair, Obstetrics and Gynecology, Brown University School of Medicine; Chief, Obstetrics and Gynecology, Women and Infants Hospital of Rhode Island, Providence, Rhode Island **Mick Crowley, R.N., B.S.N.** Department Manager, Burn Care Center/Neurosurgical Unit, University of Missouri Hospital and Clinics, Columbia, Missouri **Jeffrey A. Cutler, M.D.** Hypertension Specialist and Chief, Prevention and Demonstration Research Branch, National Heart, Lung, and Blood Institute, National Institutes of Health, Bethesda, Maryland **Joseph C. D'Amico, D.P.M.** Podiatrist, New York, New York **C. Ralph Daniel III, M.D.** Clinical Professor of Medicine (Dermatology), University of Mississippi Medical Center, Jackson, Mississippi **John Staige Davis IV, M.D.** Margaret Trolinger Professor of Medicine, University of Virginia School of Medicine, Charlottesville, Virginia **Vincent A. DeLeo, M.D.** Assistant Professor of Dermatology, Columbia–Presbyterian Medical Center, New York, New York **William C. Dement, M.D., Ph.D.** Lowell W. and Josephine Q. Berry Professor of Psychiatry and Behavioral Sciences, School of Medicine, Stanford University; Director, Sleep Disorders Center, Stanford University, Stanford, California **Barbara Deskins, Ph.D, R.D.** Associate Professor of Clinical Dietetics and Nutrition, University of Pittsburgh, Pittsburgh, Pennsylvania **Becky DeSpain, R.D.H., M.Ed.** Director of the Caruth School of Dental Hygiene, Baylor College of Dentistry, Dallas, Texas **Seymour Diamond, M.D.** Founder, Diamond Headache Clinic, Chicago, Illinois **Alan M. Dietzek, M.D.** Vascular Surgeon, North Shore University Hospital, Manhasset, New York; Assistant Professor of Surgery, Cornell Medical College, New York, New York **Karl Doghramji, M.D.** Director, Sleep Disorders Center, Jefferson Medical College, Thomas Jefferson University, Philadelphia, Pennsylvania **Missy Donnell, O.T.R., C.H.T.** Occupational Therapist, The Hand Clinic, Austin, Texas **Cornelius P. Dooley, M.D.** Gastroenterologist, Santa Fe, New Mexico **Douglas A. Drossman, M.D.** Professor of Medicine and Psychiatry, Division of Digestive Diseases, University of North Carolina at Chapel Hill, Chapel Hill, North Carolina **Roland C. Duell, D.D.S., M.S.** Professor of Endodontics, Department of Oral Health Practice, University of Kentucky College of Dentistry, Lexington, Kentucky **Christine Dumas, D.D.S.** Consumer Advisor/Spokesperson, American Dental Association; Assistant Professor of Clinical Dentistry, University of Southern California, Los Angeles, California **William Dvorine, M.D.** Chief of Dermatology, St. Agnes Hospital, Baltimore, Maryland **Harry S. Dweck, M.D.** Director, Regional Neonatal Intensive Care Unit, Westchester Medical Center; Professor of Pediatrics, Associate Professor of Obstetrics and Gynecology, New York Medical College, Valhalla, New York **Johanna Dwyer, D.Sc., R.D.** Director, Frances Stern Nutrition Center, New England Medical Center Hospitals; Professor, Tufts University School of Nutrition; Professor, Tufts University Medical School, Boston, Massachusetts **Rose Dygart** Cosmetologist; Barber; Hair-Care Instructor; Manicurist; Owner, Le Rose Salon of Beauty, Lake Oswego, Oregon **Robert Eliot, M.D.** Director, Institute of Stress Medicine; Professor of Cardiology, University of Nebraska Medical Center, Omaha, Nebraska **Melvin Elson, M.D.** Medical Director, The Dermatology Center, Inc., Nashville, Tennessee; Coauthor, *The Good Look Book*; Director, Cosmeceutical Research Institute, Inc., New York, New York **Bruce Epstein, M.D.** Spokesperson, American Academy of Pediatrics; Pediatrician, St. Petersburg, Florida **William Epstein, M.D.** Professor of Dermatology, University of California at San Francisco, San Francisco, California **Victor G. Ettinger, M.D.** Medical Director, Bone Diagnostic Centres, Torrance and Long Beach, California **Andrew S. Farber, M.D., F.A.C.S.** Ophthalmologist, Terre Haute, Indiana **Richard Ferber, M.D.** Director, Center for Pediatric Sleep Disorders, Children's Hospital; Assistant Professor of Neurology, Harvard Medical School, Boston, Massachusetts **Kenneth R. Fineman, Ph.D.** Clinical Psychologist and Associate Clinical Professor of Medical Psychology, University of California at Irvine School of Medicine, Irvine, California **Alexander A. Fisher, M.D., F.A.A.D.** Author, *Contact Dermatitis*; Clinical Professor of Dermatology, New York University Medical Center, New York, New York **Rosemarie L. Fisher, M.D.** Professor of Medicine, Division of Digestive Diseases, Yale University School of Medicine, New Haven, Connecticut **Steven C. Fiske, M.D.** Past President, New Jersey Gastroenterological Society; Associate Professor of Medicine/Gastroenterology, Seton Hall University School of Postgraduate Medicine; Assistant Clinical

Professor of Medicine and Gastroenterology, University of Medicine and Dentistry of New Jersey, Newark, New Jersey **Raymond Flannery, Jr., Ph.D., F.A.P.M.** Author, *Becoming Stress Resistant*; Assistant Professor of Psychology, Department of Psychiatry, Harvard Medical School at the Cambridge Hospital, Cambridge, Massachusetts **Michael O. Fleming, M.D., F.A.A.F.P.** Family Physician, Shreveport, Louisiana **Sharon Fleming, Ph.D.** Associate Professor of Food Science, Department of Nutritional Sciences, University of California at Berkeley, Berkeley, California **Patricia Fosarelli, M.D.** Assistant Professor of Pediatrics, Johns Hopkins School of Medicine, Baltimore, Maryland **Jonti Fox** Former Associate Program Director, Colorado Outward Bound School, Denver, Colorado **Raven Fox, R.N., I.B.C.L.C.** Registered Nurse and Lactation Consultant, Evergreen Hospital Medical Center, Kirkland, Washington **Phyllis Frey, A.R.N.P.** Nurse Practitioner, Bellevue, Washington **Lawrence S. Friedman, M.D.** Associate Professor of Medicine, Jefferson Medical College, Thomas Jefferson University, Philadelphia, Pennsylvania **Patrick C. Friman, Ph.D.** Clinical Psychologist, Father Flanagan's Home for Boys, Boys Town, Nebraska; Associate Professor of Pediatrics, University of Nebraska Medical School; Associate Professor of Human Communication and Otolaryngology, Creighton University Medical School, Omaha, Nebraska **Clifton T. Furukawa, M.D.** Past Chairman, Professional Education Council, American Academy of Allergy and Immunology; Clinical Professor of Pediatrics, University of Washington School of Medicine, Seattle, Washington **Kathleen Galligan, D.C.** Chiropractor, Lake Oswego, Oregon **Glenn B. Gastwirth, D.P.M.** Deputy Executive Director, American Podiatric Medical Association, Bethesda, Maryland **Michael E. Geisser, Ph.D.** Assistant Professor, Department of Clinical and Health Psychology, University of Florida, Gainesville, Florida **Hugh Gelabert, M.D.** Assistant Professor of Surgery, Section of Vascular Surgery, University of California at Los Angeles School of Medicine, Los Angeles, California **Ruby Ghadially, M.D.** Assistant Clinical Professor, Department of Dermatology, University of California at San Francisco, San Francisco, California **David N. Gilbert, M.D.** Director, Chiles Research Institute; Director, Department of Medical Education, Providence Medical Center, Portland, Oregon **J. Christian Gillin, M.D.** Professor of Psychiatry, Director, Mental Health Clinical Research Center, University of California at San Diego; Staff Psychiatrist, Veterans Administration Medical Center; Adjunct Professor in the Department of Psychology, San Diego State University, San Diego, California **Donald Girard, M.D.** Head, Division of General Internal Medicine, Oregon Health Sciences University, Portland, Oregon **W. Paul Glezen, M.D.** Pediatrician, Influenza Research Center, Professor of Microbiology and Immunology, Professor of Pediatrics, Chief Epidemiologist, Baylor College of Medicine, Houston, Texas **Billy Glisan, M.S.** Director, Injury Prevention Program, Texas Back Institute, Dallas, Texas **Alan H. Gluskin, D.D.S.** Associate Professor and Chairperson, Department of Endodontics, University of the Pacific School of Dentistry, San Francisco, California **David Golden, M.D.** Chair, Insect Committee, American Academy of Allergy and Immunology; Assistant Professor of Medicine, Johns Hopkins University, Baltimore, Maryland **Howard Goldin, M.D.** Clinical Professor of Medicine, The New York Hospital–Cornell Medical Center, New York, New York **Gary H. Goldman, M.D.** Assistant Attending Physician, The New York Hospital–Cornell Medical Center, New York, New York **Cary Goldstein, D.M.D.** Special Lecturer in Esthetic Dentistry, Emory University School of Dentistry, Atlanta, Georgia **Irwin Goldstein, M.D.** Professor of Urology, Boston University School of Medicine; Codirector, New England Male Reproductive Center at University Hospital, Boston, Massachusetts **Philip Gormley, W.E.M.T.** Operations Director, Wilderness Medical Associates, Bryant Pond, Maine **Arthur I. Grayzel, M.D.** Senior Vice-President for Medical Affairs, Arthritis Foundation, Atlanta, Georgia **Barbara Greene** Clinical Psychology Doctoral Candidate, State University of New York, Albany, New York **Arnold J. Greenspon, M.D.** Clinical Professor of Medicine, Director of the Cardiac Electrophysiology Laboratory, Thomas Jefferson University Hospital, Philadelphia, Pennsylvania **Sadja Greenwood, M.D.** Assistant Clinical Professor, Department of Obstetrics, Gynecology, and Reproductive Sciences, University of California at San Francisco, San Francisco, California **Fredric Haberman, M.D.** Author, *The Doctor's Beauty Hotline* and *Your Skin: A Dermatologist's Guide to a Lifetime of Beauty and Health*; Teaching Faculty, Montefiore Medical Center–Albert

Einstein School of Medicine, New York, New York **Jon M. Hanifin, M.D.** Professor of Dermatology, Oregon Health Sciences University; Board Member, Eczema Association for Science and Education, Portland, Oregon **Terry L. Hankey, M.D.** Clinical Associate Professor of Family Practice, University of Wisconsin School of Medicine, Madison, Wisconsin **Richard E. Hannigan, M.D.** Specialist in Internal Medicine, Helotes, Texas **Ernest L. Hartmann, M.D.** Professor of Psychiatry, Tufts University Medical School; Director, Sleep Disorders Center, Newton–Wellesley Hospital, Boston, Massachusetts **Jack Harvey, M.D.** Coauthor, *Coaching Young Athletes*; Chief of Sports Medicine, Orthopaedic Center of the Rockies, Ft. Collins, Colorado **Peter Hauri, Ph.D.** Author, *No More Sleepless Nights*; Professor of Psychology, Director, Mayo Clinic Insomnia Program, Rochester, Minnesota **Gregory F. Hayden, M.D.** Professor of Pediatrics, Attending Pediatrician, University of Virginia Health Sciences Center, Charlottesville, Virginia **Sandra Hazard, D.M.D.** Managing Dentist, Willamette Dental Group, Inc., Oregon **Robert P. Heaney, M.D.** John A. Creighton University Professor, Creighton University, Omaha, Nebraska **James A. Hearn, M.D.** Assistant Professor of Medicine, University of Alabama at Birmingham, Birmingham, Alabama **E.M. Hecht, M.D.** General Practitioner, New York, New York **Michael B. Heller, M.D., F.A.C.E.P.** Associate Professor of Medicine, Division of Emergency Medicine, University of Pittsburgh School of Medicine, Pittsburgh, Pennsylvania **Michael J. Henehan, D.O.** Director of the Sports Medicine Department, Stanford/San Jose Family Practice Residency Program, San Jose, California **Mindy Hermann, R.D.** Spokesperson for the American Dietetic Association **Sherman Hess, B.S., R.Ph.** Registered Pharmacist and Manager, Hillsdale Pharmacy, Portland, Oregon **Claudia Holland, M.D.** Assistant Clinical Professor of Obstetrics and Gynecology, Columbia–Presbyterian Medical Center, New York, New York **John W. House, M.D.** Associate Clinical Professor, Department of Otolaryngology, Head and Neck Surgery, University of Southern California at Los Angeles; President, House Ear Institute; Otologist–Neurotologist, House Ear Clinic, Los Angeles, California **Ellen Nona Hoyven, P.T.** Owner and Director, Ortho Sport Physical Therapy P.C., Clackamas, Oregon **Rose Hust** Osteoporosis Coordinator, Knoxville Orthopedic Clinic, Knoxville, Tennessee **Joseph Iannotti, M.D., Ph.D.** Assistant Professor of Orthopedic Surgery, Chief of Shoulder Service, University of Pennsylvania, Philadelphia, Pennsylvania **Pascal James Imperato, M.D.** Professor and Chairman, Department of Preventive Medicine and Community Health, State University of New York Health Science Center, Brooklyn, New York **Janna Jacobs, P.T., C.H.T.** President, Section on Hand Rehabilitation, American Physical Therapy Association (APTA) **Katherine Jeter, Ed.D., E.T.** Executive Director, Help for Incontinent People (HIP), Union, South Carolina **John C. Johnson, M.D.** Past President, American College of Emergency Physicians; Director, Emergency Department, Porter Memorial Hospital, Valparaiso, Indiana **Lanny L. Johnson, M.D.** Clinical Professor of Surgery, Michigan State University, East Lansing, Michigan **Conrad Johnston, M.D.** Chief, Division of Endocrinology and Metabolism, Indiana University School of Medicine, Indianapolis, Indiana **James F. Jones, M.D.** Professor of Pediatric Medicine, University of Colorado School of Medicine; Staff Member, National Jewish Center for Immunology and Respiratory Medicine, Denver, Colorado **Stephen R. Jones, M.D.** Chief of Medicine, Good Samaritan Hospital and Medical Center; Associate Professor of Medicine, Oregon Health Sciences University, Portland, Oregon **Judy Jordan, M.D.** Spokesperson, American Academy of Dermatology; Dermatologist, San Antonio, Texas **Donald B. Kamerer, M.D., F.A.C.S.** Professor, Department of Otolaryngology, University of Pittsburgh School of Medicine; Staff Physician, Pittsburgh Eye and Ear Hospital, Pittsburgh, Pennsylvania **Chrissy Kane, L.P.T.** Physical Therapist, Outpatient Physical Therapy Department, Providence Medical Center, Portland, Oregon **Marcia Kielhofner, M.D.** Clinical Assistant Professor of Medicine, Baylor College of Medicine, Houston, Texas **Pamela Kirby, O.T.R./L., C.H.T.** Occupational Therapist, Certified Hand Therapist, The Hand Center, Greensboro, North Carolina **Alan D. Klein, M.D.** Spokesperson, American Academy of Dermatology; Teaching Staff, Ventura County Medical Center, Ventura, California **Albert M. Kligman, M.D., Ph.D.** Emeritus Professor of Dermatology, University of Pennsylvania School of Medicine, Philadelphia, Pennsylvania **Matthew J. Kluger, Ph.D.** Professor of Physiology, University of Michigan Medical School, Ann Arbor, Michigan **Albert B. Knapp, M.D., F.A.C.P.** Adjunct Assistant Attending Physician, Lenox Hill Hospital, New York, New York; Instructor in Medicine, New York Medical College, Valhalla, New York **Elizabeth Knobler, M.D.** Assistant Clinical Professor of Dermatology, Columbia–Presbyterian Medical Center, New York, New York **Sefra Kobrin Pitzele** Author, "We Are Not Alone: Learning to Live with Chronic Illness" **Daniel P. Kohen, M.D.** Director, Behavioral Pediatrics Education Program, Minneapolis Children's Medical Center, Minneapolis, Minnesota **Zeb Koran, R.N., C.E.N., C.C.R.N.** Director, Educational Services, Emergency Nurses Association, Chicago, Illinois **Denise Kraft, M.D., F.A.A.F.P.** Family Practitioner, Bellevue, Washington **Kermit E. Krantz, M.D.** University Distinguished Professor, Professor of Gynecology and Obstetrics, Professor of Anatomy, University of Kansas Medical Center, Kansas City, Kansas **Stephen Kriebel, M.D.** Family Physician, Forks, Washington **Daniel Kuriloff, M.D.** Associate Director, Department of Otolaryngology–Head and Neck Surgery, St. Luke's–Roosevelt Hospital Center; Associate Professor, Columbia University College of Physicians and Surgeons, New York, New York **Myron M. LaBan, M.D.** Director, Department of Physical Medicine and Rehabilitation, William Beaumont Hospital, Royal Oak, Michigan; Clinical Professor of Physical Medicine and Rehabilitation, Wayne State University, Detroit, Michigan; Clinical Professor of Health Sciences, Oakland University, Rochester, Michigan **Raymond Lam, M.D., F.R.C.P.** Assistant Professor, Department of Psychiatry, Psychiatrist, Mood Disorders Program, University of British Columbia, Vancouver, British Columbia, Canada **Jerold Lancourt, M.D.** Orthopedic Surgeon, North Dallas Orthopedics & Rehabilitation, P.A., Dallas, Texas **Robert P. Langlais, D.D.S., M.S.** Spokesperson for the American Academy of Oral Medicine; Professor, Department of Dental Diagnostic Science, University of Texas Health Science Center at San Antonio School of Dentistry, San Antonio, Texas **Daniel M. Laskin, D.D.S., M.S.** Professor and Chairman, Department of Oral and Maxillofacial Surgery, Director, TMJ and Facial Pain Research Center, Medical College of Virginia, Richmond, Virginia **Ira J. Laufer, M.D.** Clinical Associate Professor of Medicine, New York University School of Medicine; Medical Director, The New York Eye and Ear Infirmary Diabetes Treatment Center, New York, New York **Andrew Lazar, M.D.** Assistant Professor of Clinical Dermatology, Northwestern University School of Medicine, Chicago, Illinois **Paul Lazar, M.D.** Professor of Clinical Dermatology, Northwestern University School of Medicine, Chicago, Illinois **Harold E. Lebovitz, M.D.** Professor of Medicine, Chief of Endocrinology and Diabetes, Director, Clinical Research Center, State University of New York Health Science Center, Brooklyn, New York **Mark Lebwohl, M.D.** Medical Advisor, National Psoriasis Foundation; Director of Clinical Dermatology, Mount Sinai School of Medicine, New York, New York **David J. Leffell, M.D.** Assistant Professor of Dermatology, Chief of Mohs Surgery, Yale University School of Medicine, New Haven, Connecticut **George Lefkovits, M.D., F.A.C.S.** Assistant Professor of Surgery, New York Medical College, Valhalla, New York **Theodore Lehman, M.D.** Associate Clinical Professor of Surgery (Urology), Oregon Health Sciences University; Director, The Oregon Impotence Center, Portland, Oregon **Suzanne M. Levine, D.P.M.** Podiatrist, New York, New York **Alan S. Levy, D.D.S.** Clinical Instructor, University of Southern California School of Dentistry, Los Angeles, California **Gary R. Lichtenstein, M.D.** Assistant Professor of Medicine, University of Pennsylvania School of Medicine, Philadelphia, Pennsylvania **Joseph A. Lieberman III, M.D., M.P.H.** Chairman, Department of Family and Community Medicine, Medical Center of Delaware, Wilmington, Delaware **Jerome Z. Litt, M.D.** Author, *Your Skin: From Acne to Zits*; Assistant Clinical Professor of Dermatology, Case Western Reserve University School of Medicine, Cleveland, Ohio **Allan L. Lorincz, M.D.** Professor of Dermatology, University of Chicago Medical Center, Chicago, Illinois **Lawrence Magee, M.D.** Coordinator, Sports Medicine Clinic, University of Kansas, Lawrence, Kansas **Mark Mahowald, M.D.** President, American Sleep Disorders Association; Director, Minnesota Regional Sleep Disorders Center, Hennepin County Medical Center, Minneapolis, Minnesota **Irwin D. Mandel, D.D.S.** Professor Emeritus of Dentistry, Columbia University School of Dental and Oral Surgery, New York, New York **Sanford M. Markham, M.D.** Assistant Professor of Obstetrics and Gynecology, Georgetown University Medical Center, Washington, D.C. **Allan D. Marks, M.D.** Associate Professor of Medicine, Director, Hypertension Clinic, Temple University Health Sciences Center, Philadelphia,

Pennsylvania **Andy Marshall** Scuba Instructor, Portland, Oregon **Michael Martindale, L.P.T.** Physical Therapist, Sports Medicine Center, Portland Adventist Medical Center, Portland, Oregon **Robert Matheson, M.D.** Dermatologist, Portland, Oregon **Mitchell Max, M.D.** Chief, Clinical Trials Unit, Pain Research Clinic, National Institute of Dental Research, National Institutes of Health, Bethesda, Maryland **Raymond Merkin, D.P.M.** Podiatrist, Rockville, Maryland **Elliot Michael, D.P.M.** Director, Residency Program for Podiatric Medicine, Holladay Park Hospital, Portland, Oregon **V.E. Mikkelson, M.D.** Retired General Practitioner, Hayward, California **Marilyn C. Miller, D.D.S., F.A.G.D.** Codirector, Princeton Dental Resource Center, Princeton, New Jersey **Gabe Mirkin, M.D.** Author, "The Mirkin Report," a monthly newsletter on health, fitness, and nutrition; Associate Professor, Georgetown University Medical School, Washington, D.C. **Monica L. Monica, M.D., Ph.D.** Ophthalmologist, New Orleans, Louisiana **Anthony Montanaro, M.D.** Associate Professor of Medicine, Division of Allergy and Immunology, Oregon Health Sciences University, Portland, Oregon **H. Christopher Moore III, M.D.** Assistant Professor, Department of Otolaryngology/Head and Neck Surgery, University of California at Irvine, Irvine, California **Gregg R. Morris, D.C.** Chiropractor, Beaverton, Oregon **Michael S. Morris, M.D.** Otolaryngologist and Assistant Professor, Georgetown University School of Medicine, Washington, D.C. **Alan N. Moshell, M.D.** Director, Skin Disease Program, National Institute of Arthritis and Musculoskeletal and Skin Diseases, National Institutes of Health, Bethesda, Maryland **Willibald Nagler, M.D.** Anne and Jerome Fisher Physiatrist-in-Chief, Chairman of the Department of Rehabilitation Medicine, The New York Hospital–Cornell Medical Center, New York, New York **Charlie Nardozzi** Horticulturist, National Gardening Association, Burlington, Vermont **National Waterbed Retailers' Association** Chicago, Illinois **Luis Navarro, M.D.** Author, *No More Varicose Veins*; Founder and Director, Vein Treatment Center, New York, New York **Harold Neu, M.D.** Professor of Medicine and Pharmacology, Columbia University College of Physicians and Surgeons, New York, New York **Michael G. Newman, D.D.S.** President of the American Academy of Periodontology; Adjunct Professor of Periodontology, University of California at Los Angeles School of Dentistry, Los Angeles, California **Noreen Heer Nicol, M.S., R.N., F.N.C.** Senior Clinical Instructor, University of Colorado Health Sciences Center School of Nursing; Dermatology Clinical Specialist/Nurse Practitioner, National Jewish Center for Immunology and Respiratory Medicine, Denver, Colorado **Linda Niessen, D.M.D., M.P.H.** Associate Professor and Chair, Geriatric Oral Medicine, Department of Community Health and Preventive Dentistry, Baylor College of Dentistry, Dallas, Texas **German Nino-Murcia, M.D.** Founder and Medical Director, Sleep Medicine and Neuroscience Institute, Palo Alto, California **Lawrence A. Norton, M.D.** Clinical Professor of Dermatology, Boston University School of Medicine, Boston, Massachusetts **Nelson Lee Novick, M.D.** Author, *Super Skin: A Leading Dermatologist's Guide to the Latest Breakthroughs in Skin Care*; Associate Clinical Professor of Dermatology, Mount Sinai School of Medicine, New York, New York **Edward J. O'Connell, M.D.** Past President, American College of Allergy and Immunology; Professor of Pediatrics, Allergy/Immunology, Mayo Clinic, Rochester, Minnesota **William O'Donohue, Ph.D.** Assistant Professor of Psychology, Northern Illinois University, De Kalb, Illinois **Dan Oren, M.D.** Senior Clinical Investigator, National Institute of Mental Health, National Institutes of Health, Bethesda, Maryland **Richard Ottaviano** President, Covermark Cosmetics, Moonachie, New Jersey **Carole Palmer, Ed.D., R.D.** Associate Professor and Cochair, Division of Nutrition and Preventive Dentistry, Tufts University School of Dental Medicine, Boston, Massachusetts **Mary Papadopoulos, D.P.M.** Podiatrist, Alexandria, Virginia **Frank Parker, M.D.** Professor and Chairman, Department of Dermatology, Oregon Health Sciences University, Portland, Oregon **Nalin M. Patel, M.D.** Author of *The Doctor's Guide to Your Digestive System*; Clinical Instructor, University of Illinois at Urbana–Champaign, Champaign, Illinois **Richard J. Paulson, M.D.** Associate Professor of Obstetrics and Gynecology, Director, In Vitro Fertilization Program, University of Southern California School of Medicine, Los Angeles, California **Hillard H. Pearlstein, M.D.** Assistant Clinical Professor of Dermatology, Mount Sinai School of Medicine, New York, New York **Jeannette M. Pergam, M.D.** Assistant Professor of Pediatrics, University of Nebraska Medical Center, Omaha, Nebraska **Stephen W.**

Perkins, M.D., F.A.C.S. Facial Plastic Surgeon, Indianapolis, Indiana **Henry D. Perry, M.D.** Clinical Associate Professor of Ophthalmology, Cornell Medical College, New York, New York **John H. Phillips, M.D.** Lassen Professor of Cardiovascular Medicine, Tulane University School of Medicine, New Orleans, Louisiana **Robert A. Phillips, M.D., Ph.D.** Director, Hypertension Section, Associate Director, Cardiovascular Training Program, Division of Cardiology, Mount Sinai Medical Center, New York, New York **Sandra H. Phipps, P.T.** Physical Therapist, Slippery Rock University, Slippery Rock, Pennsylvania **Neville R. Pimstone, M.D.** Chief of Hepatology, Division of Gastroenterology, University of California Davis, Davis California **Rock G. Positano, D.P.M., M.Sc., N.P.H., F.A.C.P.R.** Codirector, Foot and Ankle Orthopedic Institute, Hospital for Special Surgery, New York, New York **David Posner, M.D.** Assistant Professor of Medicine, University of Maryland School of Medicine, Baltimore, Maryland **Glenn M. Preminger, M.D.** Associate Professor of Urology/Internal Medicine, University of Texas Southwestern Medical Center, Dallas, Texas **Orvalene Prewitt** President, National Chronic Fatigue Syndrome Association, Kansas City, Missouri **Richard Price, D.M.D.** Consumer Advisor/Spokesperson, American Dental Association **Arnold Prywes, M.D.** Head, Glaucoma Clinic, Long Island Jewish Medical Center, New Hyde Park, New York; Assistant Clinical Professor of Ophthalmology, Albert Einstein Medical College, New York, New York; Chief of Ophthalmology, Mid-Island Hospital, Bethpage, New York **Deborah Purcell, M.D.** Past Chair, Department of Pediatrics, St. Vincent Hospital and Medical Center, Portland, Oregon **Gayle Randall, M.D.** Assistant Professor of Medicine, Department of Medicine, University of California, Los Angeles, School of Medicine, Los Angeles, California **David Rempel, M.D.** Assistant Professor of Medicine, Director, Ergonomics Laboratory, University of California at San Francisco, San Francisco, California **Basil M. Rifkind, M.D., F.C.R.P.** Chief, Lipid Metabolism and Atherogenesis Branch, National Heart, Lung and Blood Institute, National Institutes of Health, Bethesda, Maryland **Margaret Robertson, M.D.** Staff Physician, St. Vincent Hospital and Medical Center, Portland, Oregon **Robert S. Robinson, M.D.** General Practitioner, Metter, Georgia **Charles A. Rockwood, Jr., M.D.** Past President, American Academy of Orthopaedic Surgeons; Past President, American Shoulder and Elbow Surgeons; Professor of Orthopedics, University of Texas Medical School, San Antonio, Texas **Gary Rogers, M.D.** Associate Professor of Dermatology and Surgery, Boston University School of Medicine, Boston, Massachusetts **James Rogers, M.D.** Adolescent and Sports Medicine Physician, Virginia Mason Medical Center; Clinical Associate Professor of Pediatrics, University of Washington School of Medicine, Seattle, Washington **Paul Rosch, M.D.** President, The American Institute of Stress, Yonkers, New York **Suzanne Rose, M.D.** Assistant Professor of Medicine, University of Pittsburgh Medical Center, Pittsburgh, Pennsylvania **Richard B. Rosenbaum, M.D.** Clinical Associate Professor of Neurology, Oregon Health Sciences University, Portland, Oregon **Lynda E. Rosenfeld, M.D.** Associate Professor of Medicine and Pediatrics, Yale University School of Medicine, New Haven, Connecticut **Norton Rosensweig, M.D.** Associate Clinical Professor of Medicine, Columbia University College of Physicians and Surgeons, New York, New York **Thomas Roth, Ph.D.** Chief, Division of Sleep Disorders Medicine, Henry Ford Hospital, Detroit, Michigan **Donald Rudikoff, M.D.** Assistant Clinical Professor of Dermatology, Mount Sinai School of Medicine, New York, New York **John D. Rugh, Ph.D.** Professor, Department of Orthodontics, Director of Research for the Dental School, University of Texas Health Science Center at San Antonio, San Antonio, Texas **William F. Ruschhaupt, M.D.** Staff Physician, Department of Vascular Medicine, Cleveland Clinic Foundation, Cleveland, Ohio **Paul S. Russell, M.D.** Past Officer, American Academy of Dermatology; Clinical Professor of Dermatology, Oregon Health Sciences University, Portland, Oregon **David A. Sack, M.D.** Associate Professor, School of Public Health, Director, International Travel Clinic, Johns Hopkins University, Baltimore, Maryland **Peter K. Sand, M.D.** Associate Professor of Obstetrics and Gynecology, Northwestern University School of Medicine; Director, Evanston Continence Center, Evanston Hospital, Evanston, Illinois **Joel R. Saper, M.D.** Director, Michigan Headache and Neurological Institute, Ann Arbor, Michigan **Marty Sawaya, M.D., Ph.D** Assistant Professor of Dermatology and Biochemistry, State University of New York at Brooklyn, Brooklyn, New York **Gordon Scarbrough** Owner and Instructor, Moler Barber

College, Portland, Oregon **Richard K. Scher, M.D.** Professor of Clinical Dermatology, Columbia University School of Medicine, New York, New York **Raul C. Schiavi, M.D.** Professor of Psychiatry, Director, Human Sexuality Program, Mount Sinai School of Medicine, New York, New York **Andrew Schink, D.P.M.** Past President, Oregon Podiatric Medical Association **Robert C. Schlant, M.D.** Professor of Medicine (Cardiology), Emory University School of Medicine, Atlanta, Georgia **Alexander Schleuning, M.D.** Professor and Chairman, Department of Otolaryngology/Head and Neck Surgery, Oregon Health Sciences University, Portland, Oregon **Neil Schultz, M.D.** Dermatologist, New York, New York **Marvin Schuster, M.D.** Professor of Medicine with Joint Appointment in Psychiatry, Johns Hopkins University School of Medicine; Chief, Division of Digestive Diseases, Francis Scott Key Medical Center, Baltimore, Maryland **Alan R. Shalita, M.D.** Chairman, Department of Dermatology, State University of New York Health Science Center at Brooklyn, Brooklyn, New York **Gary Y. Shaw, M.D.** Associate Professor of Otolaryngology, Head and Neck Surgery, University of Kansas Medical Center, Kansas City, Kansas **James Shaw, M.D.** Chief, Division of Dermatology, Good Samaritan Hospital and Medical Center; Associate Clinical Professor of Medicine, Oregon Health Sciences University, Portland, Oregon **James E. Sheedy, O.D., Ph.D.** Associate Clinical Professor, School of Optometry, University of California at Berkeley, Berkeley, California **Fred D. Sheftell, M.D.** Director and Founder, The New England Center for Headache, Stamford, Connecticut **Ronald Shelton, M.S.** Certified Athletic Trainer, Rockford Clinic, Rockford, Illinois **Martyn Shorten, Ph.D.** Former Director, NIKE's Sports Research Laboratory **Louisa Silva, M.D.** General Practitioner, Osteopath, Acupuncturist, Salem, Oregon **Herbert Silverstein, M.D.** President, Ear Research Foundation and Florida Otologic Center, Sarasota, Florida **Peter A. Simkin, M.D.** Professor of Medicine, Department of Medicine, University of Washington, Seattle, Washington **Anne Simons, M.D.** Coauthor, *Before You Call the Doctor*; Family Practitioner, San Francisco Department of Public Health **Richard Simonsen, D.D.S., M.S.** Editor-in-Chief, *Quintessence International*; Professor, College of Dentistry, University of Tennessee, Memphis, Tennessee **Karl Singer, M.D., F.P., I.M.** Family Practitioner and Internist, Exeter, New Hampshire **The Skin Cancer Foundation** New York, New York **Donald Skwor, D.P.M.** Past President, American Podiatric Medical Association; Podiatrist, Memphis, Tennessee **Sharon Snider** Spokesperson, U.S. Food and Drug Administration **Alvin Solomon, M.D.** Associate Professor of Dermatology and Pathology, Emory University School of Medicine, Atlanta, Georgia **Elyse Sosin, R.D.** Supervisor of Clinical Nutrition, Mount Sinai Medical Center, New York, New York **Frank Spano, M.D.** Internist, Bridgeport, Connecticut **Thomas J. Stahl, M.D.** Assistant Professor of General Surgery, Georgetown University Medical Center, Washington, D.C. **James Stankiewicz, M.D.** Professor and Vice-Chairman, Department of Otolaryngology–Head and Neck Surgery, Loyola University Medical School, Maywood, Illinois **Michael R. Stefan, M.D.** Internist, Los Angeles, California **Jonathan S. Steinberg, M.D.** Director, Arrhythmia Service, St. Luke's–Roosevelt Hospital Center, New York, New York **Don Stewart, M.D.** Chairman, Family Practice Department, Overlake Hospital and Medical Center, Bellevue, Washington **Felicia Stewart, M.D.** Coauthor, *My Body, My Health* and *Understanding Your Body*; Gynecologist, Sacramento, California **William E. Straw, M.D.** Team Physician, San Francisco Giants; Clinical Associate Professor of Medicine, Stanford University School of Medicine, Stanford, California **Owen Surman, M.D., C.M., F.A.P.A.** Associate Professor of Psychiatry, Massachusetts General Hospital, Boston, Massachusetts **Mark Tager, M.D.** Coauthor, *Working Well*; President, Great Performance, Inc., Beaverton, Oregon **Jeffrey L. Tanji, M.D.** Associate Professor of Family Practice, Director, Sports Medicine Program, University of California Davis Medical Center, Davis, California **David M. Taylor, M.D** Author, *Gut Reactions: How to Handle Stress and Your Stomach*; Assistant Professor of Medicine, Emory University, Atlanta, Georgia; Assistant

Professor of Medicine, Medical College of Georgia, Augusta, Georgia **Joseph Tenca, D.D.S., M.A.** Past President, American Association of Endodontists; Professor and Chairman, Department of Endodontics, Tufts University School of Dental Medicine, Boston, Massachusetts **Abba I. Terr, M.D.** Clinical Professor of Medicine, Director, Allergy Clinic, Stanford University Medical Center, Stanford, California **Regan Thomas, M.D.** President, American Academy of Facial Plastic and Reconstructive Surgery; Director, Facial Plastic Surgery Center; Assistant Clinical Professor, Washington University School of Medicine, St. Louis, Missouri **Roger Thurmond, M.D.** Dermatologist, Fairbanks, Alaska **Meredith Titus, Ph.D.** Senior Psychologist, The Menninger Clinic, Topeka, Kansas **William R. Treem, M.D.** Associate Professor of Pediatrics, University of Connecticut School of Medicine; Pediatric Gastroenterologist, Division of Pediatric Gastroenterology and Nutrition, Hartford Hospital, Hartford, Connecticut **George Triadafilopoulos, M.D.** Associate Professor of Medicine, University of California Davis; Staff Physician, VA Northern California Systems of Clinics, Venicia, California **Thomas F. Truhe, D.D.S.** Codirector, Princeton Dental Resource Center, Princeton, New Jersey **Nina L. Turner, Ph.D.** Research Physiologist, National Institute for Occupational Safety and Health **Joan Ullyot, M.D.** Author, *Running Free* and *Women's Running*; Sports Medicine Physician, World-Class Runner, San Francisco, California **Frank J. Veith, M.D.** Professor of Surgery, Chief, Vascular Surgical Services, Montefiore Medical Center–Albert Einstein College of Medicine, New York, New York **Ken Waddell, D.M.D.** Dentist, Tigard, Oregon **Douglas C. Walta, M.D.** Gastroenterologist, Portland, Oregon **John R. Ward, M.D.** Professor of Medicine, University of Utah School of Medicine, Salt Lake City, Utah **Kimra Warren, R.D.** Outpatient Dietitian, St. Vincent Hospital and Medical Center, Portland, Oregon **Jack J. Wazen, M.D.** Associate Professor of Otolaryngology, Director, Department of Otology and Neurotology, Columbia University College of Physicians and Surgeons, New York, New York **Michael Wechsler, M.D.** Assistant Professor of Clinical Urology, Columbia–Presbyterian Medical Center, New York, New York **Miles M. Weinberger, M.D.** Director, Pediatric Allergy and Pulmonary Division, University of Iowa Hospitals and Clinics, Iowa City, Iowa **Allan M. Weinstein, M.D.** Asthma and Allergy Specialist, Washington, D.C. **Thelma Wells, Ph.D., R.N., F.A.A.N., F.R.C.N.** Professor of Nursing, University of Rochester School of Nursing, Rochester, New York **Sally Wenzel, M.D.** Assistant Professor of Medicine, National Jewish Center for Immunology and Respiratory Medicine, Denver, Colorado **Philip R. Westbrook, M.D., F.C.C.P.** Past President and Member of the Board of Directors, American Sleep Disorders Association; Director, Sleep Disorders Center, Cedars–Sinai Medical Center, Los Angeles, California **Spencer White** Director of Research Engineering, Reebok International Ltd., Stoughton, Massachusetts **William Whitehead, Ph.D.** Professor of Medical Psychology, Johns Hopkins University School of Medicine, Baltimore, Maryland **Ted Williams, M.D.** Media spokesperson, American Academy of Pediatrics; Pediatrician, Dothan, Alabama **Mark Winston, Ph.D.** Author, *Killer Bees: The Africanized Honey Bee in the Americas*; Professor of Biological Sciences, Simon Fraser University, Burnaby, British Columbia, Canada **Ronald Wismer, D.M.D.** Past President, Washington County Dental Society; Dentist, Beaverton, Oregon **Susan Woodruff, B.S.N.** Childbirth and Parenting Education Coordinator, Tuality Community Hospital, Hillsboro, Oregon **Virginia L. Woodward, R.D.H.** Past President, American Dental Hygienists' Association; Private Practice Clinician, Louisville, Kentucky **Stuart Young, M.D.** Director of Allergy Fellows, Clinical Education, Mount Sinai Medical Center, New York, New York **John Youngblood, M.D.** Associate Professor, University of Texas Health Science Center, San Antonio, Texas; President, Austin Ear Clinic, Austin, Texas **Carol Ziel, M.D.** Ophthalmologist, Wausau, Wisconsin **Harold Zimmer, M.D.** Obstetrician and Gynecologist, Bellevue, Washington **Jane Zukin** Author, *The Dairy-Free Cookbook* and *The Newsletter for People with Lactose Intolerance and Milk Allergies*

◆ CONTENTS ◆

FOREWORD 11

ACNE:
15 Skin-Clearing Solutions 12

ALLERGIES:
29 Ways to Feel Better 16

ARTHRITIS:
44 Coping Strategies 21

ASTHMA:
28 Ways to Breathe Easier 27

ATHLETE'S FOOT:
21 Strategies to Beat Athlete's Foot 32

BACK PAIN:
21 Ways to Keep Back Pain at Bay 36

BAD BREATH:
6 Refreshing Fixes 40

BELCHING:
8 Ways to Squelch the Belch 42

BITES:
19 Ways to Fight Bites 43

BLACK EYE:
6 Care Tips 46

BLADDER INFECTION:
15 Self-Care Techniques 48

BLISTERS:
18 Ways to Treat—and Beat—Them 51

BODY ODOR:
6 Steps to Sweet-Smelling Success 53

BOILS:
8 Ways to Foil Boils 54

BREAST DISCOMFORT:
6 Soothing Strategies 56

BREAST-FEEDING DISCOMFORT:
19 Ways to Beat the Breast-feeding Blues 58

BRONCHITIS:
7 Ways to Bear the Battle 63

BRUISES:
14 Tips for Coping with the Color Purple 65

BURNS:
26 Skin-Saving Strategies 68

BURSITIS:
10 Ways to Ax the Ache 70

CANKER SORES:
9 Soothing Strategies 72

CARPAL TUNNEL SYNDROME:
24 Tips for Protecting Your Wrists 74

CHAFING:
13 Ways to Snub the Rub 77

CHAPPED HANDS:
12 Steps to Softer Hands 79

CHAPPED LIPS:
7 Tips for Smoother Lips 82

CHRONIC FATIGUE SYNDROME:
20 Coping Strategies 83

COLDS:
11 Tips for Fighting the "Cold" War 87

COLD SORES:
6 Ways to Foil Cold Sores 91

COLIC:
15 Ways to Help You and Your Baby Cope 92

CONJUNCTIVITIS:
7 Soothing Suggestions 96

CONSTIPATION:
11 Ways to Keep Things Moving 98

CORNS AND CALLUSES:
22 Steps to Relief 101

CUTS AND SCRAPES:
9 Ways to Care for Your "Boo-Boo" 104

DANDRUFF:
11 Ways to Shake the Flakes 106

DENTURE DISCOMFORT:
9 Ways to Stop Denture Discomfort 108

DERMATITIS AND ECZEMA:
25 Ways to Fight Them 110

DIABETES:
28 Ways to Live Well with Diabetes 115

DIAPER RASH:
10 Ways to Get Rid of It—for Good 121

DIARRHEA:
15 Ways to Go with the Flow 123

DRY HAIR:
11 Tips for Taming It 127

DRY SKiN:
12 Ways to Fight Moisture Loss 129

EARACHE:
7 Sound Ways to Head Off Pain 132

EAR INFECTION:
9 Tips for Prevention and Treatment 134

EARWAX:
4 Ways to Help Your Ears 136

EXCESSIVE HAIR GROWTH:
7 Ways to Cope with the Problem 137

◆ CONTENTS ◆

EXCESSIVE PERSPIRATION:
8 Dry Ideas　　139

EYE REDNESS:
7 Ways to Look Bright-Eyed　　141

EYESTRAIN:
20 Eye Savers　　143

FEVER:
7 Ways to Manage the Ups and Downs　　146

FINGERNAIL PROBLEMS:
14 Tips for Healthier Nails　　149

FISSURES:
7 Soothing Strategies　　153

FLATULENCE:
11 Ways to Combat Gas　　155

FLU:
6 Ways to Cope with the Flu-Bug Blahs　　157

FLUID RETENTION:
29 Ways to Stop Swelling　　160

FOOD POISONING:
8 Coping Tips　　164

FOOT ACHES:
22 Ways to Ease the Agony　　166

FOOT ODOR:
13 Steps to Sweeter-Smelling Feet　　169

FROSTBITE:
25 Ways to Deal with Jack Frost　　171

GENITAL HERPES:
17 Home-Care Hints　　174

GINGIVITIS:
16 Hints for Healthier Gums　　178

GOUT:
6 Ways to Tame the Pain　　181

GRINDING TEETH:
11 Ways to Conquer the Daily Grind　　183

HAIR LOSS:
6 Ways to Fight It　　185

HANGOVERS:
8 Tips to Get You Back on Your Feet　　187

HEADACHES:
16 Ways to Keep the Pain at Bay　　189

HEARTBURN:
21 Ways to Beat the Burn　　194

HEART PALPITATIONS:
7 Ways to Control Them　　197

HEAT EXHAUSTION:
21 Ways to Regulate Your Thermostat　　200

HEMORRHOIDS:
14 Ways to End the Torment　　203

HICCUPS:
13 Techniques Worth a Try　　207

HIGH BLOOD CHOLESTEROL:
21 Heart-Healthy Ways to Lower It　　209

HIGH BLOOD PRESSURE:
13 Ways to Reduce It　　214

HIVES:
14 Methods for Relieving Them　　218

HYPERVENTILATION:
12 Ways to Catch a Breath　　220

IMPOTENCE:
17 Ways to Improve Your Sex Life　　222

INCONTINENCE:
20 Steps to Greater Security　　226

INFERTILITY:
14 Tips to Help You Get Pregnant　　230

INGROWN HAIR:
10 Ways to Get It Straight　　234

INGROWN TOENAILS:
13 Ways to Curb Them　　235

INSOMNIA:
21 Ways to Sleep Tight　　237

IRRITABLE BOWEL SYNDROME:
15 Tactics for Taming It　　241

KIDNEY STONES:
11 Ways to Avoid Them　　244

KNEE PAIN:
21 Knee-Saving Strategies　　246

LACTOSE INTOLERANCE:
10 Ways to Manage It　　251

LARYNGITIS:
18 Ways to Tame a Hoarse Throat　　254

MENOPAUSE:
11 Tips for Coping with "the Change"　　256

MENSTRUAL CRAMPS:
6 Ways to Tackle Them　　260

MORNING SICKNESS:
13 Ways to Ease the Queasiness　　262

MOTION SICKNESS:
13 Ways to Still the Savage Beast　　264

MUSCLE PAIN:
23 Steps to Relief　　266

NAUSEA AND VOMITING:
9 Soothing Strategies　　270

NECK PAIN:
16 Ways to Ease It　　271

NIGHT TERRORS:
8 Tips to Calm Them　　274

◆ CONTENTS ◆

NOSEBLEEDS:
15 Ways to Get Out of the Red   **276**

OILY HAIR:
5 Tips for Cutting the Grease   **279**

OILY SKIN:
10 Ways to Cope   **280**

OSTEOPOROSIS:
17 Ways to Combat Brittle Bones   **282**

POISON IVY, OAK, AND SUMAC:
11 Prevention and Treatment Tips   **286**

POSTNASAL DRIP:
9 Ways to Slow the Flow   **289**

PREMENSTRUAL SYNDROME:
11 Ways to Ease the Discomforts   **292**

PSORIASIS:
25 Coping Techniques   **294**

RESTLESS LEGS SYNDROME:
14 Ways to Squelch the Squiggles   **298**

RINGING IN THE EARS:
9 Sound Strategies to Quiet It   **300**

SCARRING:
6 Ways to Minimize It   **302**

SEASONAL AFFECTIVE DISORDER (SAD):
9 Ways to Stave Off the Sadness   **304**

SENSITIVE TEETH:
5 Tips to Keep You Smiling   **308**

SHAVING DISCOMFORT:
13 Ways to Nip the Nicks   **310**

SHINGLES:
10 Ways to Handle the Pain   **312**

SHINSPLINTS:
10 Ways to Say Goodbye to the Pain for Good   **315**

SIDE STITCH:
9 Ways to Stop It   **317**

SINUSITIS:
5 Ways to Head It Off   **319**

SLEEPWALKING:
13 Ways to Handle It   **321**

SLIVERS:
5 Ways to Remove Them Safely   **324**

SNORING:
9 Ways to Turn Down the Volume   **325**

SORE THROAT:
10 Steps for Quick Relief   **327**

STAINED TEETH:
8 Ways to Keep Them Whiter   **329**

STINGS:
14 Ways to Avoid and Treat Them   **331**

STOMACH UPSET:
23 Ways to Tame Your Tummy   **334**

STRESS:
14 Ways to Combat It   **336**

STY:
6 Treatment and Prevention Tips   **339**

SUNBURN PAIN:
12 Ways to Soothe the Sizzle   **340**

SWIMMER'S EAR:
5 Ways to Sidestep It   **345**

TARTAR AND PLAQUE:
16 Tips to Control Them   **347**

TEETHING:
9 Tips to Ease Baby's Discomfort   **352**

TEMPOROMANDIBULAR JOINT SYNDROME (TMJ):
6 Strategies to Ease TMJ Discomfort   **354**

TENDINITIS:
17 Ways to Take Care of Your Tendons   **356**

THUMB SUCKING:
10 Ways to Help Your Child Kick the Habit   **358**

TOOTHACHE:
9 Ways to Ease the Pain   **360**

TRAVELER'S DIARRHEA:
20 Ways to Battle It   **362**

ULCER:
7 Care Tactics   **365**

VARICOSE VEINS:
16 Coping Techniques   **367**

WARTS:
11 Ways to Wipe Them Out   **371**

WEIGHT GAIN:
37 Ways to Fight the Battle of the Bulge   **375**

WRINKLES:
5 Ways to Fight Them   **380**

YEAST INFECTIONS:
12 Strategies to Beat Them   **382**

INDEX   **386**

◆ FOREWORD ◆

The Home Remedies Handbook is a comprehensive health advisory manual. It is holistic, in the correct sense of the word—it offers preventive medicine tips as well as sound nutrition, medical, mental, dental, cosmetic, and stress-reduction advice.

The home remedies that are described in this book are not "miracle" cures or risky alternative therapies done over your doctor's objections, nor are they meant to take the place of the advice and treatments prescribed by your health-care providers. Rather, they are safe, practical actions that you can take to help yourself with your own health care. They are designed to help you prevent, cope with, and/or treat more than 100 common health problems. They can save you money on health-care costs. They can help to keep you healthy, wealthy, and wise.

How much this book helps you, however, depends on how you use it. As you read and use this book and as you take more responsibility for your own health care, keep the following important points in mind:

• Remember that there are no doctor "secrets" in this book. All of the physicians and health-care providers openly and easily shared their recommendations without payment or promise. Discuss these ideas with your own doctor to see if he or she thinks these are valid for you. Use this book to improve communication with your health-care providers. This book is loaded with practical ideas. Your doctor will be interested in your use of them.

• Be careful of "self" diagnosis. Work with your doctor on your diagnosis. Even a doctor has a "fool for a patient" if he treats himself.

• Don't try every remedy listed for your condition on every condition you have. Especially, don't put everything listed *for* your skin *on* your skin—you could end up with a new medication rash. Go slowly; use common sense.

• Heed the warnings included with the remedies. These warnings are carefully written to help you avoid harm or quackery. Pay special attention to the boxes labeled "Hello, Doctor?" These include special warnings and can help alert you to conditions and symptoms that require a doctor's attention.

The Home Remedies Handbook has been carefully compiled. It contains information currently held to be true and helpful. As medicine and scientific experience grow, we may learn to do some things differently. Learn along with us. Continue to practice good, safe, self-help techniques based on scientific opinions and facts. Continue to maintain an open dialogue with your health-care providers. Continue to read, to ask questions, and to be an active, informed participant in your own health care.

John H. Renner, M.D.
President
Consumer Health Information Research Institute
Kansas City, Missouri

◆ ACNE ◆

15 Skin-Clearing Solutions

Acne. If you're a teenager, you can't wait to get rid of it. If you're an adult, you can't believe it's back. Fortunately, improvements in acne treatments over the last decade mean you don't have to put up with it anymore.

The major determining factor in who gets acne is genes, according to Albert M. Kligman, M.D., Ph.D., emeritus professor of dermatology at the University of Pennsylvania School of Medicine in Philadelphia. In other words, you may have inherited a skin characteristic that makes you more likely to develop acne.

You have thousands of oil glands in the skin on your face, chest, and back that lubricate the skin by producing sebum, or oil, explains Alan D. Klein, M.D., a member of the teaching staff at Ventura County Medical Center in California and a spokesperson for the American Academy of Dermatology. "You have as many as 2,000 oil glands per square inch in the central part of your face," he says. The oil from the glands flows through tiny ducts to the skin surface.

Sometimes, these oil ducts become plugged with sebum, bacteria, and dead skin cells that are shed from the lining of the duct. That's acne. The condition often appears during adolescence because of changing hormone levels, which enlarge the oil glands and encourage them to produce more oil. Although the process is not well understood, the increase in oil appears to fuel acne, perhaps by stimulating the production of "sticky" skin cells that, when shed, tend to plug the duct. The situation usually settles down by the end of the teen years or during the early 20s.

So why do adults develop acne? There are a variety of reasons, among them:

• **Hormones.** "Premenstrual acne is real," Kligman says. Pregnancy, changes during the menstrual cycle, and birth control pills can cause fluctuations in hormone levels and subsequent fluctuations in acne in women. In some women, low-dose oral contraceptives improve acne; in others, they make acne worse. If you have acne along with menstrual irregularities, you may want to see a physician to see if abnormal hormone levels are to blame.

• **Stress.** Dermatologists agree that high levels of stress can affect hormone levels.

• **Cosmetics.** Wearing heavy, oily makeup may clog pores and cause acne.

• **Occupational exposure.** If you're a mechanic or you're standing over the deep-fat fryer at the local fast-food joint, your face may be getting assaulted by oils, some of which may cause acne. Numerous chemicals in the workplace can also cause acne.

• **Certain medications.** Some drugs, such as Dilantin (which is used in the treatment of epilepsy), can cause acne, says Alan N. Moshell, M.D., director of the Skin Disease Program at the National Institute of Arthritis and Musculoskeletal and Skin Diseases.

No matter what's causing your acne, there are steps you can take to help clear up your skin.

◆◆ Who Gets Acne? ◆◆

Nearly every teenage boy and around 80 percent of teenage girls will suffer from acne. (Blame those male hormones.) Boys are also more likely than girls to have severe acne during adolescence.

In contrast, women are much more likely than men to have acne in their 20s, 30s, and 40s. Some doctors say it's because of cosmetic use and birth control pills. Women may also be more likely to visit a dermatologist for treatment.

Do no harm. In other words, don't pick, press, rub, or otherwise manipulate those pimples, warns Kligman. "You risk spreading the bacteria and increasing the chances for scarring," explains Klein. Vincent A. DeLeo, M.D., assistant professor of dermatology at Columbia–Presbyterian Medical Center in New York, gets even more descriptive: The plug at the top of the pore is like a balloon. You can pop it, but below the surface, the sebum, bacteria, and skin cells may leak into the surrounding tissue, causing inflammation.

Use benzoyl peroxide. A number of over-the-counter products contain this ingredient, which helps break up the plug of dead skin cells, bacteria, and oil in pores and cuts down on the bacteria 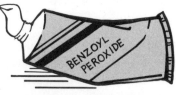 as well. Start with the lowest concentration, and work your way up, especially if you have sensitive skin, because the higher the concentration, the more irritating it may be. Use it once or twice a day. If it dries the skin too much, Kligman suggests applying a mild moisturizer.

Give one of the other over-the-counter products a shot. Other acne products contain sulfur or resorcinol, which help unplug oil glands by irritating the skin, Klein says. Most dermatologists, however, believe that benzoyl peroxide is the most effective over-the-counter ingredient for acne.

Apply over-the-counter products for prevention. "Don't just spot the product on existing acne," DeLeo says. "Put it on acne-prone areas." That can include your entire face (avoiding the lips and eyes, however), back, and chest.

Go easy on your face. "Kids with oily skin use hot water, a washcloth, and a drying soap and think they can wash their acne away," Kligman says. "But they can't." DeLeo points out, "You can

Acne Rosacea

If you're over 40 and suddenly develop severe acne, you could be suffering from acne rosacea, which is a different disease from acne vulgaris, the medical name for your garden variety of acne.

How can you tell the difference? Acne rosacea is characterized by redness, inflammation (swelling), and dilated blood vessels. Further clues: You don't have any blackheads, the acne is located mainly on the central part of your face (your nose and cheeks), and you have a lot of pustules (pus-containing pimples). You're more likely to suffer from this type of acne if you're light-skinned.

Unfortunately, there's not much you can do on your own for acne rosacea, says Vincent A. DeLeo, M.D., although you should be especially careful about avoiding the sun, since sun exposure can worsen the condition. Acne rosacea can, however, be treated by a dermatologist.

wash your face ten times a day and still have acne. It has nothing to do with cleanliness." Washing removes oils from the surface of the skin, not from within the plugged ducts. And adults can certainly suffer from both acne and dry skin, says Klein. In fact, if you're too aggressive in your quest for cleanliness, you may very well end up drying out or irritating the sensitive skin on your face.

Wash properly. How do you do that? Use a mild soap. DeLeo recommends Dove Unscented, Tone, Basis, or Neutrogena. Rub lightly with your fingertips and warm water. Do not use a

◆◆◆ Acne Glossary ◆◆◆

Most of us think of pimples when we think of acne. We don't bother dividing up the different annoying spots we see on our face. But dermatologists have broken pimples down into the following categories:

Comedo (pl. comedones). An oil duct plugged up with oil, dead skin cells, and bacteria.

Whitehead. A closed comedo, or a comedo with skin covering the top. It looks like a tiny, white bump.

Blackhead. An open comedo, or a comedo that does not have skin covering it. It appears black not because it contains dirt, as is commonly believed, but because the material has been exposed to oxygen.

Papule. A ruptured comedo in which there is inflammation and secondary infection. It looks like a small, hard, red bump.

Pustule. A ruptured comedo in which there is inflammation and secondary infection. In contrast to the papule, the pustule has more pus near the surface, giving it a yellowish center.

Nodule (sometimes called a cyst). A ruptured comedo that is generally larger, deeper, and more painful than a pustule and is more likely to result in scarring. This type of lesion marks the most severe form of acne.

washcloth. If your skin is oily, use a soap with benzoyl peroxide for its drying properties, suggests Klein. And wash once or twice a day.

Don't exfoliate. That refers to removing the top layer of dead skin cells. Some dermatologists recommend using a rough washcloth or specially designed product to do just that. "But your skin is already irritated if you have acne," says Kligman. Don't use brushes, rough sponges, cleansers with granules or walnut hulls, or anything else of that nature on the delicate facial skin, says Klein. For the back and chest, where skin is less sensitive, you can try one of the acne scrub pads along with soap that contains benzoyl peroxide, he adds.

Watch out for oily products. That goes for oily pomades on your hair, heavy oil-based moisturizers, and even oily cleansers. "The classic that I hear from women is that they use only cold cream on their face," says DeLeo. "They think they're avoiding wrinkles, but dry skin doesn't cause the skin to age, exposure to the sun does."

Use water-based makeup. If you're not sure—and DeLeo says some cosmetic labels are misleading—set the bottle of makeup on the counter. If it separates into water and powder, it's water-based, he says. If it doesn't, it contains oil. He also advises that you opt for powder blushes and loose powders. Eye makeup and lipstick are OK because you don't generally get acne in those areas.

Forego the facial. DeLeo warns that most people giving facials aren't trained to treat acne-prone skin properly and may end up doing more harm than good.

Don't rest your chin on your hands. Try not to constantly touch your face. "People who do a lot of telephone work will get chin-line acne," DeLeo says. It causes trauma to acne, just like picking the pimples does. Tight sweatbands and chin straps from sports equipment can have the same effect.

Soak up the oil. Some cosmetic companies make a paper product that can be pressed onto the skin to soak up oil, says Kligman. "It's a very simple procedure," he says. "It doesn't help the acne, but it helps relieve the oiliness, which is disagreeable."

Screen out the sun. At one time, sun exposure was believed to help acne, says Klein. However, too much sun can lead to skin cancer and premature aging, making the risks outweigh the benefits. He suggests protecting the skin with a sunscreen that has a sun protection factor (SPF) of 15 or higher. "Look for one that's oil-free or noncomedogenic," he says. Unfortunately, many waterproof products are too likely to clog oil glands to use on the face, so you'll need to be diligent about reapplying the sunscreen often.

Don't worry about diet. Chocolate, french fries, and other foods have not been proven to have anything at all to do with causing teenage acne. "It doesn't matter what you eat," says Kligman. Eating chocolate, nuts, or greasy foods is not to blame when it comes to the zits on your face. On the other hand, if you notice a correlation between something you eat and your face breaking out, most dermatologists agree that you should avoid the offending food. "Maybe one out of 100 or even 1,000 patients will have some relationship of acne to certain foods," says Moshell.

Watch out for iodine. This is still somewhat controversial, but some doctors believe that high levels of iodine, found in some multiple vitamins and in iodized salt, may encourage acne. ◆

◆◆ What Does a Doctor ◆◆ Do for Acne?

With today's drugs, there's no reason for anyone to put up with serious acne, says Albert M. Kligman, M.D., Ph.D.

"Persistent acne can affect self-esteem and confidence," Kligman says. "The psychological, social, and sexual effects of acne are very, very prominent, and the social consequences can be severe." He suggests children be treated fairly young if they start showing signs of acne, especially if their parents suffered from severe acne.

When should you see a dermatologist for your acne? Most dermatologists answer that by saying "when it bothers you." Severity is in the eye of the beholder in this case.

Vincent A. DeLeo, M.D., gives some additional guidelines for when professional treatment is called for. See a dermatologist if you:

• Use benzoyl peroxide products for six to eight weeks and still have problems

• Have pustules larger than a match head

• Have nodules the size of the end of your little finger

• Have any scarring from your acne

It's extremely important to see a dermatologist before scarring occurs.

Today's arsenal of treatments includes topical and oral antibiotics and a class of medications called retinoids. It's the latter that have "revolutionized" acne treatment, says Alan D. Klein, M.D. Tretinoin (Retin-A) is applied to the skin, while isotretinoin (Accutane) is taken orally. Pregnant women should not take isotretinoin; it has been shown to cause birth defects. It's considered a last-ditch treatment, but it's especially effective for cystic acne. One course of this treatment generally is enough, says Alan N. Moshell, M.D.

◆ ALLERGIES ◆

29 Ways to Feel Better

Spring's pollens. Summer's smog. Autumn's falling leaves. Winter's house dust. For millions of Americans, each change of season brings its own brand of allergens and irritants. For people with common hay fever and allergies, these pollutants can bring on symptoms ranging from a continuous, annoying postnasal drip to a full-scale, coughing-sneezing-itchy-eyed allergy attack. For other allergy sufferers, such as those with allergic asthma or an allergy to bee stings, attacks can be fatal.

In many cases, allergy symptoms are difficult to differentiate from the symptoms of other disorders and illnesses, such as a cold, a deformity of the nose, or a food intolerance. For this reason, many doctors suggest that allergies be properly diagnosed by a board-certified allergist (a medical doctor who treats allergies) to avoid the self-administration of inappropriate medications or other remedies. Also, many allergy sufferers can benefit from today's wide range of available treatments, such as new prescription antihistamines that don't cause drowsiness, nasal corticosteroids, and allergy injections that can provide immunity to a specific allergen (an allergen is the name for any substance, such as pollen, that causes an allergic reaction). If you don't go to the doctor, you may be missing out on a treatment that may be of great help to you.

However, many mild allergies, such as seasonal hay fever or an allergy to cats, can be treated with a combination of properly used, over-the-counter antihistamines and a wide range of strategies to reduce or eliminate your exposure to particularly annoying allergens.

The following tips are designed to help reduce the discomfort caused by the most common allergies. They may be used in combination with an allergist's treatment or, if your allergies are mild, by themselves.

◆◆ Hello, Doctor? ◆◆

If your allergies are causing you to cough, wheeze, and have trouble breathing, you should see an allergist, says Abba I. Terr, M.D., a clinical professor of medicine and director of the Allergy Clinic at Stanford University Medical Center in California. "You may have allergic asthma, which really has to be supervised by a doctor," he says. People with allergic asthma, which is sometimes mistaken for bronchitis, must often be prescribed inhalers and other medications. Trying to self-treat may be dangerous, Terr says.

Avoid the culprit. Sometimes, the best way to reduce the discomfort of an allergy is to avoid exposure to the allergen as much as possible, according to Edward J. O'Connell, M.D., professor of pediatrics at the Mayo Clinic in Rochester, Minnesota, and past president of the American College of Allergy and Immunology. "Take all practical measures," he says. For example, if you are allergic to cats, avoid visiting the homes of friends who own them. If you must be around a cat, make the visit as short as possible and avoid touching or picking up the animal, he says.

Rinse your eyes. If your eyes are itchy and irritated and you have no access to allergy medicine, rinsing your eyes with cool, clean water may help soothe them, O'Connell says. Although not as effective as an antihistamine, this remedy certainly can't do any damage.

Try a warm washcloth. If sinus passages feel congested and painful, a washcloth soaked in warm water may make things flow a little easier, according to O'Connell. Place the washcloth over the nose and upper-cheek area and relax for a few minutes, he suggests.

Use saline solution. Irrigating the nose with saline solution may help soothe upper-respiratory allergies by removing irritants that become lodged in the nose, causing inflammation, according to Anthony Montanaro, M.D., associate professor of medicine in the Division of Allergy and Immunology at Oregon Health Sciences University in Portland. "The solution may also remove some of the inflammatory cells themselves," he adds.

Wash your hair. If you've spent long hours outdoors during the pollen season, wash your hair after you come inside to remove pollen, suggests Clifton T. Furukawa, M.D., clinical professor of pediatrics at the University of Washington School of Medicine in Seattle and past chairman of the Professional Education Council for the American Academy of Allergy and Immunology. The sticky stuff tends to collect on the hair, making it more likely to fall into your eyes.

Take a shower. If you wake up in the middle of the night with a coughing, sneezing allergy attack, a hot shower may wash off any pollen residues you've collected on your body throughout the day, says Furukawa. The warm water will also relax you and help you go back to sleep, he adds.

Wear sunglasses. On a windy day in pollen season, a pair of sunglasses may help shield your eyes from airborne allergens, according to O'Connell. For extra protection, try a pair of sunglasses with side shields or even a pair of goggles.

Beware of the air. "Air pollution may augment allergies and may actually induce people to have allergies," Montanaro says. He recommends staying outside as little as possible on smoggy days

Is It a Food Allergy?

Do you feel congested after you eat dairy products? Does red meat make you feel sluggish? Does sugar give you a headache? If you answered "yes" to any of these questions, you probably don't *have a food allergy.*

"There's a big difference between what the public perceives as a food allergy and what is really a food allergy," says Anthony Montanaro, M.D. "The distinction is important, since a real food allergy can kill you and a food intolerance can't."

If you are truly allergic to a food, the reaction will be almost immediate, occurring from within a few minutes to two hours after you eat it, according to Abba I. Terr, M.D. The most common symptoms, he says, are hives, diffuse swelling around the eyes and mouth, or abdominal cramps. A less common symptom is difficulty breathing. In severe cases, extremely low blood pressure, dizziness, or loss of consciousness may result. In these instances, a call for an ambulance or other emergency medical assistance is warranted.

or wearing a surgical mask, especially if you exercise outside. "The mask won't remove everything, but it will help," he adds.

Make your house a no-smoking zone. "Don't allow smoking in your house or apartment," O'Connell says. Tobacco smoke is a notorious irritant, either causing or aggravating respiratory allergies.

Keep the windows shut. Most Americans, except for those who have jobs that keep them outdoors, spend most of their time inside. During pollen season, this can be a terrific advantage for those with pollen allergies, according to O'Connell. "The bottom line, for pollen allergies, is keeping the windows shut," he says. "Closed windows will keep pollen out of the house or apartment. For pollen sufferers, during the pollen season, there is really no such thing as fresh air." Air purifiers may help eliminate indoor pollen, but they tend to stir up dust, he adds.

◆◆◆ Bust the Dust ◆◆◆

The following tips from Edward J. O'Connell, M.D., can help you rid your bedroom of dust mites—microscopic insects that live in dusty, humid environments. The feces and corpses of the mites are thought to be the irritating components in dust. Allergists believe that since we spend most of our time at home in the bedroom, that's the most important place to allergy-proof.

Encase pillows and mattresses. *Invest in airtight, plastic or vinyl cases or special covers that are impermeable to allergens for your pillows and mattresses (except for waterbeds). Pillows and mattresses contain fibrous material that is an ideal environment for dust-mite growth. These cases are usually available at your local department store or through mail-order companies. You can also contact the Asthma and Allergy Foundation of America for more information on where to purchase cases and covers.*

Wash your bedding. *Down, kapok, and feather comforters and pillows are out for people with allergies. The feathers have a tendency to leak and can wreak havoc with your respiratory tract. Comforters and sheets should be washed every seven to ten days in as hot water as they'll tolerate. Wash your mattress pads and synthetic blankets every two weeks.*

Clean once a week. *Putting off cleaning for longer than this may allow an excessive amount of dust to collect, O'Connell says. However, since cleaning raises dust, it's best not to clean more than once a week. If necessary, you can spot dust with a damp cloth more often, he says.*

Avoid overstuffed furniture. *"If the bedroom's decor lends itself to it, add more wood and vinyl furniture and avoid overstuffed furniture," O'Connell says. Since carpeting makes an excellent dust-mite lair, opt instead for bare floors or ask your doctor about a prescription product for killing dust mites in carpets.*

Choose washable curtains. *If possible, invest in curtains that can be washed, since their fabric is often a place where dust mites hide.*

Vacuum the venetians. *The slats of venetian blinds are notorious dust collectors. If you can't replace your venetian blinds with washable curtains, at least run the vacuum lightly over them or dust them well during your thorough weekly cleaning.*

Don't use the bedroom as storage space. *Stored items tend to collect dust and have no place in an allergy-proof bedroom. If the bedroom is the only storage space you have, wrap items tightly in plastic garbage bags.*

Clean out your air conditioner and heating ducts. *Every month or so, clean out the vents on your heating and air-conditioning units, or have someone clean them for you. These ducts are breeding grounds for mold, dust mites, and bacteria. If you let such nasties collect, they'll be blown into the room each time you turn on your appliance.*

Filter your vacuum. "It is very important to not recycle the allergy factors back into your home as you clean," says Furukawa. "For example, you're not doing much good if your vacuum cleaner allows small particles of dust to be blown back into the air as you vacuum." He recommends putting a filter on the exhaust port of your vacuum, if your machine is the canister type (uprights don't usually have an exhaust port). If dust really bothers you and you've got the money, you can invest in an industrial-strength vacuuming system, Furukawa says. Some allergists recommend a brand called Nilfisk, he adds, which has an excellent filtering system and retails for about $500. To find out where you can purchase filters or special vacuums, talk to your allergist or write to the Asthma and Allergy Foundation of America, Department CG, 1125 15th Street NW, Suite 502, Washington, D.C., 20005.

Dust with a damp cloth. Dusting at least once a week is important—but if done improperly, it may aggravate respiratory allergies, O'Connell says. He recommends avoiding the use of feather dusters, which tend to spread dust around, and opting instead to contain the dust with a damp cloth. Dusting sprays may give off odors that can worsen allergies, he adds.

Don't dust at all. If dusting aggravates your allergies, don't do it. Instead, ask a spouse or family member to do the dirty work, or hire a housekeeper, if possible, O'Connell recommends.

Dehumidify. "Dust mites (microscopic insects that are usually the allergy culprits in dust) grow very well in humid areas," O'Connell says. He recommends investing in a dehumidifier or using the air conditioner, which works equally well. A dehumidifier can also help prevent mold, another allergen, from growing. When cooking or showering, take advantage of the exhaust fan— another way to help keep humidity to a minimum.

Think before you burn. Although it is common to burn household and construction refuse, this may not be such a wise idea, says Furukawa. "Wood that is treated with heavy metals or other chemical-laden materials will irritate everybody, but the person who is allergic or asthmatic will have proportionately more difficulty," he says. "Also, pay attention to what you are throwing in the fireplace." Of course, your best bet is to stay away from the fireplace when it's in use.

Cut through the smoke. Many people with respiratory allergies find that wood smoke poses a particular problem, Furukawa says. With wood stoves, the biggest problem is "choking down" the stove, or decreasing the amount of oxygen in order to cool down the fire, he explains. Choking down throws irritating toxins into the air, which will be breathed in by you and your neighbors.

Leave the lawn mowing to someone else. During pollen season, a grass-allergic person is better off letting someone else—anyone else—mow the lawn, Montanaro says. "Find out when the pollination season in your area is," he advises. "Here in the Northwest, I tell people not to mow between May and the Fourth of July."

Wash your pet. A little-known trick for cat or dog owners who are allergic to fur: Bathe your pet frequently. "There is strong evidence that simply bathing the animal in warm water substantially reduces the amount of allergen on the animal's fur," Furukawa says. "Animals secrete substances from their sweat glands and their saliva—it is water soluble and you can rinse it off." If you're a cat owner and can't imagine bathing your beloved feline for fear of being scratched near to death, take heart: Furukawa says that in an informal survey that he conducted, he discovered that one out of ten cats will purr when bathed. If they are started as kittens, chances are higher that bath time will be a harmonious experience, he says. He recommends a bath in warm water, with no soap, once every other week.

In addition to bathing your pet, try to wash your hands soon after you've had direct contact with your furry friend.

Make sure your final rinse really rinses. Chemicals in detergents and other laundry products can cause skin irritation in many people, O'Connell says. "There really are no mild detergents," he explains. "It's important that the final rinse cycle on your machine thoroughly rinses the detergent from your clothes."

Call ahead. When planning a vacation or business trip, call ahead to find a room that will be easier on your allergies. Ask for a room that's not on the lower level, because a room on the lower level may have been flooded in the past and may still be a haven for mold growth. Shop around for a hotel or motel that doesn't allow pets, so you won't be subject to the leftover dander of the last traveler's dog or cat. If possible, bring your own vinyl- or plastic-encased pillow. ◆

◆◆ Choosing and Using ◆◆ an Over-the-Counter Antihistamine

If you've got your doctor's OK to use them, over-the-counter antihistamines can be an economical way to relieve your allergy misery. However, many people misuse these drugs, believing them to be an on-the-spot fix for whenever they feel itchy-eyed or sneezy.

"The problem with antihistamines is, most people wait until they're miserable, then take one and don't find they work," says Miles M. Weinberger, M.D., director of the Pediatric Allergy and Pulmonary Division at the University of Iowa Hospitals and Clinics in Iowa City. "If you have classical ragweed hay fever, you'll get the maximum benefit from antihistamines if you start taking them a week or two before the allergy season begins." (When the season begins depends on where you live.)

As for what type of antihistamine to use, Weinberger recommends chlorpheniramine maleate, which is found in many over-the-counter preparations. Chlorpheniramine maleate is one of the oldest, safest allergy drugs with a proven track

record, he says. It can take care of symptoms such as sneezing; itchy, runny nose; and itchy eyes. (If you also have nasal stuffiness, says Weinberger, you might try a combination product that contains chlorpheniramine and pseudoephedrine, a nasal decongestant.) He suggests starting with a dose of perhaps one-fourth of what the package recommends, then slowly building up to 24 milligrams per day (12 milligrams in the morning and 12 milligrams in the evening), providing you can maintain that dosage without drowsiness. Since drowsiness tends to go away in a week or two, Weinberger recommends starting with evening doses, then adding a morning dose as you begin to tolerate the medication. (Be sure to avoid operating a motor vehicle or heavy machinery if the medication makes you drowsy.) "Approximately 75 percent of the people with pollen symptoms will get quite adequate relief with a 24 milligram dosage," he says.

Edward J. O'Connell, M.D., agrees that antihistamines work best when they are used as preventive medicine. For people with pet allergies who know they will be exposed to someone else's cat or dog, he recommends taking antihistamines beginning 10 to 14 days in advance.

◆ ARTHRITIS ◆

44 Coping Strategies

An estimated 37 million Americans are caught in the grip of some form of arthritis or rheumatic disease. And few of us will make it to a ripe old age without joining the fold. If one of these diseases has a hold on you, read on. While there are no cures, there are steps you can take to ease discomfort and get back more control over your life. There are more than 100 different forms of arthritis and rheumatic disease, with a host of causes, according to the Arthritis Foundation in Atlanta. Among the more widely known afflictions are osteoarthritis, rheumatoid arthritis, gout, and lupus.

Osteoarthritis is primarily marked by a breakdown and loss of joint cartilage. Cartilage is the tough tissue that separates and cushions the bones in a joint. As cartilage is worn away and the bones begin to rub against each other, the joint becomes aggravated. In osteoarthritis, this breakdown of cartilage is accompanied by minimal inflammation, hardening of the bone beneath the cartilage, and bone spurs (growths) around the joints. "It will eventually affect virtually everyone in old age," says John Staige Davis IV, M.D., professor in the Division of Rheumatology at the University of Virginia School of Medicine in Charlottesville.

Rheumatoid arthritis, on the other hand, is not an inevitable aspect of the aging process. For reasons unknown, the synovial membrane, or lining, of a joint becomes inflamed, so pain, swelling, heat, and redness occur.

In the case of gout, needle-shaped uric acid crystals collect in the joints, due to a fault in the body's ability to metabolize, or process, purines. Purines are naturally occurring chemicals found in certain foods, such as liver, kidney, and anchovies. The disease primarily affects overweight, fairly inactive men over the age of 35 (see GOUT).

Lupus, on the other hand, affects many more women than men. It is a condition in which the body's own immune system attacks healthy cells. The symptoms are wide-ranging, from joint pain to mouth sores to persistent fatigue.

Researchers are beginning to understand what may predispose some people to arthritis. One clue to the puzzle: "There are indications that collagen, which helps form the body's cartilage, may be defective in some people," says Arthur I. Grayzel, M.D., senior vice-president for Medical Affairs at the Arthritis Foundation.

While you cannot cure your condition, you can adopt a variety of coping techniques that will leave you more active and in control of your life.

EASING STIFFNESS AND DISCOMFORT

Here are some tips to help relieve discomfort and get you back into the swing of things.

Keep moving. Maintain movement in your joints as best you can. This can help keep your joints functioning better for a longer amount of time and, at the same time, brighten your outlook on life. "Every patient should keep active," says John R. Ward, M.D., professor of medicine at the University of Utah School of Medicine in Salt Lake City. "And remember that even small movements mean a lot. If all you can tolerate is a little housecleaning or gardening, for instance, that's OK, too."

Exercise, exercise, exercise. "Exercises work best when inflammation has calmed down," notes Janna Jacobs, P.T., C.H.T., physical therapist, certified hand therapist, and president of the Section on Hand Rehabilitation of the American Physical Therapy Association (APTA).

There are a few different types of exercises that are used to help arthritis sufferers. The simplest, easiest exercises that can be done by almost any arthritis sufferer are called range-of-motion exercises. They help maintain good movement by putting the joints through their full range of motion. You'll find several range-of-motion exercises recommended by the Arthritis Foundation in "Exercises for Arthritis."

Isometrics, in which you create resistance by tightening a muscle without moving the joint, can help to strengthen muscles. Weight-bearing exercises, such as walking, also build muscle strength. While strengthening exercises can be beneficial for the arthritis sufferer, however, they should only be done under the supervision and care of a therapist or physician, says Grayzel. And, "anyone with any type of cardiovascular disease should not do multiple resistance exercises for a sustained amount of time," warns Ward.

Stretching, which helps make the muscles more flexible, is often recommended as the first step in any exercise regime. Likewise, warming up your joints before beginning any exercise makes them more flexible. Massage your muscles and/or apply hot or cold compresses or both—whichever your health-care practitioner recommends or you prefer. A warm shower is another way to warm up. (See "Heat or Cold: Which Is Best?")

Give your hands a water workout. Try doing your hand exercises in a sink full of warm water for added ease and comfort, suggests Jacobs.

Don't overdo it. Ward has come up with a "useful recipe" you can use to see if you've overdone your exercise routine. See how you feel a few hours after you exercise and then again after 24 hours. If your pain has increased considerably during that period

◆ Exercises for Arthritis ◆

These exercises are recommended by the Arthritis Foundation. For best results, carry out the exercises in a smooth, steady, slow-paced manner; don't bounce, jerk, or strain. Don't hold your breath; breathe as naturally as possible. Do each exercise five to ten times, if possible. If any exercise causes chest pain, other pain, or shortness of breath, stop. When your joints are inflamed, it's best to skip the exercises and rest. If you have any questions, contact your therapist or physician. And remember: It may be some time before you feel the benefits of regular exercise, so be patient with yourself.

Shoulders: *Lie on your back and raise one arm over your head, keeping your elbow straight. Keep your arm close to your ear. Return your arm slowly to your side. Repeat with the other arm.*

Knees and hips: *Lie on your back with one knee bent and the other as straight as possible. Bend the knee of the straight leg and bring it toward the chest. Extend that same leg into the air and then lower the straightened leg to the floor. Repeat with the other leg.*

Hips: *Lie on your back with your legs straight and about six inches apart. Point your toes up. Slide one leg out to the side and return, keeping your toes pointing up. Repeat with the other leg.*

Knees: *Sit on a chair that's high enough so you can swing your legs. Keep your thigh on the chair and straighten out your knee. Hold a few seconds. Then bend your knee back as far as possible to return to the starting position. Repeat with the other knee.*

Ankles: *Sit on a chair and lift your toes off the floor as high as possible while keeping your heels on the floor. Then return your toes to the floor and lift your heels as high as possible. Repeat.*

Fingers: *Open your hand with your fingers straight. Bend all the finger joints except the knuckles. Touch the top of the palm with the tips of your fingers. Open and repeat.*

Thumbs: *Open your hand with your fingers straight. Reach your thumb across your palm until it touches the base of the little finger. Stretch your thumb out again and repeat.*

of time, then it's time to cut back on the frequency and amount of exercise that you're doing, he says. Of course, if the activity brought relief, you've found a worthwhile exercise. Tailor your routine to include the exercises that give you the most relief—and the most enjoyment.

Play in a pool. If you find even simple movements difficult, a heated pool or whirlpool may be the perfect environment for exercise (unless you also have high blood pressure, in which case you should avoid whirlpools and hot tubs). Try a few of your simpler exercises while in the water. The buoyancy will help reduce the strain on your joints. And, "the warm water will help loosen joints and maintain motion and strength," says Ward. Even a warm bath may allow you some increased movement. In a pinch, a hot shower may do: Running the stream of water down your back, for instance, may help relieve back pain.

Don't overuse over-the-counter creams. These pain-relieving rubs give temporary relief by heating up the joints. However, "frequent use may activate enzymes that can break down the cartilage in the joints," says Davis.

Put on a scarf. Not around your neck, but around the elbow or knee joint when it aches. "A wool scarf is your best bet," says Jacobs. Be careful not to wrap it too tightly, however; you don't want to hamper your circulation.

Pull on a pair of stretch gloves. "The tightness caused by the stretchy kind may, in fact, reduce the swelling that often accompanies arthritis," says Ward. And the warmth created by covered hands may make the joints feel better. "Wearing thermal underwear may have the same warming effect on joints," says Grayzel.

Get electric gloves. Hunters use these battery-operated mitts to keep their hands toasty on cold mornings in the woods. "The gloves just may do the trick to keep your hands warm and pain-free," says Jacobs. She recommends keeping them on all night while you sleep.

Try a water bed. According to the National Water Bed Retailers' Association in Chicago, many owners claimed in a study that their rheumatoid arthritis "was helped very much by a water bed." And Earl J. Brewer, Jr., M.D., former head of the Rheumatology Division of Texas Children's Hospital in Houston, believes he knows why. "The slight motions made by a water bed can help reduce morning stiffness," he says. "And a heated water bed may warm the joints and relieve joint pain."

Slip into a sleeping bag. If a water bed is out of the question, you might consider camping gear. "The cocoonlike effect of a sleeping bag traps heat, which can help relieve morning aches and pains," reports Brewer. He learned of its therapeutic effects when many of his patients told him that they got relief by sleeping in their sleeping bags on top of their beds.

Get "down." Brewer tells the story of a doctor from Norway who happened to stay in a bed-and-breakfast while on business in New York. The doctor, who was suffering from arthritis pain, slept peacefully each night in the B&B's bed and woke each morning pain-free. The bed was outfitted with a goose-down comforter and pillow. According to Brewer, the bedding's warmth and minute motion brought on the relief. For those who are allergic to down, an electric blanket may bring some relief.

Watch your weight. Being overweight puts more stress on the joints. As a matter of fact, a weight gain of 10 pounds can mean an equivalent stress increase of 40 pounds on the knees. So if you are carrying excess 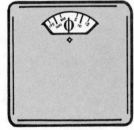 pounds, losing weight can help improve joint function. "People who lose weight can slow the progress of their osteoarthritis," says Grayzel.

Question any cure-all. Frustrated by the chronic pain of arthritis, some sufferers pursue a litany of promises for 100 percent relief—whether from a so-called miracle drug, a newfangled diet, or another alternative treatment. Unfortunately, at this time, arthritis has no cure. So, before you jump at the next hot-sounding testimonial, proceed with caution. Get all the facts. Consult your physician or other health-care provider. Even age-old techniques, such as wearing a copper bracelet, should be viewed with skepticism, agree most experts. And remember, if something sounds too good to be true, it probably is.

PROTECTING YOUR JOINTS

In addition to easing discomfort, you can learn to live well with arthritis by protecting your joints. What's more, with a little planning and reorganizing, you can learn to do daily tasks more efficiently, so that you'll have more energy to spend on activities you enjoy. Here are some tips from the Arthritis Foundation that can help.

Plan ahead each day. Prepare a realistic, written schedule of what you would like to accomplish each day. That way, you can carry out your most demanding tasks and activities when you think you'll have the most energy and enthusiasm—in the morning, for instance.

Spread the strain. As a general rule, you want to avoid activities that involve a tight grip or that put too much pressure on your fingers. Use the palms of both hands to lift and hold cups, plates, pots, and pans, rather than gripping them with your

---

◆◆◆ Heat or Cold: ◆◆◆ Which Is Best?

There are no hard and fast rules when it comes to deciding which—heat, cold, or a combination of the two—will give you the best results. The bottom line, says John R. Ward, M.D.: "Do whichever feels the best." Here are some guidelines that may help you decide.

Heat relieves pain primarily by relaxing muscles and joints and decreasing stiffness. In some instances, however, heat may aggravate a joint that's already "hot" from inflammation, as is sometimes the case with rheumatoid arthritis. On the other hand, osteoarthritis causes minimal inflammation and may respond well to heat application. If you find that your compress cools down quickly, you may want to try methods that offer more consistent heating. An electric blanket or heating pad can provide sustained dry heat. A warm shower, bath, or whirlpool can keep the wet heat coming. And using some method of warmth to loosen up the muscles before exercise can help them perform better.

Cold is ordinarily used to reduce pain in specific joints. Cold application should not be used with vasculitis (inflammation of the blood vessels) or Raynaud's phenomenon (a condition, characterized by spasms of the arteries in the fingers and toes, that may occur in conjunction with rheumatoid arthritis) without a doctor's approval, however. There are many ways to make a cold pack: Fill a plastic bag with crushed ice, use a package of frozen peas or frozen unpopped popcorn, or use a package of blue ice, for example. Apply the cold pack, wrapped in a thin towel, to only one or two joints at a time, so you don't get a chill.

You may find that alternating heat and cold gives you the most relief. For the best results, the Arthritis Foundation recommends the contrast bath: Soak your hands and feet in warm water (no more than 110 degrees Fahrenheit) for about three minutes, then soak them in cold water (about 65 degrees Fahrenheit) for about a minute. Repeat this process three times, and finish with a warm-water soak.

24

fingers or with only one hand. Place your hand flat against a sponge or rag instead of squeezing it with your fingers. Avoid holding a package or pocketbook by clasping the handle with your fingers. Instead, grasp your goods in the crook of your arm—the way a football player holds the ball as he's running across the field—and you won't be tackled by as much pain.

Avoid holding one position for a long time. Keeping joints "locked" in the same position for any length of time will only add to your pain and stiffness. Relax and stretch your joints as often as possible.

"Arm" yourself. Whenever possible, use your arm instead of your hand to carry out an activity. For example, push open a heavy door with the side of your arm rather than with your hand and outstretched arm.

Take a load off. Sitting down to complete a task will keep your energy level up much longer than if you stand.

Replace doorknobs and round faucet handles with long handles. They require a looser, less stressful grip to operate, so you'll put less strain on your joints.

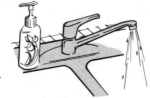

Build up the handles on your tools. For a more comfortable grip, tape a layer or two of thin foam rubber, or a foam-rubber hair curler, around the handles of tools such as brooms and mops.

Choose lighter tools. Lightweight eating and cooking utensils can keep your hands from getting heavy with hurt.

Let automatic appliances do the work for you. Electric can openers and knives, for instance, are easier to operate than manual versions. An electric toothbrush has a wider handle than a regular toothbrush.

Say no to scrubbing. Spray pots and pans with nonstick cooking spray and/or use cookware with a nonstick surface. Consider getting a dishwasher, too, to save your joints some work.

Keep your stuff within easy reach. Adjust the shelves and racks in any storage area so that you don't have to strain to reach the items you need. Buy clothes with pockets to hold things you use often and need close by, like a pair of glasses. Use an apron with pockets to carry rags and lightweight cleaning supplies with you as you do your household chores. Store cleaning supplies in the area in which they will be used. Keep the same supplies in several places, such as the upstairs bathroom and the downstairs bathroom as well as the kitchen.

Use a "helping hand" to extend your reach. For those items you can't store nearby, buy a long-handled gripper, the kind used in grocery stores to grab items from top shelves. Make household chores easier with a long-handled feather duster or scrub brush. Grab your clothes from the dryer with an extended-reach tool.

Don't overdo the housework. Plan on tackling only one major cleaning chore a day, whether it is doing the laundry or cleaning the kitchen.

Velcro is the way to go. Interlocking cloth closures on clothing and shoes can save you the frustration of buttoning and lacing.

Walk this way up and down the stairs. Lead with your stronger leg going up, and lead with your weaker leg coming down.

Bend with your knees. When reaching for or lifting something that's low or on the ground, bend your knees and keep your back straight as you lift.

Let loose with loops. You won't need quite as tight a grip if you put loops around door handles, such as those on the refrigerator and oven. Have loops sewn on your socks, too, then use a long-handled hook to help you pull them up.

Dig out that little red wagon. Heavier loads will be out of your hands if you use a wagon or cart that glides along on wheels. Use it to tote groceries or baskets of laundry, for instance.

Read with ease. Lay your newspaper out on the table rather than holding it up to read. Likewise, lay a book flat or use a book stand to give your hands a break as you read.

Sit on a stool in the tub. A specially made stool can give you a steady place to shower and can ease your way in and out of the tub.

Plant yourself on a stool in the garden. Sitting, rather than stooping, over your flower beds or vegetable garden may help reduce the stress on your back and legs.

Ask for help. Don't be afraid to ask your family members or friends for assistance when you need it. As the saying goes, many hands make light work. By sharing the load, you'll have more time and energy for the people and activities you enjoy.

Contact the Arthritis Foundation. The Arthritis Foundation can let you know of joint-friendly or energy-saving items specially made for use by arthritis sufferers. Call the Arthritis Foundation Information Line at 800-283-7800, Monday through Friday, 9:00 A.M. to 7:00 P.M. Eastern time, to talk to a skilled operator who can answer your questions about arthritis. ◆

◆ ASTHMA ◆

28 Ways to Breathe Easier

If you have asthma, you know the dreaded choking sensation, the faintness, the anxiety. It's as if someone made you run around the block, then pinched your nose shut and forced you to breathe through a straw. And you know all too well that once an asthma attack starts, it won't go away by itself.

Asthma sufferers make up an estimated five to ten percent of the population. And while no two persons with asthma are alike in the subtle characteristics of the condition, they do have one thing in common: They have trouble breathing properly. The reason is that their lungs are supersensitive and easily provoked into constriction by a wide variety of outside factors, called triggers.

As you have probably discovered, perhaps the hard way, many things can set an asthma attack into motion—someone's perfume, a smoke-filled room, a friendly dog, a flowery garden, a strong wind, or even a good laugh. (Asthma, however, is a hereditary condition, so unless a person is genetically predisposed, nothing will *make* asthma happen.) Triggers can be allergic or nonallergic, and reactions can be immediate or delayed.

While there is no cure for asthma, the good news is that asthma—whether mild, moderate, or severe—can be managed. Doctors who specialize in treating asthma can be very helpful. Every patient with asthma should see a doctor to be sure another cause of wheezing is not present and, if true atopic asthma is present, to develop a therapeutic program for managing the disorder.

In addition to working with your doctor, you can take measures to help control your asthma. The key is to track down the triggers and, as completely as possible, eliminate them from your life. In short, you can help counter an asthma attack before it happens. Here's how:

Smite the mite. "Dust mites are microscopic insects that thrive on food debris and high humidity," says Allan M. Weinstein, M.D., an asthma/allergy specialist in private practice in Washington, D.C. "Since they are among the most common allergic asthma triggers, dustproofing is a must." His suggestions:

• Enclose your mattress in an airtight, dustproof cover, then cover it with a washable mattress pad. Keep a bedspread on the bed during the day.

• Wash your sheets in hot water every week, wash your mattress pads and synthetic blankets every two weeks, and wash your pillows every month.

• Use polyester or dacron pillows, not those made of kapok or feathers, and enclose them in airtight, dustproof covers.

• Avoid carpeting, which is difficult to clean; stick to bare floors with washable area rugs.

• Choose washable curtains instead of draperies.

• Avoid dust-catchers (such as knickknacks) all over the house, especially in the room where you sleep; the less clutter the better. If possible, avoid storing out-of-season clothing or bedding in the bedroom; never store things under the bed.

• Try not to do heavy cleaning, but if you must, use only a vacuum cleaner and damp cloth to clean; dust mops and brooms stir up the dust. Always use *hot* water. "Cold water is like a day in the sun to a dust mite," says Weinstein.

• Wear a mask over your mouth and nose while cleaning, and leave the room when you're done.

• Run an air conditioner or dehumidifier in warm weather, especially in spring and fall when mites multiply. Aim to keep the humidity level in your home under 40 percent but above 25 percent.

• Consider using an air purifier in the bedroom to keep the room free from dust particles.

Minimize mold. "Fungus is a parasite that can literally 'grow on you,'" says

◆◆◆ The Quack ◆◆◆ Comes Back

If you have gone from doctor to doctor in search of a remedy for your asthma, you may feel frustrated and be tempted to explore some "alternative" treatments—cytotoxicity testing, special diets, herbal preparations, massage, and vitamins, to name a few. As tempting as these promised solutions may sound, there is one problem: They rarely work.

Cytotoxicity, for instance, is based on the premise that if the allergenic extract of a food to which you are allergic is mixed with a drop of your blood, certain cells in your blood will attack the food. Your blood cells will, therefore, be altered and, when viewed under a microscope, will be distorted. "The Asthma and Allergy Foundation of America has evaluated this test and concluded that it is unreliable," says Stuart Young, M.D.

Stuart Young, M.D., an asthma/allergy specialist in New York. "It can grow on nonliving organic material, too, in several forms—mold, dry rot, and downy mildew." Fungi reproduce by producing spores. The spores are the real problem, as millions of them float through the air to be inhaled in every breath, touching off an allergic reaction that can contribute to asthma. To stave off the spores, Young advises you to:
• Keep your windows closed, because the mold spores can come right in through the windows even if the windows have screens.
• Stay out of attics, basements, and other dank, musty places.
• Wear a face mask and give your bathroom a going-over for signs of mold. (Better yet, have a nonallergic family member do this.) The most likely spots for mold growth: dark areas, such as the backs of cabinets and under the sink.
• Examine all closets regularly to see that molds have not set up housekeeping in unused shoes and boots.
• On a regular basis, have a family member or friend investigate the inner workings of air conditioners, humidifiers, and vaporizers in your home where molds like to grow.
• Periodically check houseplants for mold growth. In fact, getting rid of mold will help your plants, as well.

Make peace with pollen. Pollen is released when plants are blooming—trees in the spring, grass in the late spring and early summer, ragweed from mid-August until the first frost. Plants that are pollinated by the wind are much more of a problem for asthmatics than are those pollinated by insects. "The goal is to learn how to live with pollen, not hide away from it," says Loomis Bell, M.D., chief of pulmonary–critical care medicine at St. Luke's–Roosevelt Hospital Center in New York. He recommends that you avoid cutting grass or even being outside while grass is being mowed. Keep your windows closed as much as possible—pollen can get through screens, too—and use an air conditioner to cool your home instead. Room air purifiers are also available that can purify recirculated air, removing particles of all sorts that are suspended in the air and further cleansing the air by passing it through a charcoal filter. After being outside in the midst of pollen, take off your clothes and wash them or at least run a vacuum over the articles of clothing. Wash yourself, too, and don't forget your hair.

Don't pet a pet. The best approach is to not have a pet that can trigger your asthma, advises Young. The problem is not the hair of the animal but the dander—the dead, dry skin that flakes off. The animal licks the skin, and the dander remains in its saliva. "If giving up a pet is impossible, the next logical step is to make very strict rules about living with an allergenic animal," Young warns. Do not allow your pet into the bedroom—ever. If the animal is in the bedroom at any time during the day, the dander will remain for hours. Leave the pet home if you are going for a car ride that would necessitate very close contact with the animal. If you do have direct contact with your pet (or any animal, for that matter), wash your hands right away. If you simply cannot keep your hands off your pet, at least keep your face away; kiss the air—your pet will still get the idea.

In addition, try bathing your dog or cat once every other week in warm water with no soap. Bathing the animal in this way significantly reduces the amount of allergen on your pet's fur, according to Clifton T. Furukawa, M.D., clinical professor of pediatrics at the University of Washington School of Medicine in Seattle.

Kick the cigarette habit. Tobacco smoke can be an irritant that triggers asthma as well as an allergen that touches off an allergic response leading to asthma. Tobacco smoke is one of the worst irritants known: It paralyzes the tiny hairlike cilia along the mucous membranes of the respiratory tract. It also reduces immune response and leaves a smoker much more susceptible to upper-respiratory infection. "There is not a single redeeming feature to cigarette smoking," cautions Weinstein. "Given the known health risks associated with smoking, asthma patients should make every effort to stop smoking—either on their own or with the help of a smoking-cessation program."

Nonsmokers who live with a smoker are no better off. So if there's someone in your household who won't quit smoking, ask that individual to take his or her habit outdoors.

Weather the weather. While each person responds to weather conditions and weather variations differently, some general trends may be noted. "Keep close watch on how the weather affects you," advises Young. (That means paying attention to factors including temperature, wind velocity, barometric pressure, and humidity.) "Then try to avoid conditions that cause you problems." For

example, you should stay indoors when it is very cold, since a blast of cold air can cause a spasm in your bronchial tubes. Stay indoors if the wind is strong, too. While gusts of wind can blow pollution and smog away, they can also blow pollen in your direction. If you enjoy walking in the rain, you're in luck, because rain tends to wash away roving allergens, pollutants, and irritants.

Watch what you eat. The question of whether foods trigger chronic asthma has yet to be answered. Some foods, such as nuts, shellfish, milk, eggs, and strawberries, can result in an array of allergic responses, including asthma symptoms. Sulfites in wine can have a similar effect. "While the information available today suggests that the chances are small that food allergies are a trigger for chronic asthma in adults, it is still wise to reduce or eliminate your consumption of certain foods that you notice make your asthma worse. But consult your doctor if you think the foods are nutritionally necessary," says Weinstein.

Allergies to certain types of food, especially milk and wheat, are more often a trigger of asthma in children. If milk and wheat seem to be causing problems for your asthmatic child, eliminate these foods. Check labels, and avoid foods that list milk, milk solids, casein, whey, or caseinate as ingredients. (Talk to your doctor about alternate dietary sources of nutrients such as calcium.)

Eating away from home can sometimes be a problem, says Weinstein. If you are invited to dinner and don't know what dinner will be, eat something at home before you leave so you won't be left hungry. If you are eating in a restaurant, inquire about the ingredients in the dish you want to order as well as the method of preparation. No matter where you have your meal, common sense suggests that you avoid overeating, eating too fast, and talking while you are eating. Steer clear of alcohol, too, especially if you are taking medications for your asthma. One final reminder: Avoid so-called cytotoxicity tests and similar methods that promise to root out hidden food allergies and cure asthma (see "The Quack Comes Back").

Stay healthy. A problem in the upper airways—such as a respiratory infection—can cause trouble in the lower airways—the bronchial tubes—and precipitate an asthma attack. "Everybody wants to be in a state of good health," says Bell. "For a person with asthma, maintaining good health can mean a dramatic lessening of symptoms." Bell suggests that you stay away from people who have a cold or the flu, drink plenty of fluids, and avoid getting overtired; otherwise, you will be more susceptible to infections. If, despite your best efforts, you do develop an infection, see your doctor; early use of antibiotics, when appropriate, can be quite helpful.

Exercise your options. For years, people with asthma have been told to avoid exercise because it would induce attacks. Research has shown, however, that the more asthmatics exercise, the more exercise they can tolerate. "If you have asthma, you should partake in regular aerobic exercise," says Bell. He recommends that you start by warming up with light exercise before a more-vigorous workout. (Young recommends using cromolyn sodium, a prescription medication, 15 to 20 minutes before aerobic exercise; discuss this with your doctor.) Begin with short workouts and gradually increase them. At least at first, keep a bronchodilator with you. If you feel tightness in your chest and can't work through it, use the device. If you are out in very cold or dry air, wear a scarf around your nose and mouth to heat the air before breathing it in. Cool down with light exercise at the end of your workout. If one type of exercise still brings on attacks, try another form of exercise. You may not be able to tolerate running, for example, but you may be able to swim regularly.

Avoid aspirin. Aspirin and certain products that contain aspirin can trigger asthma attacks in certain people. "It's just wise to stay away from the whole family of aspirin products if you have asthma," says Weinstein. "This is especially true for patients with nasal polyps, for whom aspirin ingestion can be life threatening. Even if you have not experienced an asthma flare in the past, it could occur at any time." Weinstein encourages anyone with asthma to keep aspirin out of the medicine chest by checking labels on every over-the-counter drug that is purchased. (Avoid those that list "aspirin" and those that contain the initials "ASA," "APC," or "PAC"; ask your pharmacist if you are unsure whether the medication you want to purchase contains aspirin.) If you feel that you must take aspirin, get your doctor's approval.

According to an expert report from the National Asthma Education Program, people with asthma should also stay away from certain nonsteroidal anti-inflammatory agents (ibuprofen is one such medication) that have effects similar to aspirin's. Opt instead for such "usually safe alternatives" as acetaminophen, sodium salicylate, or disalcid. You may also need to avoid tartrazine (yellow food dye #5), which is found in a number of soft drinks, cake mixes, candies, and some medications, if it aggravates your asthma.

Take a deep breath. Breathing exercises provide a form of relaxation and can be of benefit to some patients during an asthma attack. However, it would be a mistake to rely on breathing exercises alone to control an asthma flare, says Weinstein. As long as this rule is not broken, breathing exercises are fine for those patients who find them beneficial. "You can practice controlled breathing, which concentrates on slow inhalations through the nose rather than panting breathing through the mouth," says Weinstein. He suggests that before starting these breathing exercises, you blow your nose to make sure that your air passages are clear of all foreign matter. Then sit in a chair in a comfortable position. Take a deep breath and feel your breath going as far down as possible. Your abdomen should expand as you do this exercise. Exhale slowly, feeling your abdomen relax as your breath comes out of your nose. Repeat this exercise at least three times a day (but never right after eating).

Keep your weight down. "Unfortunately, some asthma medications can result in weight gain. An overweight person has to breathe more heavily, and the heart works harder to pump blood all around the body. Weight reduction is very important," says Bell. If you are overweight, you and your doctor should work together to establish a diet plan that will reduce your calorie intake without depriving you of necessary nutrients.

Mind your mind. The notion that asthma is "all in your head" has gone the way of many medical myths. Asthma is an illness with both physical and emotional aspects. For example, asthma attacks can be triggered by emotional changes, such as laughing or crying, or by stress. "The human body interacts with the mind," says Young, "so by putting your mind at ease, you can dramatically reduce the panicky feeling that can make an already existing attack worse." He recommends developing an upbeat mind-set by committing yourself to feeling better. A positive attitude works wonders to enhance your other coping methods. In addition, be forthright about your asthma; others will respect your directness and, in most cases, try to make things easier for you.

Learn to relax. Since stress and emotional upsets can trigger asthma attacks, it may be helpful to set aside time each day—preferably the same time—to practice some form of relaxation. ◆

◆ ATHLETE'S FOOT ◆

21 Strategies to Beat Athlete's Foot

Blame the advertising man who misnamed it in the 1930s, but athlete's foot has nothing to do with athletes. It's a fungal infection of the feet. Also known as *tinea pedis,* or "ringworm of the feet," it has nothing to do with worms either. The *Trichophyton* fungus that causes the redness, itching, cracking, and scaling of athlete's foot can also infect the scalp, where it causes hair loss and scaly patches; the body, where it causes round, red, scaly patches that itch; and the groin, where the so-called "jock itch" causes itching and thickening of the skin.

Athlete's foot is the most common fungal infection of the skin. It affects more men than women, probably because men typically wear heavy, often airtight shoes, and the fungus loves hot, dark, moist environments.

Contrary to popular myth, athlete's foot fungus isn't just found in locker rooms, although the moist locker-room environment is perfect for fungal growth. "The fungus is probably present in your bathroom and in your shoes all the time," says Andrew Schink, D.P.M., a podiatrist in private practice and past president of the Oregon Podiatric Medical Association.

Frank Parker, M.D., professor and chairman of the Department of Dermatology at Oregon Health Sciences University in Portland agrees. "There's no good way to avoid exposure to the athlete's foot fungus," he says, "because it's everywhere where there's moisture."

In fact, most people harbor the fungus on their skin, but it's kept in check by bacteria that live on the skin. So if the fungus is commonly present, why do some people develop an athlete's foot infection, while other people don't? Doctors aren't really sure, but they believe some people are genetically more prone to developing athlete's foot, and people with certain health conditions, such as eczema, asthma, and hay fever, have more

difficulty getting rid of the infection. "Some people are simply more susceptible to getting it than others," explains James Shaw, M.D., chief of the Division of Dermatology at Good Samaritan Hospital and Medical Center in Portland, Oregon. "Some people have chronic athlete's foot problems and others are never bothered by it. It may have to do with genetic factors or with exposure—being in places where there are numerous feet in moist environments."

Most cases of athlete's foot cause only bothersome redness, itching, flaking, and scaling on the soles of the feet and between the toes. In severe cases, however, blisters form on the soles of the feet; fissures, or cracks, that weep fluid can also open between the toes. These fissures are vulnerable to secondary infection. When the infection involves the toenails, it can cause the nails to become discolored and thick. Also, if left untreated, athlete's foot can infect other parts of the body.

Doctors don't agree on exactly how athlete's foot is spread, but most believe it's passed by direct contact with an infected person or with a contaminated surface, such as the floor of a shower stall. But Shaw says the real determinants of whether or not you'll get the infection are how susceptible you are and how dry you keep your feet.

While some severe cases of athlete's foot require a doctor's care, most can be effectively treated at home. The following strategies can help you soothe and heal athlete's foot and keep it from cropping up in the future.

Move away from moisture. When you think about athlete's foot fungus, remember that it likes moist, warm, dark environments. All of your treatment and prevention strategies should center around keeping your feet as dry as possible.

Dry between your toes. "Don't just use your damp bath towel to dry between your toes," says Schink. "Use a thin, dry hand towel and thoroughly dry between each toe." If you can't get your feet dry enough with a towel, try drying them with a hand-held hair dryer on the "warm" setting.

Wash those feet. Twice a day, wash your feet in soap and water, and dry them thoroughly, says Shaw.

Kick off your shoes. Go barefoot or wear open-toed sandals whenever you can. "Going barefoot is good for the feet and great for treating and preventing athlete's foot," says Schink.

Of course, it's not always possible to go barefoot, especially at work. But you may be able to sneak off those shoes during lunch, at break time, or when you're sitting at your desk.

Medicate 'em. Over-the-counter antifungal preparations are very effective for most cases of athlete's foot, says Parker. These products come in creams, sprays, or solutions and contain tolnaftate (Tinactin), miconazole (Micatin), or undecylenic acid (Desenex). Creams seem to be more effective, but powders can help absorb moisture. Parker recommends washing and drying the feet, then applying the medication thoroughly twice a day.

"Experiment. If one product doesn't work, try another. Different products seem to work better for different people," says Margaret Robertson, M.D., a board-certified dermatologist in private practice and a staff physician at St. Vincent Hospital and Medical Center in Portland, Oregon.

Be persistent. Too often, people stop using the antifungal preparations as soon as the symptoms of athlete's foot infection go away. The fungus, however, may still be present. "Fungus is slow-dividing," Robertson explains. "You have to be persistent and use the medication for three to six weeks to see improvement." Once the infection has

◆ How Contagious Is It? ◆

We've all heard stories about someone picking up athlete's foot in public showers and locker rooms. While it's true that such moist places probably do harbor fungus, your bathroom probably does, too. Relax and forget about trying to scrub all of the fungus from your life. It's everywhere, and you're not going to avoid it no matter how much you scrub and clean.

Does it mean you have to suffer with athlete's foot? Not necessarily, says Margaret Robertson, M.D. "It's a matter of genetics and exposure," she explains. "Some people are more susceptible to the fungus, and some strains of fungus are more infectious than others."

Robertson says that the type of athlete's foot fungus that causes red, weepy lesions is more infectious than the type that creates a white scale. Being exposed to the more infectious type doesn't mean you're going to get it, however. "My husband has battled chronic athlete's foot for 20 years," confesses Robertson, "and I've never been infected."

"It's not really all that contagious, like many of the other skin infections," says James Shaw, M.D. "If you have it, you don't have to worry too much about infecting others." Follow these simple tips to reduce the risk of infecting others:

• After bathing, wash out the tub or shower with an antiseptic cleaner like Lysol.

• Don't share your towel.

• Wash your socks twice in extra-hot water to kill fungal spores.

• Wear thongs in public showers.

• Keep your feet dry, and use the over-the-counter medications and treatments already discussed to clear your infection up quickly.

cleared, keep using the antifungal cream, powder, or lotion once a day or once a week—whatever keeps your feet fungus-free.

Make tea for toes. To help dry out the infection and ease the itching that accompanies athlete's foot, Schink advises soaking your feet in a quart of warm water containing six black tea bags. "The tannic acid in the tea is very soothing and helps kill the fungus," he says.

Soak them in Betadine. If the infection has caused redness and cracks between the toes, the fungal infection may be compounded by a bacterial infection. Robertson suggests soaking your feet once a day for 20 minutes in two capfuls of Betadine (available over-the-counter at pharmacies) to one quart of warm water. After the Betadine soak, dry your feet well, and apply antifungal medication.

Don't bleach. While the idea is to dry out the infection, avoid home remedies that involve strong chemicals and solvents, such as bleach, alcohol, and floor cleaners. "Many people are tempted to use what's at hand to treat their problem," says Shaw. "But harsh chemicals won't necessarily kill the fungus, and they can really damage your skin."

Tan your tootsies. Ultraviolet light can help dry up the infection and kill active fungus on your skin. Kick off those shoes and let the sun shine on your feet for a little while. Avoid extensive sun exposure, however, since it can promote wrinkling and skin cancer. Be careful not to burn the tops of your feet, or your dogs will really have something to bark about.

Treat your shoes. If you have fungus on your feet, you've got fungus in your shoes. To keep from reinfecting yourself every time you put your shoes

---

◆◆◆ Hello, Doctor? ◆◆◆

While most cases of athlete's foot can be effectively treated with home remedies, you should see a doctor if:

• You develop cracks in the webs between your toes. Studies have shown that toe-web cracking may indicate cellulitis, an inflammation of the connective tissue, which must be treated by a doctor, says Margaret Robertson, M.D.

• Your athlete's foot infection doesn't respond to home remedies within two to three weeks. If your condition isn't responding to treatment, it may indicate that you have some other problem, says James Shaw, M.D. "There are a whole host of things that can mimic a fungal infection," he says. Robertson agrees. "Often, fungal infections mimic other problems, like eczema and psoriasis," she says. Your doctor can perform a simple test to determine if athlete's foot is really the problem, she adds.

• Your infection is getting worse despite treatment. Some strains are hardier and are able to resist over-the-counter medication. Robertson says the antifungal medications available by prescription, such as ketoconazole and griseofulvin, are stronger and can knock out more-persistent infections.

• One or both feet swell.

• Pus appears in the lesions.

• The fungus spreads to your hands. Robertson says that when athlete's foot travels to the hands, it's called "two-foot, one-hand disease" because it often affects only one hand. Treatment may require prescription oral medication.

• The toenails appear thick and discolored. This indicates the toenails have become infected with the fungus. "Fungal infections of the toes are very difficult to treat," says Robertson. "Most of the over-the-counter topical medications that are supposed to treat fungus of the toenails don't work, because the nail is so thick."

on, Schink recommends treating your shoes with Lysol spray or an antifungal spray or powder every time you take off your shoes.

Air 'em out. On sunny days, Schink advises taking the laces out of your shoes, pulling up their tongues, and setting them in a sunny, well-ventilated place. The heat and sunshine will help dry out the shoes, eliminate odors, and kill the fungus.

Alternate shoes. Switch shoes at least every other day, advises Schink. Wear one pair for a day, while you treat the other pair with sunlight and an antifungal spray or powder.

Some people's feet are simply more prone to sweating, according to Robertson. If you're one of those "sweaty feet types," you may have to change your shoes a couple of times a day to keep your feet dry.

Choose shoes with care. When you have to wear shoes, opt for sandals or other opened-toed shoes, if possible. "Choose shoes that don't make your feet sweat," says Robertson. Avoid shoes made of plastic or rubber or shoes that are watertight. These shoes trap perspiration and create the warm, moist conditions perfect for growing a new crop of fungus. When you must wear closed-toed shoes, opt for natural, "breathable" materials like leather.

Exercise your sock options. Socks made of natural fibers, such as cotton and wool, help to absorb perspiration and keep the feet dry. However, recent research suggests that acrylic socks may do an even better job of keeping the feet dry by wicking moisture away from the feet. So what kind of sock should you choose? Try a pair of natural-fiber socks and a pair of acrylic, and see which one keeps your feet drier and more comfortable.

If your feet naturally sweat a lot or if you're participating in activities like sports that make your feet sweat more than usual, change your socks two or three times a day.

Wear thongs. When you're in a public place likely to harbor athlete's foot fungus, like the locker room of your favorite gym, wear thongs to limit your exposure to fungus, says Shaw.

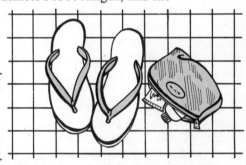

Although this technique isn't foolproof, it will decrease your risk of athlete's foot, and it may prevent you from picking up other nasty foot maladies, such as plantar warts. ◆

◆ BACK PAIN ◆

21 Ways to Keep Back Pain at Bay

Maybe you lifted something heavy or swung a golf club a little too enthusiastically. Or maybe you've been sitting in an uncomfortable desk chair for two weeks, sweating over a deadline. Whatever the reason, now you're flat on your back, wishing for something—anything— that will put an end to the agony.

Take heart—you're not alone. Almost every American suffers from back pain at some point in his or her life. The bad news is that unless you have a major injury or disc problem, your doctor may not be able to do much for you other than prescribe some pain medication and advise you to rest. The good news is that by following some simple steps, you can be on your feet again in just a few days. Even better, you can avoid having to endure similar discomfort in the future.

EASING THE PAIN

The following remedies are appropriate for anyone who is suffering from back pain as a result of tight, aching muscles or a strain. However, if you are experiencing pain, weakness, or numbness in the legs or a loss of bowel or bladder control, see a doctor without delay.

Go to bed. "Bed rest is a way of removing the strain from the muscles," says Daniel S. J. Choy, M.D., director of the Laser Laboratory at St. Luke's–Roosevelt Hospital Center and an assistant clinical professor of medicine at Columbia University College of Physicians and Surgeons in New York. "The back muscles' job is to hold you erect. If you lie down, it takes the stress off of the muscles." The best way to lie is flat on your back with two pillows underneath your knees. Never lie facedown, Choy says, since this position forces you

to twist your head to breathe and may cause neck pain. Make an effort to get up and start moving around after three days, since longer periods of bed rest may make the muscles weaker and more prone to strain, he adds.

Ice it. Applying an ice pack to the painful area within 24 hours of the injury can help keep inflammation and discomfort to a minimum, according to Willibald Nagler, M.D., Anne and Jerome Fisher Physiatrist-in-Chief and chairman of the Department of Rehabilitation Medicine at The New York Hospital–Cornell Medical Center in New York. "Ice does one thing—it decreases the nerve's ability to conduct a painful stimulus," he says. Nagler suggests wrapping ice cubes in a plastic bag, then applying the bag on top of a thin towel that has been placed on the skin. Leave the ice pack on for 20 minutes, take it off for 30 minutes, then replace it for another 20 minutes, he says.

Take a hot bath. If more than 24 hours have passed since the injury occurred, ice will not help reduce pain or inflammation. After that time, heat may help increase the elasticity of the muscles by about ten percent, Nagler says. Jerold Lancourt, M.D., an orthopedic surgeon at North Dallas Orthopedics & Rehabilitation, P.A., in Dallas, tells his patients to soak in a hot bath for 20 minutes or more. Pregnant women, however, should not sit in a hot bath for too long, since raising the body temperature over 100 degrees Fahrenheit for long periods may cause birth defects or miscarriage.

Invest in a new mattress. A soft, sagging mattress may contribute to the development of back problems or worsen an existing problem, according to Henry J. Bienert, Jr., M.D., an orthopedic surgeon at Tulane University School of Medicine in New Orleans. If a new mattress is not in your budget, however, a three-quarter-inch-thick piece of plywood placed between the mattress and box spring may help somewhat. "The verdict's not back yet on water beds," he adds. In any case, try to sleep on your back with two pillows underneath your knees.

Get a massage. If you're lucky enough to have an accommodating spouse, friend, or roommate, ask him or her to give you a rubdown. "Lie face-down and have someone knead the muscles," Choy says. Local massage therapists may also make house calls. You can check the yellow pages for listings or ask a friend for a referral.

Relax. Much back pain is the result of muscles made tight by emotional tension, Lancourt says. He recommends that his patients practice relaxation and deep-breathing exercises, such as closing their eyes, breathing deeply, and counting backward from 100.

Take two aspirin. Taking an over-the-counter analgesic such as aspirin, acetaminophen, or ibuprofen may help relieve your pain. However, be aware that not all medications—not even nonprescription ones—are for everyone. Pregnant women, for example, should not take any medication without first checking with their doctor. And people with ulcers should stay away from analgesics containing aspirin, according to Lancourt. "Any medicine should be taken with knowledge of its side effects," he says. "Make sure to get the advice of your doctor."

PREVENTING FUTURE PAIN

Many of the activities you engage in each day—sitting, lifting, bending, carrying—can put a strain on your back. By learning new ways of going about these activities, you can help prevent back pain and ensure the health of your back for years to come. The tips that follow can help.

Put your arm behind your back. If you have to sit for long periods in a chair that doesn't support your lower back and you don't have a cushion, try rolling up a towel or sweater so that it has about

the same circumference as your forearm. Then slide the rolled-up cloth between your lower back and the chair, recommends Billy Glisan, M.S., an exercise physiologist and the director of injury prevention programs for the Texas Back Institute in Dallas. In a pinch, you can simply slide your forearm between your lower back and the back of the chair to ease the strain on your back. Even with the best back support, however, sitting is still stressful on your back, so try to make small adjustments in the curvature of your lower back every few minutes or so, advises Glisan.

Use a cushion. "The seats of most cars and trucks are not well designed," Choy says. "They should support the small of your back." If your seat doesn't, Choy suggests that you buy a small cushion that can be fitted to provide the missing support. He adds that the most desirable sitting position is not one in which your back is straight up and down. It's better to be leaning back at an angle of about 110 degrees. If you sit for long hours, Choy also recommends that you periodically get up and walk around.

Swim. Swimming is the best aerobic exercise for a bad back, according to Choy. Doing laps in the pool can help tone and tighten the muscles of the back and abdomen. Walking is second best, he says. You can also try the "Back-Saving Exercises."

Lift with your knees bent. The large muscles of your legs and buttocks are better equipped to bear heavy weights than your back muscles are, according to Bienert. "Pretend you have a goldfish bowl filled with water on the top of your head," he says. "When you squat down to pick something up, don't spill a drop." Bienert also recommends strengthening leg and buttock muscles to facilitate squatting.

Carry objects close to your body. When picking up and carrying heavy objects, pull in your elbows and hold the object close to your body, Choy recommends. "If you have to reach something on a shelf, get right under it and rest it on your head," he says. "Then, the weight is carried by the erect spine, and you don't ask as much of your muscles."

Stay alert. Careless activity is the number-one cause of back injury, according to Lancourt. "If you have had previous back pain, be very careful," he says. "Avoid bending and twisting and lifting. Avoid being caught off guard. Sometimes it's better to hire somebody to do things, such as yard work or carrying heavy suitcases, than to hurt yourself and miss three months of work."

Watch your weight. Maintaining your ideal weight may help take the strain off the back muscles, according to Bienert. "The less you have to carry, the less load you have," he says. "Secondly, when you gain weight in your abdomen, you may become sway-backed, which can accentuate back pain." ◆

◆ Back-Saving Exercises ◆

The following back exercises were provided by exercise physiologist Billy Glisan, M.S. For best results, do the exercises daily, and don't discontinue them, even after the pain gets better, since strength and flexibility can only be maintained through consistent exercise. Stretches may be done twice a day. Although these exercises are safe and effective for most back pain caused by muscle strain or spasm, Glisan cautions that people with disc or other structural problems should not engage in any type of exercise without advice from their doctor.

Single Knee-to-Chest: *Lie on your back with your knees bent and your feet on the floor. Grasp the back of one thigh with both hands; gently and slowly pull toward your chest until you feel mild tension—not to the point of pain. Hold to the count of ten, without bouncing, then release. Repeat four to five times with the same leg, then switch sides. This exercise stretches muscles in the hips, buttocks, and lower back—all muscles that become shortened and tight after a long day of sitting or standing. It is a good warm-up to the other exercises.*

Double Knee-to-Chest: *Lie on your back with your knees bent and your feet on the floor. This time, grasp both thighs, and gently and slowly pull them as close to your chest as you can. Again— pull only to the point of slight tension, and don't bounce. Hold to the count of ten, then* release. Repeat four or five times before proceeding to the next exercise.

Lumbar Rotation: Lie on your back with your hips and knees bent, your feet flat on the floor, and your heels touching your buttocks. Keeping your knees together and your shoulders on the floor, slowly allow your knees to rotate to the right, until you reach a point of mild tension. Hold for a count of ten, then return to the starting position. Repeat four to five times on the right side, then switch to the left.

Partial Sit-Up: Lie on your back with your knees bent, your feet flat on the floor, and your hands gently supporting your head. Slowly curl up just to the point where your shoulders come off the floor. Avoid bending your neck. Hold for a few counts, then roll slowly back down. Remember to breathe as you do the exercise. Repeat 10 to 15 times. This exercise strengthens the abdominal muscles; strong abdominal muscles help you maintain good posture and reduce the possibility of back injury.

Active Back Extension: Lie on your chest on the floor. You can put a pillow under your stomach (not under your hips) if that feels comfortable. Put your arms at your sides, with your hands next to your buttocks. Slowly extend your head and neck and raise your upper body slowly off the floor. Hold for five to ten counts. Slowly lower yourself back to the starting position. Remember to breathe as you do the exercise. Repeat five to ten times.

Posture Enhancer: Stand with the back of your head, your shoulders and shoulder blades, and your buttocks held firmly against a wall. Your heels should be about six inches away from the wall. Do not allow your lower back to curve excessively. Start with the back of your hands against the wall at thigh level. Slowly slide the backs of your hands up the wall, without allowing your elbows, head, heels, buttocks, or shoulder blades to lose contact with the wall. (The movement is similar to making angels in the snow.) Stop at the point where your arms are so high that the above-mentioned body parts cannot stay against the wall. Repeat five times.

Office Exercises: If you spend many hours a day hunched over paperwork at a desk, chances are your lumbar, or lower, spine is being stretched and pulled in the wrong direction. (The lower spine's natural curve is slightly inward, toward the abdomen. Hunching forward causes the lower spine to be curved outward, toward the chair.) Poor sitting posture puts stress on the ligaments and other tissues. To give your lower back a break, periodically get up to a standing position, with your feet shoulder-width apart and your hands on your hips. Slowly lean back to a point of mild tension and hold for a count of ten. Repeat four to five times.

You should also practice getting out of your chair properly with your feet shoulder-width apart, your head up, your eyes focused straight ahead, and your buttocks stuck out. Use the strength of your arms, legs, and buttocks, instead of your back, to help you rise.

◆ BAD BREATH ◆

6 Refreshing Fixes

"Halitosis is better than no breath at all," jokes one dentist. But the problem of halitosis, or bad breath, has plagued mankind for centuries, leaving few people laughing about it. To conquer bad breath, the ancient Greeks reputedly rinsed with white wine, anise seed, and myrrh, while the Italians mixed up a mouthwash of sage, cinnamon, juniper seeds, root of cypress, and rosemary leaves, according to the Academy of General Dentistry.

Today, Americans spend more than half a billion dollars for mouthwashes that often contain little more than alcohol and flavoring. But people worry about their breath. Indeed, *New York Times* health columnist Jane E. Brody has written that she receives more questions about bad breath than about any other common medical problem.

Maybe one explanation is the simple fact that you can't really tell whether you've got bad breath. This is a time when you have to depend on the honesty and kindness of friends to let you know. "We're immune to our own breath," says Linda Niessen, D.M.D., M.P.H., associate professor and chair of geriatric oral medicine in the Department of Community Health and Preventive Dentistry at Baylor College of Dentistry in Dallas.

What if you're on your way to that important meeting and you simply *must* know if your breath will precede you through the door? You can try breathing into a handkerchief or running floss between your teeth, suggests Erwin Barrington, D.D.S., professor of periodontics at the University of Illinois at Chicago.

Fixing bad breath depends on what's causing it. In 80 to 90 percent of cases, it's due to something in the mouth. Most often, bad breath is the result of nothing more serious than a dirty mouth. Plaque, the nearly invisible film of bacteria that's constantly forming in your mouth, is often responsible. Other dental culprits include cavities and gum disease. "Tooth decay by itself doesn't smell bad, but the trapped food does," explains Niessen.

Occasionally, bad breath is due to something in the lungs or gastrointestinal tract or to a systemic (bodywide) condition. "Eating a garlicky meal is one of the most common causes," says Niessen.

What About Mouthwash?

Madison Avenue has played to our fears of bad breath in advertising claims for mouthwashes. But do they really work?

"Mouthwashes will cover odors," says Linda Niessen, D.M.D., M.P.H. The effects, however, are short-lived: Dental researchers agree that commercial mouthwashes mask odors only temporarily (from about 20 minutes to about 2 hours). These products don't prevent bad breath, either, says Erwin Barrington, D.D.S. While they may be able to kill bacteria that contribute to bad breath, a new batch of bacteria crops up fairly quickly.

If you do decide to use a mouthwash, Niessen recommends choosing a product with fluoride for its cavity-fighting potential or one that is accepted by the American Dental Association for removing plaque.

The strong odors of foods like garlic, onions, and alcohol are carried through the bloodstream and exhaled by the lungs. Another big loser when it comes to turning your breath sour—and harming your health—is tobacco.

In addition, some health problems, such as sinus infections or diabetes (which may give the breath a chemical smell), can cause bad breath, points out Barrington.

Figuring out the cause of bad breath is the first step, obviously, in doing something about it. Here's what you can do to keep your breath as fresh as possible:

Keep your mouth clean. "That's the key thing," stresses Sebastian G. Ciancio, D.D.S., professor and chairman of the Department of Periodontology and clinical professor of pharmacology at the School of Dental Medicine at the State University of New York at Buffalo. That means a thorough brushing twice a day. It also means flossing regularly. Food and bacteria trapped between teeth and at the gum line can only be removed with floss; if it's left to linger, it's not going to smell nice.

Clean your tongue, too. Bacteria left on your tongue can certainly contribute to less-than-fresh breath, so be sure to brush your tongue after you've polished your pearly whites.

Wet your whistle. A dry mouth can equal smelly breath. Saliva helps clean your mouth; it has a natural antibacterial action and it washes away food particles, says Ciancio. (It's the reduced saliva flow at night that explains morning breath, by the way.)

Try chewing sugarless gum or sucking on sugarless mints to stimulate saliva production.

Rinse. If nothing else, at least rinse your mouth with plain water after eating, recommends Virginia L. Woodward, R.D.H., past president of the American Dental Hygienists' Association.

◆◆ Hello, Doctor? ◆◆

Persistent bad breath may be due to a treatable cause, such as an undiagnosed cavity or periodontal (gum) disease. Sometimes, a broken filling can trap food particles. If you visit the dentist and are given a clean bill of health, you may want to investigate further and talk to your physician about other possible causes.

Swishing the water around in your mouth may help to remove some of the food particles left in the mouth after a meal.

Munch on parsley. That green sprig of parsley that came with your meal can do more than decorate your plate. While munching on parsley or spearmint won't cure bad breath, the scent of the herb itself can help temporarily cover up offending oral odor. (You're basically trading an offensive odor for a more acceptable one.)

Eat to smell sweet. Foods that help fight plaque may also help fight mouth odor, says Woodward. Opt for celery, carrots, peanuts, or a bit of low-fat cheese if you want something to snack on. "A healthy diet will help your teeth as well," Barrington points out. ◆

◆ BELCHING ◆

8 Ways to Squelch the Belch

In certain cultures, a belch after dinner is traditionally considered a compliment to the cook. In the Western world, if an adult belches after dinner—or at any time, for that matter—it is considered a breach of manners.

Babies burp, and it is certainly a satisfying sound to the mother or father who has been patting or rubbing the baby's back. Children belch, too, because they think it's a funny game, and sometimes the competition gets noisily intense. Over the years, however, such child's play can turn into a habit of frequently and unconsciously swallowing air—a habit that can result in belching.

If you suffer from aerophagia—the medical name for repetitive belching—you have probably endured the embarrassment of an unexpected outburst at precisely the most inelegant moment. But your habit can easily be broken if you just become aware of when and how you swallow air and stop doing it. Here's how:

Stifle it. "Chronic belchers may force themselves to belch because it provides temporary relief," says Lawrence S. Friedman, M.D., associate professor of medicine at Jefferson Medical College in Philadelphia. In fact, it has been demonstrated that repeated belching produces more of the same. On a fluoroscope (a special type of X ray used to visualize a body part in motion), a belching person can be seen forcing air into the mouth and esophagus. So if you're a chronic belcher, you need to make a concious effort to squelch that belch.

Don't smoke. Here is yet another reason to give up smoking if you remain in the ever-dwindling population that still engages in the habit. "By inhaling on cigarettes, cigars, or pipes, you are swallowing excessive amounts of air—much more than the belch can let out," says Gayle Randall, M.D., assistant professor of medicine in the Department of Medicine at the University of California at Los Angeles School of Medicine. And if you are counting on chewing gum or sucking on hard candy to help you kick the habit, think again; these activities stimulate air swallowing, too.

Mind your manners. Mom was right again when she told you not to talk with your mouth full. "This habit allows air into the mouth, which is then swallowed with the food," says Thomas Stahl, M.D., assistant professor of general surgery at Georgetown University Medical Center in Washington, D.C. Anyway, he adds, it's an unappealing form of behavior.

Eat slowly. People who gulp down food and beverages are, for one thing, swallowing excessive amounts of air. They're also crowding the stomach with too much to digest, which causes a gaseous buildup. "Once you take a mouthful, put down your fork and chew your food well before taking another bite," advises Randall.

Relax. Anxiety and stress can cause you to swallow more often, which increases the amount of air taken in. "You'll have to make a conscious effort to minimize air swallowing even though you may feel that your mouth is dry, because you'll only complicate your stress with stomach gas," says Stahl.

Don't catch cold. One sure thing about a cold is that it brings along postnasal drip, which will probably make you swallow much more frequently. So try to blow your nose to clear your nasal passages. Better yet, you should try to protect yourself from exposure to cold viruses.

Avoid bubbly beverages. Drinking carbonated beverages, including beer, creates air in the stomach. "Stay away from these drinks," advises Randall.

Go strawless. Drinking through a straw will only increase the amount of air you swallow. ◆

◆ BITES ◆

19 Ways to Fight Bites

Bites can range from itchy to painful to life threatening. And you needn't live out in the wilderness to run the risk of getting one. In fact, one of the most dangerous kinds of bites can be inflicted in your very own home—a bite from a fellow human being! (Doctors agree that humans have more bacteria in their mouths than most wild animals, no matter how often we brush our teeth.)

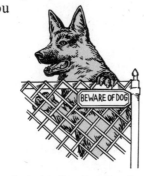

Many bites can be treated at home, although others, like a human bite, require an immediate visit to the doctor or emergency room. The trick is distinguishing the dangerous from the benign.

The following is a guide to treating the most common types of bites, as well as a few tips on how to avoid getting bitten in the first place. Of course, if you have had a run-in with a creature that you suspect is dangerous, whether or not it is discussed here, don't attempt self-treatment. See a doctor without delay. The same advice holds true if you experience any signs of illness (such as fever, loss of consciousness, nausea, dizziness, or vomiting) following a bite.

Ice an itch. Itchy mosquito bites may benefit from an ice-cold compress, according to Karl Singer, M.D., F.P., I.M., a physician in Exeter, New Hampshire. "Ice decreases the inflammation and stops the pain and itching," he says. He recommends icing the bite for 20 minutes at a time every few hours. The same goes for nonpoisonous spider bites, which can also leave an itchy welt.

Try an old fail-safe. When you had a mosquito bite as a child, your mother probably used calamine lotion—a thin, chalky, pink liquid—to stop the itch. Sold over the counter (and quite economical,

too, compared with alternatives such as hydrocortisone), it is just as effective today, says Michael R. Stefan, M.D., a physician specializing in internal medicine in Los Angeles.

Give an antihistamine a try. Over-the-counter antihistamines can also help an itchy bite, since the itch is really a mild allergic reaction, says Singer. Of course, antihistamines should not be used by sensitive individuals, pregnant women, people with allergies to ingredients in the products, or those who are taking conflicting medications. Check with your doctor or pharmacist if you are in doubt.

Recognize the signs of a severe reaction. The bite from a venomous spider can cause a severe allergic reaction. It is important, therefore, to recognize the signs of an allergic reaction before it is too late, according to Lawrence H. Bernstein, M.D., a family physician in Storrs, Connecticut. Symptoms of anaphylaxis, or severe allergic reaction, include difficulty breathing, hives all over the body, and loss of consciousness. Anyone experiencing these warning signals should be rushed to the nearest emergency room, he says. Hospital physicians usually treat anaphylaxis with steroids, adrenaline, and antihistamines.

Don't panic if you've been bitten by a tick. Lyme disease, a tick-borne illness that can cause chills, fever, headache, and other complications, has received lots of play in the media of late. But not all ticks carry the disease, and not every Lyme-carrying tick will transmit it to you if you happen to be bitten. Generally, a tick must remain on the skin for 24 to 48 hours in order to transmit the organism that causes Lyme disease, according to Bernstein. "The best thing to do, if you're in a place where there might be ticks, is to check yourself on a daily basis," he says. If you remove a tick from your skin (using the directions that follow), Bernstein recommends saving it in a small jar of alcohol, so that if a suspicious infection develops, the tick can be analyzed for Lyme disease. There is no need to see a doctor unless you notice any signs of swelling or redness around the bite (a sign of infection), a bull's-eye-shaped rash (often a symptom of Lyme disease), a fever, or a skin rash, Bernstein says.

Remove ticks with care. To remove a tick from your skin, grasp the insect's mouthparts with tweezers as close as possible to your skin and slowly pull straight upward. Do not attempt to pull the tick's body or head, as it may break off, leaving the

mouthparts underneath your skin, Bernstein says. Use the tweezers to remove any remaining parts of the tick. Next, apply a local antiseptic, such as alcohol or an antibiotic ointment, to the bite.

Stop the bleeding. If an animal bite has caused severe bleeding, apply pressure to the area with the palm of your hand, says Michael O. Fleming, M.D., F.A.A.F.P., a family physician in Shreveport, Louisiana. If the wound is large, tie a scarf, towel, or T-shirt tightly around the site to create pressure over a larger area (not tightly enough to cut off circulation). Immobilize the

◆◆ Handling Snakebites ◆◆

If you've been bitten by a snake that you suspect is poisonous, the best thing to do is to hightail it to the nearest emergency room. Some snakebites, most notably those from rattlesnakes such as the Eastern diamondback, can be fatal. However, hospital emergency units stock very effective antivenoms that will have you feeling better in no time, says Michael R. Stefan, M.D.

One fact that may make you less nervous is that snakes only envenomate, or inject their venom, between 25 percent and 75 percent of the time, according to Richard E. Hannigan, M.D. The rest of the time they leave nothing more than fang holes and a frightened victim.

If you are far from medical attention, Hannigan recommends taking the following steps while help is being sought or while you are on the way to the hospital:

• Have someone catch the snake and kill it—if the capture can be accomplished without excessive danger. Put the corpse in a bag, and take it to the hospital with you. This way, hospital staff can accurately identify the snake and will be sure to administer the correct antivenom.

• Stay quiet, still, and warm. Do your best not to panic. Getting upset stimulates the heart to pump more blood, which means that more venom will be circulated throughout your system. Taking a couple long, slow, deep breaths may help.

• If you have been bitten on a limb, remove any rings, bracelets, shoes, or socks, since the extremity may swell. If possible, immobilize the limb and let it rest at a level below the heart.

• You may tie a scarf, tie, belt, or piece of fabric above the level of the fang mark, but do not make it tight enough to cut off circulation. A good guideline is to make sure that you can slide at least one finger underneath the band.

• If you have a venom-extractor kit with you, apply the suction device for 30 to 40 minutes, or until you get to the hospital.

• Do not apply ice, cut the snakebite with a knife, or attempt to suck venom from the wound. These are outdated methods of treatment that may actually cause more harm than good.

• Ask for help. If you have been envenomated, you may begin to feel dizzy or ill. Do not attempt to drive yourself to the hospital.

area. If the bite is on a limb, elevate the limb above the level of the heart. See a physician pronto.

Don't treat a puncture like a scratch. A bite that leaves a scratch but doesn't really break the skin may simply be washed with soap and water, then covered with an antibacterial cream or ointment. Not so for a bite that breaks or punctures the skin, according to Bernstein. The latter needs the expertise of a doctor, he says. "You need to establish whether the animal is rabid or not," he advises. "Observe the animal carefully. With wild animals, if the animal is particularly placid—for example, if you can walk up to a squirrel and feed it—there's something wrong with that animal. It's sick." He suggests calling a doctor or veterinarian to find out if there have been any reported outbreaks of rabies in wild or domestic animals in your area.

Get a tetanus booster. If you've been bitten by a wild or domestic animal and the bite has broken the skin, it's probably wise to contact your doctor to see if you need a tetanus booster shot (whether or not you need one depends, in part, on the type of wound and the timing of your last tetanus shot). "Animal bites and human bites are easily infected," Fleming says. "All animals have a very large number of bacteria that live in their mouths." He also advises watching for signs of infection, such as redness and swelling.

Report an animal to the authorities. If you've been bitten by an animal in your community, call your local Society for the Prevention of Cruelty to Animals (SPCA) or animal catcher (check your local phone directory for the number) to report the incident. If the animal was wild or a stray, the proper agency may want to track it down and capture it for observation, especially if rabies is suspected. If the animal belongs to a neighbor, report it to the pet's owner, and, if you choose, to the authorities (many communities have laws concerning pet bites).

Don't get bitten in the first place. Perhaps the most sensible way to treat a bite is in advance—before you get bitten—Stefan says. Stay away from wild animals, even if they let you approach, and don't pester snakes, spiders, bees, or anything else that looks threatening. "Most animals and insects will not attack you unless you are bothering them," he says. Even animals that do not look threatening, such as ground squirrels, may be trouble, Stefan adds, since they may carry fleas that can transmit diseases. Insect and tick repellents may also help you avoid bites when spending long periods of time outdoors.

Know your local fauna. It's best to keep abreast of the insects and animals in your area, so that you know what to watch out for. For example, you may live in an area where there has been an outbreak of rabies among domestic animals or a large number of Lyme-carrying ticks, according to Richard E. Hannigan, M.D., an internist in private practice in Helotes, Texas. Likewise, you should know if rattlesnakes, poisonous spiders, or scorpions are likely to take up residence around your neighborhood. If you live in an area, such as the Southwest, that is home to poisonous snakes and scorpions, learn how to recognize them by sight and avoid them like the plague, Hannigan recommends. ◆

◆ BLACK EYE ◆

6 Care Tips

This morning's racquetball game was going so well—until your opponent hit that unbelievable shot that bounced off the wall and hit you right in the eye. After he finished apologizing profusely and the pain subsided somewhat, you picked up your ego and went home. But now you're beginning to resemble a prizefighter who lost the prize! Your eyelid is nearly swollen shut, the area around your eye is turning black and blue, and the throbbing pain is back in full force. You're starting to wonder if there's more to this injury than meets the eye.

As horrifying as a black eye can look—and as embarrassing as it can be to explain—it is usually nothing that will cause lasting or serious damage. "A black eye is simply a hemorrhage around the eye. The blood underneath the skin comes through as a purplish color. While there are many diseases and conditions that can cause black eyes [see "Other Causes of Black Eyes"], a true shiner is most often the result of trauma to the eye caused by a fistfight or a sports injury," says Jon H. Bosland, M.D., a general ophthalmologist in private practice in Bellevue, Washington. "If the swelling comes down rapidly and your vision is good, it is not likely that there is any serious damage to the eye," he says.

Still, Bosland urges anyone with a black eye to see a doctor in order to rule out damage to the eye itself. (It is especially important to see a doctor without delay if there is any change in vision.) Once you are sure everything is all right, there are some steps you can take at home to care for your shiner. There are also some preventive measures that you can take to help keep your eyes out of the black in the future.

Ice the area. "This will reduce the swelling and numb some of the initial pain," says Carol Ziel, M.D., an ophthalmologist with the Eye Clinic of Wausau in Wisconsin. Hold an ice pack or some ice cubes wrapped in a washcloth on the eye. "Putting crushed ice in a plastic bag and placing the bag on top of a cold washcloth over the eye also works well," says Charles Boylan, M.D., a pediatric ophthalmologist at A Children's Eye Clinic of Seattle.

Pack it in popcorn or peas. A bag of frozen, unpopped popcorn kernels or frozen peas placed over a washcloth on the affected eye can also help cool the area and bring some relief.

Clean it up. Clean any small lacerations with mild soap and water. "Then continue to keep them clean and dry," says Ziel. This will help to keep the area from becoming infected with bacteria. "Sometimes, the tissue around the eye can actually split because the soft tissue is being pushed against a hard surface of underlying bone. You can get a considerable hemorrhage from this, which can leave a bit of a lump afterward," adds Bosland.

Avoid pressing on the eye itself. The area has already been traumatized enough, and pressing on it will only cause further trauma, says Bosland. So be gentle when you apply an ice pack or clean the area.

Keep your chin up. OK, so you look and feel a little like Rocky Balboa. Be thankful you can see yourself in the mirror, and try to resign yourself to the added color for a while. "The discoloration tends to last one to two weeks," says Bosland. It will lessen during that time, but it won't fade completely for a couple of weeks or so.

Wear goggles. As is true with so many injuries, the best treatment is prevention. While you may not necessarily like the way you look in goggles, wearing them can help you ensure that you'll be able to *see* the way you look.

Any sport that involves close contact with other individuals and/or the use of a small ball of some sort is likely to put you at risk for a black eye. "The majority of black eyes we see are caused by the eye being hit by an elbow, hand, or knee or by an object small enough to fit inside the bony structure around the eye," says Boylan. Tennis doesn't really qualify because the ball is too big. But squash, racquetball, and skiing (the end of the pole can hit

the eye) are particularly dangerous to the eye. And basketball, where arms and legs are flying in close quarters, can also leave you vulnerable to a nasty black eye.

To protect your eyes, Boylan suggests that you wear protective eye wear, such as goggles or even glasses with shatterproof glass or plastic lenses. "Anyone with only one good eye should always wear protective eye wear if there is a chance of being hit with anything," stresses Boylan.

As far as how to choose the right goggles or glasses, it's not too difficult. "Make sure the lenses are shatterproof and the glasses or goggles fit comfortably," says Boylan. "The goggles worn by squash and racquetball players often don't contain any lenses, and that's OK. The frame itself will keep the ball away from the eye," he continues. Most sporting goods stores, as well as eye-wear stores, carry protective eye wear for sporting events. If you can't locate any, consult your eye doctor. ◆

◆ Other Causes of ◆ Black Eyes

In addition to trauma, there are several other reasons that the tissue around the eyes can become blackened. "The skin of the eyelid itself is very loose and flexible and contains no subcutaneous fat. As a result, the muscles and blood vessels around the eye are quite close to the surface of the skin," explains Jon H. Bosland, M.D. "So you can get vascular congestion around the eyes that will cause them to look kind of dark and purplish," he continues. For this reason, it is not uncommon for people with severe allergies and long-lasting allergic swelling to experience what is referred to as an "allergic shiner" in one or both eyes.

You can also get a black eye from distant injuries such as a skull fracture. "In this instance, the

fracture initiates back behind the eyes but the blood migrates up into the tissue around the eyes," explains Bosland.

And we've all felt the pressure around our eyes when we've been continually sneezing, coughing, or vomiting. This pressure can cause black eyes as well. "I once saw a girl come in with two black eyes, and the only history we had on her was that she had a very bad case of the flu and was vomiting extensively," says Bosland. "That broke some blood vessels back behind the eyes and the blood migrated out to the surface of the skin," he explains.

A variety of other serious illnesses can also cause the eyes to appear blackened. So as with a black eye caused by trauma, you should take your shiner to the doctor just to be on the safe side.

◆ BLADDER INFECTION ◆

15 Self-Care Techniques

You have to go, and you have to go *now*. Come to think of it, it seems like you've had to go every 15 minutes since you woke up this morning. And each time, it's been the same story. Not much comes out, but it burns like crazy. What in the world is going on?

If you have pain or burning on urination, the frequent urge to urinate, and/or blood in your urine, chances are you have a bladder infection (also called cystitis, urinary tract infection, or UTI). These symptoms may also be accompanied by lower abdominal pain, fever and chills, and an all-over ill feeling.

Bladder infections are caused by a bacterial invasion of the bladder and urinary tract. "The urine in the bladder is normally sterile," explains Amanda Clark, M.D., assistant professor of obstetrics and gynecology at Oregon Health Sciences University in Portland. "However, if it becomes contaminated with bacteria, a bladder infection can develop."

If you're a woman who suffers from bladder infections, you're not alone. "Women tend to suffer more bladder infections than men because the female urethra, the tube leading from the bladder to the outside of the body, is only about one-and-a-half inches long—a short distance for bacteria to travel," says Sadja Greenwood, M.D., a women's health specialist and assistant clinical professor in the Department of Obstetrics, Gynecology, and Reproductive Sciences at the University of California at San Francisco. (A man's urethra is about eight inches long.) Frequently, the urinary tract becomes contaminated with *Escherichia coli*, bacteria that are normally present in the bowel and anal area. In 10 to 15 percent of cases, bladder infections are caused by another organism, such as *Chlamydia trachomatis*.

Women also suffer more bladder infections because sexual intercourse can irritate the urethra and contribute to the transport of bacteria from the anal area and vagina into the bladder. "We don't really know exactly why intercourse increases the risk of bladder infections," says Clark. "We think it might make the bladder tissues a little more receptive to having an infection or it may cause more bacteria to move up the urethra."

Women who use the diaphragm for birth control have a greater risk of bladder infections, too, says Clark. The diaphragm presses against the neck of the bladder, which inhibits normal urination, she says. As urine flow decreases, pressure within the bladder increases, and the bladder is unable to completely empty itself. The pooled urine then acts as a growth medium for bacteria.

Pregnant women are also more likely to suffer from bladder infections. The changing hormones of pregnancy and the pressure exerted by the enlarged uterus on the bladder and ureters (the two tubes that carry urine from the kidneys to the bladder) put pregnant women at greater risk.

Men can also suffer from this malady. In men, bladder infections are almost always secondary to an infection of the prostate gland (prostatitis), according to Theodore Lehman, M.D., a urologist in private practice and director of The Oregon Impotence Center in Portland. "Primary infection of the bladder in men just doesn't happen, because the bladder is well protected," explains Lehman. "But the prostate sits right in front of the bladder, and bacteria can get into it—through sexual intercourse, trauma like bouncing on a bicycle seat, or some kind of blockage—and it stirs up an infection in the prostate. Then the prostate infection can 'move upstream,' if you will, and infect the bladder."

In men, prostate infection usually feels like "you're sitting on a brick," says Lehman. When the infection extends to the bladder, the symptoms of irritation, urinary frequency, and pain and burning on urination join the achy-bottom feeling.

Bladder infections can often be treated at home with the self-care tips that follow. However, if your symptoms persist for more than 24 hours, if they don't respond to home remedies, or if you suspect that your symptoms may be due to a sexually transmitted disease or other infection, see your physician.

Load up on fluids. At the first sign of bladder infection, start drinking water and don't stop. During the first 24 hours, Greenwood recommends drinking at least one eight-ounce glass of water every hour. People who suffer from recurrent bladder infections usually don't drink enough liquids. So even when you don't have an active infection, you should make a habit of drinking eight tall glasses of water every day.

According to Lehman, drinking lots of fluid not only dilutes the urine, giving bacteria less to feed on, it also has a "washout" effect on bacteria. "The more bacteria you can wash out," says Lehman, "the less there will be to reproduce."

Clark warns, however, that people who suffer from urinary leakage (incontinence) probably shouldn't increase their fluids. She says it can make the bladder infection and the incontinence worse.

Have a cranberry cocktail. If you've never developed a taste for the sweet tanginess of cranberry juice, now's the time. Cranberry juice (without added sugar) may make urine more acidic and less hospitable for bacterial growth, says Clark. Drinking cranberry juice is also a way to increase your fluid intake.

Go, go, go. Lehman advises both men and women to avoid what he calls "L.A.-freeway-driver bladder." "Many people don't urinate when they first get the urge because it's inconvenient or there isn't the time or place," he says. "Take a guy who gets off work, has a couple of cups of coffee or a couple of beers, and gets on the freeway in rush-hour traffic. He feels the urge to urinate, but he can't get off the freeway. When he finally gets home

and urinates, it's difficult and it burns. By the next day, he's calling his doctor with a prostate infection."

Holding urine allows it to concentrate in the bladder, creating a perfect medium for bacterial growth. In older men, holding urine can cause congestion, inflammation, and obstruction of the prostate and can eventually lead to a prostate infection or sometimes a bladder infection.

Not urinating at the first urge also causes the bladder to distend and stretch. "Essentially, the bladder is a hollow muscle," says Lehman. "If you repeatedly stretch it, then it won't void completely and creates a place for bacteria to grow."

Heat it up. For lower abdominal pain, use a heating pad or hot-water bottle or take a hot bath, advises Greenwood. Lehman says that heat not only relieves the symptoms, it also brings more blood with white blood cells and other infection-fighting blood products to the affected area. (Pregnant women, however, should not sit in a hot bath or hot tub for too long, since raising the body temperature above 100 degrees Fahrenheit for long periods may cause birth defects or miscarriage.)

Take a bath. If you have a lot of burning, a warm "sitz" bath (sitting in three to four inches of water) can ease the pain.

Take a break. Rest in bed, especially if you have a fever. You'll conserve energy and speed healing.

Wear cotton underwear. Cotton underwear, cotton-lined panty hose, and loose clothing will allow the genital area to breathe and stay dry. For men, boxer-type shorts rather than jockey-style shorts are better if prostate and bladder infections are a problem.

Avoid alcohol. Alcohol is a urinary tract irritant for both men and women and should be avoided during a bladder infection.

What about spicy foods, tea, and coffee? Clark says, "They really shouldn't hurt a bladder infection." However, the caffeine in coffee, tea, and colas does stimulate the kidneys to produce more urine and makes the bladder fill up faster during a time when urination is painful. If caffeine seems to make your symptoms worse, avoid it until the infection goes away.

Take a pain reliever. Bladder infections can be painful. Acetaminophen, ibuprofen, or aspirin, especially if taken at bedtime, can ease the pain.

Wash up, lovers. Both partners should wash up before intercourse.

Urinate after lovemaking. If you suffer from recurrent bladder infections, urinate immediately before and after intercourse, advises Clark. This can help flush out bacteria that may have entered the urinary tract.

Switch birth-control methods. Women who use a diaphragm and suffer from recurrent infections should try switching to condoms or a cervical cap. "If you have recurrent bladder infections, see your doctor to have your diaphragm's fit rechecked," says Clark. "You may do better with a smaller diaphragm or a cervical cap."

Keep a bladder-infection diary. If you suffer from recurrent bladder infections, keep a diary to discover what patterns precede an attack. Some people find that their infections are related to stress, menstruation, lovemaking, or other factors. Once you discover what precipitates your infections, you can make changes to alter those patterns.

Wipe from front to back. Most women wipe from back to front, which moves bacteria from the rectum dangerously close to the urethra.

Use condoms. Prostate infection, which can lead to bladder infection, is more common among men with multiple sex partners. Practice safe sex, and always use condoms with partners. ◆

◆◆ Hello, Doctor? ◆◆

In many cases, bladder infections can be successfully treated at home with the remedies described here. However, call your doctor if you:

- *Have a personal history of kidney disease*

- *Are diabetic*

- *Are pregnant or may be pregnant*

- *Have shaking spells or have vomited within the last 12 hours (may indicate kidney infection or septicemia, a bacterial infection in the blood that can be fatal)*

- *Have symptoms and fever that increase after 48 hours of home treatment*

- *Have blood in your urine*

- *Have had an abdominal or back injury within two weeks prior to the onset of your symptoms (may indicate kidney injury)*

- *Have high blood pressure*

- *Are male and over age 50*

- *Have or suspect that you have a sexually transmitted disease*

◆ BLISTERS ◆

18 Ways to Treat—and Beat—Them

Yου just couldn't resist a bargain. Those shoes looked great with your new outfit, even if they didn't feel so great on your feet. "They'll stretch out," you told yourself, and then patted yourself on the back for getting such a good deal. Unfortunately, you got more than you bargained for—namely, painful blisters to go with your new shoes.

Blisters are tender spots that fill up with fluid released by tiny blood vessels in an area where delicate skin tissues have been burned, pinched, or just plain irritated. Virtually everyone has experienced friction blisters, the kind caused by hot, sweaty, or ill-fitting shoes. If you have one now, read on to find out how to take care of it. Then continue reading to learn how you can help protect your tender tootsies in the future.

TREATING YOUR BLISTER
A blister is your body's way of telling you that skin and tissues are being injured. So while you take steps to relieve the discomfort, you also need to protect the injured area.

Make a tent. Instead of simply placing an adhesive bandage right on top of the blister, "tent" the bandage by bringing in its sides so the padding in the middle of the bandage raises up a bit. "This will not only protect the blister but allow air to circulate, which will aid in healing," says Nelson Lee Novick, M.D., associate clinical professor of dermatology at the Mount Sinai School of Medicine in New York.

Use a double-duty bandage. Another type of bandage, available in pharmacies, contains a gel and antiseptic to cushion and "clean" the blister, says Wilma Bergfeld, M.D., head of clinical research in the Department of Dermatology at the Cleveland Clinic Foundation in Ohio. Ask your pharmacist about it.

Let it breathe. Some physicians believe that a blister should not be covered at all for maximum aeration. Jerome Z. Litt, M.D., assistant clinical professor of dermatology at Case Western Reserve University School of Medicine in Cleveland, is one such doctor. He even suggests slipping your shoe off while you sit at your desk at work in order to give your blister some air.

Smear on an ointment. Whether you decide to cover your blister or not, you should apply an antibacterial/antibiotic ointment to it. Doctors generally recommend Bacitracin or Polysporin, which may be less likely to cause an allergic reaction or sensitivity than other over-the-counter ointments.

Pad it. When a blister is in a particularly annoying spot, like the bottom of the foot, padding might provide more of a cushion than just a bandage would, advises Bergfeld. She suggests using the circular pads made of foam adhesive found in the foot-care aisle of drug- and beauty-aid stores. "Pharmacies also carry sheets of padding that you can cut to size for a more exact fit," says Bergfeld. Cut the padding in the shape of a donut, and place it on the skin surrounding the blister so that the blister fits in the hole in the opening of the donut. Then gently cover the blister with an antibacterial ointment and bandage.

Put it up. Elevating the blistered area can help relieve the pressure, advises Bergfeld.

Be patient. Expect it to take about a week to ten days for the blister's fluid to be reabsorbed by the body.

Drain it. While some doctors believe that a blister should never be popped because of the risk of infection, most agree that a blister causing extreme pressure—such as one on a finger or toe or under a nail—is a candidate for draining.

If you should decide to pop it, first wipe the blister and a sewing needle with alcohol. "Never sterilize a needle over a flame," says Novick. "It can create soot on the tip of the needle, which can 'tattoo,' or dirty, the blister." Prick the blister once or twice near its edging; then slowly and gently press out the fluid.

Keep the roof on it. Once you have popped the blister and drained the fluid, do not remove the deflated top skin. This skin, called the blister's roof, protects the blister from infection and forms a "bridge" for new cells to migrate across on their journey to heal the site.

Soak first. To drain a blister on a tough-skinned area, such as the sole of the foot, Litt suggests first soaking the blister in Burow's solution, available from pharmacies in packets or tablets (follow the directions on the package). He recommends soaking the blister for 15 minutes, three to four times a day. A day or two of this will soften the blister and make draining easier.

Watch for signs of infection. Redness, red streaks, or pus in an intact or a "popped" blister should be treated by a doctor.

PREVENTING BLISTERS

Here are ways to prevent friction blisters, according to Glenn B. Gastwirth, D.P.M., Deputy Executive Director of the American Podiatric Medical Association in Bethesda, Maryland:

Buy shoes in the afternoon. "Over the course of the day, your feet may swell by as much as half a shoe size," says Gastwirth. When trying on shoes, wear the same type of socks that you plan to use with the shoes.

Look for leather. Unlike nonporous vinyl and plastic materials, leather has microscopic pores that allow air to circulate, keeping the foot drier. In the same way, so do the clusters of perforated holes primarily found on many styles of sports footwear. A dry foot is less likely to develop blisters.

Don't exercise at midday. The heat of midday, especially in the summer, can make the feet perspire more, making them more blister-prone.

Never wear wet shoes. The wetness can cause more "dragging" between the foot and shoe and can result in blisters. If you jog twice a day, for instance, you may want to buy a second pair of running shoes for your second run each day.

Protect "hot spots." If you have a chronic "hot spot," or place where blisters tend to develop, apply petroleum jelly to it, then slip on your sock. Foam or felt pads, used alone, can also absorb the friction and protect a hot spot. For best results, make sure the padding covers more area than you think a blister would take up, since the neighboring areas can become irritated, too.

Wear the right socks. Specially made sport socks with extra padding in hot spots can help prevent blisters. Natural fibers such as cotton and wool tend to keep the feet dry by absorbing moisture. However, according to Gastwirth, recent research suggests that acrylic fibers may, through a wicking action, actually move moisture away from the foot, keeping it drier and making it less prone to blistering. Your best bet? Try them both and see which type of fiber keeps your feet drier and more comfortable. In addition, make sure the sock fits your foot, so there is less chance of it bunching up inside the shoe and causing a blister.

Try a sprinkle. Foot powders may aid in keeping the foot dry and preventing painful blisters from forming. ◆

◆ BODY ODOR ◆

6 Steps to Sweet-Smelling Success

Let's face it, in the United States, a pungent body aroma is not going to make you the life of the party. So powerful is our cultural distaste for body odor that every day, some 95 percent of all Americans over the age of 12 reach for one product or another that will enable them to feel safe and secure in the company of others.

Body odor begins with sweat. The body has two types of sweat glands, and both types produce sweat that is made up largely of water. The eccrine glands, which are located on almost every part of the body, produce the sweat that cools the body. The apocrine glands, which are located in the armpits, around the nipples, and in the groin, produce sweat whose function, at least in modern times, is not clear. One thing is obvious, however. The sweat from the apocrine glands can make you stink, because it contains a substantial amount of oil, which provides food for bacteria. It's this bacterial feeding frenzy that causes the offensive odor. Here's what the experts recommend you do to come up smelling like roses:

Keep it clean. "The best way to prevent body odor is to wash away the sweat that forms on the skin in the area of the apocrine glands and reduce the number of bacteria waiting there to feed upon it," says Donald Rudikoff, M.D., assistant clinical professor of dermatology at Mount Sinai School of Medicine in New York. So, clean the underarm and groin area with soap, preferably a deodorant soap, and water at least once a day.

Bathe your britches. Sweat that seeps into your clothing may remind you of its presence at very inopportune times. What's more, dried, bacteria-containing sweat can damage the fibers of your clothing. "You should wash your washable clothing each time you wear it," advises Rudikoff.

Try a deodorant. For milder cases of body odor, a deodorant may help. Deodorants are considered cosmetics. Most contain a substance that helps kill the bacteria that are waiting to feed on your sweat. They may also help mask body odor by substituting a more acceptable scent.

Get tough with an antiperspirant. Since body odor begins with sweat, one of the best ways to control it is to reduce the amount of sweat. "You can probably reduce perspiration by as much as 50 percent with an antiperspirant," says Allan L. Lorincz, M.D., professor of dermatology at the University of Chicago Medical Center.

Antiperspirants are classified as over-the-counter drugs because they are intended to alter a natural body function—they decrease production of eccrine sweat. (While apocrine sweat contains the oil upon which bacteria feed, neither an antiperspirant nor a deodorant can decrease apocrine sweat.) By decreasing production of eccrine sweat, antiperspirants help keep you drier, thus reducing the moisture that creates a breeding ground for bacteria. Antiperspirants usually also contain an antibacterial agent that fights odors. (For tips on choosing an antiperspirant, see EXCESSIVE SWEATING.)

Beat irritation and odor. If you've tried antiperspirants and deodorants and found that they irritate your skin, you might instead try an antibacterial soap such as chlorhexidine (Hibiclens) or an over-the-counter antibiotic ointment. Other options for sensitive skin include using talcum powder or baking soda in place of an antiperspirant or deodorant.

Quiet your diet. Certain foods, such as hot peppers, can affect the amount of sweat an individual produces. And the aroma of other pungent foods, such as garlic, can be carried in your sweat. "If your aim is to prevent body odor, cut out foods like onions, garlic, hot spices, and beer," suggests Rudikoff. ◆

♦ BOILS ♦

8 Ways to Foil Boils

Yesterday you noticed a slight redness on your arm, but thought you had simply bumped it against something. Today, the red spot has turned into a painful, red, swollen lump that looks and feels awful. Chances are, what you're looking at is a boil.

"Most boils occur when a hair follicle is infected with staphylococcus, a bacteria that is present in many areas of the body and is often carried on the skin," says Vincent A. DeLeo, M.D., assistant professor of dermatology at Columbia–Presbyterian Medical Center in New York. "The size of the boil depends on the depth of the infection, or the depth of the infected hair follicle. The deeper the infection, the larger the boil," he continues. A small, more superficial boil looks like a little pimple on the surface of the skin.

Boils can occur on any part of the body that has hair follicles, which would exclude the lips, palms, and soles of the feet. Boils are more common in men than in women and tend to occur most often on the neck, waist, buttocks, and thighs.

Most boils are caused by some sort of trauma to the hair follicle, which allows staph bacteria to set up shop. "This could mean using a greasy ointment on your skin that blocks the follicle or wearing tight clothing that rubs against the hair follicle," explains DeLeo. But he goes on to say that some people are simply staph carriers and are more prone to develop staph infections in the hair follicles.

Unfortunately, there is not too much you can do to treat a boil once it appears. "The treatment for a boil is drainage, so if you can get it to drain on its own, you probably won't need antibiotics," says Denise Kraft, M.D., a family practitioner in Bellevue, Washington, and a Fellow of the American Academy of Family Physicians. Most boils simply need to run their course. What you can do is try to speed this process up a bit. Here are some suggestions:

Heat it up. Apply warm compresses to the boil a few times a day. "This home remedy is designed to help the boil come to a head and open up or be absorbed internally," says Neil Schultz, M.D., a dermatologist in private practice in New York. "The way you do this is to run a washcloth under warm (not hot) water and put it on the area for five minutes, three to four times a day. The heat increases the blood supply in the area, which better enables the body to deal with the toxins and clean out the infection," explains Schultz. "A warm bath or a heating pad will do the trick as well," says Kraft.

Don't burst the bubble. If the boil comes to a head, resist the urge to break it open yourself, especially if it is located on your nose or cheek. "If it's coming to a head, you don't have to poke it with anything. You just keep soaking it in warmth, and it will spontaneously drain," says Kraft. "Picking at the boil and trying to force the infection out only makes it worse," adds DeLeo.

Give it a gentle squeeze. When the boil does finally rupture, squeeze it gently to get the remaining pus out. "Don't force it—just sort of help it along by milking it a little bit," says Schultz. Once the boil ruptures, it usually dries up and goes away in a couple of days.

Cover it up. Put a bandage over the boil once it ruptures. "This will keep the draining fluid from getting all over your clothes and will also protect the opening from becoming reinfected," says Schultz.

Skip the solutions. Avoid over-the-counter solutions that claim to draw out the fluid. "These preparations only tend to further irritate the skin," warns DeLeo. Drawing ointments are meant to irritate the boil, causing it to form pus at a faster rate than it normally would. The pus accumulation then increases the pressure inside the boil and causes it to burst and eventually drain on its own. But the increased pressure created by these ointments also forces the pus and bacteria down deeper into the skin and possibly into the bloodstream. Once these bacteria get into the blood, they can infect any organ of the body. Topical antibiotics are also ineffective against boils because the infection is already too deep, according to DeLeo.

Use an antibacterial soap or solution. "If you're especially prone to boils, wash your skin with one of these solutions regularly," recommends DeLeo. "Betadine solution and deodorant soaps have antibacterials in them and work rather well," he says. According to Kraft, "pHisoDerm cleanser also works well." These soaps and solutions are available without a prescription.

Choose moisturizers with care. Avoid oil-based moisturizers, which have a tendency to clog the hair follicles and leave them prone to infection.

Loosen your collar. Tight-fitting clothing can rub against and irritate hair follicles, increasing the chance that a boil will develop. Opt for looser-fitting garments whenever possible, especially on areas where you've had a boil before. ◆

◆◆ Hello, Doctor? ◆◆

Whether or not you've tried home treatment, seek immediate *medical attention if you:*

• *Notice an expanding area of redness around the boil*

• *Have pain in the lymph glands near the boil*

• *Notice a red streak radiating from the area of the boil*

"All of these signs are indications that the infection is spreading into your lymphatics or even into your bloodstream," warns Vincent DeLeo, M.D. "You will either need antibiotics or will need to have the boil opened and drained to get the infection out," he says. "Boils are not usually very serious, but they can be, and you need to be concerned. And anyone with a chronic illness, such as cancer or kidney problems, should be even more concerned," says DeLeo.

It's also wise to skip self-treatment and see a doctor if you have:

• *More than one boil on your body*

• *A boil on your nose or cheek*

• *A boil that is larger than a quarter*

• *A boil that lasts more than seven days*

◆ BREAST DISCOMFORT ◆

6 Soothing Strategies

For many women, breasts are a source of sensual pleasure. For breast-feeding mothers, they are a part of the bonding between mother and baby and a way of nurturing a new life. But at certain times in a woman's life, breasts can be uncomfortable or downright painful. They may even become the focus of worry and anxiety.

Breast discomfort is a normal part of being a woman. It is almost always not a sign of breast cancer. Breasts are mammary glands that are responsive to natural hormonal changes, especially fluctuations in estrogen, that occur at menstruation, menopause, and pregnancy. Hormonal changes can cause breasts to become hot, swollen, tender, and painful to the touch. "Breast discomfort is really common for women," says Amanda Clark, M.D., assistant professor of obstetrics and gynecology at Oregon Health Sciences University in Portland. "We see it a great deal during early pregnancy, with menstruation, and during early hormone therapy at menopause."

All of the hormonal changes that occur just before menstruation and during pregnancy prepare the woman's breasts for breast-feeding. With the onset of menstruation, estrogen levels fall and the breasts return to normal.

With pregnancy, the hormonal changes continue, and the breasts begin producing milk for the baby. Lactating breasts present their own special problems and challenges. Sometimes, a mother's milk comes in too early or too heavily and causes a painful condition called engorgement. Nursing nipples can become sore. Milk ducts may become backed up and can lead to a painful infection called mastitis. (For more information on preventing and treating discomfort associated with breast-feeding, see BREAST-FEEDING DISCOMFORT.)

During menopause, many women opt for hormone therapy to reduce menopausal symptoms such as hot flashes and to reduce their risk of developing the bone-thinning disease osteoporosis. However, it often takes a while to find just the right combination and dosage of hormones for each woman. During this period, many women experience breast discomfort.

Some women also suffer from a noncancerous breast condition such as fibrocystic breasts that can cause the breasts to feel lumpy, painful, and tender. The condition is related to monthly hormonal fluctuations. As many as 30 percent of all women suffer from fibrocystic breasts, according to Sadja Greenwood, M.D., assistant clinical professor in the Department of Obstetrics, Gynecology, and Reproductive Sciences at the University of California at San Francisco. "Fibrocystic breasts were once considered a disease," she says. "But it's very common and is considered a normal—although somewhat painful—condition."

Even young girls who are just beginning to develop breasts are subject to hormonal fluctuations and can therefore experience breast tenderness. "Breast discomfort in prepubescent young women with breast budding is normal," says Deborah Purcell, M.D., a pediatrician in private practice and past chairperson of the Department of Pediatrics at St. Vincent Hospital and Medical Center in Portland, Oregon. As odd as it may sound, "even young boys can experience some enlargement of the breasts and discomfort during this growth spurt," says Purcell.

While you can't always escape the natural fluctuations in hormones, there are things you can do to make yourself and your breasts more comfortable.

Wear a supportive bra. Breasts often swell with fluid during periods of hormonal fluctuation. Susan Woodruff, B.S.N., childbirth and parenting education coordinator at Tuality Community Hospital in Hillsboro, Oregon, advises women to wear a supportive bra, especially if their breasts are large. "You may have to wear it 24 hours a day when the breasts are tender," she says. "Try one of those soft athletic bras that provide comfort and good support."

Try cutting back on caffeine. Greenwood says that the scientific evidence is mixed about whether or not eliminating caffeine helps lumpy, fibrocystic breasts. One study, reported by the National Institutes of Health, which included more than 3,000 women, found no relationship between caffeine consumption and fibrocystic disease. On the other hand, some women have reported good results from cutting back or eliminating caffeinated coffees, teas, colas, and chocolate. Try reducing your consumption of caffeine to see if your breast discomfort decreases.

Cut salt. Many women are bothered by fluid retention, particularly near the time of their menstrual period, says Clark. "Avoiding salt around this time can help minimize fluid retention," she says.

Apply heat/cold packs. Woodruff says that some women find relief from painful breasts by alternating a warm heating pad and ice packs. Try using the heating pad for 30 minutes, then the ice packs for 10 minutes, then the heating pad for 30 minutes, and so on.

Try a nonprescription pain reliever. Aspirin, ibuprofen, or acetaminophen can ease the pain of premenstrual breasts, says Clark. For fibrocystic breasts, Purcell recommends ibuprofen.

Hello, Doctor?

While some causes of breast discomfort can be effectively treated at home, see a doctor if you have any of the following symptoms:

- *A lump or firmness*

- *Soreness in only one breast*

- *A change in your breast self-exam*

- *Nipple discharge on one side (Lactating breasts may secrete white/yellow discharge for up to a year after nursing is discontinued.)*

In addition, be sure to examine your breasts monthly, regardless of whether you are having any discomfort or not. Self-examination of the breasts is an effective way to detect cancerous changes early. The best time to perform the examination is during the week following your menstrual period. If you do not know how to do a breast self-examination or are not sure if you are doing it properly, talk to your doctor.

Check out your cosmetics. Some herbal cosmetics and remedies, such as those made with ginseng, can have steroidal effects similar to estrogen. If you suspect that a product that you use may have such an effect, try avoiding the product temporarily to see if your condition improves. ◆

◆ BREAST-FEEDING ◆ DISCOMFORT

19 Ways to Beat the Breast-feeding Blues

Throughout your pregnancy, you probably fantasized about the wonderful experience breast-feeding would be for both you and your baby. All you could think about was looking down into that tiny, trusting face and feeling the closeness between you and this new little being. So naturally, when it finally came time to put baby to breast, you were excited. But now, you're in agony. Your nipples are sore, cracked, and bleeding. If your milk has already come in, your breasts may be painfully swollen. The milk may not flow when you need it to and may seem to flow uncontrollably when you most wish it wouldn't (like when you're standing in line at the grocery store or sitting at a dinner party). So where are those tender, happy moments you've seen in the magazine and television advertisements?

Well, hang in there. Those moments do actually exist, just not right off the bat. The problem is, many mothers give up breast-feeding in frustration because they don't realize that things will get better with time. They also don't realize that there are things they can do to decrease breast-feeding discomfort.

As far as what causes breast-feeding pain, it depends on what part of the breast you are talking about. Nipple pain is most often caused by the baby latching on to the nipple incorrectly. "If the baby doesn't latch on in a way that allows the nipple to get adjusted correctly in his palate, it can be very traumatic for the breast," says Phyllis Frey, A.R.N.P., a nurse practitioner with Bellegrove OB-GYN, Inc., in Bellevue, Washington. In addition, she notes, "American women tend to experience more nipple discomfort than foreign women because we always wear bras to protect that sensitive skin. Foreign women, however, go braless more often and sunbathe topless, which toughens the nipples." Pre-existing conditions, such as inverted nipples or nipple sensitivity that developed during the pregnancy, can also cause problems.

Pain in the fleshy part of the breast is most often caused by engorgement of the breast with milk when the milk first comes in. Engorgement may also make the breasts feel sore in between feedings.

While you can't escape all initial discomfort from breast-feeding, there are some tips and techniques you can use to prevent or alleviate much of the pain.

Make sure the baby latches on correctly. Despite what you may have been told, breast-feeding is a *learned* skill, and it takes time and practice to perfect. "If the baby is latching on at the very end of the nipple, he is really mashing his gums against that tender skin," says Raven Fox, R.N., I.B.C.L.C., a registered nurse and lactation consultant/educator at Evergreen Hospital Medical Center in Kirkland, Washington. "If this motion persists, the nipples can start to crack, bleed, and blister, all of which leaves them more vulnerable to infection," she continues. The key is to get the baby's mouth open wide, lift your breast from underneath, and pull the baby in close as quickly as possible. "You want to get the baby to close down on the areola (the darkened area around the nipple), rather than on the nipple itself. And if you bring him in too slowly, he will clamp down as soon as his lips touch the nipple," Fox explains. When the baby does close directly on the nipple, you'll know it. "You may feel a general tenderness when the baby first latches on, or you may experience a real sharp pain, almost as if someone had pinched you," she warns.

Use a prop. Place the baby on a pillow on your lap when breast-feeding. "Doing so lifts the baby up a little higher so that once on, he isn't further irritating the nipple area by tugging down on it," says Frey.

Treating Breast Infections

Cracked and bleeding nipples brought on by those first few days of breast-feeding can leave you vulnerable to infection of the breast, which is referred to as mastitis. While it is rarely serious, mastitis can be quite painful and cannot be cured without the use of an antibiotic.

According to Raven Fox, R.N., I.B.C.L.C., signs that you may have mastitis include a reddened area on the fleshy part of the breast that is painful to the touch and ranges from the size of a quarter to the whole side of the breast, a fever of up to 102 degrees Fahrenheit, general achiness, and chills. You may have one or two of these symptoms, or you may have all of them at once. They tend to come on very rapidly. "You may be feeling a little off at 7:30 in the morning and an hour later feel as if a truck ran over you," says Fox.

While you will need to see a doctor if you suspect a breast infection, there are a few things you should do on your own during the course of an infection.

Continue nursing, starting with the infected breast each time. *This may sound like sheer lunacy when you are in so much pain, but it helps clear the infection and will not hurt the baby. "The milk is absolutely not infected. It is the area around the milk duct that is infected," stresses Fox. She recommends nursing at least every two to three hours, and more frequently if the baby is willing.*

Prior to nursing, pack the breast in heat. *Again, use a warm towel with a plastic bag over it to maintain the heat. "Then massage and stroke the*

breast from the fleshy part down to the nipple, focusing especially on that sore spot," says Phyllis Frey, A.R.N.P.

Get in bed. *You need to go on full bed rest. This is your time to take care of yourself and let everyone else nurture you while you get over the infection. Usually, it takes only about 24 to 36 hours for the pain to pass. But Fox stresses the importance of continuing the antibiotics throughout their full 10- to 14-day course, despite the fact that you're feeling better.*

Other problems that can cause discomfort include yeast infections in the nipple and clogged milk ducts. "Yeast infections can cause ongoing discomfort in the nipple and need to be diagnosed and treated by your doctor," says Frey.

Clogged ducts, on the other hand, usually resolve themselves within 24 hours. They are characterized by a hard, uncomfortable lump in the fleshy part of the breast. It can be very tender to the touch but isn't usually accompanied by a fever. To relieve the pain of a clogged duct, pack the breast in heat before feedings, get the baby to nurse on the infected breast first, and massage the hard spot the whole time the baby is nursing in order to loosen up the milk and unclog the duct.

"If the milk is locked in the duct for more than 24 hours, it can start leaking into the breast tissue and leave a moist breeding ground for bacteria," cautions Frey. "And once it becomes infected, it is a hot spot that hurts all of the time." Fox adds that the pattern tends to be sore nipples, engorgement, clogged ducts, and mastitis. Solving the first two problems will usually prevent the latter.

Go easy at first. "It's so exciting initially to breast-feed your baby, and you often feel you don't want to interrupt him when he's finally latched on and gulping away," says Frey. "But you will pay later," she warns. She recommends limiting the breast-feeding time for the first five days of breast-feeding. Try five minutes on each breast at first. If you don't notice yourself getting tender, you can increase that time rather quickly.

Then, nurse, nurse, nurse. Once your milk comes in, let the baby nurse as long as he or she wants to. "Babies go through a marathon nursing period right as their mother's milk is coming in, and we recommend letting the baby nurse constantly during this 12- to 24-hour period. Just get it into your head that this will be your sole job for the next 24 hours," advises Fox. "We're finding that women who resign themselves to doing this are totally missing that initial engorgement period because the baby is helping to siphon off all of the excess milk the body initially produces." After all, the body automatically makes enough milk for twins; it then gradually lowers its milk production to meet one baby's needs if there is no twin. Fox goes on to say that if you trap yourself into feeding the baby every three to four hours and letting the baby sleep as long as he or she wants, your milk will come in and make your breasts look and feel as if they're going to explode. "The engorgement period should only last 36 to 48 hours, but the pain makes it seem like five years," she says.

◆◆◆ Taking the Pain ◆◆◆ Out of Weaning

Once you get through the initial discomfort of breast-feeding, nursing becomes easy and relatively painless until that fateful day when you decide it is time to wean your baby off of the breast. In addition to producing some emotional discomfort, weaning can cause physical pain. As you decrease feedings, it takes a little time for the body to catch on and produce less milk in response, so the engorgement of those early days often returns.

"Every expert is a little different in terms of their advice on how to best wean a baby," says Harold Zimmer, M.D. "Some advise you to go 'cold turkey' and some advise you to truly wean," he continues. For Mom, it is a little more comfortable to do it gradually, but some babies will decide to wean themselves and will abruptly reject the breast for good. "Generally, trying to drop one feeding about every two days is what I recommend," says Zimmer. "And the last feedings to be dropped should be the first one in the morning and the last one at night because the baby tends to be most attached to breast-feeding at these times," he explains. It is also important to never drop two feedings in a row. In other words, if you typically breast-feed your baby twice in the morning, twice in the afternoon, and twice in the evening, avoid dropping one morning feeding one day and another morning feeding two days later. Instead, try dropping one morning feeding, then an afternoon feeding, then an evening feeding.

As far as the pain of engorgement that can result, there are a few things you can do. "Tying a towel or Ace bandage around your breasts can help decrease your milk supply, because the extra pressure collapses the glands so that they can't hold as much milk," says Zimmer. "Applying ice packs to the breasts decreases circulation and further reduces the degree of engorgement and swelling," he continues. And once you have started to wean, he gives his OK to taking aspirin. "Aspirin is a good anti-inflammatory and can relieve some of the discomfort of engorgement," he says.

Whatever you do, avoid any extra stimulation to the breasts during weaning. "Anything that stimulates the breasts will promote more milk production," warns Zimmer.

Don't reach for the pump. If you do get engorged, resist the urge to express milk with a manual or electric breast pump. Unfortunately, the body doesn't know the difference between a pump and a baby's mouth. Whenever milk is drawn from the breast, the body thinks it's being used by the baby and makes more to compensate for that loss. So the more you pump, the more milk your body produces. "In essence, using a breast pump introduces a twin to your body," says Fox. The only time this advice wouldn't apply is when you are on a trip away from your baby and want to continue nursing regularly when you return, or when your baby is ill and his or her appetite is temporarily down. In these instances, you would want to pump at the baby's normal feeding times to keep up your milk supply.

Air them out. Try to expose your nipples to air whenever possible to help toughen them up. "If you finish nursing and immediately put your bra back on with a nursing pad in it, you're likely to get some milk leakage that will wet the pad and keep moisture against the nipple," says Frey. "This further softens the nipple, which is not what you want." Instead, she suggests keeping your bra flaps open (on a nursing bra) or going braless under a light T-shirt for at least 15 minutes after feeding. If you were planning to nap after a feeding, you might consider napping braless, as well.

Stand in a warm shower. This causes some milk to drip from the breasts, which can relieve some of the pressure, according to Frey. But unlike pumping the breast, this technique doesn't cause the body to produce more milk. It just provides welcome relief as long as the water is hitting directly on the breasts. "Another way to get similar relief is to fill the sink with warm water, take your bra off, lean over the sink, and splash the water up over your breasts," says Fox.

Try "cold storage." Between feedings, pack your breasts in ice, and wear a bra to hold the ice in place. "My favorite way to do this is to freeze four

Hello, Doctor?

If none of these tips seems to help much, it's time to see your doctor to rule out the possibility of a breast infection. In addition, your local chapter of the La Leche League and most hospital maternity wards can offer over-the-phone answers to your breast-feeding questions.

Ziploc bags of unpopped popcorn. The popcorn holds the cold much longer than the frozen peas and carrots many people use, and it doesn't get mushy. It also molds to the shape of your breasts so that you don't have big, bulky ice cubes lying on you," says Fox. "Usually, engorgement in between feedings lasts no more than seven to ten days after the baby's birth. This is because the mother's milk production and the baby's milk consumption are still balancing out," explains Harold Zimmer, M.D., an obstetrician and gynecologist in private practice in Bellevue, Washington.

Warm up for feedings. Fifteen minutes before feeding your baby, warm up your breasts. "Soak a bath towel in hot water, wring it out, and place it across your breasts with a plastic garbage bag over it to maintain the heat a little longer," advises Fox. Then take it off and massage the breast from the fleshy part down to the nipple to encourage the release of milk into the nipple. "Latching your baby onto an empty nipple can hurt so much more than if there is milk in the nipple," says Frey.

Try the "burp and switch" strategy. Always begin a feeding on the sorest breast or the one that seems fullest. "Once the baby is latched on, let him nurse for five minutes, and then burp him and switch him to the other side for five minutes. Continue switching him every five minutes until he is finished eating," recommends Fox. This method ensures that the baby drains both breasts sufficiently, rather than tanking up on one and leaving the other ready to explode.

Try some tea. Placing warm tea bags on your nipples a few times a day is one of the best home remedies around for nipple discomfort, according to Zimmer. Fox stresses that it has to be black tea, as opposed to chamomile or yellow tea, because black tea contains tannin, and the tannic acid is what soothes and toughens up the nipples. Soak the tea bags in warm water for a few minutes, squeeze them out, and place them on the nipples for ten minutes.

Massage the nipples with an ice cube. "This will numb the painful area and give you some temporary relief," says Zimmer. But he goes on to say that once the numbness wears off, the nipples will be just as painful as before. "It is not a healing remedy as much as it is a relief mechanism," he explains.

Wear a well-supporting bra. "You want to avoid as much additional trauma to the breasts as possible, and this is one way to protect them somewhat," says Zimmer.

Take acetaminophen if you develop a fever. It is very common to develop a low-grade fever as high as 100.2 to 100.6 degrees Fahrenheit, according to Fox. Acetaminophen should help to lower it and make you feel a little better. Be sure to check with your doctor, however, before taking any medication while you are nursing.

Take ibuprofen if you feel achy. "It is also not uncommon to feel as if a truck has run over you," warns Fox. If this is the case, ibuprofen should help relieve some of the aches and discomfort. Once again, however, check with your doctor before taking any medications. ◆

◆ BRONCHITIS ◆

7 Ways to Bear the Battle

You thought you were finally shaking that cold, but this morning your cough is worse than ever. You're coughing up phlegm by the cupful, and it feels as if someone spent the night tap-dancing on your chest. You've probably developed bronchitis, an often painful infection in the major bronchial tubes leading to the lungs.

"Bronchitis has many causes, the two most common being bacterial infections and viruses that weaken the immune system and leave the respiratory passages vulnerable to secondary infection," explains Evan T. Bell, M.D., a specialist in infectious diseases at Lenox Hill Hospital in New York. "Its hallmark symptom is a cough that is productive of thick, yellowish or greenish sputum in large amounts," he continues. But other symptoms can include a low-grade fever, chills, aches, and pains. "You may also experience some rattling noises in the lungs and chest," adds W. Paul Glezen, M.D., professor of microbiology and immunology and of pediatrics and chief epidemiologist at Baylor College of Medicine in Houston, Texas.

"Unlike cold and flu viruses, which are easily passed through respiratory excretions in the air, bronchitis tends to be particular to an individual and is rarely contagious," says Bell.

And while bronchitis sounds horrible, its bark is worse than its bite. According to Marcia Kielhofner, M.D., a clinical assistant professor of medicine at Baylor College of Medicine in Houston, Texas, the two most worrisome symptoms tend to be the characteristic burning or aching chest pain directly under the breastbone and the sometimes blood-streaked sputum produced by the cough.

Unless you have a severe underlying disease or have asthma and allergies, you may have to let bronchitis run its course. But there are some things you can do to move the process along.

Humidify your environment. Use a warm- or cool-mist humidifier to add moisture to the air. "While the cough is an irritative thing, it is the body's natural response for getting rid of the infection," says Bell. "For this reason, it is best to help it along rather than to suppress it with an over-the-counter cough remedy," he advises. Any added humidity will help to bring the sputum up and out of the body. Standing in a steamy shower with the bathroom door closed or keeping a pan of boiling water on the stove can also help loosen and bring up phlegm.

Drink plenty of liquids. Taking in extra liquids helps to keep the sputum more fluid. It doesn't really matter what type of liquid you take in, although warm liquids may feel better than cold ones. "Warm liquids, such as teas and soups, work very well to relieve the sore throat that accompanies the cough," says Kielhofner.

Gargle with warm salt water. Gargling with salt water may provide a double dose of relief by soothing the inflammation in the throat and by cutting through some of the mucus that may be coating and irritating the sensitive throat membranes, according to Bell. It only takes one teaspoon of salt in a glass of warm water; too much salt causes burning in the throat, and too little is ineffective. Gargle as often as needed for relief.

Rest, rest, rest. Since the bronchitis probably followed on the heels of a cold or the flu, you may find it hard to sit still any longer. But according to Kielhofner, you'll need to take it easy a little longer. Walking around with bronchitis will only make you feel worse.

Take aspirin or ibuprofen to relieve the chest pain. "These over-the-counter remedies are extremely helpful for relieving the discomfort resulting from the chest pain," says Kielhofner. Acetaminophen tends not to help much with the aches and pains.

Use a cough remedy as a last resort. "The best cough medicines for a productive cough contain guaifenesin to help bring up the sputum," says Bell. "If you really want to suppress it, which we generally don't recommend, look for something that contains dextromethorphan," he advises. Combination products should generally be avoided. Decongestants, antihistamines, and alcohol (common ingredients in combination products) have no role in the treatment of coughs; they may even increase discomfort by causing side effects. Most of the candy-type cough drops act as demulcents on the throat—their soothing properties are due largely to their sugar content.

Keep an eye out for complications. While letting nature take its course is generally the best treatment for bronchitis, complications can sometimes occur, and you'll need to stay alert for signs that it's time to see your doctor. The complications that are most worrisome include pneumonia, sinus infections, and ear infections, all of which need to be treated with prescription antibiotics. Signs that one or more of these complications may be present include a persistent high fever (which is not normally characteristic of bronchitis), shortness of breath, prolonged coughing spells, and severe chest pain.

In addition, Kielhofner offers the following warning: "While blood-streaked sputum is often a normal symptom of bronchitis, it can also signal several more-serious problems and should be checked out just to be safe. Any distinct change in sputum color or consistency also warrants a trip to the doctor." ◆

◆◆ Bronchitis and ◆◆ Smokers

Smoking is a habit that is continually under fire for its negative impact on a person's health. And rightly so. It has been proven to be a significant contributing factor in emphysema, lung cancer, heart disease, and several other serious illnesses. Bronchitis is no exception. Smoking leaves a person much more vulnerable to chronic bronchitis.

"Bronchitis often occurs in patients who don't tolerate respiratory infections, such as smokers," says Evan T. Bell, M.D. "As a result, smokers tend to make up the largest group of individuals who suffer from chronic bronchitis," he continues.

"Even though a bronchial infection is not in the lung tissue itself, it's getting quite close, which is always a worry," says Bell. Because the bronchial passages of smokers are already irritated, the added inflammation resulting from a bronchial infection also makes medical attention more of a necessity for these individuals, according to W. Paul Glezen, M.D.

Marcia Kielhofner, M.D., stresses that smokers who develop bronchitis should certainly take it upon themselves to refrain from smoking throughout the course of the illness. Of course, the healthiest move would be to kick the habit for good.

◆ BRUISES ◆

14 Tips for Coping with the Color Purple

When something goes bump in the night, and it's you, you may end up with the most common type of injury known to man. Bruises, those purplish blue testimonies to our physical foibles, occur when blood seeps from damaged blood vessels into the surrounding tissue. Known medically as contusions, bruises are usually caused by what doctors call direct trauma. Whether from hitting a corner of the coffee table or being kicked in the shin, the result is a painful reminder of our not-so-best moments.

Thankfully, bruises generally heal in about 10 to 14 days. Along the way, their coloring changes and fades from a dark purple to a yellowish blue. The changing colors indicate that "scavenger" white blood cells have moved into the area to break down ruptured red blood cells (called corpuscles) into iron by-products. These by-products can then be whisked away by the blood. When a greenish maroon color appears, healing is almost complete.

While your body is taking care of healing the injury, there are some things you can do to minimize discoloration, maximize pain relief, and prevent bruises from "hitting" you in the future.

Cool it down. To stop the bleeding from the damaged blood vessels, use a cold compress. "The sooner you apply ice, the better," says Wilma Bergfeld, M.D., head of clinical research in the Department of Dermatology at the Cleveland Clinic Foundation in Ohio. The cold also helps prevent swelling. Wrap the ice in a damp cloth and apply it for about 10 to 15 minutes. If your fingers or toes are bruised, plunge them into ice-cold water for quick results. Never place ice directly on the skin, however, or keep a compress on for prolonged periods of time, because an ice burn can result.

Take a load off. No matter where the injury occurred, it's important to rest the affected area.

Give it a lift. Elevation is helpful for bruises to the arms or legs, because less blood is pumped into the injured site when gravity lends a hand. Try supporting your arm on the back of a chair or propping your leg up on a few pillows for 30 minutes each hour for the first few hours after injury.

Switch to heat. About 24 hours after the injury, once the bleeding has stopped and the healing process has begun, use heat to help reduce the muscle spasms that can accompany bruising. "The muscles contract to 'splint' an injury, especially near a joint," explains Nelson Lee Novick, M.D., associate clinical professor of dermatology at Mount Sinai School of Medicine in New York. Apply lukewarm compresses for about half an hour to an hour, three to four times a day, to relax the muscles surrounding the bruise.

While either moist or dry heat can be used—whichever is most comfortable for you—many physicians say that for reasons unknown, moist heat seems to be more effective in treating bruises. "But no matter which heating method you use, the heat should never be too high," warns Bergfeld. If you use a heating pad, for example, it should be set on the lowest temperature.

Keep your aspirin in the cabinet. You may be tempted to reach for aspirin to dull the pain of the injury, but don't do it. "Both aspirin and acetaminophen contain anticoagulants, commonly known as 'blood thinning' agents, which can aggravate the bruise," says Jerome Z. Litt, M.D., an assistant clinical professor of dermatology at Case Western Reserve University School of Medicine in Cleveland. Instead, reach for ibuprofen, the other major nonprescription painkiller, which does not contain anticoagulant factors.

Put your moisturizer in the fridge. If you decide to treat the bruise with dry heat and the area becomes dry, use an emollient, preferably a hypoallergenic one, to help smooth and soothe the affected area. Gently pat—do not rub—it on, a few times a day. "By keeping the lotion in the refrigerator, it will feel pleasantly cool on your hot, tender skin when you use it," says Bergfeld.

Be a teetotaler. Alcoholic beverages, whether wine coolers, beer, or hard liquor, can dilate (open up) blood vessels, which in turn can aggravate the bruising, warns Novick. Alcohol consumption is also a major contributor to accidents in the home.

Wear loose clothing. Tight, restrictive clothes will only increase the bruise's tenderness. For bruises on the legs, for example, try going without panty hose or socks for a day if you can.

Watch the way you decorate. Furniture that is more rounded or that has softer edges—such as Queen Anne-style coffee tables—may be less hazardous to your legs and hips than squared-off styles, especially in small rooms where space is tight.

Consider putting down carpeting. You might be less likely to slip on carpeting than you would on

◆ Unexplained Bruising ◆

If you find a bruise or multiple bruises that seem to have appeared spontaneously or from the slightest touch, you should consult your family physician or dermatologist. These types of bruises may be the result of other problems or factors, such as the following:

Senile purpura. Many older people suffer from this condition, which loosely means "bruises of the elderly." As people age, the collagen (elastic fiber) that gives the skin and blood vessels their suppleness becomes thinner and frayed, allowing blood to seep through the vessel walls. The result: oversized bruises that can cover the entire length of an arm or leg. While the appearance of these colossal bruises may be frightening, the condition is an unfortunate part of the aging process and not life threatening. "It's fairly common," says Nelson Lee Novick, M.D. "I see patients with senile purpura all the time in my practice." The home-

treatment procedure for senile purpura is the same as that for common bruises; however, a physician should be consulted for a proper diagnosis, since large-scale bruising may indicate other diseases.

Drugs. Besides aspirin and acetaminophen, hundreds of over-the-counter and prescription medications can cause adverse reactions, which can lead to or aggravate bruising. Among the culprits: cortisone-like medications, often used to treat inflammation; some antibiotics; and certain heart medications. Check with your doctor or pharmacist if you suspect that your bruises may be related to a medication you are taking.

Blood disorders. Hematological, or blood-related, problems, such as a low platelet count, may show up first as bruising. (Platelets are the blood cells that aid in blood clotting.) Leukemia, or cancer of the blood, may also be indicated by bruises.

Vitamin K deficiency. Vitamin K is essential for proper blood clotting. A lack of the vitamin may reveal itself as bruising.

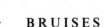

linoleum or tile, and if you do happen to fall, the carpet may help to prevent more serious injury by acting as a cushion.

Tack down area rugs. Those small throw rugs, often found in entry halls, bathrooms, and kitchens, frequently slide around or bunch up, leaving you open to an unexpected trip and a potentially bruising fall. To remedy the problem, use adhesive tape or specially made tacking to adhere them to the floor.

Light the way to safety. Night lights or lights set on timers are a relatively low-cost way to illuminate your path for late-night trips to the kitchen or bathroom. You might also try keeping a small flashlight on your nightstand so you can take it along when navigating dark hallways or stairways. Motion sensor fixtures, which turn on when movement is detected nearby, are great for outdoor use because they will instantly light up your driveway or sidewalk as you approach.

Improve your footing in the tub. Put a rubber mat in your bathtub or shower stall to help prevent slipping. You might even consider installing a handrail to decrease your risk of slipping while getting in or out of the tub.

Put everything in its place. Clutter can be hazardous to your health. Just think about the times you found a missing item by literally tripping over it. ◆

◆ BURNS ◆

26 Skin-Saving Strategies

It can take just an instant: A harried cook grabs the pan of burning food out of the oven; a cup of hot coffee comes tumbling down over the side of the table onto a curious child; a toddler manages to turn on the hot-water faucet during bath time.

Many burns are minor and can be treated at home. The injured skin turns red; that's known as a first-degree burn. Sometimes, tiny blood vessels may be damaged and may leak fluid, causing swelling and a weepy appearance. If blisters appear, the burn is classified as second degree. In third-degree burns, blisters do not form, and the skin turns white instead of red. "Usually, the deeper the burn, the less the pain," says Mick Crowley, R.N., B.S.N., department manager of the Burn Care Center/ Neurosurgical Unit at University of Missouri Hospital and Clinics in Columbia.

TREATING A BURN
Here's what to do when a burn occurs:

Put out the fire first. If your clothes are on fire, your first concern is to put out the flame. "Drop and roll," says Crowley. If a hot object is responsible, remove it.

Know when to seek medical help. There are times when first-aid methods at home just won't be enough. Get medical attention immediately if you have burns on your hands or face or over a joint, like the elbow; if your burns blister or you suspect that you have a third-degree burn; or if you've suffered chemical or electrical burns. Electrical burns can be "very, very tricky" says Crowley, because the damage often occurs out of sight, below the surface of the skin. In addition, consult your doctor before applying any products to burned skin.

Cool the burn. For minor burns, gently run cool water over the burned area, use cool compresses, or place the area in a bowl of cool water. "Don't

---

◆ The Butter Myth ◆

Some folk remedies have merit. And some can be downright dangerous. Applying butter to a burn is "just stupid," according to Patricia Fosarelli, M.D.

Why? Butter isn't sterile. "It will also insulate the area and hold the heat in," says Mick Crowley, R.N., B.S.N. The salted kind will irritate broken skin.

---

turn the faucet on full force," warns Patricia Fosarelli, M.D., assistant professor of pediatrics at Johns Hopkins School of Medicine in Baltimore. You risk further injury to the skin. "And use cool, but not ice-cold, water." The coolness will stop the burn from spreading by eliminating the thermal energy, says Terry L. Hankey, M.D., clinical associate professor of family practice at the University of Wisconsin School of Medicine in Madison.

Leave the ice in the freezer. Just because cool water is good for a burn doesn't mean ice is better. "Putting ice on the burn will restrict the blood flow," says Crowley.

Don't worry about dirt. Most first-degree burns aren't dirty, Fosarelli says. If, for some reason, yours is, then gently clean it with soap and water. "Gently is the operative word," she cautions. "Don't rub."

Bandage the burn for a child. If the burn occurs in an area that could be injured again or where a child might pick at it, you may want to cover the burn with some gauze or a bandage. Forgo any covering if it's an open, weeping wound, however, because the bandage will stick to the wound, says Crowley.

Don't pop any blisters. If a blister does develop, keep your hands off of it. "It's the body's way of keeping the burn sterile," explains Fosarelli. "Don't rub, poke, or break it."

PREVENTING BURNS IN CHILDREN

Even the best remedy can't beat prevention. Take the following steps to help protect your child from burns:

Turn handles in on the stove. Probably the most common cause of indoor accidents that burn children is a pan of something hot falling (or being pulled) off the stove.

Put coffee out of reach. You're sitting on the couch, relaxing, your cup of steaming hot coffee nearby on the aptly named coffee table. Before you know what's happening, your toddling little boy grabs the cup and dumps it on himself.

Lower the thermostat on the hot-water heater. Set it for under 120 degrees Fahrenheit, recommends Fosarelli. "A second-degree burn can happen in seconds in water over 120 degrees."

Keep a watchful eye. Never, ever leave a child unattended in a room with a fireplace (even if it has a screen in front of it), a wood-burning stove, a kerosene heater, or any kind of space heater. "Not even for a minute," warns Fosarelli. Don't leave a young child alone in the bathroom, either.

Plug electrical outlets. Cover all electrical outlets with specially made caps.

Don't run electrical cords across the floor. "A child reaches down and bites the cord and that spells tragedy," says Fosarelli.

Keep matches away from young children. That goes for lighters, too. And don't leave them in your purse, where children can find them, either.

Have fire drills. That means you need to establish escape routes in your house and demonstrate to your child how to follow them.

◆ Protect Yourself ◆

Some common-sense advice for adults:

• *Don't spray lighter fluid on charcoal that's already lit.*

• *Don't smoke in bed.*

• *Let the engine cool before you open the radiator cap.*

• *Don't prime the carburetor with gasoline.*

• *Keep oven mitts and pot holders handy when cooking.*

• *When opening a package of microwaved popcorn, keep the package directed away from your face.*

Tell your child about "911." "Even a four-year-old can learn to dial this, especially if you have it programmed on your phone," says Fosarelli.

Get fire extinguishers. Keep them accessible and in good repair. Explain to your children that a fire extinguisher, not water, should be used on a grease fire in the kitchen.

Make the stove off-limits. Keep younger children away from the stove, especially when you're cooking, and discourage older kids from cooking when you're not around.

Keep smoke alarms in working order. Check them monthly, if not more often.

Protect against sunburn. See SUNBURN PAIN for tips on preventing this type of burn. ◆

◆ BURSITIS ◆

10 Ways to Ax the Ache

Bursitis has some funny nicknames. It's called Housemaid's Knee, Clergyman's Knee, and Baker's Cyst, among others. But anyone who's experienced the pain of bursitis knows that it's no laughing matter.

The bursa is a fluid-filled sac that helps protect muscle, ligaments, tendons, or skin that rubs across bone. There are bursae throughout our bodies, but the ones where inflammation most commonly occurs are at the shoulder, elbow, knee, and heel.

The painful inflammation of a bursa is called bursitis. It's caused by bumping or bruising, repeated pressure, or overuse. It can develop after an activity you're not used to doing or after increasing a familiar activity. "If you haven't been in the garden, and you start hoeing several rows, that one exposure may give you acute bursitis," says Jack Harvey, M.D., chief of sports medicine at the Orthopaedic Center of the Rockies in Fort Collins, Colorado. "Conversely, swimmers who swim 5,000 yards a day may do fine until they up their workout to 7,500 yards a day."

Sometimes, bursitis can flare up without a clue as to its cause. All you know is, it hurts. "It can occur spontaneously with no real clear precipitating event, or doing an activity that you've done a million times," says Joseph P. Iannotti, M.D., Ph.D., assistant professor of orthopedic surgery and chief of Shoulder Service at the University of Pennsylvania in Philadelphia.

The good news is, once you tone down your activity, the symptoms begin to disappear. Here's how to speed your recovery along:

Give it a rest. The pain of bursitis may disappear completely after a few days of resting the joint. This doesn't mean ceasing all movement, warns Harvey. Particularly in a shoulder, immobilization could "freeze" the joint with fibrous tissue and scar tissue. Just take it easy and try to avoid the activity that brought on the pain.

◆ Don't Shrug Off ◆ Shoulder Pain

Don't be too quick to label your shoulder pain as bursitis, especially if your condition doesn't improve after a few days of rest. There are many conditions for which shoulder pain is a symptom, but absolutely none for which pain and swelling should be ignored.

Orthopedic surgeons who specialize in shoulder problems say that treatment shouldn't be left to the patient or even to nonspecialist doctors. A physical examination by an expert, usually followed by X rays, is the first step in proper treatment of the condition.

"I think if a person has significant shoulder pain, if it's interfering with their activities or their sleep, then in my view it's best to be examined early by a physician," says Lanny L. Johnson, M.D.

Get new shoes. If you have bursitis on your heel, you probably got it because of improperly fitting shoes. The solution is simple: Toss the shoes and put on a better-fitting pair.

Make a change. If you have bursitis on your elbow or your knee, change the activity that caused it or wear protection. "Change the shoe, wear knee pads, wear elbow pads—or don't lean on your elbow or crawl on your knees," advises Lanny L. Johnson, M.D., orthopedic surgeon and clinical professor of surgery at Michigan State University in East Lansing.

Deflate the inflammation. Take two five-grain aspirin four times a day to reduce the swelling of the bursa. Ibuprofen is another option. But avoid these if you're taking blood pressure medicine or you have kidney problems, says Iannotti.

Skip the acetaminophen. Unlike aspirin and ibuprofen, this over-the-counter pain reliever isn't an anti-inflammatory, so it doesn't do as much for bursitis. "Many people, in their mind, translate aspirin to Tylenol," says Harvey. "So I tell them plain aspirin, just to avoid confusion."

Put it on ice. Ice brings down swelling by slowing down the blood flow into the area. Leave an ice pack wrapped in a thin towel on the joint for about 20 minutes—twice as long if your bursitis is deep in your shoulder, says Harvey.

Warm it up. After the initial swelling has been brought down, heat from a heating pad or heat pack will not only feel good but will get rid of excess fluid by increasing circulation. "The heat increases the blood flow, picks up the excess fluid, and carries it away," says Charles A. Rockwood, Jr., M.D., professor of orthopedics at the University of Texas Medical School in San Antonio.

Get in the swing of things. Retaining range of motion in the joint is important, so certain exercises are a necessary part of treatment. "They're to maintain motion in the least strenuous way," says Iannotti. While most of these exercises should be prescribed by a doctor, there are a couple that you can do on your own, says Iannotti. One effective exercise for bursitis in the shoulder is the pendulum swing. To do this exercise, bend at the waist, and support your weight by leaning your good arm against a desk or chair back. Swing your sore arm back and forth and then in clockwise and counterclockwise circles.

Play "itsy bitsy spider." Another exercise you can do to restore your shoulder's range of motion is to have your hand crawl up the wall, like a spider. Make it a laid-back spider, however. Anything other than slow, gradual movement may do more harm than good.

Use a stepladder. Overhead reaching or pushing and pulling at or above shoulder level may worsen shoulder pain, says Iannotti. His advice: Use a stepladder, or better yet, have someone else reach that top shelf for you. ◆

◆ CANKER SORES ◆

9 Soothing Strategies

It may only be the size of a pencil eraser, but a canker sore can be hard to ignore. You know it's there—and it hurts like the dickens, especially whenever you eat or drink something.

Fortunately, a canker sore is usually a fairly short-lived misery, and there are a few things you can do to find some temporary relief.

First, however, you need to be able to tell the difference between a canker sore and what's called a cold sore, or fever blister, which is caused by the herpes virus. A cold sore often begins as several tiny blisters that eventually form one larger sore. They appear most often on the lips and face.

In contrast, canker sores usually travel alone. And unlike a sore caused by the herpes virus, a canker sore is not contagious. A canker sore has a yellow or white-gray center with a well-defined red border. It generally measures three to five millimeters in diameter (approximately the size of a pencil eraser) and is usually located on the inside of the lip or cheek or, less commonly, on the tongue.

What causes canker sores? No one knows for sure, says Robert P. Langlais, D.D.S., M.S., professor in the Department of Dental Diagnostic Science at the University of Texas Health Science Center at San Antonio. "Being run down or tired, or suffering from stress or poor nutrition may contribute."

"You see them in students around finals," says Alan S. Levy, D.D.S., clinical instructor at the University of Southern California School of Dentistry in Los Angeles. He points out that they may also occur as a result of a minor injury in the mouth, such as from a slip of the toothbrush or a jab from a taco shell. Certain foods, such as spicy dishes and citrus fruits, have also taken some of the blame.

About 20 percent of the population seems to get canker sores occasionally, and women are more likely than men to suffer from them. Some women tend to get canker sores at certain times during their menstrual cycle.

Here's what you can do for relief. Keep in mind, though, that "a canker sore will last seven days with treatment and one week without treatment," Levy says. A canker sore can take up to two weeks to heal; if one sticks around longer than that, see your dentist.

Get out the styptic pencil. Many a barber has used a styptic pencil to stem bleeding from minor nicks and cuts. Used on a canker sore, it will numb the nerve endings, temporarily reducing the pain.

Make your own remedy. It may sound like a strange combination, but several dentists swear by this homemade remedy. Mix together equal amounts of Milk of Magnesia or Kaopectate and Benylin or Benadryl. Milk of Magnesia and Kaopectate both contain ingredients that coat wet tissues, such as those in the mouth. Benylin and Benadryl contain ingredients that act as mild topical anesthetics and antihistamines (which reduce inflammation). Apply the mixture to the canker sore using a cotton swab. Be careful not to swallow the stuff; you could end up anesthetizing (numbing) the reflex that keeps the windpipe closed when you swallow, warns Langlais.

Go over-the-counter. Use an over-the-counter product like Orabase with Benzocaine. "It's like an oral bandage," says Becky DeSpain, R.D.H., M.Ed., director of the Caruth School of Dental Hygiene at Baylor College of Dentistry in Dallas. "It covers up the surface." If you use something that keeps the sore coated, you'll help prevent a secondary infection, says Levy. Products with xylocaine, a local anesthetic, can also dull the pain.

Take two aspirin. You can take aspirin, acetaminophen, or ibuprofen to help relieve the pain, especially before meals if the canker sore interferes with eating, says Langlais.

Stick to cool foods. Stay away from foods that are hot—in terms of temperature and spiciness. They'll burn and sting tender canker sores, says DeSpain.

Be gentle. Wield that toothbrush extra carefully to avoid irritating a canker sore. You may want to avoid rough, scratchy foods such as chips for the time being as well.

Stop bad habits. Alcohol and smoking can irritate a canker sore, says Richard Price, D.M.D., consumer adviser/spokesperson for the American Dental Association. A little abstinence may provide a lot of relief.

Check out your diet. One old wives' tale blames canker sores on tomatoes. Experts admit some sort of allergic reaction to foods may be to blame, but others point out that food allergies can cause lesions that resemble canker sores. If you're plagued with frequent canker sores, pay attention to your diet and notice whether an outbreak seems to be linked with any particular food. Likely offenders: nuts, shellfish, chocolate, and tomatoes. What to do if you discover a connection? You guessed it—avoid the offending food.

Learn to handle stress. That's the best advice for preventing canker sores. Try to find some method of relieving or coping with stress. Examples that you might try include engaging in a hobby, an exercise program, yoga, or meditation. ◆

◆ Hello, Doctor? ◆

If you are suffering from frequent canker sores, talk to your dentist about them. Same goes if you have a canker sore that is an inch in diameter or leaves a scar when it heals. And definitely get to your dentist or physician if you develop a fever; a fever may indicate that the canker sore has become infected (from poor oral hygiene, dirty fingers in the mouth, or chewing tobacco), in which case you would likely need an antibiotic.

If you've got a sore that doesn't go away or has been around indefinitely, see your dentist. "Don't think that because it doesn't hurt, it's not serious," says Alan S. Levy, D.D.S. Ironically, while a canker sore hurts and stings, "lesions that are oral cancer rarely cause pain." And while a canker sore will usually disappear in seven to ten days, a cancerous lesion will not. More than 30,000 cases of oral cancer are diagnosed each year, says Levy.

Other conditions can also cause mouth ulcers that resemble canker sores, says Robert P. Langlais, D.D.S., M.S. These include iron deficiency anemia, pernicious (vitamin B_{12} deficiency) anemia, folic acid deficiency, gluten intolerance, celiac disease, and Crohn's disease.

◆ CARPAL TUNNEL ◆ SYNDROME

24 Tips for Protecting Your Wrists

If, for you, working nine to five means tapping a computer keyboard, punching cash-register keys, working a jackhammer, or doing any other repetitive motion with your hands, you may be at risk for a painful condition called carpal tunnel syndrome (CTS). CTS is a collection of symptoms that can include tingling, numbness, burning, and pain from the wrist to the fingers. By far the most common cause of CTS is repetitive motion with the hands. For this reason, CTS is considered a "cumulative trauma disorder." However, medical conditions such as rheumatoid arthritis, hypothyroidism (low levels of thyroid hormone), pregnancy, and overweight can also cause symptoms of CTS.

If you suffer from CTS, you're not alone. According to the United States Bureau of Labor Statistics, cumulative trauma disorders, including CTS, currently account for more than half of all occupational illnesses reported in the United States today. To understand why CTS occurs, it helps to take a look inside the wrist. The carpal tunnel is a narrow passageway that runs through the wrist. It is only about the size of a postage stamp, but it is crowded with nerves, blood vessels, and nine different tendons, packed in like strands of spaghetti, that control finger movement. Repetitive motions or medical conditions can cause the tendons to swell, decreasing blood flow and compressing the median nerve, which supplies the thumb, index finger, and middle finger. This compression can cause the numbness, pain, tingling, and burning we call carpal tunnel syndrome. If left unchecked, muscle wasting and permanent damage to nerves can result.

For most people, the key to beating this syndrome is prevention—making changes *before* CTS becomes a problem. If you're already experiencing the tingling, numbness, and pain associated with CTS, you may be able to prevent further damage and promote healing by making a few simple changes in your lifestyle. The tips that follow can help you keep your hands and wrists healthy and help reduce symptoms of CTS. If your symptoms are severe or if they don't resolve after two weeks of self-care, however, see your doctor.

Stay in shape. You'll be less likely to suffer injury if your body's circulation and repair systems work well, says Mark Tager, M.D., president of Great Performance, Inc., a company in Beaverton, Oregon, specializing in occupational health. He suggests practicing good nutrition, getting adequate sleep, taking frequent exercise breaks, and avoiding smoking (cigarette smoking cuts down circulation to all areas of the body).

Take minibreaks. Fatigue in the joints or muscles is a warning sign to change your pattern of working, says Michael Martindale, L.P.T., a physical therapist at the Sports Medicine Center at Portland Adventist Medical Center in Oregon. "The body is trying to tell you something," he says. "It's up to you to listen and take a break."

"Get up and change your activity," advises David Rempel, M.D., assistant professor of medicine and director of the Ergonomics Laboratory at the University of California at San Francisco. "A 1- to 2-minute break every 20 or 30 minutes is a good idea. Then take a longer break every hour."

Don't snooze and lose. Some people are bothered more by CTS symptoms at night. Many doctors believe this is because the fluid in the body is redistributed when you lie down, so more of it accumulates in the wrist. In addition, many people unwittingly cause wrist-nerve compression by sleeping with one hand tucked under their head, says Tager. He suggests altering your sleep position to keep your wrist from being bent or compressed.

Take some weight off. Excess weight can compress the nerves in the wrist, says Tager. He advises keeping your weight within five to ten pounds of your ideal weight by eating a low-fat diet and getting plenty of exercise.

Rotate jobs. Experts at the National Safety Council suggest that you rotate between jobs that use different muscles and avoid doing the same task for more than a few hours at a time.

Rempel offers the following example: "If your job is to tie a knot in a rope, and the guy down the line cuts the rope, see if you can modify your job so that either you switch tasks frequently or you combine tasks so you're not just doing the same thing over and over."

If your job doesn't allow rotation, talk with your supervisor or union about a change. Rotation reduces job stresses and minimizes production losses.

◆◆◆ Stay Loose ◆◆◆

"A lot of times, initial problems with the wrist are actually tendon problems that don't yet involve the nerve," says David Rempel, M.D. "Exercises may be able to help these symptoms."

Rempel says that in many work settings today, the problem is that workers don't move around enough. "You're seated in front of a computer for hours in the same position," he says. "It's bound to cause problems. Exercises can help promote blood flow and strengthen the muscles and tendons."

The National Safety Council suggests performing the following four exercises twice a day or whenever you need a break. Stop doing any exercise, however, if it makes your symptoms worse.

Wrist Circles: With your palms down and your hands out, rotate both wrists five times in each direction.

Thumb Stretch: Hold out your right hand, and grasp your right thumb with your left hand. Pull the thumb out and back until you feel a gentle stretch. Hold for five to ten seconds, and release. Repeat three to five times on each thumb.

Five-Finger Stretch: Spread the fingers of both hands far apart and hold for five to ten seconds. Repeat three to five times.

Finger-Thumb Squeeze: Squeeze a small rubber ball tightly in one hand five to ten times. Afterward, stretch the fingers. Repeat with the other hand.

In addition, Rempel suggests strengthening the wrist tendons by doing the following exercises using small hand-held weights. Once again, however, stop any exercise that makes your symptoms worse.

Palm-Up Wrist Curls: Rest your forearms on a table, with your palms facing upward and your hands held straight out over the edge of the table. With a light weight (one to two pounds) in each hand, flex your wrists up ten times. Over the course of several weeks, gradually build up to 40 repetitions. Increase the weight of the dumbbells each week by one pound to a maximum of five pounds. Don't exceed five pounds with this exercise, however, or you may traumatize the wrist.

Palm-Down Wrist Curls: Adopt the same position as in the previous exercise, but have your palms facing downward. Flex your wrists up ten times. Gradually increase the number of repetitions over several weeks.

Arm Curls: Stand and hold the weights at your sides, palms facing forward. Slowly curl your arms up, keeping your wrists straight. Do 10 curls, and over several weeks, build up to 40 curls.

Keep it in "neutral." "Work with your body and your wrists in a comfortable, neutral position," advises Rempel. For wrists, a "neutral" position is straight, not cocked. Check the height of your computer screen (it should be at eye level). Rearrange the level of your keyboard or workstation so that you don't have to strain, reach, or bend your wrists. Your wrists should always be in a straight line with your forearms. And be sure your work is within your "comfort zone" (not too close or too far away).

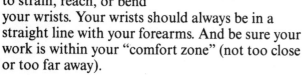

Get the right grip on it. Most of us have a tendency to grip with only the thumb, index, and middle fingers, which can increase pressure on the wrist. If you have to grip or twist something, such as the lid of a jar, Tager suggests you use your whole hand.

Alternate hands. Whenever possible, Martindale suggests, give your dominant hand a break.

Watch those pressure points. Too often, typists rest their wrists on the sharp edge of a desk or table as they work, which can cause excess pressure on the wrists, says Rempel. Adjust your workstation, if necessary, to keep your wrists off the edge.

Soften up and slow down. It's often powerful movements done at high speed that cause carpal tunnel problems. Martindale suggests slowing down and applying only the force needed.

Decrease bad vibes. People who use vibrating tools, such as sanders and jackhammers, for extended periods are at risk for wrist problems. If you are one of these folks, take frequent breaks and, when possible, operate the tool at the speed that causes the least vibration.

Go "ergo." Often, CTS can be prevented or treated by adopting tools and workstations that have been "ergonomically" redesigned to cause less stress on the body. Some tools have been designed to work with less force, while others now feature better grips and handles. Some knife manufacturers, for example, have redesigned knives for meat packers that require less wrist bending. Other companies have created aids such as wrist rests for computer users that can prevent or reduce CTS problems.

Look for items that can ease the strain on your wrists and hands, but be wary of miracle machines and gadgets. "Some of the ergonomic aids can be really helpful," says Rempel. "But I tell people to be careful about devices that make medical claims that say they'll cure CTS."

Watch for symptoms, and take action. Pay attention to early warning signs of CTS, such as morning stiffness in the hands or arms, clumsiness, inability to make a fist, or thumb weakness, and take preventive and self-care action immediately, says Tager.

Ice it. If you're having CTS symptoms, use ice to reduce swelling and inflammation. Place an ice pack on the wrist and forearm for 5 to 15 minutes two or three times a day, advises Rempel. At the same time, however, be sure to take steps to eliminate the cause of the trauma to your wrist.

Take the heat off. Heat can worsen CTS. "Heat may be good for loosening sore muscles, but you should never use heat with a nerve problem," says Rempel. "Heat causes the tissue to swell, which can make the problem worse."

Nix flimsy splints. Wrist splints prescribed by physicians can help CTS; too often, however, people who develop CTS symptoms rush to the pharmacy for a wrist splint as a home remedy. Rempel says these splints can do more harm than good. "The wrist splints you buy at the pharmacies are pretty flimsy," he says. "They often allow the wrist to move. If people put them on and don't take them off for long periods of time, they can cause muscle shrinking (atrophy)."

Reach for over-the-counter relief. For minor pain and swelling, take aspirin or ibuprofen. ◆

♦ CHAFING ♦

13 Ways to Snub the Rub

Does your skin—or your clothing—rub you the wrong way? If so, you're probably suffering from a condition called chafing. While chafing is rarely a serious problem, nothing can take the spring out of your step like sore, irritated, chafed skin.

Chafing is a condition in which the skin's normal balancing act is disturbed. Normally, the body constantly sheds skin cells, a few at a time, and replaces them with new skin. "During chafing, persistent friction against the skin rubs off more of the skin's outer layer than the skin is able to replenish," says Rodney Basler, M.D., dermatologist and assistant professor of internal medicine at the University of Nebraska Medical Center in Omaha.

Redness and irritation are the first telltale signs of chafing. As the problem worsens, so does the pain and aggravation to the skin. "Left untreated, or if the area becomes wet through constant sweat or wetting, the skin may split and ooze or even bleed," says William Dvorine, M.D., dermatologist and chief of dermatology at St. Agnes Hospital in Baltimore. Ultimately, infection may set in. Fortunately, chafing rarely gets that bad.

Those most prone to this bothersome condition are overweight people and athletes. Why these two groups? "If there's greater areas of skin touching skin [as with heavy or very muscular people], then it's more likely that friction injuries will develop," says Basler, who is also chairman of the Task Force on Sports Medicine for the American Academy of Dermatology. When athletes are in motion, the movement of skin against skin is increased. What's more, they may wear rough fabrics that can further irritate the skin.

Target zones for chafing include the upper, inner thighs; under the arms; beneath the breasts in women; and, surprisingly, men's nipples (see "Joggers Beware"). Joggers often experience chafing between the thighs, but Basler says it's largely a male problem. He chalks up this difference between the sexes to the angle of the hips.

♦♦ Joggers Beware ♦♦

Despite its rather odd-sounding name, "joggers' nipple" is actually a common chafing condition among runners, especially those who go long distances. "At the end of a marathon, you will see a number of people running with bloodstains on the front of their jogging shirts," says Rodney Basler, M.D. Caused by rough fabric, you see it "ten to one in men over women, who are protected by bras," says Basler.

The following tips from Basler should help you avoid joggers' nipple.

For Women:
• *When running, wear a soft, supportive, well-fitting bra.*

For Men:
• *If weather permits, run without a shirt.*

• *Choose shirts of soft, natural material, such as cotton, rather than more-irritating synthetic fabrics.*

• *Before running, put a thick cream on your nipples for lubrication.*

• *If all else fails, apply an adhesive strip, cut so it just covers the nipple and areola (the dark area surrounding the nipple). Scaling down the size of the bandage in this way will help prevent tape burn and painful hair pulling.*

Whether you're a man or a woman, chafing doesn't have to cramp your style. Here are several simple steps you can take to alleviate the problem and prevent it from happening again:

◆ Hello, Doctor? ◆

Chafing can usually be taken care of at home, but in some cases it requires professional help. According to William Dvorine, M.D., here are some red flags that should send you to the doctor:

• *Your chafing gets worse despite using the powder/cream treatment for a week.*

• *Your skin is oozing and cracking.*

• *You have fever or chills and a feeling of heat on the skin.*

Keep your clothes clean. This is especially important for the outfits you jog or exercise in. "Dirt and sweat can accumulate in fabric and act as an irritant," says Dvorine. Choose a mild cleanser, and wash clothes frequently.

Go easy on the bleach. Bleach can irritate chafed skin. "I've seen this particularly in people who do martial arts," says Dvorine. "They will often wash their uniforms in bleach and may not wash the bleach out thoroughly enough." Avoid bleaching your clothes, or at least make sure the bleach is thoroughly rinsed out.

Rinse your suit. The chlorine used in swimming pools can also irritate chafed skin, so after a swim in a chlorinated pool, be sure to rinse off your suit and your skin.

Sprinkle with powder. Powder, applied to chafed areas during the day or before a workout, can act as a buffer and cut down on friction. "Using powder may prevent a mild case of chafing from progressing into a more serious one," says Dvorine.

Most any powder will do, but you may be wise to look for one with talc or cornstarch, suggests Hillard H. Pearlstein, M.D., assistant clinical professor of dermatology at Mount Sinai School of Medicine in New York. "They are excellent drying agents that absorb water and moisture," says Pearlstein.

If you're chafed in the groin area and you've had a fungal infection such as jock itch in the past, an over-the-counter antifungal powder may be in order. "That gives you the added benefit of not only cutting down on the friction but killing any fungus that might be present," says Dvorine.

Dab on some cream. Applying 0.5 percent or 1 percent hydrocortisone cream (available without a prescription) to the chafed area can provide soothing relief. "Cortisone quiets down the inflammatory response in the skin and allows the skin to heal itself, which it will do if just given half a chance," says Dvorine. You can apply the cream during the day or, if you find that too messy, you can put it on only at night. If you apply it in the evening, Dvorine suggests removing the cream with mineral or baby oil in the morning and using the powder by day. He advises against using soap and water to wash off the cream, as that can further irritate chafed skin.

Give your underarms a break. Hold off on deodorants or antiperspirants—or at least use them sparingly—if your underarms are chafed. Until the condition clears, don't shave or trim the hair in your armpits, either, says Dvorine. These practices will only further aggravate the skin.

Wear "bun huggers." "The advent of the bun huggers in the last five years has been wonderful for eliminating chafing," says Basler. These sports briefs with tight-fitting legs that end about midthigh are great for runners.

Cut back. While most cases of chafing don't get this bad, you may find it is simply too painful to do whatever activity caused the chafing. In that case, Basler suggests you take a few days off from the activity and let the skin heal. Then, when you're ready to begin again, protect your skin: Before each workout, smooth thick cream on areas where you usually get chafed. ◆

◆ CHAPPED HANDS ◆

12 Steps to Softer Hands

Suffering from dry skin is bad enough. But sometimes dry skin gets so bad it becomes chapped skin—red, rough, scaly, and even cracked and bleeding. The hands are common victims for such distress, taking the abuse we dish out each day as we wash them over and over, subject them to harsh chemicals and cleansers, and expose them to the elements. Whether you're a postal carrier, a cannery worker, a bartender, or a new parent changing diapers countless times a day, your hands are probably getting left high and dry.

To understand why your hands get such a raw deal, it helps to take a look at the skin itself. "Think of your skin as continuous layers of oil and water," says Paul Lazar, M.D., professor of clinical dermatology at Northwestern University School of Medicine in Chicago. The top layer of the skin, called the stratum corneum, is made up of 6 to 12 layers of cells. Those layers contain lipids, or fats, that act as a barrier to keep the moisture in your skin, explains Ruby Ghadially, M.D., assistant clinical professor in the Department of Dermatology at the University of California at San Francisco. "Because the air around you is drier than the body, that barrier stops you from losing water from the inside out," she says.

Unfortunately, the constant wetting and drying that our skin undergoes during the course of an average day can remove the protective oils that help seal in moisture. It can also damage the skin by drying it out, says Jerome Z. Litt, M.D., assistant clinical professor of dermatology at Case Western Reserve University School of Medicine in Cleveland. When you combine moisture loss and the removal of the skin's natural protective barrier, you end up with dry skin that can quickly become chapped and painful.

Winter is the time that you are most likely to suffer from dry, chapped hands. That's because a combination of factors are at work. Indoor heating decreases the humidity in the air, making it more

◆◆◆ The Power of ◆◆◆ Petrolatum

It's thick and heavy and "gunky," says Albert M. Kligman, M.D., Ph.D., but it may be the most effective (and probably the cheapest) product on the market when it comes to treating dry, chapped skin.

Until recently, most doctors believed that petrolatum's healing properties came solely from its "occlusiveness." In other words, it seals in the skin's moisture, preventing evaporation. They figured that the petrolatum, unlike other moisturizing products, merely sat on the top layer of the skin.

A study published in 1992, however, revealed that petrolatum does more than coat the skin after all. In the study, the researchers applied acetone to remove the lipids in the skin of both human volunteers and a breed of hairless mice, thus causing dry skin. Petrolatum was then applied. According to Ruby Ghadially, M.D., a coauthor of the study, the petrolatum actually penetrated the top layers of cells and replaced the missing lipids, or fats. The fats in these outer layers of cells normally act as a barrier to keep the moisture in your skin from evaporating. The petrolatum was most effective at protecting the skin when it was applied soon after damage had occurred.

◆ Hello, Doctor? ◆

"If chapped skin persists, maybe it's not chapped skin," says Paul Lazar, M.D. Look for these signs that indicate your hands are more than chapped:

- *Itchy skin*

- *Swollen or inflamed skin*

- *Weeping, oozing blisters*

- *Silver scales (a sign of psoriasis)*

Irritant contact dermatitis, a rash that occurs from overexposure to chemicals, detergents, and other irritants, may be to blame for your "chapped" skin. An allergy to substances ranging from poison ivy to nickel in costume jewelry can also cause a rash. In addition, intense scratching can lead to a bacterial infection that will require a prescription antibiotic to clear up. If you suspect your hands are more than chapped, see your doctor.

likely that water will be pulled from your skin. At the same time, the cold, dry air and wind outdoors rob precious moisture from your skin.

And the older you are, the more likely your skin is to get dry, points out Albert M. Kligman, M.D., Ph.D., emeritus professor of dermatology at the University of Pennsylvania School of Medicine in Philadelphia.

Unfortunately, dry or chapped skin is more than just uncomfortable. It can actually make your skin more susceptible to other types of damage, such as bacterial infections, or more likely to suffer the effects of irritating substances such as detergents, says Ghadially.

Here's what the experts recommend for protecting and repairing dry, chapped hands.

Wear gloves or mittens outside. Your mother probably used to tell you this each time you made a move to the door in winter. Well, she was right again. Keep your hands covered to protect them from cold, windy, dry weather.

Dress your hands for work. Wear vinyl gloves "as much as practical" when you're washing dishes, scrubbing the tub, or otherwise exposing your hands to chemicals and cleansers, says Lazar. Vinyl gloves are a better choice than rubber gloves because they don't cause 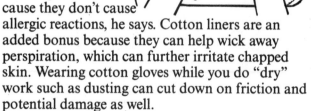 allergic reactions, he says. Cotton liners are an added bonus because they can help wick away perspiration, which can further irritate chapped skin. Wearing cotton gloves while you do "dry" work such as dusting can cut down on friction and potential damage as well.

Protect against sunlight. The sun's ultraviolet rays damage the skin and only worsen dryness and chapping, says Kligman. So be sure to wear a sunscreen with a sun protection factor (SPF) of at least 15 on all exposed skin when you're going outdoors in daylight.

Smear on the petrolatum. Petrolatum, or petroleum jelly, is the most effective for treating chapped skin, agree the experts. One way to get results without getting the petrolatum all over everything: Rub it on at night, before you go to bed, and cover your hands with a pair of cotton gloves. You might also consider doing this before you sit down to read the newspaper or watch television, says Lazar. According to Kligman, one week of regular petrolatum use will result in soft skin.

Use moisturizers. If you don't like the greasy feel of petrolatum, use a product you do like. Among the products recommended by dermatologists: Eucerin, Nivea, Lubriderm, Moisturel, and Aquaflor. Remember that a cream works better than a lotion at protecting your skin because it is thicker and heavier. No matter which product you choose, however, be sure to apply it several times a day, especially after bathing or washing your hands.

Don't worry about lanolin. As for lanolin, an ingredient that some people say is highly allergenic: Both Kligman and Lazar disagree that it causes as many allergic reactions as some claim. Kligman blames false-positive readings from patch testing (a type of skin test used to determine if a substance causes an allergic reaction) for the claims that it's highly allergenic. "It's about as sensitizing as water," he adds.

Leave the "magic" ingredients on the shelf. In other words, "you don't need something with vitamin A, E, or C or mink oil," says Kligman.

Give your pocketbook—and your hands—a break. "The higher the price, the less likely it's useful," Kligman says.

Avoid fragrances. Although fragrances are responsible for few allergic reactions, they can cause an allergic rash in some susceptible individuals, says Ghadially.

Use a mild soap. Ivory has a reputation for purity, but it's far from gentle to your skin, says Kligman. Choose a superfatted soap or even a liquid cleanser. Some choices: Dove, Basis, Eucerin, Aquanil, S.C. Lotion, or Moisturil. Cetaphil cleanser is touted by dermatologists as one of the mildest products you can buy and is recommended for problem skin. Stay away from deodorant soaps, except for Lever 2000, says Kligman.

Stay out of hot water. The hotter the water temperature, the better it is at removing oil— whether it's the grease from your dishes or those valuable oils from your skin. Use warm water for baths and hand washing.

Humidify your house. It's not as efficient at protecting against dry skin as are other measures, says Lazar, but humidifying the air in your home can help. ◆

◆ CHAPPED LIPS ◆

7 Tips for Smoother Lips

If puckering is painful and pursing is too much to bear, you're probably suffering from chapped lips. Harsh winter weather, dry indoor heat, a habit of constantly licking your lips—all of these factors can help dry out the skin of your lips by causing the moisture in the skin to evaporate. The result: Rough, cracked, sensitive lips that leave you little to smile about.

Protecting your lips from chapping is not only important for appearance and comfort, but for health. Cold sores, bacterial infections, and other problems are more likely to strike lips that are already damaged by chapping. Here's what you can do to keep your lips soft and moist:

Don't lick your lips. The repeated exposure to water actually robs moisture from the lips, causing them to become dry. "People feel better if they lick their lips, but it just aggravates the problem," says Paul Lazar, M.D., professor of clinical dermatology at Northwestern University School of Medicine in Chicago.

Use a lip balm. Numerous products are available over the counter. Pick one that you like so you'll use it frequently. Most lip balm products are waxy or greasy and work by sealing in moisture with a protective barrier.

Try petrolatum. Plain old petrolatum is good, too, says Jerome Z. Litt, M.D., assistant clinical professor of dermatology at Case Western Reserve University School of Medicine in Cleveland.

Wear lipstick. "If you look at old men and old women, you'll see a difference in their lips, especially the lower," says Albert M. Kligman, M.D., Ph.D., emeritus professor of dermatology at the University of Pennsylvania School of Medicine in Philadelphia. He attributes that difference to the "moderately helpful" properties of lipstick in moisturizing and protecting against the sun's ultraviolet rays. Be careful of cosmetics made outside of the United States, however, since the purity of such products may vary.

Screen out the sun. The sun's ultraviolet rays can damage and dry the sensitive skin on your lips. Indeed, the lips are a common site for skin cancer. "Your lips don't contain melanin [the pigment, or coloring, that can help protect skin from the sun] and they sunburn easier," points out Ruby Ghadially, M.D., assistant clinical professor in the Department of Dermatology at the University of California at San Francisco. Certain skin cancers that appear on the lips may be more serious and more likely to spread, she says. So if you'll be out in the sun, use a lip balm that contains sunscreen. Choose a product that has a sun protection factor (SPF) of 15 or higher.

Check out your toothpaste. An allergy—to your toothpaste or mouthwash—could be to blame for the rough, red skin on your lips, says Litt. Try switching brands of toothpaste and going without the mouthwash for a few days to see if the problem clears. Rinse well after brushing.

Watch what passes between them. When your lips are chapped, they're more sensitive, and certain foods can irritate them. Lazar recommends holding off on pepper, mustard, barbecue sauce, orange juice, and alcoholic beverages to give your lips a break as they heal. ◆

CHRONIC FATIGUE SYNDROME

20 Coping Strategies

Chronic fatigue syndrome (CFS) has become one of medicine's most recent mysteries. First dubbed the Yuppie flu in the 1980s by the media because it seemed to strike the young and the ambitious, especially women, the condition continues to perplex and frustrate patients, physicians, and researchers.

CFS sufferers are plagued with a debilitating fatigue that can persist indefinitely. Their flulike symptoms—fatigue (lack of energy), malaise (feeling bad), muscle aches, sore throat, low-grade fever, and swollen lymph nodes—often continue long after what they thought was merely a bout with the flu, mononucleosis, or some other infectious illness. Depression, a common companion to many chronic conditions, can accompany the other symptoms of CFS. So can cognitive problems, like confusion and forgetfulness, as well as sleep disorders.

Theories abound as to the cause of CFS, but so far, no one has come up with a definitive answer. Is it a virus? Is it encouraged by a genetic tendency? Is it triggered by stress? Is it a malfunction of the immune system? No one knows.

Even the diagnosis of CFS is murky, with no available blood tests or X rays to say "Yes, this patient has CFS." Instead, it remains a diagnosis of exclusion—that is, your doctor must rule out other conditions, such as anemia, multiple sclerosis, thyroid disorders, lupus, and even cancer, that can cause similar symptoms.

"The symptoms of CFS are so similar to those of other conditions," says James F. Jones, M.D., professor of pediatric medicine at the University of Colorado School of Medicine and staff member at National Jewish Center for Immunology and Respiratory Medicine in Denver. Indeed, chronic fatigue is one of the most common complaints doctors hear from patients.

Some news reports have hinted at epidemics of CFS. Yet there have been few cases of CFS spreading through a family, Jones says. He, along with many other researchers, doubts that the condition is highly contagious. "In fact, the condition may not be due to a specific infectious agent but to a host factor [something within the person who gets the illness], which allows the condition to occur," he explains.

If you suffer from CFS, what can you do? There is no cure. No one can tell you how long you'll be sick. The disease does not get progressively worse, and it's not fatal. In fact, you're usually sickest during the first year, often before you're even diagnosed.

"You have to learn how to cope with the disease," says Orvalene Prewitt, president of the National Chronic Fatigue Syndrome Association, based in Kansas City, Missouri. "If a cure comes down the road, that's wonderful, that's icing on the cake. But in the meantime, if you've mastered how to live with this condition, you've done what you could."

And sometimes, patients recover, points out Jones. "I've had patients who were sick three to five years and then get well. It can happen fairly fast sometimes."

Here are the coping strategies recommended by the experts—physicians, psychotherapists, and patients. Some deal with the physical side of the condition, some with the emotional side of living with chronic illness, and some are simply practical tips. Together with your doctor's advice and care, they can help you live day to day with CFS.

Establish a partnership with your health-care team. "Interview your doctor and see if it's a good match," recommends Meredith Titus, Ph.D., senior psychologist at The Menninger Clinic in

The Difficulty of Diagnosis

Comedienne Gilda Radner was mistakenly diagnosed with chronic fatigue syndrome, which delayed the discovery of the ovarian cancer that eventually killed her. That's one of the worst-case scenarios that can occur with CFS. So if you suspect you may have CFS, you want to be sure your physician has ruled out any other condition that can cause similar symptoms.

Because there's no diagnostic test for CFS, the Centers for Disease Control established guidelines in 1988 for its diagnosis. According to the guidelines, you must have suffered from debilitating fatigue that has reduced your activities by 50 percent for at least six months. And you should have at least eight of the following symptoms:

- *Mild fever or chills*
- *Sore throat*
- *Generalized muscle weakness*
- *Muscle discomfort or pain*
- *Fatigue that lasts at least 24 hours after exercise that's normal to the individual*
- *Headaches that differ from those before the illness began in their type, severity, or pattern*
- *Joint pain without swelling or redness*
- *Forgetfulness, confusion, or inability to concentrate*
- *Sleep problems, such as insomnia*
- *Rapid onset of symptoms, usually within a few hours or days*

Topeka, Kansas. "Ask when he'll take phone calls, when he returns them. Trust your intuition." Learn about your illness, too, and don't be afraid to ask questions.

Do what you can for your body. Practice the basics of healthy living: Eat a nutritious diet, get enough rest, and participate in a mild exercise program, even if it's just a five-minute walk.

Grieve for what you've lost. "You have to accept the fact you have a chronic illness," explains Sefra Kobrin Pitzele, author of *We Are Not Alone: Learning to Live with Chronic Illness.* "That means giving up who you used to be and accepting who you are now."

Let yourself feel your feelings. "You have to go through the feelings of loss, of grief, anger, sadness when you learn you have a chronic illness," says Titus.

Don't blame yourself. It's not your fault you're sick. "We're programmed in this country to believe we can overcome anything if we work hard enough," says Jones. "You can't let yourself feel guilty because you have this illness."

Find support. "It really helps to talk to other patients," says Judy Basso, a CFS patient and president of the Chronic Fatigue Syndrome Association of Minnesota in Minneapolis. "You don't have to explain a lot of things, and you can't go through this feeling totally alone." She calls joining a support group "a lifesaver" that helped her get direction for her life. "You learn a lot from other people, and it also helps keep you from dumping on your family and friends all the time." She warns against some support groups that use the gatherings as a sales meeting for alternative products.

You might also want to consider seeking professional counseling, since depression often accompanies any chronic condition. "With chronic fatigue syndrome, it can be hard to distinguish between the feelings of tiredness and the helplessness and hopelessness of depression," says Titus. Talking to a therapist may help.

◆◆ Alternative Therapies ◆◆

Janet Bohanon, who became ill with CFS in 1975, estimates she spent $30,000 to $40,000 in search of relief during the first ten years she was sick.

Her "treatments"—none of which worked—included herbal remedies, vitamin B_{12} shots, bee pollen, hair analysis, oral doses of hydrogen peroxide, a fasting diet of water and aloe vera juice, a three-year drug regimen based on the theory that a supersensitivity to yeast was to blame, acupuncture, a potassium supplement that tasted like "motor oil," and a $200 appliance that propels negatively charged ions into the air. She's also tried replacing her aluminum and Teflon cooking pans with glassware. She's had her water supply checked for lead. She's converted to hypoallergenic products. She's still sick.

"Like a lot of CFS patients, I was vulnerable and I was desperate and I was willing to believe anything," Bohanon says. "Since cofounding the National CFS Association in 1985, I've learned how important it is to check out these supposed cures and treatments."

She's not alone in turning to desperate measures. "It's such a frustrating illness," says John H. Renner, M.D., president of the Consumer Health Information Research Institute in Kansas City, Missouri, and a member of the board of directors of the National Council Against Health Fraud. "It's the perfect condition for the quacks to exploit. People get frustrated with the medical community because doctors can't offer a cure, and they feel like they have no control over their own health," says Renner. "Then someone comes along who says he has a cure, and he's warm and understanding, and the patient feels like, at last, somebody cares," he adds.

Yet, ironically, many of the so-called treatments for CFS have merely been recycled from other incurable illnesses. "Some of the products once sold for cancer were then supposed to cure AIDS when it came along," says Renner. "Now they're supposed to cure chronic fatigue syndrome as well."

He cites immune boosters, hydrogen peroxide, hyperthermia (a procedure that involves taking blood, warming it, and injecting it back into the body), and nutritional supplements.

Some products may harm you only by emptying your pocketbook, while others endanger your health. "A nonfatal illness like CFS can turn into a disaster if you're not careful," Renner cautions. "Or you can worsen the symptoms." For example, taking the herb ginseng causes fatigue.

How can you protect yourself? Be suspicious if:

• The claims made for a product sound too good to be true. "If it sounds too good to be true, it probably is," Renner points out.

• Testimonials rather than scientific studies are used to prove the product's worth. A disease can go into remission or the patient may feel better because of the placebo effect (a beneficial effect that occurs but that cannot be attributed to any special property of the substance).

• You're told that "you're one of the lucky few to know about this product." Or it's a "secret" cure that medical professionals don't want to share with the public. "If a 'secret' cure for cancer existed, no doctor or member of a doctor's family would die of cancer," says Renner.

• Accompanying information warns against telling your doctor about using the product.

• The product is sold through a multilevel marketing scheme.

• Phrases like "oxygenate your body," "detoxify your system," or "cleanse your body of numerous poisons" are used.

• The practitioner is clearly profiting from the product. For example, your doctor insists you buy vitamin supplements from his or her office rather than at your local pharmacy.

James F. Jones, M.D., asks, "How can you treat something when you don't even know what's causing it? That's the crux of the whole issue. Relying on these alternative therapies is like playing the lottery."

Spend your energy wisely. Several patients talk of using their precious stores of energy like coins from a piggy bank. "You carefully ration every ounce of energy," explains Basso.

Set reasonable goals. "If you're having a bad day, maybe your goal shouldn't be to get groceries, but to take a shower, get dressed, make a sandwich, and do the dishes," suggests Pitzele. "You may have to lower your expectations, but then you can be successful in meeting your goals."

Be energy efficient. "I sit down on a stool in the kitchen, I don't stand," says Basso. "When I take laundry down to the basement, I take a book or the newspaper along and I stay down there on a couch, so I don't have to go up and down the stairs several times." Get a handicapped parking sticker; have your groceries delivered; hire someone to clean the house. Pitzele divides her groceries when she shops so the sack with canned goods can sit in the car for a few days until she can bring it in.

Schedule rest periods. "One woman I know takes what she calls 'power naps' instead of power lunches so she can get through the day at work," says Basso. "It's critical that you schedule rest before and after activities." You have to learn, too, to listen to your body. "Lie down before it's screaming," says Pitzele.

Set priorities. "Make a list of what you must do, would like to do, and what doesn't matter," says Pitzele. As patient Brian Lutterman writes in "Long Night's Journey: Coping with Chronic Fatigue Syndrome," published by the CFS Association of Minnesota, "When all your living must be done in a few hours a day, and with only a small amount of energy, you begin to realize what is truly important."

Learn to adapt. "Maybe you're too sick to go to a movie, but you can ask a friend to bring over some Chinese food and watch a movie on the VCR," suggests Basso. "People who really love you don't care if you cook them a gourmet meal or send out for fried chicken," says Pitzele.

Keep work and home schedules on the same calendar. "You don't want to have a big meeting with your boss and a birthday party for your three-year-old scheduled on the same day," says Titus.

Realize you have limits. "Remember that everyone—even healthy people—can't do everything," says Basso. Try to be realistic about what you expect from yourself.

Have fun. "Keep your social outlets," says Titus. "Maybe you can't entertain your friends the way you'd like, but that doesn't mean you don't have something to share with them." Pitzele adds that it's "crucial" to make time for play. "If you have three hours of energy—work two of them, but spend one having coffee with a friend or taking a short walk. Keep the balance in your life."

Keep a journal. "You don't have to write in it every day," Titus says, but "it will help you see the patterns. You'll realize how awful you felt on the darkest days, but that you moved past that and felt good again."

Don't ignore your sexuality. You may have to schedule sex for when you feel good, says Pitzele. "Night is not the best time—you probably feel better at lunch or in the morning before you get out of bed."

Remember you still have choices. "Exercise your choices," says Titus. "Those feelings of control help fight any feelings of depression."

Keep your sense of humor. "The movies I watch, the books I read, are more upbeat these days. I'm dealing with enough difficulty and pain on a day-to-day basis," says Basso.

Live for today. "CFS patients are living with the unknown, and living with the unknown is frightening because it reminds us we're out of control," Titus explains. "So maximize the known. If you feel good, then enjoy today. Live in the now." ◆

◆ COLDS ◆

11 Tips for Fighting the "Cold" War

Headache. Stuffy nose. Cough. Fever. Itchy eyes. Sore throat. Muscle aches. If you're like most people, you know the symptoms of the common cold all too well. Although Americans spend more than $5 billion annually on doctor visits and cold remedies—everything from tissues and vitamin C to over-the-counter decongestants and herb teas—there is no cure for the common cold.

Colds, also called upper respiratory infections, are caused by hundreds of different viruses, according to David N. Gilbert, M.D., director of the Department of Medical Education at Providence Medical Center in Portland, Oregon. "But we don't have any drugs that can kill or inhibit these viruses," he says. "We have to depend on the body's natural defenses."

During a cold, virus particles penetrate the mucous layer of the nose and throat and attach themselves to cells there. The viruses punch holes in the cell membranes, allowing viral genetic material to enter the cells. Within a short time, the virus takes over and forces the cells to produce thousands of new virus particles.

In response to this viral invasion, the body marshals its defenses: The nose and throat release chemicals that spark the immune system; injured cells produce chemicals called prostaglandins, which trigger inflammation and attract infection-fighting white blood cells; tiny blood vessels stretch, allowing spaces to open up to allow blood fluid (plasma) and specialized white cells to enter the infected area; the body temperature rises, enhancing the immune response; and histamine is released, increasing the production of nasal mucus in an effort to trap viral particles and remove them from the body.

As the battle against the cold virus rages on, the body counterattacks with its heavy artillery—specialized white blood cells called monocytes and lymphocytes; interferon, often called the "body's own antiviral drug"; and 20 or more proteins that circulate in the blood plasma and coat the viruses

and infected cells, making it easier for the white blood cells to identify and destroy them.

The symptoms you experience as a cold are actually the body's natural immune response. In fact, says Michael Castleman, author of *Cold Cures,* by the time you feel like you're coming down with a cold, you've likely already had it for a day and a half.

Many people believe the old adage, "Do nothing and your cold will last seven days. Do everything and it will last a week." While we may not be able to cure the common cold, the simple self-care techniques that follow can help you feel more comfortable and speed healing.

Drink plenty of fluids. "Fluids keep the mucus thin," says Gilbert. Donald Girard, M.D., head of the Division of General Internal Medicine at Oregon Health Sciences University in Portland, agrees. "Colds can make you somewhat dehydrated and you don't even know it," says Girard. Drink at least eight ounces of fluid every two hours.

Cook up some chicken soup. One of the most beneficial hot fluids you can consume when you have a cold is chicken soup. It was first prescribed for the common cold by rabbi/physician Moses Maimonides in twelfth-century Egypt and has been a favorite folk remedy ever since. In 1978, Marvin Sackner, M.D., of Mount Sinai Hospital in Miami Beach, Florida, included chicken soup in a test of the effects of sipping hot and cold water on the clearance of mucus. Chicken soup placed first, hot water second, and cold water a distant third. Sackner's work has since been replicated by other researchers. While doctors aren't sure exactly why chicken soup helps clear nasal passages, they agree "it's just what the doctor ordered."

Rest. Doctors disagree about whether or not you should take a day or two off from work when you come down with a cold. However, they do agree that extra rest helps. Staying away from the work site may be a good idea from a prevention standpoint, too. Your coworkers will probably appreciate your not spreading your cold virus around the office. If you do decide to stay home, forgo those chores and take it easy, read a good book, take a nap.

Girard adds that you should skip your normal exercise routine when you've got a cold. In fact, he says, if you're feeling pretty bad, you should just head for bed.

Stay warm. "I usually recommend people stay indoors and stay warm when they have a cold," says Girard. If nothing else, staying warm may make you feel more comfortable, especially if you have a fever.

Use a saltwater wash. The inflammation and swelling in the nose during a cold is caused by molecules called cytokines, or lymphokines, which are made by the lymphocytes, explains Stephen R. Jones, M.D., chief of medicine at Good Samaritan Hospital and Medical Center in Portland, Oregon. "Recent evidence has shown that if we can wash out those cytokines, it reduces the swelling and fluid production." Jones recommends filling a clean nasal-spray bottle with dilute salt water (one level teaspoon salt to one quart water) and spraying each nostril three or four times. Repeat five to six times per day.

Gargle. Girard says gargling with warm salt water (a quarter teaspoon salt in four ounces warm water) every one to two hours can soothe your sore throat. "Salt water is an astringent that is very soothing to the inflamed tissues, and it tends to loosen mucus," he says.

♦♦♦ Don't Pass It On ♦♦♦

Unfortunately, modern medicine hasn't invented a cold vaccine that will protect us from becoming infected by the hundreds of cold viruses just waiting for an opportunity to take up residence and multiply. As a result, getting at least one cold a year is "pretty inevitable," says Stephen R. Jones, M.D. But if you get a cold, you don't have to pass it on. By learning some simple techniques, you can keep your cold to yourself.

Most authorities on the common cold are now convinced that cold viruses are passed in two ways—by direct contact and by viral-filled droplets from the nose being inhaled by others (the so-called "aerosol method"). The direct-contact method works something like this, says David N. Gilbert, M.D.: "You get a virus in your nose, then blow your nose, which contaminates your fingers with the virus, and then you shake hands with someone. They touch their noses and get the cold."

Viruses can also live on inanimate objects such as telephones, doorknobs, and cloth handkerchiefs. But no one is really sure just how long they live. To avoid spreading your cold to others by direct contact, Gilbert advises washing your hands frequently and using paper tissues instead of a cloth handkerchief. Be sure to dispose of the tissues promptly after use.

People can also get your cold by directly inhaling viral particles. While most of us feel uncomfortable around someone who is sneezing and coughing, the truth is that those symptoms are late-stage and usually come on when the person is least infectious. Most people spread their colds to others during the first few days when their throat feels sore and they're just coming down with a cold. To avoid giving your cold to others, you may want to stay away from coworkers and friends for a day or two during the onset of a cold. "Avoid crowded places if you can, and cover your nose when you cough or sneeze," says Jones.

Consider vitamin C. Although studies suggest that vitamin C may boost the body's immune system, the use of this vitamin in treating colds is still controversial. Many physicians don't recommend vitamin C as a cold remedy. Others, including cold researcher Elliot Dick, Ph.D., chief of the Respiratory Virus Research Laboratory at the University of Wisconsin–Madison, have found

◆◆◆ What About "Cold ◆◆◆ Medicines?"

When cold season arrives, doctors' offices fill up with people searching for a "cold cure." Unfortunately, modern medicine doesn't have any medication that is effective against viruses, including the more than 100 viruses that can cause the common cold. Antibiotics, such as penicillin, don't work against cold viruses. "The first thing you shouldn't do," says David N. Gilbert, M.D., "is go to the doctor's office and get a penicillin shot. They're ineffective, expensive, and they expose you to unnecessary side effects."

OK, if the doctor can't help, what about all those "cold remedies" touted on television and radio? Surely they must work.

Not really. Some cold experts believe that popular cold remedies may actually inhibit the body's immune responses as they suppress cold symptoms. All of your cold symptoms are part of your body's natural response in its battle against the viral invaders. To stop or suppress those responses may actually make your cold hang on longer.

For example, cold experts say a mild fever—below 102 degrees Fahrenheit—enhances the body's ability to fight the cold virus. Gilbert, therefore, suggests forgoing aspirin and acetaminophen to lower a mild fever. (If you're over 60, have heart disease, or have any immune-compromising health condition, however, contact your physician at the first sign of a fever.)

Another example of potentially counter-productive cold remedies is antihistamines, which are common ingredients in multisymptom cold formulas. Antihistamines stop the runny nose, but they may do more harm than good. "Antihistamines dry up mucous membranes, which are already irritated," says Gilbert. "They thicken the nasal mucus so you feel like you need more decongestant, and they can cause an irritated cough."

One over-the-counter cold remedy that can bring symptomatic relief is pseudoephedrine, a decongestant ingredient found in products such as Sudafed, says Stephen R. Jones, M.D. "This ingredient effectively shuts down the swelling and fluid production and promotes drainage," he says. People who have high blood pressure or heart disease, however, should avoid this over-the-counter drug.

Cough syrups that contain glyceryl guaiacolate (but not dextromethorphan) can help loosen thick sputum, making it easier to cough up, according to Donald Girard, M.D.

If you think you need over-the-counter remedies to cope with your cold, most authorities recommend single-action remedies rather than the "shotgun" approach of multisymptom products. Most people get their cold symptoms serially—sore throat first, cough last. But multisymptom cold remedies say they cure all your cold symptoms at once, even the ones you don't have. Why take drugs and risk their side effects when you don't need them?

"These multisymptom cold remedies don't really do anything," Jones says. "The reason people like the nighttime cold remedies is that many of them contain large amounts of alcohol. They're expensive and ineffective. I tell my patients to avoid them."

Hello, Doctor?

While most colds can be effectively treated at home, you should call your doctor if:

• *You have a headache and stiff neck with no other cold symptoms. (Your symptoms may indicate meningitis.)*

• *You have a headache and sore throat with no other cold symptoms. (It may be strep throat.)*

• *You have cold symptoms and significant pain across your nose and face that doesn't go away. (You may have a sinus infection, which requires antibiotics.)*

• *You have a fever above 101 degrees Fahrenheit (adults), you've taken aspirin, and the fever isn't going down.*

• *Your child has a fever above 102 degrees Fahrenheit.*

• *Your cold symptoms seem to be going away, but you suddenly develop a fever. (It may indicate pneumonia, which is more likely to set in toward the end of a cold.)*

Vaporize it. The steam from a vaporizer can loosen mucus, especially if the sputum is thick, says Girard. It may also raise the humidity in the immediate area slightly, which may make you feel more comfortable.

Stop smoking. "Smokers have colds longer in duration than nonsmokers," says Gilbert. "If you chronically irritate the bronchial tubes while you have a cold, you're more likely to develop a complication like pneumonia."

In addition to irritating the throat and bronchial tubes, smoking has been shown to depress the immune system. Since you have to depend on your own immune system rather than medicine to cure a cold, you'll want it to be in the best condition possible to wage the "cold" war.

Stay away from "hot toddies." While a hot alcoholic beverage might sound good when you're feeling achy and stuffy, Gilbert says it increases mucous membrane congestion. "If you want to minimize your discomfort," he says, "stay away from alcohol."

Maintain a positive attitude. Although mind-body science is in its infancy, some researchers suggest that a positive I-can-beat-this-cold attitude may actually stimulate the immune system. "If you give up, so does your immune system," says Castleman. "Buoyancy and self-confidence help rev up the immune system or at least keep it from collapsing while it fights your cold."

Jones isn't as convinced about the connection between the mind and the immune system. He says the evidence directly linking one's thoughts with immunity is "interesting, but inconclusive." But, he admits, "a positive attitude is always best and certainly couldn't hurt your cold." ◆

that taking 2,000 milligrams or more of vitamin C daily can lessen the severity of cold symptoms.

If you do decide to try boosting your vitamin C intake during a cold, don't overdo it. While vitamin C has been found to be relatively safe at doses of up to 10,000 milligrams per day, some people find vitamin C causes diarrhea at or above the 10,000-milligram level. Perhaps the safest way to get more vitamin C is to choose vitamin C-rich foods more often. For example, since you'll need to increase your fluid intake while you have a cold, fill some of that requirement with orange juice.

◆ COLD SORES ◆

6 Ways to Foil Cold Sores

It never fails. Every time you have a big meeting coming up or an important presentation to give, you develop an unsightly cold sore on your lip. You wake up with a small cluster of tiny, harmless-looking, white blisters, which quickly explode into a painful sore the size of Rhode Island (OK, so maybe it just *looks* that big to you).

"True cold sores, the ones that occur on the lips, are caused by the herpes simplex virus I," says Evan T. Bell, M.D., a specialist in infectious diseases at Lenox Hill Hospital in New York. "Herpes viruses presumably lie dormant in certain nerve cells of the body lifelong, until something like stress, strain, a cold, or excessive exposure to the sun causes them to manifest. In the case of herpes simplex virus I, it happens to be on the lip," he explains. The sores last from 7 to 14 days.

Although many use the terms "cold sore" and "canker sore" interchangeably, they are different. Unlike cold sores, canker sores are oral lesions that are characterized by small, round, white areas inside the mouth surrounded by a sharp halo of red. And, while cold sores are highly contagious, canker sores are not.

Unfortunately, attempting to camouflage the little buggers with makeup often produces an even worse effect. Still, while you can't do much about the way they look, you can do a few things to help decrease discomfort, speed healing, and keep them from coming back. You can even take steps to prevent passing on your cold sore to others. Here's how:

Cover it with a protective petroleum-based product. "This will protect it from infection and help it to heal a little quicker," says Marcia Kielhofner, M.D., clinical assistant professor of medicine at Baylor College of Medicine in Houston, Texas.

Reach for aspirin, acetaminophen, or ibuprofen. "These sores can be quite painful because they are in an area that tends to be easily and continually irritated," says Kielhofner. "An over-the-counter painkiller can greatly reduce this discomfort."

Hello, Doctor?

"Many people choose to leave cold sores alone and let them go their own way since they are usually not severe or life-threatening," says Evan T. Bell, M.D. And doing so certainly won't hurt you.

On the other hand, if you have frequent or severe cold sores, see your doctor. "There is a prescription drug called acyclovir that works actively against initial outbreaks of herpes simplex viruses," says Bell. Although the drug tends to be less effective for recurrences, you and your doctor may decide that it's worth a shot.

Avoid salty or acidic foods. Things like potato chips or citrus fruits can further irritate cold sores and add to the pain, according to Kielhofner.

Apply an over-the-counter anesthetic. Putting a local anesthetic ointment containing benzocaine on the cold sore can help numb the pain temporarily.

Protect your lips from the sun. Applying sunscreen to your lips may help prevent sun-induced recurrences of cold sores, according to a study by the National Institutes of Health. Look for a sunscreen, designed especially for the lips, that has an SPF of 15 or higher. Some colored lipsticks now also contain sunscreen; check the cosmetic counter at your local department store.

Keep it to yourself. One important thing to keep in mind with cold sores is that they are extremely contagious. While you have a cold sore, avoid kissing and sharing cups, towels, or other such items. And wash your hands frequently. ◆

◆ COLIC ◆

15 Ways to Help You and Your Baby Cope

How Much Does a Normal Baby Cry?

In 1962, the famous pediatrician T. Berry Brazelton, M.D., published a study of the crying patterns of 80 normal, middle-class infants. He found that their crying lasted for about two hours a day at two weeks of age, increased to a peak of almost three hours a day by six weeks of age, and then gradually decreased to about one hour a day by the time they had reached three months of age.

The generally accepted medical definition of colic is a young infant who is otherwise healthy and well fed, but who has bouts of irritability, fussing, or crying lasting for a total of more than three hours a day on more than three days of the week, according to William B. Carey, M.D. Sometimes, doctors add the stipulation that the baby's excessive crying continue for a period of more than three weeks to be considered colic.

Carey emphasizes this simple point: Normal babies cry—a lot. So don't assume that just because your child is putting up a fuss for three hours a day, he or she is abnormal. More than likely, it's just your baby's way of letting you know that he or she is healthy, energetic, and alive. Lastly, take solace in the fact that by three months of age, you're likely to have a lot more peace and quiet around the house.

When you brought your new baby home from the hospital, he seemed so quiet, so sweet, so well behaved. Suddenly, about two weeks after your child's arrival, Mommy's angel turned into a crying, squalling, red-faced little devil. At times, the child may have appeared to be in pain: He drew his legs up to his belly and appeared to pass gas more frequently. Perhaps you took your child to the pediatrician for a diagnosis, or maybe you were able to recognize the symptoms yourself—the demon of colic had invaded your once-peaceful home. By now, you've probably reached the end of your rope. You feel frustrated and tired. You may have started to doubt your ability to parent your child properly. You may have even considered packing up your bags and leaving home.

The first step to take is to relax in the knowledge that your feelings are perfectly normal. Parents are often conditioned to believe that if their child is crying, something is wrong—something that they should be able to fix. Fortunately, you can take solace in the fact that your child is probably otherwise healthy. Colic does not indicate the presence of a serious medical problem. And a certain amount of crying is normal and healthy, says William B. Carey, M.D., a clinical professor of pediatrics at the University of Pennsylvania School of Medicine and director of Behavioral Pediatrics in the Division of General Pediatrics at Children's Hospital, both in Philadelphia. Still, to set your mind at ease, it may be helpful to take your child to the pediatrician to ensure that his or her crying is not a sign of a medical problem, says Carey. It can also be reassuring to keep in mind that most cases of colic go away by the time the child has reached three months of age.

The bad news is that doctors still don't know what causes colic, what the disorder really is, or how to cure it. They don't even know if colicky babies really are in pain. However, there are some tried-and-true ways of helping to soothe your baby, even if you can't curb his or her crying completely. These are included in the tips that follow. Another important component to the well-being of your colicky baby and to you is your sanity. So some of the tips below are designed to help you cope.

Set the baby in motion. As most parents can attest, mild repetitious motion, such as that of a moving car or a rocking chair, can calm a cranky baby. With a colicky child, that knowledge is doubly important, according to Cheston M. Berlin, Jr., M.D., a professor of pediatrics 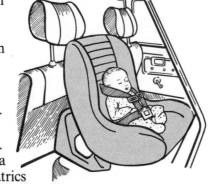 and of pharmacology at Pennsylvania State University College of Medicine's Milton S. Hershey Medical Center in Hershey. "Motion is the best thing for children who are having so much trouble," he says. If taking the child out in the car is too inconvenient, he recommends putting the child in a safety seat and placing it atop a running dryer (don't leave the baby unattended).

There are also devices on the market that will rock or vibrate the baby's crib, Berlin says. Some of these devices even have sound sensors that will start the motion only when the baby starts crying and will stop after it senses that the baby has calmed down or gone to sleep. One device even simulates the motion of a car moving at 55 miles per hour. Some physicians find it effective, while others feel that it makes little difference.

Let the baby sleep. Many parenting books and pediatricians would have you believe that you should pick the baby up every time he or she cries, says Carey. However, babies often cry because they are tired. If this is the case, picking up the child only stimulates him or her further. "I think some of the time you should be leaving the baby alone," Carey says. "If you pick up a tired baby, he'll cry more."

To assess whether your child is crying because of fatigue, try everything else first: feeding, burping,

changing, cuddling. Then, if the baby is still crying, put him or her down to sleep, and walk away. Often, the child will settle down within five minutes, Carey says.

Stay calm. "It is important to emphasize that colic is a benign disorder," Berlin says. "It has never been known to cause or represent any serious medical problem." With that knowledge in mind, understand that this is just a stage in your child's development—an unpleasant stage that will soon pass.

Take your baby off cow's milk. Some studies have shown an improvement in colic after dairy products have been removed from babies' diets, according to Ronald G. Barr, M.D.C.M., an associate professor of pediatrics and psychiatry at McGill University and director of the Child Development Program at Montreal Children's Hospital, both in Montreal. The culprit seems to be a protein in cow's milk, which is present in many infant formulas and is also found in the milk of breast-feeding mothers who eat dairy products, Barr says. The protein may be responsible for colic in about five to ten percent of babies who suffer from the condition. Changing the baby's formula (there are many soy-based formulas available) or staying off dairy products yourself if you are breast-feeding, is worth a try. If your baby's crying does not seem to improve after two weeks, you can assume that the milk was not the problem.

Try peppermint water. Although it has never been definitively proven to be effective, peppermint-flavored water is a century-old remedy for colic, according to Berlin. "It was very recently discovered that the active ingredient in peppermint oil is a calcium-channel blocker, a substance that may relax the gut," he says. He recommends soaking a piece of a peppermint stick in water, then feeding a bottleful of the flavored water to the baby. Do not use straight peppermint oil, he says, as this may be too strong for the baby.

Add fiber to your baby's formula. Some studies have shown that colic seemed to improve in certain infants when fiber was added to their formula,

Colic Medications and Babies: A Poor Combination

Several colic medications have been tried throughout the years, with varying degrees of success. However, recent studies out of the Southwest SIDS (Sudden Infant Death Syndrome) Research Institute in Lake Jackson, Texas, and Children's Hospital in Camperdown, New South Wales, Australia, have found that colic medications may prove dangerous and even fatal.

The Texas researchers studied eight infants who were experiencing life-threatening respiratory and gastrointestinal symptoms. All of the babies had previously been given a premixed colic medication containing Dramamine, a popular antihistamine used to relieve motion sickness, and Donnatal, a drug prescribed for irritable bowel syndrome and other intestinal disorders. Donnatal contains, among other things, phenobarbital, a barbiturate used as a sedative. In an article published in the journal Clinical Pediatrics, *the researchers wrote that the possibility that the drug can lead to respiratory and gastrointestinal problems in certain infants "requires serious consideration and further evaluation."*

according to William R. Treem, M.D., a pediatric gastroenterologist in the Division of Pediatric Gastroenterology and Nutrition at Hartford Hospital in Connecticut and associate professor of pediatrics at the University of Connecticut School of Medicine. "Some babies seemed to be dramatically better when we added fiber to their formula," he said. "We used Citrucel, a bulking agent that draws water into the stool. We have added anywhere from one-half teaspoon three times a day to one-half teaspoon six times a day. I think it's best to start small and build up to the higher doses." Although not the answer for every baby, adding fiber is certainly safe and is definitely worth a try, Treem says.

Take a shower. If your baby's crying has driven you to the point of near madness, it's time to stop and take a break, Berlin says, since an overly frustrated parent can be of no help to anyone. "I recommend 20 to 30 minutes in a warm shower," he says, adding that the sound of the water can successfully mask the baby's crying. (Be sure the baby is in a safe place, such as a crib).

Keep a calendar. A record of your baby's weight and the frequency and length of crying bouts may be of help in tracking his or her progress, Barr says. It can also be a handy record to take to the pediatrician's office, he says. A useful bonus of the charting is that it reminds you that your baby does cry a lot, but that there are breaks in between. "Parents tend to feel like the baby just cries all the time," Barr says.

Be realistic. "The babies that you see in magazines and books—the babies who are neat, clean, and happy—well, you can expect your baby to be like that for about 30 minutes out of every 24 hours," says Edward R. Christophersen, Ph.D., professor of pediatrics at the University of Missouri at Kansas City School of Medicine and chief of the Behavioral Pediatrics Section at Children's Mercy Hospital in Kansas City, Missouri. "Keep in mind that the only exercise babies get is crying and nursing." In other words, don't be discouraged: Your baby is not abnormal just because he or she cries a lot.

Soothe, don't stimulate. Since crying, colicky babies are already overly stimulated, try soothing the baby instead of bouncing or rocking him or her, says Carey. Some time-honored tools: a hot-water bottle, filled with warm—not hot—water and placed on a towel on the child's back or stomach; a pacifier; or the use of repetitious sounds, such as the noise of a fan or humidifier.

Maintain as much direct contact as possible. Pediatricians often recommend carrying and cuddling a colicky baby as much as possible. However, studies have failed to show that carrying actually causes a reduction in crying. On the other hand, carrying the baby more frequently before colic ever sets in may prevent the condition from developing in the first place, says Barr. He mentions a study where the caretakers of 99 normal infants increased their carrying of the infants by the age of three weeks. The result? The babies cried 43 percent less than other babies of the same age. "The carrying prevented the crying peak from ever occurring in those infants," Barr says. He also describes studies of a tribe of Botswanian hunter-gatherers, the !Kung San, whose infants cry as often as North American babies, but only for about half as long. Mothers in the tribe spend significantly more time with their babies held close to their bodies than North Americans do, he says.

Feed more often. One reason that the !Kung San spend so much time holding their babies is that they feed them almost continuously, Barr says. "They feed very frequently—approximately four times per hour, four minutes per feed," he says. This type of feeding schedule may be partly responsible for the reduced crying of the !Kung San infants, according to Barr. "Parents do have

the option to feed more frequently," he says. "I think there is lots of room for changing the frequency of feeding that is within the range of what is normal." Even if continuous feeding does not fit into your schedule, adding a few extra feedings still may help, Barr says.

Put your baby on a schedule. Some children cry excessively because they simply don't know how to calm themselves down enough to go to sleep, says Christophersen. Since babies under the age of 12 weeks often fall asleep while being fed, it is sometimes difficult for them to fall asleep without feeding, he says. He suggests starting your baby on a regular schedule of sleeping and waking and trying to get him or her to fall asleep without your assistance. "Kiss them, hug them, sing them songs, then let them fall asleep on their own," he says. "This way, they learn to make their own transition from the alert, crying state to the sleeping state."

Touch base with your pediatrician. Your pediatrician can be an invaluable source of ideas, experience, and reassurance, says Christophersen. "Parents can get very discouraged with a colicky child," he says. He recommends taking advantage of all support systems that are available to you.

Wait it out. If all else fails, take solace in the fact that colic generally stops by three months of age, Berlin says. The longest you'll have to wait is until the baby reaches six months, although colic this long-lasting is rare. Unfortunately, "there's no dramatic cure," he says. ◆

◆ CONJUNCTIVITIS ◆

7 Soothing Suggestions

If it feels like someone threw sand in your eyes, but you haven't been anywhere near a beach or sandbox lately, you may have conjunctivitis. Conjunctivitis is an inflammation of the conjunctiva, the mucous membranes that line the inner surface of the eyelids and the front of the eyeball.

"Conjunctivitis usually involves both eyes and doesn't affect vision," says Jon H. Bosland, M.D., a general ophthalmologist in private practice in Bellevue, Washington. "Symptoms can include routine burning or itching, extreme sensitivity to light, and tearing. The eyes get red and the lids and surface of the eye can become swollen," he continues. There may also be a watery, mucus secretion or, in the case of bacterial infection, a thick discharge coming from the eyes. The discharge may be so thick that you wake up in the morning with a crust over your eyes and the feeling that your eyes are "glued" shut.

The causes of conjunctivitis are as numerous as the types. Infectious types of conjunctivitis, which are highly contagious, can be caused by viruses or by bacteria, such as pneumococcus, streptococcus, and staphylococcus. "The eyes are continually bombarded with germs all of the time. But the blink reflex and the tearing reflex are amazingly effective at fighting off most of these germs," explains Bosland. "And if a particularly aggressive set of germs attacks the eye, the backup defense mechanisms come into play. The blood vessels dilate to bring more bacteria-killing white blood cells to the area, and the eye begins discharging the infection," he continues. These defensive maneuvers by the body result in the symptoms of conjunctivitis.

Noninfectious types of conjunctivitis tend to be caused by foreign bodies getting under the lid, exposure to ultraviolet light, and allergies. Wind, smoke, and other types of air pollution, as well as the chlorine in swimming pools, can irritate the conjunctiva. The chronic condition of "dry eye" can also cause conjunctivitis, according to Bosland.

"Allergic conjunctivitis is most often associated with itching and swelling of the white part of the eye, which can sometimes be so severe that the white part of the eye looks like a balloon sticking out between the lids," says Charles Boylan, M.D., a pediatric ophthalmologist at A Children's Eye Clinic of Seattle. "Young children often get this when they play out in the grass and weeds in the summertime and get pollen on their hands and then into their eyes. In this instance, the eye can swell up in a matter of minutes," says Boylan.

Whatever the cause, conjunctivitis can be painful and irritating. As with most symptoms or conditions involving the eyes, it is important to see a doctor for correct diagnosis and treatment. Although a viral or bacterial conjunctivitis will usually go away on its own, it will go away much quicker with the use of proper antibiotics and antiviral agents, says Carol Ziel, M.D., an ophthalmologist with the Eye Clinic of Wausau in Wisconsin. Bosland adds that if an infectious conjunctivitis lasts longer than two or three weeks, it can start to turn into chronic conjunctivitis. "In this instance, the bacteria get into the outer corners of the eyelid and spill over into the eye, infecting it as well. And these mixed infections involving the eyelid and the eye can go on for quite a long time," he cautions. In addition to seeing a doctor and following his or her advice, you can take some simple steps at home to help relieve discomfort and, if you have infectious conjunctivitis, to keep from spreading the infection around.

Cool the itch of allergic conjunctivitis. "If there is any itching in relation to the conjunctivitis, cool compresses will really help to reduce it," says Ziel. Simply wet a washcloth with cool water and hold it against the eyes.

Ice the swelling. Applying an ice pack to the eyes can help bring down any swelling from allergic conjunctivitis. "Try to keep the ice on long enough to reduce the swelling to the point where the eyelid can close down over the cornea," says Boylan. (The cornea is the transparent circular covering in front of the eyeball that helps to focus light entering the eye.) "Otherwise, the cornea could dry out, which is another problem in itself," he adds. "You rarely see this type of conjunctivitis not improve with ice packs and a little bit of time. Often, by the next morning, the swelling is almost completely gone."

Apply heat to fight a bacterial infection. "Hot compresses can help the infection quite a bit because the heat dilates the blood vessels, bringing fresh blood to the area, and raises the temperature up above what is optimum for the germ to survive," explains Bosland. "The heat also relaxes the muscles around the eye, which can be quite soothing," he continues. Applying a washcloth soaked in hot water (provided it is not hot enough to burn the skin) or using a hot-water bottle works very well.

Drop in some relief. For minor allergic conjunctivitis, over-the-counter eye drops may provide soothing relief. "Any of these eye drops are fine to use provided there is nothing seriously wrong with the eye and provided you use them on a short-term basis only," says Boylan. For safety's sake, and especially if you are also using prescription eye medication, ask your doctor if it's OK to use over-the-counter eye drops.

Be selfish. Conjunctivitis caused by bacteria or viruses is very contagious, so you'll need to keep from sharing towels, washcloths, pillows, and handkerchiefs with others. "The fluid draining from the eyes could get on the towel or pillow and infect someone else," warns Ziel.

Keep your hands off. "Because conjunctivitis can be quite contagious, it's good to keep the germs off of your hands," says Ziel. If you have infectious conjunctivitis, try not to rub your eyes, and be sure to wash your hands after wiping your eyes or applying eye medication.

Shield your eyes. Conjunctivitis can make your eyes extremely sensitive to light and other irritants. So do all you can to give them a break. If you're going outdoors, put on a pair of sunglasses to help shield your eyes from wind and sunlight. Put off mowing the lawn or working in the garden until your conjunctivitis has cleared, or at least wear a pair of goggles to keep pollen and dust out of your eyes. Take time off from swimming, or wear a pair of well-fitting swimming goggles. And, when possible, close your eyes to give them a rest. ◆

◆ CONSTIPATION ◆

11 Ways to Keep Things Moving

Irregularity is one of those things that no one likes to talk about. It's personal and, well, a little embarrassing. But if you're one of the millions of people who's ever been constipated, you know it can put a real damper on your day.

The first thing to realize when you're talking about constipation is that "regularity" is a relative term. Everyone has his or her own natural rhythm. Ask four people to define regularity, and you're likely to get at least four different answers. Normal bowel habits can span anywhere from three bowel movements a day to three a week, according to Marvin Schuster, M.D., professor of medicine with a joint appointment in psychiatry at Johns Hopkins University School of Medicine and chief of the Division of Digestive Diseases at Francis Scott Key Medical Center, both in Baltimore.

"One of the most common forms of constipation is imaginary or misconceived constipation," says Schuster. It's based on the idea that if you don't have the "magical" one bowel movement a day, then something's wrong. Constipation has a lot to do with a person's comfort level, says Peter Banks, M.D., director of Clinical Gastroenterology Service at Brigham and Women's Hospital and lecturer on medicine at Harvard Medical School, both in Boston. People who are constipated often strain a lot in the bathroom, produce unusually hard stools, and feel gassy and bloated.

Schuster calls it "constipation" if you have fewer than three bowel movements a week or if you experience a marked change in your normal bowel patterns. A sudden change in bowel habits merits a visit to your doctor to rule out any more serious underlying problems (see "Hello, Doctor?"). But for the occasional bout of constipation, here are some tips to put you back on track:

Get moving. Exercise seems not only to boost your fitness but to promote regularity as well. "The thinking is that lack of activity puts the bowels to rest," says Banks. That may partially explain why older people, who may be more sedentary, and those who are bedridden are prone to becoming constipated. "We encourage people to get up and be more active," says Banks. So gear up and get moving. You don't have to run a marathon; a simple walking workout doesn't take much time and can be very beneficial. When it comes to regularity, even a little exercise is better than none at all.

Raise your glass. Drinking an adequate amount of liquids may help to alleviate constipation or prevent it from happening in the first place. The reason for this is simple. "If you dehydrate yourself or drink too little fluid, that will dry out your stool as well and make it hard to pass," says Schuster.

On the other hand, some people have the misconception that if you drink far more than you need, you can treat constipation. Schuster disagrees, saying the excess fluid will just get urinated out.

To achieve a balanced intake of liquids, a good rule of thumb is to drink eight cups of fluid a day, says Mindy Hermann, R.D., a registered dietitian and spokesperson for the American Dietetic Association. (This rule of thumb doesn't apply, however, if you have a kidney or liver problem or any other medical condition that may require restricting your intake of fluid.) Drink even more when it's hot or when you're exercising. Hermann suggests that athletes weigh themselves before and after a workout. Any weight lost during the activity reflects water loss. To replace it, they should drink two cups of liquid for every lost pound of body weight.

For those who are constipated, all liquids are not created equal. Avoid drinking a lot of coffee or other caffeinated drinks, urges Elyse Sosin, R.D., a registered dietitian and the supervisor of clinical nutrition at Mount Sinai Medical Center in New York. Caffeine acts as a diuretic, taking fluid out of your body when you want to retain it. She suggests sticking with water, seltzer, juice, or milk instead.

Don't fight the urge. Often, because people are busy or have erratic schedules or because they don't want to use public bathrooms, they suppress the urge to have a bowel movement. "If they do this over a period of time, it can block the urge so it doesn't come," explains Schuster. If at all possible, heed the call when you feel it.

Take advantage of an inborn reflex. As babies, we're all born with a reflex to defecate a short time after we're fed, says Schuster. With socialization, we learn to control our bladders and bowels and we inhibit this reflex. Schuster suggests that you try to revive this reflex by choosing one mealtime a day and trying to have a movement after it. "Very often, people can program the colon to respond to that meal." Schuster does point out that this works better with younger people than with the elderly.

Know your medications. A number of prescription and over-the-counter medications can cause constipation. If you are currently taking any medication, you might want to ask your doctor or pharmacist whether it could be causing your constipation. Among the drugs that can cause constipation are calcium-channel blockers taken for high blood pressure, beta-blockers, some antidepressants, narcotics and other pain medications, antihistamines (to a lesser degree), certain decongestants, and some antacids. Antacids that contain calcium or aluminum are binding and can cause constipation. When choosing an antacid, Schuster suggests you keep in mind that the names of most of those with aluminum start with the letter "a." Those that start with the letter "m" contain magnesium, which does not constipate. If you are unsure, check the label or ask your pharmacist.

Bulk up. Many times, adding fiber or roughage to your diet is all that's needed to ensure regularity. Fiber, the indigestible parts of plant foods, adds mass to the stool and stimulates the colon to push things along. Fiber is found in fruits, vegetables, grains, and beans. Meats, chicken, fish, and fats come up empty-handed in the fiber category. The

◆◆ Laxative Alert ◆◆

Laxatives seem like an easy solution for constipation woes, but they can cause many more problems than they solve. Indeed, these tablets, gums, powders, suppositories, and liquids can be habit forming and produce substantial side effects if used incorrectly.

Laxatives work in many different ways, and "each one has its problems," says Marvin Schuster, M.D. Some lubricate, others soften the stools, some draw water into the bowel, and still others are bulk forming. One real danger is that people can become dependent on them, needing ever-increasing amounts to do the job. Eventually, some types of laxatives can damage the nerve cells of the colon until the person can't evacuate anymore. Some laxatives inhibit the absorption or effectiveness of drugs. Those with a mineral-oil base can prevent the absorption of vitamins A, D, K, and E. Still others can damage and inflame the lining of the intestine.

"I think laxatives ought to be avoided if at all possible and only used under a doctor's care," says Schuster. In the long run, you'll be much better off to depend on exercise, adequate fluid intake, and a high-fiber diet to keep you regular.

current recommendations for daily dietary fiber are 20 to 35 grams. "Most people eat between 10 and 15 grams," says Hermann. So there's plenty of room for improvement. Fiber supplements may be helpful, but most doctors and dietitians agree that it's preferable to get your fiber from food (see "Laxative Alert").

Add fiber slowly. People assimilate high-fiber foods into their diet more easily if they do it gradually. "You need to add one high-fiber food at a time, start with small amounts, and wait a couple of days before adding something else so you don't throw your system into chaos," says Hermann. Sosin agrees and also stresses the need to "drink an adequate amount of fluids with the fiber."

Eat at least five servings of fruits and vegetables daily. Select a variety of fruits and vegetables, recommends Hermann, some that are high in fiber and others that aren't so high. Potatoes (white and sweet), apples, berries, apricots, peaches, pears, oranges, prunes, corn, peas, carrots, tomatoes, broccoli, and cauliflower are all good choices.

Eat 6 to 11 servings of grain products daily. That's in addition to the five servings of fruits and vegetables just mentioned. Grain products include 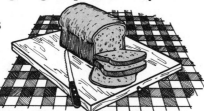 cereals, breads, and starchy vegetables (such as corn, green peas, potatoes, and lima beans). "I tell people to start out the day with a high-fiber cereal because it's easy to do and it immediately knocks off a big chunk of the amount of fiber they should be getting during the day," says Hermann. Check the labels on cereal boxes; anything with more than five or six grams of fiber per serving qualifies as high fiber. If you don't like any so-called "high fiber" cereals, line up the boxes of cereal that you would be willing to eat and pick the one with the most fiber, suggests Hermann.

Read labels when choosing breads as well. "Just because a bread is brown doesn't mean it has a lot of fiber in it," says Hermann. Find a bread that has at least two grams of fiber per slice. Watch the portion size, too, when looking for high fiber foods. "Sometimes they will give you a very large size that's unrealistic for one serving," says Sosin.

Bring home the beans. Dried beans and legumes—whether pinto, red, lima, navy, or garbanzo—are

Hello, Doctor?

Constipation can be a symptom of a more serious problem, such as an underactive thyroid, irritable bowel syndrome, or cancer, to name a few. See your doctor if you have any of these symptoms:

- *A major change in your bowel pattern*

- *Constipation lasting for several weeks or longer*

- *Blood in your stool*

- *Severe pain during bowel movements*

- *Unusual stomach distention*

excellent sources of fiber. Many people don't like them because of the gassiness they may cause. Cooking beans properly can ease this problem considerably. Hermann's technique for cooking less "explosive" dried beans: Soak the beans overnight, then dump the water out. Pour new water in, and cook the beans for about 30 minutes. Throw that water out, put in new water, and cook for another 30 minutes. Drain the water out, put new water in, and finish cooking.

Cut back on refined foods. You can bump up your fiber intake by switching from refined foods to less-refined foods whenever possible. Switch from a highly processed cereal to a whole-grain cereal, move from heavily cooked vegetables to less-cooked vegetables, and choose whole-grain products over products made with white flour. A glass of orange juice, for instance, provides 0.1 grams of fiber, while eating an orange gives you 2.9 grams. And while a serving of potato chips has only 0.6 grams of fiber, a serving of popcorn supplies 2.5 grams. "As soon as you start juicing something or straining it or taking the pulp out, you're taking out the fiber," says Hermann. ◆

◆ CORNS AND CALLUSES ◆

22 Steps to Relief

You may refer to your feet as tootsies or dogs, but the fact remains that feet are highly sophisticated structures. The human foot is a miracle of engineering designed to stand up under a lot of wear and tear. It's a good thing, too: Your feet are the most used and abused parts of your body. According to the American Podiatric Medical Association, the average American walks 115,000 miles in a lifetime—a distance that would take you all the way around the earth four times. Your feet support the weight of your body, plus clothing and whatever extras you might be carrying. And in an average day of walking, your feet are subjected to a force equal to several hundred tons.

Despite how well designed your feet are, however, things can go wrong. In fact, an estimated 87 percent of all American adults have some type of foot problem. Among the most common of these problems are corns and calluses.

Although both corns and calluses are patches of toughened skin that form to protect sensitive foot tissue against repeated friction and pressure, they are different in some ways. Hard corns are usually found on the tops of the toes or on the outer sides of the little toes, where the skin rubs against the shoe. Sometimes, a corn will form on the ball of the foot, beneath a callus, resulting in a sharp, localized pain with each step. Soft corns, which are moist and rubbery, form between toes, where the bones of one toe exert pressure on the bones of its neighbor. Both hard and soft corns are cone shaped, with the tip pointing into the foot (what you see is the base of the cone). When a shoe or another toe puts pressure against the corn, the tip can hit sensitive underlying tissue, causing pain.

Calluses, on the other hand, generally form over a flat surface and have no tip. They usually appear on the weight-bearing parts of the foot—the ball or the heel. Each step presses the callus against underlying tissue and may cause aching, burning, or tenderness, but rarely sharp pain.

There are some things you can do to relieve the discomfort associated with these two conditions. Try the tips that follow. If, despite trying these strategies, your corn or callus continues to cause discomfort, see a podiatrist. In addition, if you have diabetes or any other disorder that affects circulation, do not attempt to self-treat any foot problem; see your podiatrist right away.

Play detective. "Corns and calluses develop for a reason," says Suzanne M. Levine, D.P.M., a podiatrist in private practice in New York. "Abnormal amounts of dead, thickened skin form at certain spots on your feet to protect them from excess pressure and friction." Obviously, the real solution to corns and calluses is to track down and eliminate whatever is causing the pressure and friction. "The place to start is with your shoes," advises Levine. See "If the Shoe Fits" for tips on choosing well-fitting shoes.

Trim those toenails. Toenails are designed to protect the toes from injury. However, the pressure of a shoe on a toenail that is too long can force the joint of the toe to push up against the shoe, forming a corn. To take the pressure off, keep your toenails trimmed. Cut each toenail straight across so that it doesn't extend beyond the tip of the toe. Then, file each toenail to smooth any rough edges.

Take a soak. While eliminating the source of the problem is essential, sometimes you need immediate relief from the sharp pain of a corn. Levine suggests soaking the affected foot in a solution of Epsom salts and warm water, then smooth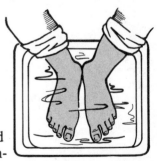ing on a moisturizing cream, and wrapping the foot in a plastic bag. Keep the bag on for a couple

◆ Over-the-Counter ◆ Corn and Callus Removers

Salicylic acid is the only over-the-counter drug that is safe and effective for treating calluses and hard corns, according to the Food and Drug Administration (FDA). For medicated disks, pads, or plasters, the recommended concentration of salicylic acid is 12 percent to 40 percent. A concentration of 12 percent to 17.6 percent is recommended for liquid forms.

Many podiatrists, however, advise against the use of these products as home remedies, mainly because the active ingredient is an acid that can burn healthy skin as well as the dead skin of a callus or corn. If you do decide to try one of these products, follow the package directions carefully and be sure to apply the product only to the area of the corn or callus, avoiding the surrounding healthy tissue (one way to do this is to spread petrolatum in a ring shape around the corn or callus). If your corn or callus does not improve within two weeks, stop using the product and see a podiatrist. If you are diabetic or have any medical condition that hinders circulation, do not try one of these products at all; see a podiatrist at the first sign of any foot problem.

The following ingredients are not *generally recognized as being safe and effective for removing corns and calluses, according to the FDA: iodine, ascorbic acid, acetic acid, allantoin, belladonna, chlorobutanol, diperodon hydrochloride, ichthammol, methylbenzethonium chloride, methyl salicylate, panthenol, phenyl salicylate, and vitamin A.*

of hours. Then remove the bag and gently rub the corn in a sideways motion with a pumice stone. "This will provide temporary relief—and I stress temporary," says Levine.

Ice a hard corn. If a hard corn is so painful and swollen that you can't even think of putting a shoe on your foot, apply ice to the corn to help reduce some of the swelling and discomfort.

Don't cut. There are a myriad of paring and cutting items to remove corns and calluses available in your local drugstore or variety store, but you should ignore them all, in the best interest of your feet. "Cutting corns is *always* dangerous," says Mary Papadopoulos, D.P.M., a podiatrist in private practice in Alexandria, Virginia. "You can expose yourself to an infection, or you may cause bleeding that is not easily stopped."

Soft step it. "You can give yourself temporary relief from corns and calluses with shielding and padding," says Joseph C. D'Amico, D.P.M., a podiatrist in private practice in New York. What you want the padding to do is transfer the pressure of the shoe from a painful spot to one that is free of pain. Nonmedicated corn pads, for example, surround the corn with material that is higher than the corn itself, thus protecting the corn from contact with the shoe.

A similar idea applies when padding a callus. Cut a piece of moleskin (available at your local drugstore or camping supply store) into two half-moon shapes and place the pieces on opposite sides of the area to protect it.

Separate your piggies. To relieve soft corns that form between toes, keep the toes separated with lamb's wool or cotton. A small, felt pad, like those for hard corns, may also be used for this purpose.

Baby your soft corn. In addition to separating your toes, sprinkle a little cornstarch or baby powder between them to help absorb moisture.

Mix your own callus concoction. For calluses, Levine suggests mixing up your own callus softener. Make a paste using five or six aspirin tablets and a tablespoon of lemon juice, apply it to the callus, wrap your foot in a plastic bag, and wrap a warm towel around the bag. Wait ten minutes, then unwrap the foot and gently rub the callus with a pumice stone.

Invite your feet to tea. Soaking your feet in chamomile tea that has been thoroughly diluted has a soothing effect and, according to Levine, will help dry out sweaty feet (excessive moisture can contribute to foot problems). The chamomile will stain your feet, but the stain can be easily removed with soap and water.

Coat your feet. If you expect to be doing an unusual amount of walking or running, coat your toes with a little petroleum jelly to reduce friction. ◆

◆◆ If the Shoe Fits... ◆◆

"When corns and calluses form, the real underlying problem is one of mechanics—the foot inside the shoe is not functioning properly. But poor-fitting shoes may precipitate the problem," says Joseph C. D'Amico, D.P.M.

Here are some guidelines to getting a better fit:

• Have the salesclerk measure each foot twice before you buy any pair of shoes. Don't ask for a certain size just because it's the one you have always worn; the size of your feet changes as you grow older.

• Be sure to try on both the left and the right shoe. Stand during the fitting process, and check to see that there is adequate space (three-eighths to one-half inch) for your longest toe at the end of each shoe. Remember, your longest toe may not be your big toe; in some people, the second toe extends the farthest. Likewise, your feet may not be the exact same size. If one foot is slightly larger than the other, buy the shoes for the larger foot and use padding, if necessary, for a better fit on the smaller foot.

• Make sure that the shoe fits snugly at the heel.

• Make sure the ball of your foot fits snugly into the widest part of the shoe—called the ball pocket.

• Shop for shoes at the end of the day, when your feet are likely to be slightly swollen.

• Walk around the store in the shoes to make sure they fit and feel right as you stride along.

• Don't buy shoes that feel too tight, expecting them to stretch out. If they don't feel right in the store, they will never fit comfortably. They should not need to be stretched.

• If you are not sure about the fit, check into the store's refund policy. If possible, take the shoes home, wear them on a rug for an hour, and if they don't feel good, take them back.

• When buying shoes for everyday use, look for ones with fairly low heels.

• Make sure the material of the upper is soft and pliable.

• Have several different pairs of shoes so that you do not wear the same pair day after day. Alternating your shoes is a wise move, not only for your feet but for the shoes.

You may discover, as most people do, that your left and right foot are not exactly the same size. Or you may have a high instep, a plump foot, or especially long toes. While these characteristics may make it somewhat difficult to step into every pair of shoes you try on, they do not mean that you must resign yourself to never finding a pair of shoes that fit. All it takes is a little time and the determination to walk in comfort.

One last reminder: Like Cinderella, who was the only one able to fit into the glass slipper, the person who buys a pair of shoes is the only one who should wear them.

◆ CUTS AND SCRAPES ◆

9 Ways to Care for Your "Boo-Boo"

You're hurrying along and the front of your shoe catches on a crack in the cement, sending you tumbling to the ground. When you get up, you find that not only is your ego bruised, but you've managed to peel away the skin on your elbows and knees. You've got yourself a collection of painful scrapes.

You scramble home to prepare the appetizer tray for the guests who will be arriving any minute. You have just one more carrot to slice when, "Ouch!"—your knife slips and slices not the carrot, but your finger. You've got a cut.

"A cut is an incision into the skin," explains Robert Matheson, M.D., a dermatologist in private practice in Portland, Oregon. "It's a vertical slice into the skin that affects only a limited number of nerves. In contrast, a scrape involves the traumatic removal of skin in a horizontal fashion. It scrapes away the skin's surface and exposes a larger number of nerves, usually making it more painful than a cut."

An amazing number of things happen when you cut or scrape yourself. When you disrupt the skin, a clear, antibody-containing fluid from the blood, called serum, leaks into the wound. The area around the cut or scrape becomes red, indicating that more blood is moving into the wound site, bringing with it nutrients and infection-fighting white blood cells. Nearby lymph nodes may swell. After a few days, pus (which contains dead white blood cells, dead bacteria, and other debris from the body's inflammatory response to infection) may form. And finally, a scab develops to protect the injury while it heals.

Even being extra careful, you can't always avoid the scrapes and cuts of life. But you can learn how to care for them and speed their healing (be sure to read "Hello, Doctor?" on the following page to determine if your injury needs a doctor's care):

Stop the bleeding. When you get a cut or scrape, the first thing to do (after admonishing yourself for being so clumsy) is to stop the bleeding. "Apply pressure with a clean cloth or tissue to stop the blood flow," says Louisa Silva, M.D., a general practitioner in Salem, Oregon, who sees plenty of cuts and scrapes in her private practice.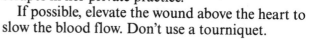

If possible, elevate the wound above the heart to slow the blood flow. Don't use a tourniquet.

Wash up. One of the most important things you can do in treating a cut or scrape is to make sure you cleanse it thoroughly. "Wash it thoroughly with soap and water," says dermatologist Paul Contorer, M.D., chief of dermatology for Kaiser Permanente in Beaverton, Oregon, and clinical professor of dermatology at Oregon Health Sciences University in Portland.

Matheson says soap and water is usually sufficient, but you can also use over-the-counter cleansers like Hibiclens that don't sting. If the wound is really dirty, he recommends using hydrogen peroxide to bubble out debris. Apply it carefully, since it can damage surrounding skin.

Bring on the antibacterial ointment. Contorer says antibacterial ointments can be very helpful. Polysporin, Neosporin, and Bactine are examples of antibacterial ointments available without a prescription. Matheson says he prefers Polysporin to other ointments because it contains fewer ingredients that may cause allergic reactions.

Close the skin. Properly closing the skin is important in cuts that are an eighth to a quarter inch wide. Matheson says closing makes the cut heal faster and reduces the chances of scarring. Be sure that you have thoroughly cleansed the cut before attempting to close it. Line up the edges of the cut, then apply butterfly strips or an adhesive bandage to keep the cut closed.

Cover it. "It's important to keep a cut or scrape covered," says Silva, "to keep the wound clean and protected." Instead of covering with plain gauze, which tends to stick to wounds, Silva recommends using Telfa, a coated, gauze-type bandage. Adhesive bandages often have Telfa on them, she says, but you can also buy larger pieces of Telfa in the pharmacy and cut them to fit. Cover the wound with the Telfa pad, and use adhesive tape to hold the pad in place.

Keep it clean. The initial washing isn't enough to prevent infection, says Matheson. You'll need to remove the bandage and wash the wound every day with soap and water. Then re-cover it with a clean bandage.

Don't let it dry out. One of the myths about cuts and scrapes is that a thick, crusty scab is good. Not so, says Matheson. "Don't let your wound get dry and crack," he says. "If you keep it relatively moist, you'll speed healing and minimize scarring."

If a scab forms, don't pick at it; this disrupts the skin and can introduce bacteria. Instead, Matheson recommends soaking off crusty scabs with a solution of one tablespoon of white vinegar to one pint of water. The mildly acidic solution is soothing and helps kill bacteria.

Contorer advises patients to use a water/petrolatum regimen at night before retiring. "I have them wash the wound thoroughly and then cover it with a little Vaseline to seal in the moisture," he says.

Both doctors emphasize that a certain amount of air circulation is important to wound healing. You want the bandage or covering to be tight enough to protect, but not so tight that it seals out all air and causes the wound to become too moist.

◆◆ Hello, Doctor? ◆◆

Many cuts and scrapes can be safely treated at home, but see your doctor if:

• *You notice signs of infection (redness, red streaks, swelling, pus, enlarged lymph nodes).*

• *The injury is located on the face.*

• *The cut or scrape is very deep or is too dirty to clean.*

• *The cut is wider than a quarter inch or is too ragged to close evenly.*

• *You can't stop the bleeding.*

• *The injury occurred in the area of tendons and nerves, and you can't feel the area or you can't move it.*

Don't get locked up. Silva says it's important to have a tetanus shot within 72 hours if you haven't had one in the last five years. Tetanus bacteria, which causes "lockjaw"—a condition that can involve stiffness in the jaw and other joints, paralysis, and even death—exists in our soil, she says. "It's still very much a threat in this country."

Protect it from sunlight. To avoid the skin darkening that often occurs when a cut or scrape heals, Contorer says to avoid sun exposure during the healing process and apply over-the-counter hydrocortisone to the wound.

Matheson suggests using a good sunscreen for several weeks on areas where you've had a wound. Look for a sunscreen with a sun protection factor (SPF) of 15 or higher. (Of course, to shield your skin from damaging ultraviolet light and protect your skin from sunburn and skin cancer, it's wise to wear sunscreen on all exposed skin when you go outside during the day, especially if you are fair skinned.) ◆

◆ DANDRUFF ◆

11 Ways to Shake the Flakes

Don't toss out all those dark suits. There's a better way to deal with dandruff. As a matter of fact, you may be able to simply wash it away.

If you are like most people, you have always thought of those unsightly flakes as dry skin. In reality, though, dandruff is usually a condition of oily skin and an oily scalp.

The process that causes dandruff—the shedding of dead skin cells—is a natural one that goes on continually all over your body. In fact, you get a whole new suit of skin about every 27 or 28 days. The old stuff just sort of flakes away. You simply may not notice the tiny skin cells dropping off your arms and legs.

You happen to see the skin cells that make up dandruff because your hair traps them before they can float off unnoticed. Then the oil from your hair and scalp clumps up the cells until they turn into those visible flakes that decorate your shoulders. Naturally, they are even more noticeable on first dates, job interviews, and other important occasions.

According to Joseph P. Bark, M.D., chairman of dermatology at St. Joseph Hospital in Lexington, Kentucky, you should be glad your scalp flakes away. "If you didn't lose that skin progressively, everybody would be carrying their scalp around in a wheelbarrow," he says. "It would be tremendously thick."

Unfortunately, few of us are brave enough to shrug off dandruff, even if it reflects a normal and necessary process. Fortunately, you can take steps to sweep those flakes away once and for all.

Shampoo each day to keep it away. What easier way to get rid of dandruff than to wash it down the drain? Often, this is all that's required, says Andrew Lazar, M.D., assistant professor of clinical dermatology at Northwestern University School of Medicine in Chicago. Getting rid of excess oils and flakes through daily shampooing may be the easiest way to tame your mane.

Switch shampoos. If your regular shampoo isn't doing the trick, even with daily washing, it's time to switch to an antidandruff shampoo. Check the ingredients for over-the-counter shampoos, says Fredric Haberman, M.D., author of *The Doctor's Beauty Hotline.* Look for a dandruff shampoo that contains zinc pyrithione, selenium sulfide, sulfur, or salicylic acid.

Switch, and switch again. Your favorite dandruff shampoo may stop working after a while. To your dismay, those little white flakes may take up residence on your shoulders again. It's not the fault of the shampoo, says Haberman. You simply may build up a resistance to the shampoo's active ingredient. Haberman recommends rotating three brands of dandruff shampoo (each with a different formulation), using each for a month. In other words, use one shampoo for a month, then switch to a second brand for a month, then to a third brand for a month, then back to the original shampoo for a month, and so on.

Lather twice. The first lathering and rinsing gets rid of the loose flakes and the oily buildup on your hair and scalp. It sort of clears the area so the second lathering can get to work. Leave the second lathering of shampoo on your hair at least five minutes before rinsing it off, advises Haberman. That gives the shampoo a chance to penetrate the skin cells and do what it's supposed to do.

Try tar. If the antidandruff shampoos aren't working, it's time to bring out the big guns, namely the tar shampoos. Tar shampoos have been a proven remedy for more than 200 years, says Bark.

The tar decreases cell turnover quite effectively. However, there are some drawbacks. Tar shampoos have a strong odor, may stain the shaft of lighter-colored hair (it can take weeks of using a milder shampoo to get rid of the discoloration), and may irritate the skin.

Rinse. If you decide to go with a tar shampoo, rinse your hair with lemon juice, a conditioner, or creme rinse to get rid of any odor lingering from the shampoo, according to Paul S. Russell, M.D., clinical professor of dermatology at Oregon Health Sciences University in Portland. Russell says that using a conditioner after washing with an antidandruff shampoo is a good idea anyway, because the medicated shampoos tend to stiffen hair and make it less manageable.

Be sensitive to your sensitivity. There are some people who just plain shouldn't use a tar shampoo. Why? Because they're so sensitive. Rather, their scalp is. Bark says the shampoo can irritate and inflame the hair follicles of some people and can cause a condition called folliculitis. The cure? Switch to a milder shampoo.

Stop those itchy fingers. Try to resist the temptation to go after those itchy patches like a dog chasing fleas. You may end up with wounds to your scalp caused by your fingernails. If you break the skin on your scalp, discontinue use of medicated shampoo for a while. Switch to a mild shampoo, such as a baby shampoo, advises Russell, and use it daily until the scratches are healed.

Shower away sweat. After exercise or strenuous work that makes you perspire, shower and shampoo as soon as possible. Sweat irritates the scalp and speeds up the flaking of skin cells, says Lazar.

Go easy on the sticky stuff. Although you needn't give up the various mousses, sprays, and gels that

---

◆◆◆ Is It Really ◆◆◆ Dandruff?

You may have something that's like dandruff, but isn't dandruff. Other possibilities that also involve flaking of the skin are seborrheic dermatitis and psoriasis.

Seborrheic dermatitis is a chronic disorder characterized by inflammation of the skin, along with scaling. It sometimes strikes the eyebrow area, the sides of the nose, the ears, and the central chest.

Psoriasis is characterized by red, scaly patches on the skin that are caused by unusually rapid turnover of cells.

Prescription medications are available to control both conditions. So if you still have trouble with dandruff after attempting the home remedies discussed here, see your doctor.

---

hold your hairstyle in place, try to use them less often, says Lazar. These hair products can contribute to oily buildup.

Be kind to yourself. People who are under a great deal of stress seem to have more dandruff, observes Haberman. He says that stress somehow contributes to the proliferation of skin cells. Although there is no known diet connection to dandruff, "poor diet can stress you out and contribute to any dermatitis condition," says Haberman. Adopting a healthier lifestyle and finding ways to relax or let off steam can make a difference. ◆

◆ DENTURE ◆ DISCOMFORT

9 Ways to Stop Denture Discomfort

Dentures have come a long way since the wooden teeth worn by George Washington. But, as anyone who has worn them can attest, dentures can cause discomfort. There are two times when dentures often cause discomfort—during the initial "adjustment" phase, when dentures are new, and after several years of wearing, when dentures may stop fitting properly.

Most people become accustomed to their new dentures within a short time. However, at first, you may have difficulty talking and eating. You may find the dentures tend to "slip," or you may develop sore spots in your mouth.

Even people who have had dentures for years sometimes develop problems with them, usually problems related to fit. "When the teeth are extracted, the dentures sit on the bony ridge that's left," says Sandra Hazard, D.M.D., a managing dentist with Willamette Dental Group, Inc., in Oregon. "Without the teeth, the stimulation to the bone is gone and, over many years, the bone is reabsorbed by the body. The plastic denture, of course, stays the same but starts to fit badly."

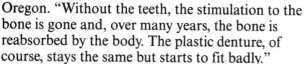

Poor fit is probably the most common cause of denture discomfort. As the bony ridge shrinks, the dentures can slip, move around, and cause sore areas. Often, people try to refit their dentures by using commercial denture adhesives. But using too much adhesive can change the relationship of the denture to the tissue and result in more soreness. Sometimes the body itself tries to solve the ill-fitting denture problem by causing tissue to overgrow in the mouth.

While dentures will never be as comfortable as your natural teeth, there are plenty of things you can do to prevent and resolve denture discomfort:

Keep those chompers clean. When you first have your teeth extracted and your new dentures fit, it's important to keep your dentures clean, because excess bacteria can retard the gums' healing process, says Hazard.

Once you're accustomed to your dentures, it's important to clean them at least twice a day. "You can brush them with toothpaste or use a special denture cleaner," says Hazard.

Jack W. Clinton, D.M.D., associate dean of Patient Services at Oregon Health Sciences University School of Dentistry in Portland, prefers plain old soap and water to keep dentures sparkling. "Using a hand brush and soap and water works great," he says.

Brush the gums. Don't forget to brush your gums, too. "You can help maintain the health of the tissues that lie underneath the dentures by brushing the gums twice a day with a soft brush," says Ken Waddell, D.M.D., a dentist in private practice in Tigard, Oregon.

Brushing the gums, palate, and tongue not only stimulates the tissues and increases circulation, it also helps reduce bacteria and removes plaque.

Baby your mouth. At least at first, your gums will need time to adjust to the compression created by the dentures. Hazard advises patients to eat soft foods during the denture adjustment period to avoid damaging the tender tissues.

Once the gums have healed and your dentist has refit your dentures properly, you'll be able to chew more normally. But Waddell says some foods, such as apples and corn on the cob, are probably best avoided by people who wear dentures. "Advertisements show people with dentures eating all kinds of hard foods," he says. "But hard foods cause the denture to traumatize the gums and bone of the upper jaw. Cut up your apples and take the corn off the cob."

Take an over-the-counter pain reliever. During the initial break-in of your dentures, your mouth is likely to feel sore. Over-the-counter pain relievers, including aspirin, ibuprofen, and acetaminophen, can take the sting out of the pain, says Hazard.

However, if you have persistent pain or if you've worn dentures for several years and pain develops, see your dentist.

Take them out. When you develop a sore area in your mouth from dentures, Clinton says to do what comes naturally—take them out. "If you're uncomfortable, you probably have a soft tissue injury," says Clinton. "Take the denture out and leave it out for an hour or so. In most cases, that takes care of it."

If you develop a red spot, Clinton advises going dentureless for 24 hours. Then, if it doesn't clear up or if the soreness returns when you start using your dentures again, see your dentist.

Rinse with salt water. If you're in the adjustment phase of wearing dentures or if you're a denture veteran who has developed a sore area in your mouth, Clinton advises rinsing the mouth with warm salt water (half a teaspoon of salt to four ounces of warm water). "Take out your dentures and rinse your mouth every three to four hours with the salt water," he says. "Not only does the salt water help clean out bacteria, it also helps toughen the tissue."

Try hydrogen peroxide. Rinse your mouth out once a day with oral three percent hydrogen peroxide, advises Ronald Wismer, D.M.D., past president of the Washington County Dental Society in Oregon. Mix the peroxide half and half with water, swish for 30 seconds or so (don't swallow), and spit. The hydrogen peroxide helps clean out bacteria.

Don't self-adjust. Too often, people who have worn their dentures for a while and develop a fit problem try to "adjust" their dentures themselves with a pocket knife or other tool. This can cause

---

◆◆ Hello, Doctor? ◆◆◆

While some denture discomforts can be handled at home, Jack W. Clinton, D.M.D., says you should see your dentist if:

• *You develop soreness that doesn't improve within a week.*

• *You have an area on the gum that bleeds spontaneously or is filled with pus.*

• *There's extra tissue growing, particularly between the upper lip and the gum.*

• *You have a white sore for more than one week.*

• *You have a sore that doesn't heal completely within 10 to 14 days.*

---

more harm, says Clinton, because it can break down the dentures, change the dentures' "bite," and alter how the dentures fit against the gum.

Also, don't try to "fill the space" between the denture and the gum tissue with over-the-counter adhesive. If your dentures begin to slip or don't feel like they're fitting properly, see your dentist, who can reline them.

Take time out. "I tell people their dentures should be out of their mouths half the time," says Clinton. "It gives the soft tissues time to recover."

Always take your dentures out at night, Clinton advises. "You don't sleep with your shoes on," he says. "It's the same with your dentures." ◆

◆ DERMATITIS ◆
AND ECZEMA

25 Ways to Fight Them

Dermatitis, which is sometimes also called eczema, can create a vicious cycle. Your skin itches, so you scratch it. It becomes red and swollen, and then tiny, red, oozing bumps appear that eventually crust over. You keep scratching because the itching is unbearable, so the rash gets even more irritated and perhaps even infected.

All too often, you don't even know what's causing the itching. It could be an allergy to the soap you use in the shower each morning. It could be irritation due to a chemical you're exposed to at work. It could be atopic eczema—a mysterious itchy rash common to people with a history of allergies and most prevalent in children.

Dermatitis is sometimes used as a catch-all term for any inflammation or swelling of the skin. The term eczema is used interchangeably with dermatitis by some experts, while others differentiate between the two as separate types of inflammation.

Regardless of what kind of dermatitis you're suffering from, however, some general rules apply when you're seeking relief. There are also some treatment and prevention tips that are specific to the type of dermatitis that you have. So first, we'll give you some basic strategies for relief—no matter which type of dermatitis has you scratching. Then we'll give you some specific helpful hints to protect your skin from some of the most common types of dermatitis.

RELIEF FROM THE ITCH

Determining what's causing your dermatitis is important in treating it, but if you can't think of *anything* but the itching at the moment, here are some steps you can take for fast relief.

Cool the itch and swelling. You can do this with cool compresses. Jerome Z. Litt, M.D., assistant clinical professor of dermatology at Case Western Reserve University School of Medicine in Cleveland, recommends using a folded handkerchief or a piece of bed linen folded eight layers thick. Dip the clean cloth into cool water or Burow's solution (available over the counter at your pharmacy) and place it on the rash for 10 to 15 minutes every hour. Wet compresses are appropriate when weeping, oozing blisters are present; you'll actually dry up the rash by using water on it.

Litt also says whole-milk compresses are effective. "The protein in the milk helps relieve itching."

Apply calamine lotion. This old standby can help relieve the itch. Apply it in a thin layer, so that the pores aren't sealed, two to three times a day. "The problem with calamine lotion is that it's visible, so it's not very elegant," says Col. Ernest Charlesworth, M.D., assistant chief of allergy and immunology at Wilford Hall U.S. Air Force Medical Center in San Antonio. At least one manufacturer, however, has come out with a version of calamine lotion that will leave you a little less "in the pink." Check your local pharmacy.

Use an over-the-counter hydrocortisone cream. The one percent formulation is more effective, but it won't help a bacterial or fungal infection (two other common causes of rashes). "Hydrocortisone cream is the dermatologist's equivalent of 'take two aspirin and call me in the morning,'" says Litt. Hydrocortisone seems to be more effective on allergic rather than irritant dermatitis, points out Alan N. Moshell, M.D., director of the Skin Disease Program at the National Institute of Arthritis and Musculoskeletal and Skin Diseases in Bethesda, Maryland.

Stay away from products that end in "-caine." These can often cause allergies in sensitive individuals.

Charlesworth tells about a pharmacist's wife who treated a bad sunburn with a product containing benzocaine and ended up with an allergic contact dermatitis on top of her burn.

Don't try topical antihistamines. Again, these products can cause allergic reactions. "You should swallow an antihistamine," emphasizes Litt. "Don't ever rub it on your skin. I've seen too many horror stories—you can end up with a rash squared to the second power."

Take an oral antihistamine. Try an over-the-counter product like Benadryl to relieve itching. Such products cause drowsiness, but that may help at night when itching is most severe. If you take it during the day and it makes you drowsy, avoid driving or operating heavy machinery.

Don't scratch. By scratching the affected area, you can break the skin and cause a secondary infection, warns Alexander A. Fisher, M.D., F.A.A.D., clinical professor of dermatology at New York University Medical Center in New York. Litt recommends rubbing the itch with your fingertips instead of scratching with your nails.

Take a soothing bath. Adding oatmeal or baking soda to bathwater will make it more soothing, says Litt, although it won't cure your rash. Buy an 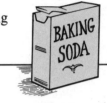 over-the-counter colloidal oatmeal bath treatment (the oatmeal is ground up so it dissolves better) or add a cup of baking soda to warm, not hot, bathwater.

◆◆ Condom Dermatitis ◆◆

More and more people are exposed to latex these days. More people are using condoms in their practice of safe sex. And physicians and dentists routinely wear latex gloves when examining patients.

As a result, more people are showing signs of allergies to latex. Around ten percent of health personnel are now allergic to rubber gloves, says Alexander A. Fisher, M.D., F.A.A.D. Between one and two percent of the general population is allergic.

That could add up to a lot of reactions, considering that 500 million condoms were sold in 1986, Fisher says. As far as condom dermatitis is concerned, you may react to a protein in the rubber itself, to some of the antioxidizing chemicals (which help keep the rubber from breaking down) contained in the rubber, or even to preservatives like paraben used in the "wet" condoms. (Most of the lubricated condoms in the United States, Fisher says, use a silicone-based lubricant that's dry.)

Symptoms of condom dermatitis include vaginal burning, redness and swelling in the groin, an

eczemalike rash on the inner thighs, or a rash around the mouth.

You may be able to switch to another brand of condom for relief. Another option: Use a condom made of processed sheep's intestine. This type, however, does not protect against the AIDS virus, so Fisher suggests combining the latex condom with one of sheep's intestine. The order they're worn, of course, depends on which partner suffers from the allergy.

If you're allergic to latex, you may also notice problems when you visit the doctor. "The patient goes to the gynecologist and afterwards has a vaginal itch," Fisher says, "because of the doctor's gloves during the exam. Or the rubber dam used by some dentists can cause allergies."

You can test yourself by wearing a rubber glove, or just the fingers of the glove, on your damp hand for 15 to 30 minutes and then looking for any reaction. Remember, if you react to latex on your hands, any part of your body will react to latex.

Hope for the future: the condom for women, since it's made of polyurethane instead of latex.

◆◆◆ Ear Piercing ◆◆◆ Alert

If you decide to get your ears pierced, make sure those first earring studs have stainless steel posts, warns Col. Ernest Charlesworth, M.D. Also make sure that the needle used is of stainless steel rather than nickel plated. Otherwise, they may contain nickel, and you'll risk becoming sensitized to this common allergen. The downside: It won't just be your earlobes that react the next time you're exposed to nickel. A watchband, ring, or belt buckle that touches the skin could set off an allergic reaction—and an itchy rash—in the future.

ALLERGIC CONTACT DERMATITIS

Some people sneeze when confronted with ragweed pollen or dander from cats. And some people break out in a rash, known as allergic contact dermatitis, when confronted with substances that are normally harmless to other people, like ingredients in costume jewelry or makeup.

Confounding the issue: You have to be exposed at least once to become "sensitized," or allergic, to the substance in question. That means you might be able to wear your grandmother's ring for years before it brings on any symptoms or be able to try a new makeup for weeks before it causes a reaction.

Add to that the time delay in which a reaction occurs. An airborne allergen, like ragweed or animal dander, usually elicits sneezing or a runny nose within 15 minutes of exposure. But it may take up to 72 hours before a reaction shows up on your skin. That can make identifying the culprit pretty tough.

The most common allergen in allergic contact dermatitis is poison ivy, which can cause reactions in at least half of the people ever exposed to it (see POISON IVY).

The next most common allergen that causes this type of dermatitis is nickel, a metal commonly used in costume jewelry. Even 14-karat gold jewelry has some nickel in it. Up to ten percent of the population may suffer an allergic reaction to this metal, says Charlesworth. You're safest with 24-karat gold, which is pure gold, says Litt, or jewelry made of platinum or stainless steel.

Other possible causes of allergic contact dermatitis:
• Neomycin or benzocaine in topical anesthetics
• Leather
• Formaldehyde, which is used in shampoo, detergent, nail hardeners, waterless hand cleaners, and mouthwashes
• Cinnamon flavor in toothpaste and candies
• PABA, the active ingredient in some sunscreens
• Chemicals found in hair dyes
• Preservatives in cosmetics

How can you handle allergic contact dermatitis?

Ferret out the cause. If the rash recurs or won't go away, you're going to have to play detective to find out what's causing it. If you're having trouble pinning down the cause, a dermatologist or allergist can help. Either can do a test using common allergens (called a patch test) and ask you the right questions to detect the culprit. "It can be difficult," Charlesworth warns. "Some of these chemicals are present in such small amounts." What's more, we use so many different products. Paul Lazar, M.D., professor of clinical dermatology at Northwestern University School of Medicine in Chicago, points out that the average woman uses 17 different products on her scalp and head each morning.

Don't sweat it. Wearing nickel-containing jewelry in a hot, humid environment may worsen the allergy, says Charlesworth, because perspiration leaches out some of the nickel. So before you start a workout or go out into the heat, take off any nickel-containing jewelry.

Don't depend on the "hypoallergenic" label. That's a "very ambiguous" term, says Charlesworth, like "low-fat" or "high-fiber" on a box of cereal. The only requirement to use the term, he says: The product has to have been tested on 200 rodent ears and not caused a reaction.

Coat nickel jewelry. Paint the surfaces that come in contact with your skin with clear nail polish.

Protect your skin. "If you're working in the garden, wear work gloves and a long-sleeved shirt," says Lazar.

IRRITANT CONTACT DERMATITIS

Some things in this world are so harsh that prolonged exposure to them can result in a rash known as irritant contact dermatitis. Numerous chemicals in industry cause problems for workers, but the household is not without its share of hazards to your skin. Soaps, detergents, oven cleaners, bathroom cleaners, and a whole multitude of products can irritate the skin by removing the skin's protective oils, explains Fisher.

What's the difference between irritant and allergic contact dermatitis? Soap, for example, can cause either one. But it's repeated exposure to soap that causes irritation, while a brief exposure to the perfume or an antibacterial agent in the soap can set off an allergic reaction, explains Moshell.

Clues to the culprit: Where is the rash on your body, and what could have touched the skin in that area?

If you suspect that an irritant has caused your red, itchy, bumpy rash, there's one very important thing you should do:

Avoid exposure to the irritant. Until you manage to do that, you'll keep subjecting the skin to the irritant, and the rash will continue. If exposure to household cleansers is the problem and it's your hands that are suffering, wear vinyl gloves, rather than those made of rubber, when handling products such as oven cleaners or when washing dishes or doing other chores that expose your

Hello, Doctor?

When should you see a doctor for your rash? "When you feel uncomfortable with what's going on," says Paul Lazar, M.D. "Patients worry they come in too soon, when many of them come in too late because a simple problem has ended up turning into a chronic disease." He adds that if you're worried about your rash, you need to seek medical attention.

hands to water, soap, and chemicals. "No one's allergic to vinyl," Fisher points out. Wearing cotton liners with the gloves will help keep perspiration from further irritating your skin, although this can be a bulky combination.

ATOPIC DERMATITIS

This one takes its name from atopy, the term for an inherited condition that can show up as dermatitis, as allergies to airborne substances such as pollens, or as asthma. If any other family members have any one of these conditions, you may be at risk for atopic dermatitis.

Infants and children are most likely to be plagued, and a majority of the cases will end by adulthood. If you or your child suffers from this chronic rash, you'll need the care of a physician, most likely a dermatologist or allergist.

It's characterized by intense and miserable itching. The key to coping with this condition is to reduce irritation to the skin, says Noreen Heer Nicol, M.S., R.N., F.N.C., a dermatology clinical specialist/nurse practitioner at National Jewish Center for Immunology and Respiratory Medicine and senior clinical instructor at the University of Colorado Health Sciences Center School of Nursing, both in Denver. Here's her advice:

Wash new clothes before wearing. This will help remove formaldehyde and other potentially irritating chemicals that are used to treat fabrics and clothing.

Rinse twice. Even if you use a mild laundry detergent, it's a good idea to rinse your clothes twice to make sure that all of the soap is removed.

Wear loose, natural-fabric clothing. You want your skin to be able to "breathe," so choose loose-fitting, open-weave, cotton or cotton-blend clothes.

Keep temperatures constant. Abrupt temperature changes—hot to cold or vice versa—can irritate the skin, so try to avoid them whenever possible. Try to maintain constant humidity levels in your home, too.

Keep your fingernails trimmed. It's hard to scratch effectively—and therefore hard to cause further damage to your sensitive skin—if your fingernails are short.

Hydrate your skin with a bath or shower. Use warm, not hot, water, and soak or shower for at least 15 or 20 minutes. Nicol recommends avoiding the use of a washcloth, except for cleaning the genital area, because it's abrasive.

Use soap only where necessary. Choose a gentle soap, such as Dove, Oiltum, Alpha Keri, Neutrogena, Purpose, or Basis; a nonsoap cleanser, such as Aveeno or Emulave; or a liquid cleaner, such as Moisturel, Neutrogena, or Dove. Rinse thoroughly, gently pat away excess moisture, and then apply moisturizer to your still-damp skin to seal in the water. Plain petrolatum is the best after-bath sealant.

Use moisturizer throughout the day. This is extremely important in atopic dermatitis, says Moshell, to prevent excessive dryness of the skin. Nicol recommends Aquaphor ointment, Eucerin cream, Moisturel cream or lotion, D.M.L. cream or lotion, Lubriderm cream or lotion, Neutrogena emulsion, Eutra, Vaseline Intensive Care lotion, or LactiCare lotion.

Protect your skin from the sun. A sunburn is only going to irritate the skin further. Whenever you go outside during the day, use a sunscreen with a sun protection factor (SPF) of 15 or more on all exposed areas of skin.

Wash after swimming. The chlorine and other chemicals found in most swimming pools can irritate the skin. So soon after you've finished your swim, take a shower or bath and use a mild soap all over. Don't forget to reapply your moisturizer as well.

Check out your diet. Some physicians believe food allergies may play some role in atopic dermatitis, while others say it hasn't been proven. If you suspect a food aggravates your rash, omit it from your diet for a few weeks. If your rash clears up, and then you eat the food again and the rash returns, you should probably eliminate it, suggests Fisher. ◆

◆ DIABETES ◆

28 Ways to Live Well with Diabetes

Each day, some 12 million diabetics in this country walk a tightrope between too little sugar in the bloodstream and too much. Too little—which may come from a complication of medication—and they may quickly be overcome by dizziness, fatigue, headache, sweating, trembling, and, in severe cases, loss of consciousness and coma. Too much—which can happen after eating too much, especially if the person is older and overweight—and the person may experience weakness, fatigue, excessive thirst, labored breathing, and loss of consciousness. Left untreated, the picture is bleak: Blindness, kidney disease, blood vessel damage, infection, heart disease, nerve damage, high blood pressure, stroke, limb amputation, and coma may result.

Because the initial symptoms (fatigue, weakness, frequent urination) are usually mild, half of all diabetics do not realize that they have the disease. And that's a real shame, because with early diagnosis and treatment, the chances of living a long and productive life are higher than if the disease creeps along undetected until irreversible problems set in.

If you'd like some proof that diabetes is clearly a disease you can live with, take a look at these prolific diabetics: jazz musician Dizzy Gillespie, singer Ella Fitzgerald, actress Mary Tyler Moore, baseball Hall of Fame great Jim (Catfish) Hunter. Even before treatment was as sophisticated as it is today, author Ernest Hemingway and inventor Thomas Edison, both of whom were diabetic, managed to leave their marks on history.

If you are one of the lucky ones whose diabetes has been diagnosed by a doctor, you have an idea of what has gone awry in your body. The disorder stems from the way your body processes carbohydrates, which you take in through food. Normally, these foods are converted into a form of sugar called glucose, which floats along in the bloodstream until the pancreas, a large gland located behind the stomach, goes into action. The pancreas produces insulin, a hormone that signals body cells to soak up the glucose. Once inside the cell, the glucose is either used to produce heat or energy or is stored as fat. A person with diabetes produces little or no insulin or else becomes resistant to the hormone's action and can't compensate. Either way, the glucose can't get into the cells; it accumulates in the blood and is later expelled in the urine. In short, blood sugar rises while cells starve.

Early Warning Signs

Early diagnosis and treatment is extremely important in helping diabetics live healthier, longer lives. If you notice the early warning signs listed below or suspect that you may have diabetes, see your doctor.

Some of the early warning signs of Type I diabetes are:
- *Frequent urination accompanied by unusual thirst*
- *Extreme hunger*
- *Rapid weight loss with easy tiring, weakness, and fatigue*
- *Irritability, nausea, and vomiting*

Some of the early warning signs for Type II diabetes are:
- *Frequent urination accompanied by unusual thirst*
- *Blurred vision or any change in sight*
- *Tingling or numbness in the legs, feet, or fingers*
- *Frequent skin infection or itchy skin*
- *Slow healing of cuts and bruises*
- *Drowsiness*
- *Vaginitis in women*
- *Erectile dysfunction in men*

Changing Your Ways

As any dieter knows, losing weight takes more "won't" power than willpower, says John Buse, M.D., Ph.D. Sometimes, people just make it too easy for themselves to fail. Here are some tips to help you succeed:

Learn what triggers your eating. *If the sight of a bakery window sets off a craving for cake, make it a habit to walk on the other side of the street. Become aware of any cues like this, and learn to control them.*

Don't keep large amounts of food on hand. *For some overweight people, the fact that food is within reach means that it must be eaten. Buy only enough for a few meals at a time.*

Prepare your meals from scratch rather than relying on take-out. *For one thing, take-out foods are likely to be high in calories because of the methods used in preparation. And you might easily order too much and thereby overeat.*

Only about one-tenth of all diabetics have the severe form of the disease, called Type I, which usually affects children and young adults and requires daily injections of insulin. Most have what doctors refer to as Type II, or adult-onset diabetes. While about one-third of Type II diabetics do require insulin to control blood sugar, and another one-third use medications to increase insulin production, the remaining Type II diabetics rely on nonmedical measures (such as diet, weight loss, and exercise) alone to control their disease. No matter which group you fall into, you can benefit from taking an active role in your treatment. But don't make a move without consulting your doctor first. He or she will call the shots; then it's up to you to carry through. Here's how:

Dish up a special diet. "The goal of dietary intervention for Type I diabetes is to help minimize short- and long-term complications by normalizing blood sugar levels. The goal of dietary intervention in Type II diabetes is to help the patient achieve and maintain normal body weight," says John Buse, M.D., Ph.D., assistant professor in the Department of Medicine, Section of Endocrinology, at the University of Chicago and director of the Endocrinology Clinic at the University of Chicago Medical Center.

Both Type I and Type II diabetics should follow the guidelines offered by the American Diabetes Association (ADA), which were revised in 1986 based on new research findings. (See "Choose One from Column A . . .")

Know your carbohydrates. The traditional dogma for diabetics was this: Avoid simple carbohydrates, or simple sugars (such as table sugar), because they raise blood sugar quickly, and choose complex carbohydrates (such as the starches and fiber found in grains, potatoes, beans, and peas), because they raise blood sugar more slowly. But this dogma has given way recently to newer rules, which really aren't rules at all in the strictest sense.

"Diabetic meal planning must account for many factors," says Harold E. Lebovitz, M.D., professor of medicine, chief of the Division of Endocrinology and Diabetes, and director of the Clinical Research Center at State University of New York Health Science Center at Brooklyn. "A food eaten alone may affect blood sugar differently than when it is eaten with another food. The same variations can be noted with cooked foods versus raw foods and even with different brands of foods. And not least, different foods affect blood sugar differently in different people."

Consequently, while complex carbohydrates like lentils, soy beans, peanuts, and kidney beans are still best for causing the slowest and lowest rise in blood sugar after a meal, present evidence suggests that sucrose (table sugar) may not be "off limits" for Type II diabetics if blood glucose levels stay normal after their ingestion. "Experimenting with 'forbidden foods' may be possible with a doctor's consent," says Lebovitz. "But before you start bingeing on bonbons, it's important to be prepared to see what happens in terms of the blood-glucose response."

Get fond of fiber. The key to the effectiveness of complex carbohydrates may lie in the fiber content. "While the cause and effect of fiber in control of Type II diabetes has yet to be established, we do know that such foods are very satiating and can help enormously toward weight loss and maintenance," says Buse.

Understand "sweet" talk. Actually, there are a number of different kinds of sugar, and each has a potentially different effect on blood sugar levels. "The most basic form of sugar is glucose, or dextrose, which will raise blood sugar levels faster than any other kind when swallowed," says Ira J. Laufer, M.D., clinical associate professor of medicine at New York University School of Medicine and medical director of The New York Eye and Ear Infirmary Diabetes Treatment Center in New York. "Sucrose also tends to raise blood sugar almost as quickly as dextrose. But fructose, sometimes called fruit sugar, generally has a very mild effect on blood sugar. If your diabetes is in good control, dietetic desserts and candies sweetened with pure fructose are not likely to raise your blood sugar levels very much," he adds. On the other hand, fructose provides as many calories as other sugars, so it may not be the wisest choice for diabetics who need to lose weight.

Reduce your risks. To emphasize the fact that excess weight is a Type II diabetic's most serious problem, experts on diabetes are fond of saying that if you want to find out if there's a possibility of getting diabetes, just keep on eating and get fat. You can do other things, too, but the main thing is get fat. An estimated 80 percent of those with Type II diabetes are obese when diagnosed with the disease. Added weight can both accelerate the diabetes and bring on its complications, especially cardiovascular disease and stroke.

In contrast, even a modest weight loss can have dramatic effects: High insulin levels drop, the liver begins to secrete less glucose into the blood, and peripheral muscle tissues begin to respond to insulin and take up glucose better. Just as obesity

---

◆ Choose One from ◆ Column A...

These recommendations should be considered "ground rules" for a Type II diabetic. Diets must be adjusted to meet individual needs, so be sure to discuss your diet with your doctor before making any changes.

• *Raise carbohydrate intake to more than half of total calories. Every gram of carbohydrate provides four calories.*

• *Keep protein intake to 12 to 20 percent of total calories. A gram of protein provides four calories as well.*

• *Lower fat intake to less than 30 percent of total calories and make every effort to substitute polyunsaturated fat or monounsaturated fat for saturated fat. Each gram of fat provides nine calories, so go easy!*

• *Maintain cholesterol intake at less than 300 milligrams a day. Less saturated fat in the diet will automatically lead to reduced cholesterol.*

• *Include fiber in the diet; it should be part of as many meals as possible.*

---

leads to insulin resistance, so weight loss reverses the condition. When persons with Type II diabetes lose weight, they frequently are no longer diabetic. "Type II diabetics may *only* need to get and stay at an ideal body weight," says Buse. "And unless they do that, nothing else will work very well." (See "Changing Your Ways" for weight-loss tips.)

Don't "crash." Too rapid weight loss rarely works in the long run and is potentially dangerous if undertaken without a doctor's advice. Sometimes, a doctor *will,* in fact, prescribe a very-low-calorie diet to initiate weight loss, but only for a very short period of time. Generally, the best approach is to lose weight gradually with a low-fat, lower-calorie, nutritionally balanced diet combined with increased activity. Avoid the use of over-the-counter appetite suppressants that contain phenylpropanolamine (PPA).

Graze. Many experts believe that a Type II diabetic may more easily achieve normal blood sugar levels by not overloading with too much food at one time. "Three smaller meals a day—breakfast, lunch, and dinner—plus two or three snack-type meals in between is easier for the diabetic person's insulin to handle. Just be sure that you don't overshoot your calorie limit, however," advises Lebovitz.

Get a firm foothold. Neuropathy, damage to the nerves, is a common problem for diabetics. It occurs most often in the feet and legs, and its signs include repeated burning, pain, or numbness.

"Neuropathy can be dangerous if it causes a loss of feeling, because then even a minor foot injury may go undiscovered—leading to serious infection, gangrene, and even amputation of the limb," says Joseph C. D'Amico, D.P.M., a podiatrist in private practice in New York. Diabetics, therefore, need to be diligent about foot care. (See "Foot Notes for Diabetics.")

Be a sport. Regular exercise provides many benefits. It tones up the heart and other muscles, strengthens bones, lowers blood pressure, strengthens the respiratory system, helps raise HDL (good cholesterol), gives a sense of well-being, decreases tension, aids in weight control, enhances work capacity, and confers a sense of achievement. "For those with diabetes," says Laufer, "exercise bestows additional benefits. It promotes the movement of sugar from the bloodstream into cells, where it is burned for energy, and it improves the cells' ability to respond to insulin, thus decreasing their need for the hormone."

◆◆◆ Hypoglycemia: ◆◆◆ The Disease that Isn't

After eating a meal—or going too long without one—are you tired? Lightheaded? Dizzy? A little bit anxious? You may be among the thousands of people who have been told or who have convinced themselves that they have low blood sugar, or hypoglycemia—and who are wrong.

Hypoglycemia, also called "sugar blues," was a condition that appeared some years ago and was supposedly caused by eating excess sugar, which led to very high glucose levels followed by very low levels. More likely, says John Buse, M.D., Ph.D., the symptoms were caused by skipping meals, lack of sleep, or tension.

But hypoglycemia does, indeed, exist. Doctors have determined that there are two basic types. One, called fasting hypoglycemia, occurs after

missing one or more meals and develops slowly as the blood sugar gradually drops lower and lower. It commonly produces central nervous system symptoms, and its causes can be serious underlying disorders, such as tumors that produce insulin. Type I diabetics who take too much insulin for the amount of food they eat may experience the symptoms of fasting hypoglycemia.

The second type, reactive hypoglycemia, occurs about two to four hours after eating, especially if the meals are high in carbohydrates. The usual symptoms include shakiness, weakness, sweating, rapid heartbeat, and faintness, which indicate that the body is reacting to a sudden blood sugar drop by producing adrenaline, cortisol, and glucagon—hormones that aim to bring blood sugar back to normal. People in the early stages of diabetes may rarely have this type of hypoglycemia, but it is more common after extensive abdominal surgery or other surgery.

Not all exercises are for every diabetic person. If blood sugar is high, exercise will lower it; if it's low, exercise will lower it further. Those on medication must work with a doctor to make necessary adjustments. 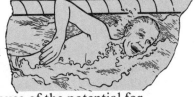 Because of the potential for neuropathy, diabetics need to protect the nerve endings in the feet and so may need to avoid high-impact activities such as jogging. Another consideration is that diabetics are particularly sensitive to dehydration. Also, intense exercise could endanger capillaries in the eyes already weakened by diabetes, leading to rupture, vision problems, and even blindness. So you will need to choose your exercise program carefully with the aid of your doctor. And, especially if you are over 40 years old, you will need to undergo a general medical examination, including a cardiovascular screening test and exercise test, before proceeding with your exercise program.

Once your doctor gives you the go-ahead to begin a program of regular exercise, you need to set up realistic goals in order to avoid too-high or too-low blood sugar levels and other problems that could result from doing too much too soon. "Someone who has not spent much time engaged in physical activity who is also overweight should not be thinking in terms of running races," advises Laufer.

Foot Notes for Diabetics

A common complaint from many people is, "My feet are killing me!" For a diabetic, the statement could be all too true. Loss of nerve function, especially on the soles of the feet, can reduce feeling and mask a sore or injury on the foot that, if left unattended, can turn into an ulcer or gangrene. "A person with diabetes must be super cautious about foot care," says Joseph C. D'Amico, D.P.M. "Remember, there's only one pair per person per lifetime."

Here's how to start at the bottom:

Look them over. *Give your feet a thorough going-over every night to make sure that you haven't developed a sore, blister, cut, scrape, or any other tiny problem that could blow up into big trouble. If your vision isn't good, have someone with good eyesight check your feet for you.*

Wash, rinse, and dry. *A clean foot is a healthy foot, with a much lower susceptibility to infection. And clean feet feel better, too.*

Avoid bathroom surgery. *Under normal circumstances, there is little danger from using a pumice stone to reduce a corn or callus. But for a diabetic, such a practice might lead to a little irritation, then a sore, then infection, and finally, a major ulcer.*

Remove "removers" from reach. *Caustic agents for removing corns and calluses can easily cause a serious chemical burn on a diabetic's skin. Never use them.*

Take care of the little things. *Any time a cut, sore, burn, scratch, or other minor injury appears on a diabetic's foot, it must be attended to immediately. "Wash the lesion with soap and water to remove all foreign matter. Cover with a protective sterile dressing. Use adhesive tape with caution, if at all, because it can weaken the skin when it is pulled off. Use paper or cloth-type tape instead," suggests D'Amico. If the sore is not healing or if you notice signs of infection, such as redness, red streaks, warmth, swelling, pain, or drainage, see a podiatrist.*

Choose shoes with care. *"Since a person with diabetes may not always be aware of the pain caused by shoes that are too tight, he or she must be very attentive to fit when buying new shoes," says D'Amico.*

Swimming, bicycle riding, and brisk walking are all recommended. Indeed, walking is the one activity that all medical experts agree is ideal for a diabetic patient. "The average Type II diabetic patient is over 50, overweight, and underactive," says Laufer. Walking is a kinder, gentler activity for such individuals. Remember, however, that the positive effects of exercise last for only a day or two, so your goal should be to exercise at least every other day.

Watch your mouth. Diabetics must be extra careful about their teeth. "Good dental hygiene is important for everyone," says Andrew Baron, D.D.S., a dentist and clinical associate professor at Lenox Hill Hospital in New York. "Because they are at increased risk for infection, diabetics should be super cautious about preventing tooth decay and periodontal disease." Keep a supply of toothbrushes so you won't have to deal with old, worn brushing aids. Brush and floss without fail after every meal and before bedtime. And see your dentist regularly for checkups and cleaning.

Check your dentures. Ill-fitting dentures or permanent bridgework cause frustration for anyone who has to live with them. For a diabetic, the consequences go far beyond annoyance. "Dentures that move around in your mouth can cause sores that don't heal," cautions Baron. "It's a shame to suffer with such problems, especially when they are so easily remedied by a dentist." If you notice sore spots in your mouth or find that your dentures are moving or slipping, see your dentist to have the problem corrected.

Take charge. How do you psych yourself up for a game that has no timeouts and that never ends? That's the question diabetics face every day. One way is to learn all you can about your illness so that you can better control it. "Diabetics are constantly learning and relearning lifestyle changes and behavior adjustments. It's like studying for a master's degree in diabetes—and, in this case, there is no graduation and no vacation," says Laufer.

It's a given that even in a diabetic whose disease appears to be totally under control, there will be occasional rapid and even violent swings in blood sugar levels, brought on by emotional or physical stresses, meals, medications, or even the time of day. But if they are anticipated and accepted, these episodes can be viewed as simply a bump in the road rather than a major detour.

Do something nice for yourself. While it's important to learn as much as you can about your diabetes and stay with your treatment regimen, you also need to keep things in perspective. "It is a rare individual who takes time to 'stop and smell the roses,' as it were," notes Laufer. "This is especially true for diabetics, who often get so caught up in their disease that it is difficult for them to focus on other, more-positive aspects of life." Make a list of all the things you would like to do if you had the time—and then *make* the time to do at least some of them. Obviously, finishing a box of chocolates should not appear on this list. While staring into space may be an ideal uplifter for one person, and napping the afternoon away does the same for another, straightening out a messy closet may do the trick for a third.

Do something nice for someone else. It's hard to think of your own problems when you are engaged in making another person's life more pleasant. In any city or town in the country, there are those who are less well-off, with more-severe problems. "You can call your local hospital or library to inquire about volunteers," says Laufer. "Or you can knock on the door of an elderly, housebound neighbor who might appreciate a visit." ◆

◆ DIAPER RASH ◆

10 Ways to Get Rid of It—for Good

Diaper rash. It's not a pretty sight for you, and your baby probably doesn't enjoy it much, either. While far from being a serious medical problem, diaper rash is just another of life's little discomforts.

There's not too much to say about how to recognize diaper rash—if your baby's got a red, sore bottom underneath his or her diaper, that's a pretty conclusive diagnosis. The good news is, you can cure that rash within a matter of days. And with some conscientious care, you can say goodbye to it forever.

The following are sure cures for diaper rash. Luckily, the same principles apply to the prevention side of the coin. In other words, the very things that make the rash go away are also what keep it away, so keep on doing them. Good riddance!

Get rid of the diaper. As its name implies, diaper rash is caused by a diaper. Say goodbye to the diaper, and—voila!—no more rash, says Gregory F. Hayden, M.D., a professor of pediatrics and an attending pediatrician at the University of Virginia Health Sciences Center in Charlottesville. "If the baby has a rash, take his diaper off whenever practical," says Hayden. "This way, stool and urine won't touch the skin." To keep any mess to a minimum, you can put the baby on a rubber mat covered with a washable cloth while you air out his or her bottom.

Change the baby often. The best way to avoid diaper rash or to cure an existing rash is to make sure that the baby is always clean and dry, says Jeannette M. Pergam, M.D., a pediatrician and assistant professor of pediatrics at the University of Nebraska Medical Center in Omaha. "The moist, warm environment under the diaper is one that is very conducive to causing skin infections," she says.

◆◆ Hello, Doctor? ◆◆

If all else fails, call the doctor. Diaper rash, if left untreated, can worsen, leaving your baby's bottom raw and painful. A good rule of thumb is to wait two to five days and, if the condition doesn't improve, head for the doctor's office, says James E. Bridges, M.D.

Avoid commercial baby wipes. Many brands of store-bought baby wipes contain alcohol and other chemicals that can dry and irritate your child's skin, says Pergam. Wet, soapy washcloths are best for cleaning baby's bottom, she says. Be sure to rinse thoroughly with a clean, wet cloth or plain water to remove any soap.

Dry that bottom. When you change your child's diapers, make sure you dry the area thoroughly with a towel, says Pergam. She also advises leaving the area exposed to air for a few minutes before putting on a new diaper. An old-fashioned way to keep baby's bottom dry is to brown a little cornstarch in a frying pan and apply it to the child's bottom, according to James E. Bridges, M.D., a specialist in family medicine in Fremont, Nebraska. He adds that commercial cornstarch baby powders probably work just as well.

Choose an ointment and use it. Many pediatricians recommend using a diaper-rash cream or ointment, such as A and D or Desitin, every time you change your baby. These heavy creams

◆ The Great Diaper ◆ Debate

Are cloth diapers or disposable diapers better at preventing diaper rash? The issue is far from clear-cut, but do take into account the results of the following studies when making your decision: A 1990 study conducted at the Department of Design at Colorado State University in Fort Collins found that diapers labeled "super absorbent" kept the skin drier and retained more moisture than cloth or conventional disposable brands. In most cases, the regular disposables were less effective than cloth diapers at keeping the skin dry. Among cloth diapers, the most effective were those that contained an inner layer of nonwoven fabric, the researchers wrote.

Another study conducted at the Department of Dermatology at the University of Rochester in New York found that babies who wore diapers containing substances to absorb urine and make it "gel" had significantly less diaper rash than babies who wore regular disposables.

create a block so that stool and urine won't irritate the skin, says Hayden. "Some people worry that the ointments will keep moisture in," he says, "but they work pretty well for most skin." A cotton ball dipped in baby oil will usually take the creams off without scrubbing.

Try baby powder, but be careful where you shake it. Dusting the baby's bottom with baby talcum powder may be another way to protect your child's skin against irritants, according to Hayden. However, studies have shown that if babies inhale the powder, it can be dangerous, even fatal.

Cornstarch-based powders may pose less of a threat, Hayden adds. When using any powder, try shaking some into your hand—away from baby's face—and then sprinkling it onto the diaper area.

Hang the diapers out to dry. "There's an old wives' tale that if you hang your baby's diapers out to dry instead of putting them in the dryer, they won't cause diaper rash," Pergam says. Although she has no explanation for the efficacy of this tip, she swears that it worked for her own children. If you have a place to hang them, you may want to give this a try to see if it helps.

Fight back against yeast. Sometimes, what appears to be an innocuous diaper rash can really be an infection of yeast, also called *Candida albicans*. It may be hard to tell the difference between the two, Hayden says, although a yeast infection may appear as little white specks dotting an area of red irritation. To cure a yeast infection, try using an over-the-counter antiyeast medication, such as Lotrimin, or see your pediatrician for a prescription.

Try vinegar solution. Urine is an extremely alkaline solution, says Bridges. It can burn the skin the same way that acid can. To balance out the equation, try adding half a cup of white vinegar to your rinse water when you wash the baby's diapers, he suggests. "That neutralizes the ammonia," he says. Pergam recommends wiping baby's bottom with a solution of eight parts water to one part vinegar—the theory is the same.

Avoid plastic pants. Plastic pants worn over a diaper keep moisture in and may cause irritation or worsen an existing infection, Hayden says. "It's better to let things evaporate and dry out." ◆

◆ DIARRHEA ◆

15 Ways to Go with the Flow

You may blame it on a 24-hour bug or something you ate, but if you're like the average American, you'll suffer once or twice this year from diarrhea—frequent, watery bowel movements that may be accompanied by painful cramps or nausea and vomiting.

Gastroenteritis—the catch-all medical term for intestinal flu, viral infection, and food poisoning—is the second leading cause of missed work time (the common cold beats it).

Diarrhea is uncomfortable and unpleasant, but generally no big deal in otherwise healthy adults. However, if diarrhea becomes a chronic condition, the situation changes. If it affects the very young, the elderly, or the chronically ill, it can be dangerous. And if you're not careful to drink enough fluids, you could find yourself complicating what should have been a simple situation.

What causes diarrhea? Because the condition generally lasts only a few days, doctors don't usually culture the stool to diagnose what started it in the first place. It's most often due to a viral infection, which antibiotics can't fight. You just have to tough it out for a couple of days. The virus has invaded the bowel, causing it to absorb excessive fluid, which leads to the watery stools. You may also experience cramping, nausea and vomiting, headache, fever, malaise, and even upper-respiratory-tract symptoms, such as a runny nose. One clue: If members of your family all get sick, but at different times, it's likely a virus that got passed around. Bacteria, which often cause traveler's diarrhea in certain parts of the world, can also be responsible for diarrhea as the result of food poisoning. "When the whole family goes on a picnic and six hours later, they're all sick, that's a classic sign of food poisoning," says Rosemarie L. Fisher, M.D., professor of medicine in the Division of Digestive Diseases at Yale University School of Medicine in New Haven, Connecticut.

Much rarer are microbes like amoebae and giardia that try to set up permanent housekeeping

---

◆◆ Hello, Doctor? ◆◆

"If you see blood in your stool, that should immediately ring a bell to see your doctor," says Rosemarie L. Fisher, M.D.

If you feel like you're getting dehydrated, get medical attention. The signs: Dizziness when you stand up, scanty and deeply yellow urine, increased thirst, dry skin. Children may cry without tears as well.

If you've got a fever or shaking chills, or the diarrhea persists past 48 to 72 hours, see the doctor.

If diarrhea occurs in the very young, the elderly (see "The Young and the Old"), or the chronically ill, a doctor should be consulted immediately.

---

in your bowel, causing diarrhea that lasts for weeks or months. You can get these from contaminated food or water, public swimming pools, and communal hot tubs.

Certain drugs, especially antibiotics, can have diarrhea as a side effect. Magnesium-containing antacids and artificial sweeteners such as sorbitol are often overlooked culprits.

Unless diarrhea persists, you usually don't find out its cause. Treatment is aimed at relieving the symptoms and at preventing dehydration, the most serious consequence of diarrhea.

So what can you do?

Ride it out. If you're not very young or old or suffering from any chronic illness, it may be safe just to put up with it for a couple of days.

"Although there's no definite proof that diarrhea is a cleansing action, it probably serves some purpose," explains Richard Bennett, M.D., assistant professor of medicine at Johns Hopkins University School of Medicine in Baltimore.

Keep hydrated. In the meantime, make sure you "maintain your fluid and electrolyte balance," as the doctors say. Obviously, you can lose a lot of liquid in diarrhea, but you also lose electrolytes, which are minerals like sodium and potassium, that are critical in the running of your body. Here's how to replace what you're losing:
• Drink plenty of fluids. No one agrees on which fluid is best—again, because of the electrolyte problem. The experts do agree you need at least two quarts of fluid a day, three if you're running a fever. Plain water lacks electrolytes, although you may want to drink this part of the time. Weak tea with a little sugar is a popular choice. Some vote for Gatorade, although Fisher points out it's constituted to replace fluids lost through sweating,

not for diarrhea, a whole different ball game. Defizzed, nondiet soda pop is recommended by some, although anything with a lot of sugar can increase diarrhea. So can caffeine. Fruit juices, particularly apple and prune, have a laxative effect, but others may be OK.
• Buy an over-the-counter electrolyte replacement formula. Pedialyte, Rehydralyte, and Ricelyte are available over-the-counter from your local drug store. These formulas contain fluids and minerals in the proper proportion.

Keep your liquids cool but not ice-cold. Whatever you choose to drink, keep it cool, suggests Peter A. Banks, M.D., director of Clinical Gastroenterology Service at Brigham and Women's Hospital and lecturer on medicine at Harvard Medical School, both in Boston. It will be less irritating that way. Sip, don't guzzle; it will be easier on your insides.

Sip some chicken broth. Or any broth, says Banks. But have it lukewarm, not hot, and add some salt.

◆◆ When Diarrhea Lasts ◆◆ and Lasts and Lasts

Sometimes diarrhea goes on . . . for weeks. That's when a more serious problem is probably responsible. Your doctor can ferret out the cause. Here are some of the possibilities:

Lactose intolerance. "If you get diarrhea every time you drink a glass of milk, you may suffer from this condition that involves an inability to digest lactose, the sugar in milk and dairy products. It's the most common reason for chronic diarrhea," says Rosemarie L. Fisher, M.D. Avoid milk, but take a calcium supplement, she suggests.

Celiac disease. In this case, you can't digest gluten, which is part of wheat.

Irritable bowel syndrome. Emotions play a big role in this one, which can include alternating

constipation and diarrhea. "The classic picture is the young adult with diarrhea on the morning of a big exam," says Fisher.

Parasitic infections. As mentioned previously, these may hang on indefinitely.

Crohn's disease or ulcerative colitis. These two conditions are similar, and no one knows their cause. But the end result of these is inflammation of the bowel and diarrhea, often accompanied by pain.

Systemic illnesses. Chronic diarrhea may be a complication of diseases such as diabetes, scleroderma, and hyperthyroidism.

Cancer. It's not a pleasant thought, but one of the warning signs of tumors in the bowel is diarrhea, especially if blood is present.

Rest in bed. Give your body a chance to fight the bug that's causing this.

Put a heating pad on your belly. Banks says it will help relieve abdominal cramps.

◆ The Young and the Old ◆

For most people, diarrhea is nothing more than a minor inconvenience. But for the very young and the elderly, it can be life threatening, even fatal.

Why is it so dangerous for these groups? "Young children have a much smaller blood volume," explains Harry S. Dweck, M.D., director of the Regional Neonatal Intensive Care Unit at Westchester Medical Center in Valhalla, New York. What constitutes "a small fluid loss in an adult can make a big difference in an infant."

Dehydration can take days to occur in an adult, hours to days for a child, and seconds to minutes in a newborn, Dweck emphasizes. That's why diarrhea has been such a killer of children in many countries around the world.

If your child has diarrhea, "call the doctor right away, with the first loose stool," Dweck stresses.

Diarrhea may be harder to recognize in infants. "Newborns may have up to 6 to 9 bowel movements a day," Dweck says. "And if they're breast-fed, it's a more liquid stool." But parents generally learn fast what their baby's normal stool looks like. If it becomes more liquid, if it's explosive, or if the odor changes, it's probably diarrhea. "The best way by far to prevent diarrhea in infants is to breast-feed," Dweck points out. The colostrum, the special kind of milk produced during the first few days of the baby's life, "is loaded with antibodies and white blood cells" that are absorbed directly into the baby's gastrointestinal tract, which will help prevent gastrointestinal infections down the road.

There's also less chance of contamination with breast-feeding, since bottles don't have to be washed. And formula itself can cause allergic reactions that include diarrhea.

Diarrhea is less serious in children over 18 months of age, but diarrhea still warrants a call to the doctor. Your physician will tell you how to treat your baby and what to give him or her to prevent dehydration and electrolyte imbalance. Once kids reach the age of eight or so, you can follow the same recommendations for treating diarrhea as you would for adults.

The elderly can't stand to lose much fluid, either, but that's because their circulatory system has changed with aging. Hardening of the arteries occurs throughout the blood vessels in the body; lowered blood pressure that occurs when fluid is lost means there's not enough pressure to force blood to circulate.

"That puts them at a high risk for stroke, heart attack, or kidney failure," explains Richard Bennett, M.D.

But when the elderly have diarrhea, it's often difficult to know when they're becoming dehydrated. "They don't recognize thirst as well," says Bennett. "Or maybe they can't get around well enough to get a drink when they are thirsty." Changes in the skin that signal dehydration also aren't apparent in aged skin. The best clue: Are they still passing urine every hour or two?

If you're older and in good health but have a history of congestive heart failure and/or are taking diuretics, you should call your physician as soon as the diarrhea starts. "The doctor may want to change your dosage of diuretics, since these drugs cause you to lose fluid," says Bennett.

Ironically, medical care can lead to some cases of diarrhea in the elderly, says Bennett. They're more likely to be on antibiotics, which can have diarrhea as a side effect. They're also prone to constipation and may self-medicate or have a physician recommend several types of laxatives, which can end up responsible for diarrhea. About half of the cases of diarrhea in the elderly are probably due to infections, the majority of which are viral.

Try yogurt. You'll want to make sure you get a product that contains *live* lactobacillus cultures, which are friendly bugs that normally live in the gut. "There are anecdotal reports but no good studies that yogurt works," says Bennett. "But there's no harm in trying."

Eat light. Soups and gelatin may go down easy. Banks recommends bland foods like rice, noodles, and bananas. Potatoes, toast, cooked carrots, soda crackers, and skinless, defatted chicken are also easy on the digestive system.

Take the pink stuff. Stopping the diarrhea with an over-the-counter medication may not be the best thing for your body. Diarrhea probably reflects your body's attempt to get rid of a troublesome bug. If you do feel it's necessary, however, Pepto-Bismol is probably the safest over-the-counter antidiarrheal medicine, says Bennett. And studies show it may have a mild antibacterial effect, which would be most useful in traveler's diarrhea, since this condition is usually bacteria related (see TRAVELER'S DIARRHEA).

Take Kaopectate or Imodium A-D. Again, you're probably better off going without antidiarrheal medication. If you absolutely need some relief, however, you can try one of these over-the-counter medications. Imodium A-D slows down the motility, or movement, of the gut; Kaopectate absorbs fluid. Bennett does not recommend these for elderly patients because decreased motility can be dangerous in an infection and can lead to worse problems.

Don't do dairy. Avoid milk or other dairy products like cheese during the time that you're having diarrhea as well as for one to three weeks afterward. The small intestine, where milk is digested, is affected by diarrhea and simply won't work as well for a while. "Milk may sound soothing," says Fisher. "But it could actually make the diarrhea worse."

Cut out caffeine. Just as it stimulates your nervous system, caffeine jump-starts your intestines. And that's the last thing you need to do in diarrhea.

Say no to sweet treats. High concentrations of sugar can increase diarrhea. The sugar in fruit can do the same.

Steer clear of greasy or high-fiber foods. These are harder for your gut to handle right now. It needs foods that are kinder and gentler. ◆

◆ DRY HAIR ◆

11 Tips for Taming it

Your hair feels like straw—dry, fly-away, unmanageable. How could you have been cursed with such a mane? You probably weren't, according to Frank Parker, M.D., professor and chairman of the Department of Dermatology at Oregon Health Sciences University in Portland. "While some people are born with hair that tends to be more dry, most dry hair problems aren't organic or genetic problems at all. They're instead due to what you're doing to your hair," he says.

That's right. Those dry locks are most likely your own fault. Exposing your hair to harsh chemicals such as hair dyes, permanent-wave solutions, and the chlorine in swimming pools and hot tubs dries out the hair. So does shampooing too often and using styling tools such as hot combs, hot rollers, and blow dryers. Even too much sun and wind can dry out your tresses.

You can learn to treat your dry hair with T.L.C. and teach it to be more manageable. Here's how:

Don't overdo the shampoo. Overshampooing is one of the most common causes of dry hair, according to Parker. "Too often, people think they have to shampoo their hair every day with harsh shampoos," he says. "It just strips away the natural oils."

On the other hand, you shouldn't go too long without a good lather. "Shampoo at least every three days," says barber, cosmetologist, and hair-care instructor Rose Dygart, owner of Le Rose Salon of Beauty in Lake Oswego, Oregon. "Gentle shampooing stimulates the oil glands."

Be kind to your hair. Dygart says dry hair is the most fragile type of hair and is subject to breakage, so it must be handled with care. "Learn to shampoo your hair very gently," she says. "Try not to pull the hair or put any tension on the hair shafts."

When lathering, avoid scrubbing with your fingernails, which can not only break the hair but can irritate your scalp. Work up a lather using your fingertips, instead.

Use a gentle shampoo. Dry hair needs a gentle, acidic cleanser, says Dygart. "Use a shampoo with a pH of between 4.5 and 6.7 for dry hair. Use a gentle cleanser you wouldn't be afraid to put on your face," she says. Some people recommend baby shampoos, but Dygart says their pH is far too high, and alkaline shampoos dry out the hair. Instead, she recommends acidic shampoos.

Pour on the conditioner. Dry hair needs conditioning, says Nelson Lee Novick, M.D., associate clinical professor of dermatology at Mount Sinai School of Medicine in New York. "Find a conditioner that has as little alcohol as possible in it, because alcohol is drying," he says. "Products that have little or no fragrance usually have less alcohol. For really dry hair, try an overnight conditioner that you put on and wear a shower cap over and rinse off the next day."

For severely dry, damaged hair, Novick recommends using Moisturel, a body lotion that contains petrolatum and glycerin, instead of a conditioner. Apply the moisturizer to damp hair, and leave it on overnight beneath a shower cap. Rinse it out thoroughly in the morning.

Pour the hot oil. "Hot oil treatments are excellent for restoring dry hair," says Dygart. She recommends using over-the-counter hot oil products that you heat and place on the hair for 5 to 20 minutes (according to package instructions). Wear a plastic bag or shower cap over your hair while the hot oil is on. Then, wash the hair thoroughly with a gentle shampoo.

Slather on the mayo. Mayonnaise is another excellent moisturizing treatment for dry hair, says Dygart. "Use old-fashioned mayonnaise, not diet or low-cholesterol types," she says. "First, shampoo your hair, then apply about a tablespoon of mayonnaise. Wrap the hair in a plastic bag for 20 to 30 minutes. Then shampoo and rinse thoroughly."

Nix the 100 strokes. Novick says that because dry hair is so fragile, too much brushing can actually fracture the hair, causing hair fall. He suggests brushing gently and never brushing the hair when it is wet.

Dygart says the type of hairbrush you use is important. She recommends boar-bristle brushes or "vent" brushes, ones with rubberized tips, that don't pull the hair excessively.

Give yourself a scalp massage. One way to stimulate the oil glands on the scalp is to gently massage the scalp during shampoos, says Dygart. "Use the tips of your fingers to very gently massage all over your scalp," she says. "It not only stimulates the oil glands, it also feels great."

Be an egghead. Dygart suggests beating an egg in a cup and, with tepid water (not hot—it cooks the egg!), lathering the egg into the hair and then rinsing it out with tepid water. There's no need to shampoo afterward. The egg not only cleans the hair but gives it a lovely shine.

Pace your hair treatments. If you perm on Tuesday, dye your hair on Thursday, and put it in hot rollers on Saturday, your hair is destined to be dry and damaged. "Think about your hair like a sweater," says Novick. "How many times can you dye it repeatedly before it begins to look terrible?" Novick says people with dry hair don't necessarily have to abandon styling practices like dyes, permanent waves, or hair straightening, but he says it's important to space those treatments out.

Hold the heat. Using hot combs, hot rollers, and blow dryers is asking for dry hair trouble, says Paul Contorer, M.D., chief of dermatology for Kaiser Permanente in Beaverton, Oregon, and clinical professor of dermatology at Oregon Health Sciences University in Portland. Hot rollers are the worst because they stretch the hair while the heat shrinks it. Hot combs also tend to stretch the hair and expose hair to heat for long periods of time.

If you must use artificial heat on your hair, Dygart suggests that you use a blow dryer on a low setting and avoid pulling or stretching the hair while drying. ◆

◆ DRY SKIN ◆

12 Ways to Fight Moisture Loss

Everyone occasionally suffers from dry skin, according to dermatologist James Shaw, M.D., chief of the Division of Dermatology at Good Samaritan Hospital and Medical Center and associate clinical professor of medicine at Oregon Health Sciences University, both in Portland. "Dry skin is largely influenced by genetics and by climate and other drying factors like taking hot showers," he says.

When there's not enough water in the skin's top layer (called the stratum corneum), the skin becomes flaky, itchy, and unsightly. In extreme cases, this layer can become rough, cracked, and scaly, and chronic dermatitis (skin irritation) can develop.

Normally, the outer layer of the skin is kept moist by fluid from the sweat glands and from underlying tissues. Oil, produced by the sebaceous glands in the skin, helps to seal in that fluid. But lots of things rob moisture from the skin's outer layer. Some people simply have an outer skin layer that doesn't hold water well. Others may have less-active sweat glands. Age is also a factor in dry skin. The older you get, the less oil the sebaceous glands produce, and the drier your skin is likely to be.

One of the greatest skin-moisture robbers is low humidity. Cold, dry air, common in many areas during the winter months, sucks water from the skin. Add the drying effects of sun and/or high altitude to low humidity and the parching is compounded. Heated or air-conditioned air in your home or office may also be dry and cause your skin to lose moisture.

Water can actually take moisture from your skin. Overbathing or bathing in hot water for long periods of time causes a repeated wetting and drying of the tissue that holds the outer layer of skin together and, over time, can make it less able to hold and retain water. "People who bathe several times a day or take lots of hot tubs are actually leaching important proteins from their skin that normally keep the skin moist," explains Frank Parker, M.D., professor and chairman of the Department of Dermatology at Oregon Health Sciences University in Portland.

Harsh soaps, detergents, household cleansers, and chemical solvents can also take their toll on the skin. These products can damage the skin's outer layer. People who must frequently wash and dry their hands, such as nurses and hairstylists, often complain of red, chapped hands, so-called "dishpan hands."

While you can't keep skin away from all of the external moisture robbers, here are some tips to keep your skin moist and youthful-looking for years to come:

Moisturize, moisturize, moisturize. Always keep a lotion or cream on your skin, especially if you tend toward dry skin, says Parker. "Apply moisturizer right after you bathe, while you're still damp," he says. *Pat,* don't rub, yourself dry-damp with a soft towel. Apply moisturizers throughout the day whenever your skin feels dry and before retiring to bed.

Which moisturizers should you use? "The more oil a product has in it, the more protection it offers, and the thicker the product, the more it seals in moisture," says Shaw. "Thin lotions are mostly water. Cold creams are thicker and have more oil and less water. And products like Vaseline [petrolatum] are all oil."

Dermatologist Margaret Robertson, M.D., a staff physician at St. Vincent Hospital and Medical Center in Portland, Oregon, advises using a thick, unscented moisturizer that doesn't automatically disappear on the skin. She says you can mix water with petrolatum to form a cream that provides good moisture protection.

Take short, cool showers and baths. Hot water actually draws out oil, the skin's natural barrier to

◆◆ Sun and Your ◆◆ Dry Skin

If you're a sun worshipper who is always "working on your tan," you're also drying out your skin and increasing your risk of developing wrinkles, age spots, and skin cancer (melanoma), warns Frank Parker, M.D. "Just as the sun dries wet clothes hanging on a clothesline, it dries out the outer layer of the skin," he says. "Over time, the damage the sun does to the skin causes it to wrinkle and develop pigmentation spots."

Even more sobering is the increased risk of developing skin cancer from excessive sun exposure. People who are fair-skinned are at greater risk of developing such cancers than are darker-skinned individuals. To avoid the dry skin, wrinkles, and increased cancer risk from sun exposure, Parker suggests these tips:

Wear sunscreen. Sunscreens are rated by their sun protection factor, or SPF. The higher the SPF number, the greater the sun protection.

Cover up. Wear a lightweight, long-sleeved shirt and a hat when you're in the sun.

Avoid the sun between 10:00 A.M. and 3:00 P.M. This is the time of day when the sun's burning rays are at their strongest, so try to plan outdoor activities for earlier or later in the day.

Use lotions. If you must sunbathe, apply cream-type lotions and occasionally "spritz" your skin with mineral water to keep it moist. Keep your tanning sessions as short as possible, and moisturize afterwards.

moisture loss, and can make itching worse, says Shaw. Bathe or shower only as often as *really* necessary and no more than once a day. If you insist on long, hot soaks, always apply a moisturizer immediately after bathing.

Use soap sparingly. Shaw advises decreasing soap and water washing. "People wash too much," he says. "Overwashing with soap and water harms the skin's outer layer."

People who suffer from chronically dry skin should take brief baths or showers and lather up only the groin, armpits, and bottoms of the feet, says Robertson. When you use soap, opt for milder, oilated or superfatted soaps such as Dove, Basis, or Aveenobar. For super-dry skin, you may have to use a soap substitute to cleanse your skin.

Don't be abrasive. Scrubbing your skin with washcloths, loofah sponges, or other scrubbing products dries your skin out even more, says Robertson. "Often, when people have dry skin, they develop scale and try to scrub it off with washcloths or sponges," she says. "But they're doing more harm than good."

Oil that bath. "Bath oils can help," says Shaw. But, he warns, if you put the bath oil in the water before you get in and get wet, the oil can coat your skin and prevent it from becoming saturated with water. Instead, he recommends adding the oil to the bath after you've been in the water for a while or applying it directly to your wet skin after bathing. (If you do add the oil to your bathwater, be sure to use extra care when getting in or out of the tub, since the oil will make the tub slippery.)

Robertson says that mineral oil makes an excellent bath oil. However, she warns not to soak, even in an oil bath, for longer than 20 minutes.

Raise the humidity. The higher the humidity, the less dry the skin. "In the tropics, where the humidity is around 90 percent, no one suffers from dry skin," says Shaw. He says once the temperature drops below 50 degrees Fahrenheit, the humidity tends to drop off too.

Sixty percent humidity is perfect for the skin. It's the point at which the skin and the air are in perfect balance and moisture isn't being drawn from the skin into the air. If you live in a dry climate or if the humidity in your office or home is less than 60 percent, consider using a home humidifier. Even a vaporizer or kettle of water on slow boil can raise the humidity in a room somewhat.

Avoid detergents, cleansers, and solvents. Common household products, such as cleansers, window cleaners, ammonia, turpentine, lighter fluid, and mineral spirits can dry and damage the skin's outer layer. Avoid directly exposing your skin to such products by wearing vinyl gloves and using less-harsh alternatives (for example, vinegar and water make a great window cleaner) whenever possible. Use a long-handled brush to keep your hands out of dishwater.

Nix alcohol-based products. Some people like to cleanse their faces with alcohol wipes or astringents. They leave the skin feeling clean and tingling, but there's a price. "Alcohol-based products have a drying effect," says Shaw.

Use cream- or oil-based makeup. If you wear foundation and blusher, choose oil-based types that help retain moisture rather than water-based products, says Robertson. In the evening, wash off makeup with mild soap. Then, rinse thoroughly, blot dry with a soft towel, and moisturize well with a heavy, cream-type moisturizer.

Cool it off. Hot environments heated by wood stoves or forced air heating systems dry out the skin. Shaw recommends keeping the air temperature a few degrees lower to keep your skin moist.

Toss off the electric blanket, pile on the comforter. The heat from electric blankets can dry out your skin, too. Shaw says that for people who have chronically dry skin, opting for an extra blanket instead of an electric one is a good idea.

Avoid too much alcohol. The effects of excessive alcohol consumption usually don't show up on the skin for several years. "We don't really know if there's a cause-and-effect relationship between drinking alcohol and dry skin," says Robertson. "But we do know that alcoholics tend to have drier, more wrinkled skin."

Each time you drink alcohol, your skin loses moisture needed to keep it young-looking. When alcohol enters the bloodstream, it lowers the water concentration of the blood. To replace the lost water, the body draws water from surrounding cells. Limit your intake to no more than two ounces per day. Better yet, avoid alcohol altogether. ◆

◆ EARACHE ◆

7 Sound Ways to Head Off Pain

Most people don't think about their ears much, unless they're self-conscious about their size. But when an earache develops, the affected ear can feel as if it has taken on monster proportions, making it difficult to think of anything else.

For all the unspeakable pain caused by earaches, they are rarely life threatening. Still, they can be serious, especially if they are caused by infection. Signs of an ear infection include ear pain and hearing loss. In a young child, clues that an ear infection may be present include rubbing or tugging at the ear, excessive crying or fussiness, fever, nausea, and vomiting. Since an untreated ear infection can lead to permanent hearing loss, and since ear pain can sometimes reflect a problem in another part of the body (see "Earaches that Aren't"), it is important to have an earache checked out by a doctor. (For information on preventing ear infections, see EAR INFECTION and SWIMMER'S EAR.)

Other than infection, the most common cause of earache is a blocked eustachian tube. The eustachian tube is a thin, membrane-lined tube that connects the inside back portion of the nose with the middle ear. The air in the middle ear is constantly being absorbed by its membranous lining, but the air is never depleted as long as the eustachian tube remains open and able to resupply air during the process of swallowing. In this manner, the air pressure on both sides of the eardrum stays about equal. However, when the eustachian tube is blocked for one reason or another, the pressure in the middle ear can't be equalized. The air that is already there is absorbed and, without an incoming supply, a vacuum occurs in the middle ear, sucking the eardrum inward and stretching it painfully taut.

This type of earache is especially common in people who travel by air, especially when they have a cold or a stuffy nose. As the plane takes off, the air pressure in the plane's cabin decreases, and as the plane lands, the air pressure in the cabin

---

Earaches that Aren't

Sometimes, diseases and disorders in other parts of the head and neck can sound an alarm in the ear. "Referred pain has its origin elsewhere but is felt in the ear," says John W. House, M.D. That's one reason it's important to have ear pain checked out by a doctor.

To otolaryngologists, the most common culprits in referred ear pain are the "five Ts:"

- *Tongue*
- *Teeth*
- *Tonsils*
- *Throat*
- *Temporomandibular joint (TMJ)*

---

increases; in each instance, the pressure change occurs very rapidly. While normally the air in the middle ear manages to equalize on its own, if there is congestion in the upper-respiratory tract, air may not be able to flow through the eustachian tube to reach the middle ear. (This type of earache can also occur as a result of pressure changes during an elevator ride in a tall building and during scuba diving.) Fortunately, there are some tricks you can try to ward off ear pain that results from the ups and downs of air travel.

Swallow hard. "The act of swallowing activates the muscle that opens the eustachian tube," says James Stankiewicz, M.D., professor and vice-chairman of the Department of Otolaryngology–Head and Neck Surgery at Loyola University Medical School in Maywood, Illinois. When the pilot announces that it's time to fasten your seat belts for landing, get your mouth set to swallow. Swallowing can also bring temporary relief from earache pain until you can get to the doctor.

Keep your mouth moving. You swallow more often when you chew gum or suck on hard candy, so pop some into your mouth just before the plane descends.

Don't stifle a yawn. It's not the company, it's the atmospheric conditions. "Yawning is the best way to keep the eustachian tube open," says John W. House, M.D., associate clinical professor in the Department of Otolaryngology, Head and Neck Surgery at the University of Southern California at Los Angeles.

Stay awake. If you're sleeping, you're not going to be swallowing. "Ask the flight attendant to wake you before descent," suggests Jack J. Wazen, M.D., associate professor of otolaryngology and director of otology and neurotology at Columbia University College of Physicians and Surgeons in New York. "It's much more pleasant than being awakened by a pain in your ear."

Hold your nose. If your ears still become uncomfortably blocked as the plane descends, the American Academy of Otolaryngology, Head and Neck Surgery suggests that you try this: With your thumb and forefinger, pinch your nostrils tightly closed and block the external opening of the unaffected ear with the forefinger of your other hand. Now, with your mouth closed, try to blow through the pinched nostrils, blowing as forcefully as you would blow your nose. Repeat if necessary. You should experience a cracking sensation or a loud pop and a relief of the pain if the maneuver works. Don't try this trick if you have a sore throat or fever, however, because the infection might be forced into your ears. And don't attempt it if you have a heart or circulatory disorder.

Reach for relief. Frequent flyers should tuck away a decongestant pill or nasal spray to use an hour or

When Your Eardrum Takes a Beating

If you feel a sudden, sharp pain in your ear following a trauma such as an explosion or a scuba-diving accident, you may have a perforated eardrum, says Jack J. Wazen, M.D.

While the pain may occur only at the time of the accident, the injury itself needs evaluation by a specialist to head off permanent disruption of the middle-ear mechanism. Most injury-related eardrum perforations are small and will heal spontaneously within a few weeks, provided middle-ear infections are prevented or controlled (which is why you still need to see a doctor even for small perforations). Large perforations may require surgery.

so before landing. This shrinks the membranes, making it easier to keep the eustachian tube open. "If you suffer from allergies or sinusitis, you must be sure to take your medication at the beginning of the flight," says Stankiewicz. Over-the-counter medications like this are not for everyone, however. People with heart disease, high blood pressure, irregular heart rhythms, or thyroid disease should avoid them. Pregnant women and individuals who are subject to anxiety should stay away from them, as well.

Take the train. If, despite all your best efforts, you still end up with an uncomfortable stuffed feeling and pain following air travel, you might consider taking the scenic route. ◆

◆ EAR INFECTION ◆

9 Tips for Prevention and Treatment

Step into a pediatrician's waiting room, and you're likely to find that one of every three children under the age of three is there because he or she has an ear infection. Some one-third of all children have more than three middle-ear infections (the medical name is otitis media) during the first three years of life, resulting in 30 million doctor visits a year.

Of course, children aren't the only ones who get ear infections. But they are, by far, the most common victims. Adults are more likely to get an infection of the outer ear, which is aptly referred to as "swimmer's ear" because it usually gets its start when water containing bacteria or fungi seeps into the ear and gets trapped in the ear canal (see SWIMMER'S EAR).

In order to understand how middle-ear infections develop, it helps to know how healthy ears function. The outer ear is connected to an air-containing space called the middle ear. The eardrum, a thin membrane, is stretched across the entrance to the space, and three sound-conducting bones are suspended within it. The pressure within the middle-ear space is equalized with the atmosphere through a narrow tube called the eustachian tube. The eustachian tube opens into a space behind the nose where air or fluid may enter or escape. The air pressure in the middle ear is equalized more than one thousand times a day—every time you swallow—usually without your noticing it. The eustachian tube also carries fluid away from the middle ear.

When a cold or an allergy is present, the eustachian tube swells and air is absorbed by the lining of the middle ear, creating a partial vacuum. The eardrum then gets pulled inward, and fluid weeps from the lining of the middle ear. Bacteria or viruses from the nose and throat can travel up the eustachian tube and infect the stagnant, warm fluid in the middle ear, which provides a perfect environment for them to live and multiply. When this happens, an infection is underway.

Children may be more prone to middle-ear infections for a variety of reasons. For example, their eustachian tubes are shorter and straighter, which may make it easier for bacteria and viruses to penetrate. Children also get colds and sore throats more often than adults.

PREVENTING EAR INFECTIONS

As a parent, there are some things you can do to decrease the chance that your child will develop a middle-ear infection.

Steer your child clear. "The entire process starts with a cold, allergic reaction, or infection of the tonsils or adenoids," says James Stankiewicz, M.D., professor and vice-chairman of the Department of Otolaryngology–Head and Neck Surgery at Loyola University Medical School in Maywood, Illinois. "If you can keep your child out of contact with children who have colds and other respiratory infections and make sure that allergies are under control, then there is a better chance of avoiding ear infection." If you are in the process of choosing a day-care facility for your child, check into the center's policy for dealing with children who are ill.

Teach proper nose-blowing technique. Once your child is old enough, teach him or her to blow his or her nose softly rather than with excessive force, so as not to drive infection into the ears. And teach your child not to stifle a sneeze by pinching the nostrils, since this, too, may force the infection up into the ears.

Don't smoke. Here's another reason not to smoke: Children who live with smokers seem to be more susceptible to middle-ear infections than are those who live in smokefree homes. Cigarette smoke irritates the linings of the nasal passages and middle-ear cavity, which interferes with the normal functioning of the eustachian tube. If you cannot quit, at least take your habit outside.

Be careful with bottle-feeding. Avoid giving a bottle of milk or formula to a baby who is lying on his or her back, because the milk can flow into the eustachian tube during swallowing and initiate a middle-ear infection.

Stay alert to the signs. It is essential to get your child to the doctor as soon as you suspect an ear infection, but to do that, you need to be aware of the symptoms that can signal an ear infection. An older child who has an ear infection may complain of ear pain or aching or a stuffiness in the ear. In a younger child who cannot yet describe an earache, you need to be alert to other signs that may signal an imminent ear infection. "One of the first signs is that the child pulls or rubs his or her ears frequently. This is before real pain sets in but indicates that something is amiss," says John W. House, M.D., associate clinical professor in the Department of Otolaryngology, Head and Neck Surgery at the University of Southern California at Los Angeles. "You may also notice that your child does not seem to hear you. Then come the real signs of infection: fever, crying and other signs of pain, nausea, and vomiting."

TREATING AN EAR INFECTION

"It is most important that a child showing signs of ear infection be taken to a doctor immediately," advises Daniel Kuriloff, M.D., associate director of the Department of Otolaryngology–Head and Neck Surgery at St. Luke's–Roosevelt Hospital Center and associate professor at Columbia University College of Physicians and Surgeons,

both in New York. If a middle-ear infection is treated promptly, it is not serious. If not treated right away, your child might suffer hearing loss and, as a result, a delay in learning and speech development. Once your child has seen the doctor, however, there are some things you can do to help make your little one more comfortable.

Follow through on the doctor's instructions. Your job doesn't end with a visit to the doctor. You will need to be sure that your child receives the medication prescribed by the doctor. The one medication that the pediatrician will almost certainly prescribe is an antibiotic. "You must be sure that your child takes the medication for the full time prescribed—usually 10 to 14 days," says Kuriloff. "Read the label on the prescription bottle carefully and follow directions." The doctor may also prescribe an antihistamine and/or a decongestant if your child has a cold or allergy. If you have any questions about the proper use or administration of the medication, call your doctor or pharmacist.

Keep your child's chin up. If your child is lying down, prop his or her head up on pillows. Elevating the head will help to keep the eustachian tubes draining into the back of the throat.

Try mild heat. Applying a heating pad set on warm—not hot—may make your child more comfortable.

Give acetaminophen. Try giving your child acetaminophen to help relieve pain and fever. Do not, however, give your child aspirin. Aspirin use in children with a viral illness has been associated with Reye's syndrome, an often-fatal condition characterized by severe, sudden deterioration of liver and brain function. ◆

◆ EARWAX ◆

4 Ways to Help Your Ears

Before you pick up a cotton swab or car key to wage war on the wax in your ears, you need to know which side of the battle you're on.

Earwax is formed in the outer part of the ear canal. Normally, earwax is good for the skin in the outer ear canal. It becomes a problem only when the ear canal is almost completely blocked by wax, preventing the entry of air and sound and preventing the escape of trapped fluid. Here's how to deal safely with earwax.

Respect its role. The skin in the ear canal has special modified sweat glands that produce earwax. This wax acts as a trap for dust and other particles that might find their way into your ear and cause injury, irritation, or infection. It also contains enzymes to help fight bacteria. In addition, it "waterproofs" the skin of the ear canal, protecting it from water damage, which would make the skin susceptible to infections such as swimmer's ear (see SWIMMER'S EAR). Earwax doesn't need to be removed under normal circumstances—it's there naturally as a barrier against injury and infection. Only when there is evidence of hearing loss or discomfort should it be attended to. "This is certainly an instance when the old adage holds true: 'If it's not broke, don't fix it,'" says Daniel Kuriloff, M.D., associate director of the Department of Otolaryngology–Head and Neck Surgery at St. Luke's–Roosevelt Hospital Center in New York. In fact, without wax, or with a diminished amount of it, the inside of your ears would become dry and itchy.

Wipe it out. Usually, wax accumulates a little at a time, gradually dries up, and rolls out of your ear on its own, carrying all the foreign matter with it. Sometimes, however, the wax moves to the outside of the ear canal more slowly. In this case, you can simply wipe off the wax once it becomes visible. "If you look in the mirror and see little dried-up bits of yellowish matter, you should take a piece of cotton moistened with water to wash it away,"

advises Jack J. Wazen, M.D., associate professor of otolaryngology and director of otology and neurotology at Columbia University College of Physicians and Surgeons in New York.

Use your elbow. One bit of wisdom that has been handed down through generations is: "Never clean your ears with anything smaller than your elbow." Unfortunately, most people never think twice about cleaning their ears as often—and with the same vigor—as they wash their face. Cotton swabs are the most popular tool, but an endless list of "cleaning" utensils have been employed, including toothpicks, paper clips, and pencil tips. "The point is, don't try to clean your ears at all. You may harm the delicate lining in the ear canal or poke a hole in your eardrum, either of which will lead to infection," says John W. House, M.D., associate clinical professor in the Department of Otolaryngology, Head and Neck Surgery at the University of Southern California at Los Angeles. "Most important, you are almost certain to poke the wax deeper into your ear canal, even up against your eardrum, where it will interfere with hearing."

Don't rush out for softening drops. Different people form different amounts and types of earwax, and in some cases, the wax may accumulate to such an extent that it interferes with hearing. If you suspect that earwax is hindering your hearing, however, don't use over-the-counter drops to soften the wax—at least not until you check with an ear doctor. These drops, although effective for some benign external ear conditions, are generally not recommended until the exact source of the hearing loss or ear discomfort is determined by a doctor. In fact, the drops can actually exacerbate certain ear problems, says Kuriloff. Wax buildup that is causing symptoms must be removed by an ear doctor. Likewise, if your ears are tender to the touch, reddened in an area that you can see, or draining fluid, don't use any kind of ear drops or medication before consulting an ear doctor. ◆

◆ EXCESSIVE HAIR ◆ GROWTH

7 Ways to Cope with the Problem

Rarely do men complain about having too much hair—even if it grows dark and dense on arms, chest, and legs. But for women, the tendency of hair to crop up in places other than the scalp can be a decided cosmetic liability. For some women, it goes beyond a cosmetic problem; it is a serious psychological handicap that can result in extreme self-consciousness and social isolation.

Women with markedly abnormal hair growth in the same distribution as that of a normal postpubertal male are called hirsute. Some eight to ten percent of all adult women in the United States face this problem.

We're not talking about vellus hair—the "peach fuzz," or downy growth, present over most of the human body. Hirsutism refers to an excess of terminal hair—thick, pigmented hair that, before puberty, is present only on the scalp, eyebrows, and eyelashes. In a hirsute woman, once she becomes sexually mature, terminal hair grows in unwanted locations, such as the upper lip and chin.

In some cases, hirsutism may reflect an abnormality that can be medically corrected (see "Hair Today, Hair Tomorrow?"). Often, however, hirsutism is simply a matter of heredity, and a problem that can be controlled cosmetically. Here are your choices:

Make up a solution. For a mild case of excess facial hair, a heavy base of cosmetics can cover up the problem. If your skin tends to be oily or is acne prone, look for foundations and blushes that are water based or noncomedogenic.

Try a close shave. The most obvious way to rid yourself of unwanted hair is to shave it away. It may not be the best choice for removing facial hair, however, since one wrong move can have you sporting a snippet of bathroom tissue over a bleeding nick. There's another drawback to shaving facial hair. "Shaving mows the hairs down at skin level and may leave an unsightly dark line," says Donald Rudikoff, M.D., assistant clinical professor of dermatology at Mount Sinai School of Medicine in New York.

Still, shaving can be a viable option for removing hair on other parts of the body. It's the easiest and cheapest method, says Rudikoff, and, contrary to popular belief, "shaving does not make hair coarser or cause it to grow faster."

Use a little pluck. Tweezing works well if the overgrowth problem is confined to a specific area, such as a few errant hairs around the eyebrows or on the chin. "It is time consuming, uncomfortable, and impractical for areas like the legs and underarms," notes Elizabeth Knobler, M.D., assistant clinical professor of dermatology at Columbia–Presbyterian Medical Center in New York.

Tweezing can hurt a bit and leave the area red and irritated for a time. New hairs may appear within 4 to 13 weeks. However, there is no medical basis for the belief that nine new hairs will grow in place of one that is plucked.

Lighten up. Bleaching to make hairs colorless and less prominent is probably the most common home treatment for unwanted facial hair. Several bleaches are sold in drugstores. Most involve mixing together a powder with a cream to activate the bleaching agent. Be sure to ask if the bleach is fresh, because it can lose strength if it has been on the shelf for several months. For women with very dark facial hair, the bleaching process may not be 100 percent successful on the first pass; a repeat bleaching will usually do the trick. As the hairs grow out, they'll have to be bleached again.

Wax it away. One technique that is similar to plucking involves the use of wax to pull hairs out by the roots. Once the wax has been heated to a fluid state, it is spread on one swath of skin at a time, then stripped off a few seconds later, taking hundreds of hairs with it. Waxing is not without its sore spots, however. "As you can imagine, this method can be painful and time consuming," says Bruce R. Carr, M.D., Paul C. MacDonald Professor of Obstetrics and Gynecology at the University of Texas Southwestern Medical Center at Dallas. Surface skin can sometimes be pulled off in the bargain, and even if the skin remains intact, the waxing can create long-lasting irritation and redness. Indeed, as Carr points out, the skin can become so irritated that infection can develop. So if you want to try waxing, be sure to follow package instructions carefully.

Cream off the crop. Drugstores offer a variety of creams and lotions that chemically remove hair; these are generally as cheap and easy to use as bleach. "Depilatories take off all the hair on the leg or lip—the dark, terminal hair and the lighter vellus hair—so regrowth feels unusually thick and stubbly. But it still holds true that only one hair will grow back where a hair was removed," says Carr. Depilatories come in different types for use on different parts of the body. Be sure you use the appropriate type for the body area you will be applying it to. Since a depilatory can irritate sensitive skin, always test it on a small patch of skin before using it on a larger area.

Get to the root of the problem. There is only one method of permanent hair removal: electrolysis. In this procedure, a trained electrologist inserts a very fine probe into the hair follicle. A small amount of electrical current is then applied through the probe to destroy the hair root and render it useless for future growth. Does it hurt? "That's relative to each individual being treated and the area being worked on," says Rudikoff. "Typically, electrolysis on the upper lip and inner thigh are most uncomfortable, while treatment on the forearms and chest area hurt least." If performed improperly, electrolysis can cause scarring and infection. When performed by a trained operator, there are generally few side effects. A slight swelling or redness may occur that should subside in a matter of hours. Occasionally, slight scabbing may appear two to four days after treatment; if left alone, it will fall off. This procedure is safe if performed by a trained operator; ask to see credentials—such as certification by the Society of Clinical and Medical Electrologists. ♦

♦♦♦ Hair Today, ♦♦♦ Hair Tomorrow?

The spectrum of abnormality of hair growth, according to Elizabeth Knobler, M.D., ranges from a woman who has only scattered patches on the face and chest to a woman with a full beard.

There are actually two types of increased hair growth. One is hirsutism, which happens as a result of increased amounts of or increased sensitivity to hormones called androgens. The causes can include menopause, pregnancy (rarely), an overactive adrenal gland, Cushing's disease, polycystic ovary syndrome, a pituitary tumor, an ovarian tumor, and the use of medication that contains androgens.

The second type of abnormal hair growth is called hypertrichosis, which has nothing to do with hormones but rather is often due to ethnic and geographic influences. Among white people, those of Mediterranean and Semitic descent tend to be hairier than Scandinavians and Anglo-Saxons. The least hairy peoples are Asians and American Indians. Hypertrichosis can also be caused by certain medications, physical factors such as chronic rubbing, and systemic (bodywide) disease.

In short, if your mother and your mother's mother kept a hairy upper lip, you probably don't have to be concerned that there is a medical problem underlying your excess hair growth. If, on the other hand, you come from a long line of sparsely whiskered folk, the appearance of a crop of dark and/or coarse hair on your face, chest, back, arms, or legs should be reported to your doctor. Often, the excess hair will disappear once the underlying condition is corrected.

◆ EXCESSIVE ◆ PERSPIRATION

8 Dry Ideas

Following a spicy dinner at your favorite restaurant, you realize that your back and chest are damp. At the end of a very important interview, you reach out to shake hands and notice that your palm is wet. After narrowly missing a collision with a car that has run a red light, you wipe the moisture from your brow.

What's going on here? In a word, it's sweat. Sweat is the byproduct of the body's diligent internal thermostat and air-conditioning system, which sometimes responds to spicy foods, anxiety, and danger in the same way that it does to excessive heat. But before you conclude that you would be more comfortable and self-confident without such sensitive reactions, remember that the system keeps you alive.

There's nothing complicated about the mechanics of sweat (or perspiration, as it is often referred to by those who would rather think they don't do it). The human body contains more than two million sweat glands (women may have more, according to some studies) of two types: eccrine glands and apocrine glands. The eccrines are located almost everywhere on the body's surface—about 400 to the square inch of skin, except in places like the palms of the hands, where as many as 3,000 may be concentrated. The eccrines are the smaller of the two types and originate deep within the skin, with narrow ducts threading to the skin's surface. The task for these glands is primarily temperature control: When things get too hot, the sweat glands go into high gear, drawing fluid from the blood to produce sweat and transporting it through the pores to the skin surface. Once on the surface, sweat evaporates, cooling the skin. This, in turn, cools the blood, which has also been rushed to the surface by temperature-control cells in the brain. The cooled blood then returns to the internal organs and muscles, cooling them.

Apocrine glands are larger, fewer in number, and attached to hair follicles in the genital area and armpits. The apocrines become active after puberty and are exquisitely sensitive to emotional stress and sexual stimulation.

Even the most inactive person sweats as much as a quart a day. Marathon runners, on the other hand, may produce up to two gallons during the course of a race. Such extreme sweat production is still considered quite normal under the circumstances; one would hardly grant it a passing thought except for the fact that it can make its presence known in most embarrassing ways (see BODY ODOR). On the other hand, if you have a body that beads up like a cold seltzer can on a hot day—even when you're sitting perfectly still in the shade—you have what is known, in medical terms, as hyperhidrosis. Here's what you can do about it:

Stay out of the midday sun. When the sun is at its highest and hottest, your body will quickly become overheated, sending your thermoregulatory response into high gear. "One of the most logical ways to avoid excessive sweating is to avoid excessive overheating," says Allan L. Lorincz, M.D., professor of dermatology at the University of Chicago Medical Center. A warm, humid day is even worse. "With high humidity, the percentage of water suspended in the air rises, reducing the amount of sweat that can be taken up by the air from the skin," adds Lorincz.

Dress right. Most synthetic materials appear to increase sweating because they do not absorb moisture. "Try wearing natural fibers such as cotton in summer months and wool during the winter," advises Donald Rudikoff, M.D., assistant clinical professor of dermatology at Mount Sinai School of Medicine in New York.

◆ EXCESSIVE PERSPIRATION ◆

Antiperspirant Primer

Here are some tips from the FDA Consumer *that will help you get more protection and less irritation from your underarm antiperspirant:*

• *Repeat applications regularly. Antiperspirants work for only a certain length of time. Check the label to see how often yours should be applied.*

• *Dry the underarms thoroughly before applying an antiperspirant. Dryness enhances penetration of the active ingredient.*

• *To avoid irritation, don't apply an antiperspirant to freshly shaved skin. (Try shaving at night, so you won't have to apply the antiperspirant until the following morning.)*

• *Try another product with a different active ingredient if one product doesn't work. What works for one person may not work for someone else.*

Stay "dry." Since alcohol stimulates blood flow to the skin, alcoholic beverages can cause increased sweating—even before you begin to feel any other effects on your body. "Stick to nonalcoholic beverages on hot, humid days," advises Rudikoff. Cold (but not ice-cold) water is best in terms of quenching your thirst and replacing fluids lost during excessive sweating.

Cut the caffeine. Caffeine is a stimulant that speeds up the heart, making it behave as it would in response to overheating. "Reduce your intake of caffeine—coffee, tea, cola drinks—it will benefit your heart as well as your peace of mind," says Rudikoff.

Watch what you eat. Eating hot, spicy foods can trigger perspiration, so it may be wise to avoid them at times when staying dry is a priority.

Slim down. If you are overweight, even the most moderate activities make your heart strain harder to pump blood around your body. "Reaching and maintaining your desirable body weight may go a long way toward easing a problem of excessive sweating," notes Lorincz.

Cool it. Increased anxiety—even if it is temporary—can cause excessive sweating. In anxiety-prone people, even the merest stress—or none at all—can bring on an anxiety attack with accompanying sweating. "If you frequently become anxious, try to divert the symptoms with physical activity, such as jogging, walking, or swimming, or relaxation exercises such as deep breathing," suggests Alan R. Shalita, M.D., chairman of the Department of Dermatology at State University of New York Health Science Center at Brooklyn.

Spray, stroke, dab. To add an extra layer of confidence, you can use an antiperspirant under your arms and even on the palms of your hands and soles of your feet (if they are trouble areas). "Antiperspirants inhibit production of eccrine perspiration," says Rudikoff. Most of these products contain an aluminum salt, which is thought to work by causing a slight swelling around the sweat-gland ducts that decreases the outflow of perspiration. Aluminum chlorohydrate is the mildest of the salts; aluminum chloride and aluminum sulfate are even more effective but are also more acidic and, when mixed with perspiration, tend to irritate the skin and stain clothing, particularly linen and cotton. ◆

140

◆ EYE REDNESS ◆

7 Ways to Look Bright-Eyed

What do a long day at the office, a night on the town, and an afternoon of gardening have in common? They can all have you seeing red—when you look in the mirror, that is.

"Eye redness can be caused by a lot of things," says Carol Ziel, M.D., an ophthalmologist with the Eye Clinic of Wausau in Wisconsin. "A red eye may simply be dry or slightly irritated, or it may be a sign of chronic or acute glaucoma, inflammation of the eye, or a conjunctivitis," she continues.

"In the case of acute glaucoma, which most often occurs in children but can also occur in adults, there tends to be red eyes in conjunction with dilated pupils, blurring of vision, and pain," says Charles Boylan, M.D., a pediatric ophthalmologist at A Children's Eye Clinic of Seattle.

"You can get red eyes from certain diseases such as chronic glaucoma, blood diseases, gout, thyroid diseases, and even a tumor," warns Jon H. Bosland, M.D., a general ophthalmologist in private practice in Bellevue, Washington. "You can also get red eyes from iritis, an inflammatory disease which is usually inside the eye. It is often associated with discomfort and increased pressure within the eye as well. And it can be very serious if not treated with cortisone," says Boylan.

For these reasons, the experts recommend that you have your eyes checked if the redness persists for more than a couple of days, if there is any pain or change of vision associated with the redness, if your eyes suddenly become sensitive to light, if you notice redness or blood over the pupil (the dark center of the eye), or if you have any discharge from one or both eyes.

For red eyes that are caused by everyday irritants—such as long hours in contact lenses, allergies, fatigue, air pollution, or dry air—there are some things you can do to help get the red out and relieve irritation.

◆◆ Eye-Drop Alert ◆◆

Sometimes, the continual use of over-the-counter eye drops can actually cause *red eyes, rather than alleviating them. According to Jon H. Bosland, M.D., there are a couple of reasons for this. "Many of the over-the-counter eye drops have preservatives in them, which can further irritate sensitive eyes," he says. "And certain decongestant eye drops that claim to whiten your eye are pretty mild but can cause a rebound effect similar to the kind you can get with nose drops," he warns. "What happens is that the decongestant in these fluids causes the little arteries to shrink up, making the eye look whiter. This works well at first, but with continued use of these drops, the arteries can become dependent on the chemical in order to stay shrunken. So when the chemical wears off, the arteries dilate again and make the eye appear red," he explains.*

While using over-the-counter eye drops for a few days to soothe and whiten eyes is generally OK, using them regularly can be counterproductive. Be sure to read the label for instructions on proper use.

Give your eyes a "lube" job. "Lubricating eye drops such as Visine can help to relieve some of the dryness and make the eye feel better," says Bosland. "But don't use them any longer than a few days at most," he adds (see "Eye-Drop Alert"). Eye drops and artificial tears can be especially helpful to older individuals. "Older people don't produce as many tears as they should, which can make the eyes red," says Boylan.

Apply cool or warm compresses. "It doesn't really matter which kind you use. Whatever feels best to you is fine," says Ziel. "A washcloth soaked in cool water feels good, as does simply cupping cool water in your hand and holding it under the eye," adds Bosland.

Use an over-the-counter antihistamine. If your red, itchy eyes are the result of an allergy, such as hay fever, then treating the allergy itself will tend to help your eyes as well, according to Bosland.

Get a good night's rest. "This is often enough to clear up red eyes that are the result of too little sleep," says Bosland. If 40 winks don't perk up your peepers, however, then the redness is probably the result of some other cause and should be checked out by a doctor.

Wear goggles in the pool. If you plan to take a splash in the pool, protect your eyes from the irritating effects of chlorine with a pair of well-fitting swimming goggles.

Use eye drops in the air. "The air in the cabin of an airplane is extremely dry and contains less oxygen, both of which can irritate and redden the eyes," says Bosland. Over-the-counter lubricating drops add moisture to the eye, which helps to keep them from getting dried out.

Sport shades. Wear a pair of good-quality sunglasses whenever you go out during the day. This is especially important if you'll be skiing, boating, or sunbathing on a bright day. "Snow blindness and ultraviolet burns can result when the eyes are unprotected in the sunlight," warns Bosland. "And both conditions can be extremely painful," he adds. "I've also seen skiers get red eyes from going down the hill without protective eye wear and ending up with extremely dry eyes from the wind," says Boylan. "Usually, it's the not-so-good skiers like myself who keep their eyes wide open on the way down so as not to hit anything," he says. ◆

◆ EYESTRAIN ◆

20 Eye Savers

You simply can't read another word. Your eyes have had it. They're tired, dry, and sore. You're suffering from eyestrain.

There are numerous causes of eyestrain—from stress to astigmatism to jaw disorders. "Most people have a tiny bit of astigmatism and do not even know they have it," says Andrew S. Farber, M.D., F.A.C.S., an ophthalmologist in private practice in Terre Haute, Indiana. "But it may show itself as eyestrain." Astigmatism is a defect in vision caused by an abnormal curvature of the cornea or lens of the eye, both of which help the eye to focus an image; it can usually be corrected with eyeglasses or contact lenses.

Tension in the neck and back muscles—from sitting at a computer all day, for instance—can also cause the eyes to tire.

Numerous diseases may show themselves as eyestrain. Glaucoma, a condition in which pressure within the eye becomes elevated, is one such condition. Even diseases not directly related to the eye may show up as eyestrain. In rare instances, the jaw disorder called temporo-mandibular joint syndrome, or TMJ, which causes facial pain (see TMJ), can lead to aching eyes.

One of the reasons eyestrain is so common is that the lens in the eye gradually loses some of its ability to change shape—and thus focus an image clearly—as we age. This condition, referred to as presbyopia, becomes most pronounced after age 40. It affects the eye's ability to focus on an image up close, which is why older individuals often need to hold reading material at arm's length.

Because there are so many causes of eyestrain, it's best to consult an eye-care professional for a complete diagnosis if you've been suffering from eyestrain for a month or more or if it seems to have become more frequent or bothersome, advises Henry D. Perry, M.D., clinical associate professor of ophthalmology at Cornell Medical College in New York. An eye examination should be performed once a year, especially for people 35 years of age and older and for anyone with a family history of glaucoma or diabetes.

Should You Exercise Your Eyes?

Eye exercises, primarily developed by a turn-of-the-century ophthalmologist, William Bates, are generally regarded as a worthless practice. The Bates Method promotes such techniques as laying warmed hands over the closed eyes and alternating blinking with squeezing to keep the eyes in shape.

Most eye-care professionals agree that instead of a workout, resting your eyes is one of the best things you can do. Your eyes work all day, every day. Giving them the relief of only having to look at the inside of your eyelids for even a few minutes can make quite a difference. And, if you can take a nap or get a sufficient amount of sleep at night, all the better for your hard-working eyes.

In the meantime, here are some ways to ease the strain on your eyes.

Make the light right. "Working in dim or harsh light won't harm the eyes, but it may be more demanding," says Farber. Too much light can result in too much glare, while too little light may simply make it too difficult to read or see clearly, says Farber. Try to keep the lighting at a comfortable level—not too dark or too bright.

Try indirect lighting. Fixtures that face upward, allowing their light to bounce off a ceiling or wall, create a comfortable, diffusely lighted environment that's not as hard on the eyes as lights that shine down directly on you.

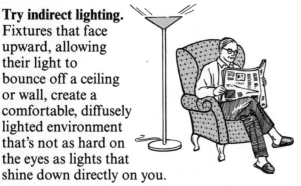

Buy a pair of reading glasses. Especially for those over 40 years of age, reading glasses may do the trick by magnifying the printed page and other close work. Reading glasses can be purchased without a prescription in drug stores and pharmacies; you simply try on several pairs until you find the magnification that provides you with the sharpest vision.

Get glare-busting glasses. Prescription lenses made with polarized ultraviolet (UV) filters reduce glare by filtering out certain wavelengths of light. These can be especially good for computer users.

Take a break. Whether you're reading, writing, sewing, or tapping away on a computer, it's a good idea to take a break from such close work or switch to a task that isn't so visually demanding for a few minutes each hour, says Farber. Take a walk, make a phone call, talk to someone, focus on objects at a distance, or just close your eyes. Taking a break will give your neck and shoulders, as well as your eyes, a rest; tenseness in these areas can aggravate eyestrain.

Try a saltwater soak. Perry recommends adding half a teaspoon of salt to a quart of warm water. Then, moisten cotton balls in the water, close your eyes, and place the cotton balls on your eyelids for about ten minutes.

Try a cool-water splash. For some people, splashing the face with cool water or laying a cool, damp towel across the eyes helps relieve eyestrain. If nothing else, it provides a break for overworked eyes.

Think to blink. Dry eyes can result from tasks such as continuous reading or computer use. "The eyes blink less frequently, so they're not getting as lubricated as they should," explains Arnold Prywes, M.D., an assistant clinical professor of ophthalmology at the Albert Einstein Medical College in New York and chief of ophthalmology at Mid-Island Hospital in Bethpage, New York. When you're doing close work or concentrating on a computer screen for long hours, remember to blink frequently.

Know your drops. Eye drops that decrease redness are not meant to be used for eyestrain, says Farber. Besides, the drops remove the redness by constricting the blood vessels in the eyes, and repeated use will actually have a rebound effect and make the eyes redder in the long run. On the other hand, if you know you're suffering from a case of dry eye, a drop or two of an over-the-counter eye lubricant, commonly referred to as artificial tears, may give you relief.

Buy a plant. Increasing the humidity in your home or office can help a case of dry eyes. Using a humidifier is an obvious way to do this. But setting a pot of water on your home radiator can also increase the humidity level in your home. Potted plants in your home or office can also act as inexpensive—and attractive—humidifiers.

Clear the air. Cigarette smoke can irritate the eyes and make them sore. So give your eyes a break and put out that cigarette for good. ◆

◆◆ How Computer Users ◆◆ Can Stop the Strain

"Computer users often find themselves in a visually demanding job in a visually unfriendly environment," says James E. Sheedy, O.D., Ph.D., associate clinical professor of the School of Optometry at the University of California in Berkeley and chief of the Video Display Terminal Eye Clinic. One result: eyestrain. Here are Sheedy's suggestions for preventing it.

Keep all light at the same level. *Ideally, the brightness of the computer screen should be the same as the light in the room.*

Get a glare-resistant screen. *These filters that fit on your computer screen help decrease eye-straining reflections and glare. "Antireflection screens made of glass are better than the ones made of meshed material for proper imagery," says Sheedy.*

Lighten the background, darken the letters. *This contrast on the computer screen is most pleasing to the eye, says Sheedy. Make the background white or near white and the letters a darker color. Although you may not be consciously aware of it, your computer screen flickers, and your eyes see this flickering. Lightening the background of your computer screen makes this flickering less discernible to your eyes.*

Place your terminal slightly lower than the top of your head. *"Your eyes should be looking at the computer at about a 15-degree angle," says Sheedy.*

The eyes are most comfortable viewing the screen at this angle rather than straight on.

Use a document holder. *These metal stands decrease eyestrain by getting your work off a flat surface and putting it in the same line of sight as your computer screen.*

Wear a visor. *This helps to block overhead light that is too strong and that interferes with your peripheral vision, which can cause eyestrain.*

Shut off a light. *Many office environments are overlit," says Sheedy. "The lighting was originally set up for people looking down at work on their desks all day. But nowadays, people are often looking straight ahead at their computers and getting too much light in their eyes." If possible, shut off every other fluorescent ceiling fixture (if there are four fixtures in a row, for example, shut off the second and the fourth one) or at least remove one or two of the four tubes from each fixture.*

Move your desk. *If you can't shut the lights off, perhaps you can rotate the position of your desk to get the too-bright lighting out of your line of sight.*

Get prescription glasses specially made for computer use. *People with bifocals and trifocals often have a problem using a computer because the section of lens they need to use to focus on the computer screen is either too high or too low for working comfortably. An optometrist can fashion lenses for computer use.*

◆ FEVER ◆

7 Ways to Manage the Ups and Downs

You're drenched in sweat. Your head is filled with a dull, throbbing ache, and, worse, you feel like someone is pressing their thumbs against your eyelids. One minute you feel afire; the next minute you are overcome with shaking chills. You put a thermometer under your tongue, and the mercury climbs to 101 degrees Fahrenheit. Yep, you have a fever.

To understand what having a fever means, and what you should or shouldn't do about it, it helps to know something about how the body controls temperature. There is quite a range in what is considered normal in body temperature. (By the way, *everyone* has a *temperature;* when it rises above what is considered normal and stays there, it is termed a *fever.*) The body's natural temperature-control system, located in a tiny structure at the base of the brain called the hypothalamus, is normally set somewhere around 98.6 degrees Fahrenheit. A normal temperature measured orally ranges from 96.7 to 99.0 degrees Fahrenheit (taken rectally, it measures one degree Fahrenheit higher). Your own temperature probably varies by more than two degrees during the course of a day, with the lowest reading usually occurring in the early morning and the highest in the evening.

Fever is not a disease in itself but a symptom of some other condition, usually an infection caused by bacteria, fungi, a virus, or parasites or even an allergic reaction. When this enemy invades, white blood cells are triggered to attack, releasing a protein called endogenous pyrogen. When endogenous pyrogen reaches the brain, it signals the hypothalamus to set itself at a higher point; if that new set point is over 100 degrees Fahrenheit, you have a fever.

When that happens, what should you do? Here's some advice:

◆◆ Hello, Doctor? ◆◆

Letting a fever run its course is not the best idea for everyone. While a fever of 102 to 103 degrees Fahrenheit is not usually dangerous in an otherwise healthy adult, it can be risky for very young children, who can develop seizures, and very elderly individuals, in whom fever can aggravate an underlying illness, such as a heart arrhythmia or respiratory ailment. Infants, young children, and very elderly individuals should be monitored carefully, and a physician should be called if the temperature continues to rise. Even in otherwise healthy adults, if a high fever (above 102 degrees Fahrenheit) lasts for more than a couple of days, a doctor should be consulted. Keep in mind, too, that if you or your child has a fever or other symptom that worries you, it never hurts to contact your doctor for advice.

Let it be. The fact is, fever may do the body some good. An untreated fever tends to be self limited, relatively benign, and—contrary to popular belief—not likely to escalate to the point that it causes harm. Nor does lowering fever mean that you are lessening the severity of the illness; indeed, fever may be the body's way of mobilizing itself against invading organisms. "Over more than a decade of research, studies show that elevated body temperatures can enhance the immune response," says Matthew J. Kluger, Ph.D., professor of physiology at the University of Michigan Medical School in Ann Arbor. This heightened immune response is brought about by pyrogen, the same protein that causes the hypothalamus to reset itself. And pyrogen also has the ability to withhold iron from the blood, which apparently keeps infectious organisms from feasting and flourishing. "By leaving a fever untreated, you may be following Mother Nature's way of dealing with infection," says Kluger. There are, however, some noteworthy exceptions to this "let it be" approach (see "Hello, Doctor?" for more information on when to call the doctor). In addition, if you are feeling truly miserable, there are some steps you can try to make yourself more comfortable when you have a fever.

Dress comfortably. Let your body tell you what to wear. If, as the fever is developing, you get the chills, bundle up until you feel more comfortable. On the other hand, if you feel uncomfortably warm, shed some clothing. With your body exposed as much as possible, your sweat glands will be better able to release moisture, which will make you feel more comfortable. "The fewer the clothes, the faster the fever will go down," says Pascal James Imperato, M.D., professor and chairman of the Department of Preventive Medicine and Community Health at State University of New York Health Science Center at Brooklyn. Avoid overbundling an infant.

Don't go under cover. Unless you have the chills, bundling yourself in bed under a pile of blankets or quilts will only hold the heat in and make you more uncomfortable. "Forget everything you've heard about 'sweating the fever out' by piling on the covers," advises Harold Neu, M.D., professor of medicine and pharmacology at Columbia

How to Read a Fever

"Feeling your forehead doesn't even give a good guess about your body temperature," says Harold Neu, M.D. "You must use a fever thermometer to get an accurate reading."

There are two basic types of glass fever thermometers, oral and rectal, with the only difference being in the shape of the bulb: thin and long on the oral and short and stubby on the rectal. Rectal temperatures are the most accurate; oral temperatures can be thrown off by breathing through the mouth, smoking, or having just had a drink of something hot or cold. Rectal readings are, in general, one degree Fahrenheit higher than oral temperatures. (If neither of these methods is convenient, temperature can also be taken by placing an oral thermometer under the armpit for at least two minutes, which will give a reading about one degree Fahrenheit lower than an oral temperature.)

Glass thermometers have several disadvantages: They may break in handling or even in the mouth.

If a thermometer breaks in the mouth, don't worry; there is only a tiny amount of mercury in the tube. Just be sure to remove any slivers of glass from the mouth. Glass thermometers also need to be shaken down to 96 degrees Fahrenheit in order to allow the body's true temperature to register. On the other hand, glass thermometers have a big advantage: They are cheap, with most selling for about three dollars.

More convenient—and somewhat more expensive (costing about seven to ten dollars)—are newer digital thermometers, which register temperatures accurately within a tenth of a degree. These thermometers are also fast. It takes less than a minute for the temperature to register as compared to three minutes with glass thermometers. Most digital thermometers run on a "button" (or hearing-aid type) battery that boasts a two- to three-year life under normal use.

Pharmacies generally carry a selection of both glass and digital thermometers.

Eat Yourself Well

As your fever breaks and you start feeling better, your appetite will improve. You may even feel ravenously hungry for a while. To restock your body's nutrient shelves, try eating a variety of foods, including fruits and vegetables, whole grains, low-fat dairy products, and low-fat meats, fish, and poultry. The more variety in your diet, the likelier it is that you will provide your body with all of the nutrients it needs.

In spite of a sudden onset of appetite, however, remember one thing: If you haven't eaten much for a few days, your digestive system may need to be reacclimated, too. Eat, but not so much that you make yourself sick.

University College of Physicians and Surgeons in New York. Once again, let your body be your guide. If a light sheet makes you feel more comfortable, don't feel that you have to bury yourself under blankets.

Dip. If you feel uncomfortably warm, sponge yourself with tepid water or sit in a tub of shallow, tepid water and splash the water over your body. Don't fill the tub with water, since it's the evaporation of the water from the skin that helps cool you down. "Make sure the water is not ice cold, which can be counterproductive, since it will cause shaking and make the fever rise again. Avoid alcohol altogether because it can be absorbed into the skin and cause intoxication and dehydration," advises Imperato.

Sip. Fever, especially if it is accompanied by vomiting or diarrhea, can lead to fluid loss and an electrolyte imbalance. "Keep yourself well hydrated," says Neu. Cool water is best, but unsweetened juices are OK if that's what tastes good. Getting a child to drink plenty of water is sometimes difficult; try Popsicles or flavored ices, which are primarily water.

Don't force food down. "Don't force yourself to eat if you don't feel like it when you have a fever," says Imperato. Your body will tell you when it's time to eat. (For your recovery diet, see "Eat Yourself Well.") Be sure, however, to keep up your fluid intake.

Take two aspirin. Drugs known as antipyretics seek out the pyrogen and put it out of commission. Aspirin and acetaminophen are both antipyretics. However, "do not give aspirin to a child who has or is suspected to have chicken pox, influenza, or even a minor respiratory illness," warns Imperato. "This may trigger a potentially fatal condition known as Reye's syndrome," he adds. Stick with acetaminophen for children, and follow package directions carefully. ◆

◆ FINGERNAIL ◆ PROBLEMS

14 Tips for Healthier Nails

Scratch an itch. Strum a guitar. Peel an orange. Your fingernails come in handy all day long, but too much use—or misuse—can cause problems ranging from nasty fungal infections to brittle, broken nails.

Your nails are made of keratin, the same type of protein that goes into your hair. Each nail actually consists of several parts, all of which play an important role in its health and growth:

• Nail plate: This is what you see as the fingernail.

• Nail bed: This lies below the nail plate; the two are attached. The capillaries in the nail bed nourish the nail and give it its pinkish color.

• Nail matrix: You don't see most of this, yet it may be the most important. It's below the cuticle at the base of the nail. Cells in the matrix produce the fingernail. If the matrix gets damaged, your nail will be distorted or may even stop growing completely.

• Lunula: This is the part of the matrix that you can see. It's the moon-shaped portion at the bottom of your nail.

• Cuticle: This fold of skin, made of dead cells, keeps foreign substances, like infection-causing bacteria, out.

• Nail fold: The nail fold is the ridge of skin around the nail.

Although plenty can go wrong with the nails, one of the most common complaints dermatologists hear is that fingernails are brittle—"whether they're soft and brittle or hard and brittle," says Lawrence A. Norton, M.D., clinical professor of dermatology at Boston University School of Medicine.

"Brittle nails can be compared to dry skin of the nails," explains Richard K. Scher, M.D., professor of clinical dermatology and nail specialist at Columbia University School of Medicine in New York. "You treat them like dry skin—use moisturizers and avoid harsh chemicals and detergents that are drying."

Stop Nail Biting

"There's not a lot that parents can do actively," says Bruce Epstein, M.D., a pediatrician in St. Petersburg, Florida, and a spokesperson for the American Academy of Pediatrics.

"You don't want to engage in a battle you can't win," he points out. His advice to parents: Tell your children that they can chew or bite on their nails all they want as long as they do it in the privacy of their bedrooms and not in front of you. That way, you've expressed your disapproval but you're not forcing your child to stop completely.

Those nasty medicines you can paint on the nails rarely work with kids, Epstein says. "They'll learn to like the taste."

Your child may eventually give up the habit, especially if peer pressure comes into play.

"Such nails are often shingling—they split like roof shingles at the end of the nail," says Norton. He blames the condition on nails dried out from indoor heat, exposure to detergents, and too frequent use of nail polish removers.

Nails that are soft and brittle, on the other hand, need to be kept dry. "You've used too much lotion or kept your hands in water too long," says C. Ralph Daniel III, M.D., clinical professor of medicine (dermatology) at the University of Mississippi Medical Center in Jackson.

◆◆◆ Nail Facts ◆◆◆

Your fingernails grow about one-eighth of an inch a month. Fingernails grow faster than toenails. Nails on the longest fingers grow the fastest. If you're right-handed, nails on that hand grow faster than on your left hand; the opposite is true for lefties. Your fingernails will also grow faster during the summer, during pregnancy, and when they are recovering from injury.

Trauma, the doctors' term for injury, is another major problem for fingernails. "You hit your fingernail with the hammer," says Daniel. If a bruise forms beneath the nail, a doctor may have to relieve the pressure that builds up.

Injuries also open the door to infections, especially fungal infections. Although these generally plague toenails more often than fingernails (because of athlete's foot), fungal infections can strike the nails on the hands, with some unpleasant consequences.

And finally, certain skin diseases, such as psoriasis, can show up in your nails.

What you don't want to occur: Separation of the nail plate from the nail bed, a condition called onycholysis. It can occur after an injury, infections, allergies to nail cosmetics, exposure to chemicals, or diseases like psoriasis. If the nail appears white, it may have separated. You'll need to see your doctor and you'll want to be careful not to aggravate the problem further. Unfortunately, once the nail separates, it won't reattach until a new nail has grown out.

You also want to take good care of the nail matrix. If this is damaged, it will start producing a deformed nail or, even worse, no nail at all.

Here's what the experts recommend you do to keep your nails as healthy and attractive as possible:

Avoid the culprits. The housewife or househusband is exposed to detergents and cleansers, the janitor to strong cleaning fluids, the bartender to citrus fruits, and so on, says Daniel. If you can't stay away from these substances, wear gloves whenever possible. Otherwise, you risk brittle nails and even nail separation, or infection, which could lead to a deformed nail or even the loss of it.

Wear vinyl gloves for wet work. That's vinyl, not latex or rubber, stresses Daniel, which will make hands sweat. In fact, Scher recommends wearing cotton gloves under the vinyl gloves.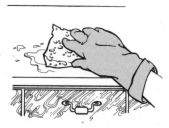

Wear cotton gloves for dry work. You'll help protect nails from damage or possible injury.

Keep your nails short. Try giving that advice to actress/singer Barbra Streisand or Olympic star Florence Griffith Joyner. But face it, the shorter your nails, the less the risk of damaging them.

◆◆◆ Protect Your ◆◆◆ Toenails, Too

Toenails are most likely to fall prey to fungal infections. That's because the fungus that causes athlete's foot can invade the toenail after it's been injured. "Use topical antifungals with clotrimazole or miconazole to decrease athlete's foot," recommends C. Ralph Daniel III, M.D. These medications are available without a prescription at your local pharmacy.

Be careful of nail bangers. Don't use your nail in place of a screwdriver, says Daniel. Try not to hit it with a hammer. You get the idea: Such actions can injure your nails, opening the door to infections, stopping nail growth, or causing bruises. "If your nail turns black and blue, go to your doctor or the emergency room," says Daniel. The pressure should be relieved on the blood vessel that's been injured underneath the nail.

Moisturize your nails. "Soak them in tepid water," says Norton. "Then massage in a moisturizer to hold the water. There's no fat in your nails to hold the moisture in." He suggests trying any product with phospholipids, urea, or lactic acid—all are "humectants," which will hold water; two he recommends are Complex 15 or Aquaderm. Daniel suggests white petrolatum or Moisturil.

Avoid moisture. Sounds like a contradiction, right? If your nail becomes infected, particularly with a yeast organism, it's important to keep it as dry as possible. The nail plate may look chalky white, yellowish, brownish, or even green when an infection has set in. The nail may separate from the bed, or the nail fold may be red and irritated looking. See your doctor if you're not sure what's happening.

Care for your cuticles. But not the way you may think. "Don't use mechanical instruments and cut them," warns Scher. Soak them first, then push them back with a moist towel. He warns against orange sticks and cuticle scissors. "When you clip cuticles, you're breaking down the normal barrier to bacteria and moisture," says Norton, "and that can lead to an infection."

Secrets Your Nails Reveal

The eyes may be the window to the soul, but your fingernails may provide a peek into the status of your health. Remember, the symptoms listed here may possibly signal the health problems listed; they do not provide definite diagnoses. But if you notice any of these, let your doctor know.

• Pale or bluish nails: This may indicate anemia.

• Pink color slow in returning when nail is squeezed: This may indicate decreased or slowed blood circulation.

• White spots: These occur as the result of an injury to the nail; they're not due to zinc deficiency, as some people believe.

• Beau's lines: These horizontal depressions occur after a traumatic event, such as a high fever. "You can actually date the event by measuring the nail and figuring in the growth rate," explains C. Ralph Daniel III, M.D.

• White lines parallel to the lunula (and not the cuticle): These indicate some sort of systemic (bodywide) insult.

• Clubbed nails: These nails are shaped like the backside of a spoon and may indicate cardiopulmonary disease or asthma.

• Spoon nails: These dip inward and could mean certain types of anemia or injury.

• Pitted nails: These punched-out looking spots may signify psoriasis.

• Anything resembling a wart around the nail: This could be a skin cancer and needs to be examined by a doctor.

• Dark spot: This could be melanoma, the most dangerous type of skin cancer. If the spot "bleeds" into the cuticle or nail folds or if you're fair-skinned, this is a serious warning sign that requires immediate medical attention.

Don't pick or tear at hangnails. Otherwise, you're opening the door to infection by making a break in the skin where bacteria can enter. Daniel suggests clipping the dry part of the hangnail with fine scissors and applying an over-the-counter antibiotic ointment. Keeping your hands, nails, and cuticles moisturized will help prevent future hangnails.

Realize the risk with nail cosmetics. Sculptured nails can hold in too much moisture, says Norton. The glues used in nail wraps can cause reactions resulting in permanent damage to the nail bed and root, says Daniel. The most common problem is separation of the nail from the bed. But if you notice any pain or tenderness, you're probably reacting to the glue, and you need medical attention, stresses Daniel.

Forget formaldehyde. Although most fingernail polishes and nail hardeners are not supposed to contain formaldehyde, some still do. And if they cause an allergy or irritation, you can end up with nail separation.

Cut down on polish remover. "Apply and remove polish no more often than once a week," advises Daniel. "The acetone in polish remover dehydrates the nails."

Don't eat gelatin hoping to build strong nails. It just doesn't work.

Ditto for calcium. "Calcium has very little, if anything, to do with how hard your nails are," Daniel says. Unless you are crash dieting or suffering from a malabsorption problem, your nails are not influenced that much by what you eat, says Scher. ◆

◆ FISSURES ◆

7 Soothing Strategies

During the summer, your skin looks radiant. All of those sunscreens and all that humidity in the air leave your skin moist and supple. But as soon as winter comes, you suffer from flaky, dry skin that often reaches the point of breaking open into painful cracks.

"Fissures, as these linear cracks are commonly referred to, can occur in many parts of the body, such as the corners of the mouth, the opening to the nose, the space between the toes, and the callused areas of the heels and hands," says Vincent A. DeLeo, M.D., assistant professor of dermatology at Columbia–Presbyterian Medical Center in New York. Once that layer of superficial skin cracks, it exposes living layers of skin, which are extremely sensitive. "The reason they hurt so much when they are on the hands is because you have more nerve endings in that one small area than you have on, say, your knee," says Denise Kraft, M.D., F.A.A.F.P., a family practitioner in private practice in Bellevue, Washington.

"Fissures most commonly occur in people with an underlying skin disorder that dries out the skin, such as eczema. It's not thought to be due to any kind of nutritional deficiency," says Kraft.

"Fissures are caused by uneven expansion of the skin. In the warm weather, the top layer of skin tends to expand with moisture. But in the winter, it loses moisture and shrinks up more than the layers beneath it, which causes it to crack," explains Neil Schultz, M.D., a dermatologist in private practice in New York. This process is often helped along by nicks and bangs to the skin. "It can happen from your doing nothing or from excessive hand washing or lack of moisturizing," says Schultz. And it usually occurs in areas where the skin is a little thicker, such as the palms, feet, and fingertips.

The best way to treat a fissure is as follows:

Lock moisture into the area. The best way to do this is to use a petrolatum-based product, says Schultz. "Spread some Vaseline over the crack and

> ### ◆◆ Hello, Doctor? ◆◆
>
> *If, after a few days to a week of home treatment, you see no improvement in a fissure, see your doctor. Signs that the area may have become secondarily infected include fever, redness around the fissure, pus draining from the fissure, or pains in the glands (lymph nodes) that drain the area of the fissure. Such an infection would need to be treated by a doctor. And if you have a fissure around the anal opening, skip the self treatment altogether, and see a proctologist.*

then put a bandage over it to lock in the moisture," he says. The petrolatum, or petroleum jelly, tends to "melt" the skin a little bit, softening it and making it easier for the skin to grow back together, explains Schultz.

DeLeo suggests soaking the area in lukewarm water for five to ten minutes before applying the moisturizer. "The moisturizer itself doesn't add moisture, it simply seals in the moisture from the water," he explains.

"If the fissure is on the hand, I recommend that my patients put the Vaseline on and then wear a glove at night," says Kraft. Wear vinyl gloves over the petrolatum, since latex can sensitize, or cause a skin reaction, in some individuals.

Try a petrolatum-based antibiotic ointment. "There are several over-the-counter versions of these, and they provide the double benefit of keeping moisture in while also protecting against infection," says Schultz.

Fight back with a steroid cream. "You can also use an over-the-counter steroid ointment to cut down on the inflammation and the redness," advises Kraft. "These ointments won't help the pain much, but they will help to recreate a barrier that prevents the outside world from getting inside of your body," she explains.

Raise the humidity. Using a commercial humidifier or simply keeping a pot of steaming water on the stove or radiator will add moisture to the air in your immediate environment and keep your skin from drying out as much, according to Schultz. "You can even set a pan of unheated water out and get a similar effect," adds Kraft. "Keeping one in the bedroom is especially good," she says.

Wear gloves in cold weather.
This advice applies to those who have fissures on the hand. "Anything that keeps the area warm and moist is helpful," says Schultz. Applying moisturizer before putting on your gloves is even better.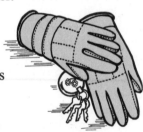

Protect your hands from harsh chemicals. Wear vinyl gloves whenever you are using strong solvents or cleaning products. These solutions are extremely drying and should never be used without protecting your skin first. They will not only encourage fissures to develop; they will cause further damage once the problem occurs, according to DeLeo.

Apply an antifungal. If the fissure is in an area prone to fungal infection (such as in the corner of the mouth or between the toes), apply an over-the-counter antifungal agent. "Your pharmacist can identify these ointments for you. They used to be prescription only but are now offered over the counter," says DeLeo. Do not, however, use these antifungal agents near the rectum. ◆

Preventing Fissures

Avoiding fissures is simply a matter of good skin care. Here are some tips:

• *Don't bathe any more than is necessary (especially in winter).*

• *When you do bathe, use a mild soap.*

• *Moisturize with a petrolatum-based product after showering, bathing, or hand washing. "I even go as far as to apply Vaseline or baby oil to my body before showering or bathing in order to protect my skin from drying out," says Denise Kraft, M.D., F.A.A.F.P.*

"Since fissures often occur on the hands, it's also a good idea to keep a good moisturizer by every sink in your house so that when you do wash your hands, you remember to moisturize afterward," advises Vincent A. DeLeo, M.D.

• *Try bath oil. Some contain lanolin or mineral oil and are specially formulated to mix with your bathwater. When you bathe in them, a thin layer of oil covers your skin and traps water there. But be careful when using these oils, because they make the bathtub very slick and could cause you to fall.*

• *Always wear vinyl gloves when using any kind of solvent or cleaning solution.*

• *Dress warmly, covering all parts of the body, when going out in the cold.*

◆ FLATULENCE ◆

11 Ways to Combat Gas

For stand-up comedians, the subject of flatulence is sure to generate lots of snickering, giggles, and guffaws. But for those who suffer from this distressing—not to mention embarrassing—problem, it's no laughing matter.

Everyone passes a certain amount of flatus—or "breaks wind," as we delicately describe it. Normally, from 400 to 2,000 milliliters of oxygen, nitrogen, carbon dioxide, hydrogen, and methane are expelled each day from the anus. Most of the time, this happens without inviting notice through sound or smell. But under some circumstances and in some people, undigested food products pass from the small intestine into the large intestine (colon), where the mass is fermented by large amounts of bacteria that are normally present there. The benign bugs of the colon are not choosy. Whatever comes their way goes right on their menu. It is the bacterially produced gas that gives flatus its characteristic odor when expelled.

If you are a stoic or a recluse, you may simply be able to ignore that gaseous excess and its audible effects. If you're neither, there are some things you can do to prevent or relieve flatulence. Here's how:

Eat to beat it. "Carbohydrates may be problematic for some people," says Lawrence S. Friedman, M.D., associate professor of medicine at Jefferson Medical College in Philadelphia. But before you cut out nutritious carbohydrates, try eliminating simple carbohydrates—those refined sugars, like fructose and sucrose, and white-flour foods that may taste good but are not very good for you, especially if you have a flatulence problem.

Minimize milk consumption. "Milk—the so-called perfect food—does cause gas for *some* people," says Sharon Fleming, Ph.D., associate professor of food science in the Department of Nutritional Sciences at the University of California at Berkeley. Some people don't have enough of the enzyme lactase in their gut or intestine to digest the milk

sugar lactose. Drinking skim milk and buttermilk instead won't solve the problem either; the lactose is in the nonfat part. Cultured buttermilk may have a little less lactose, but the taste doesn't agree with everyone. If you cut down on or eliminate milk for a few days and you still have a flatulence problem, however, you can feel assured that milk is not the cause.

Add a little enzyme. If you are lactose intolerant but don't want to give up milk, you can try one of the over-the-counter products, such as Lactaid and Dairy Ease, that contain lactase enzyme, which helps to break down lactose. Be sure to follow the package directions carefully.

Banish the offenders. "Some foods are known to be flatulogenics—or flatus producers," says Norton Rosensweig, M.D., associate clinical professor of medicine at Columbia University College of Physicians and Surgeons in New York. He recommends giving up the most common ones (see "Gassers" for a list of these) and then when you feel that the flatulence problem has been relieved, start adding the foods back one by one. If your body can tolerate small quantities, you can gradually increase your intake.

Soak your beans. Beans are a great source of fiber and protein, but for many people, eating them can be an "explosive" enterprise. Rather than give up beans, however, you can try adjusting the way you prepare them. Mindy Hermann, R.D., a registered dietitian and spokesperson for the American Dietetic Association, suggests the following technique for decreasing the flatulogenic effects of beans: Soak the beans overnight, then dump the water out. Pour new water in, and cook the beans for about half an hour. Throw that water out, put in new water, and cook for another 30 minutes. Drain the water out for the last time, put new water in, and finish cooking.

Try Beano. This over-the-counter food modifier contains an enzyme that breaks down some of the sugars that can cause gassiness. You may find that it helps make foods such as beans, cabbage, broccoli, carrots, oats, and other vegetables and legumes more tolerable. Follow the package directions.

Stay calm. Emotional stress can play a major role in worsening a flatulence problem. The gastrointestinal tract is exquisitely sensitive to anxiety, anger, and depression. A network of nerves connects this area of the body to the brain, and when you are under stress, muscles in the abdomen tighten. The results are painful spasms. "Eating while under stress also makes you swallow air, which can worsen the problem," says Friedman.

Get physical. Sometimes, flatulence is less a matter of a faulty diet than of a faulty digestive process; the smooth passage of foods down the digestive tract may be hindered. Exercise helps to regulate the process, notes Friedman, who recommends taking a walk when things get uncomfortable. You can also apply pressure to your abdomen or lie facedown on the floor with a pillow bunched up under your abdomen to help relieve discomfort. Rocking back and forth on the floor with your knees drawn up to your chest and your arms wrapped around your legs may also help. So might a heating pad placed on your abdomen.

Bust the belch. Habits that can lead to excessive belching can also cause problems with flatulence (see BELCHING).

Get activated. Activated charcoal tablets, available without a prescription, may help to absorb some excess gas and calm flatulence. If you are taking any prescription medications, however, ask your pharmacist whether the activated charcoal will interfere with them.

Reach for relief. A variety of nonprescription preparations containing simethicone (such as Mylanta and Maalox) may ease gassiness. ◆

◆◆◆ Gassers ◆◆◆

"People who suffer with chronic flatulence may be able to control the problem by eliminating foods that increase fermentation activity, thereby producing gas," says Norton Rosensweig, M.D. Here are some possible culprits:

Extremely flatulogenic:
Beans
Beer (dark)
Bran
Broccoli
Brussels sprouts
Cabbage
Carbonated beverages
Cauliflower
Onions
Milk (for those who are lactose intolerant)

Mildly Flatulogenic:
Apples (raw)
Apricots
Bananas
Bread and other products containing wheat
Carrots
Celery
Citrus fruits
Coffee
Cucumbers
Eggplant
Lettuce
Potatoes
Pretzels
Prunes
Radishes
Raisins
Soybeans
Spinach

◆ FLU ◆

6 Ways to Cope with the Flu-Bug Blahs

Yesterday, you felt fantastic. Today, you feel 100 years old and counting. Your head aches, your skin feels sore to the touch, and you're chilled to the bone even though your forehead is on fire. Welcome to the wonderful world of the flu virus.

"People use the term 'flu' to describe any viral, upper-respiratory-tract infection. But strictly speaking, influenza is a very distinctive viral agent," says Marcia Kielhofner, M.D., a clinical assistant professor of medicine at Baylor College of Medicine in Houston, Texas. "Flu viruses occur yearly and attack almost exclusively between the months of October and April," she continues.

As far as who gets the flu, it seems to occur initially in children. "We'll start to see an increasing level of absenteeism within the schools and an increasing number of children hospitalized for some sort of respiratory illness. Following that, we'll see adults being hospitalized with pneumonia or with worsening of an underlying heart or lung problem," she explains.

While there are two major strains of the flu virus—influenza A and influenza B—each strain changes slightly from year to year, so being infected one year doesn't guarantee protection against the flu the following year. "Every once in a while, we'll get what's referred to as a 'pandemic.' This is when we see an entirely new type of influenza virus that is associated with a much higher rate of infection and death. The last one reported in the United States was in 1977," says Kielhofner.

Regardless of the strain, the symptoms are generally the same. They include a high fever, sore throat, dry cough, severe muscle aches and pains, fatigue, and loss of appetite. Some people even experience pain and stiffness in the joints. Usually, the aches, pains, and fever last only three to five days. The fatigue and cough, however, can hang on for several weeks.

◆◆ Hello, Doctor? ◆◆

Signs that it's time to see your doctor include a high fever that lasts more than three days, a cough that persists or gets worse (especially if associated with severe chest pain or shortness of breath), or a general inability to recover. These things could signal a secondary bacterial infection that would need to be treated with prescription antibiotics. Marcia Kielhofner, M.D., also urges individuals with underlying lung or heart disease to consult their physician at the first sign of the flu.

The change in flu strains from year to year also makes it hard to develop 100 percent effective flu vaccines. "We tend to make vaccines that contain antibodies to the previous year's strain, which presents a real obstacle to fully protecting people from the flu each year," explains W. Paul Glezen, M.D., a pediatrician in the Influenza Research Center, a professor of microbiology and immunology and of pediatrics, and chief epidemiologist at Baylor College of Medicine in Houston. Still, flu vaccines manage to be about 80 percent effective when received before the flu season begins (ideally in September or October). So, if you really can't afford to get sick, a flu shot may not be a bad idea. And, if you fall in a high-risk group (see "Should You Get a Flu Shot?"), a flu shot is a priority.

On the other hand, if you don't manage to outrun this relentless bug, you can do a few things to ease some of the discomforts and give your body a chance to fight back.

Get plenty of rest. "This is especially important due to the high fever that accompanies the flu," says Evan T. Bell, M.D., a specialist in infectious diseases at Lenox Hill Hospital in New York. This shouldn't be hard to do considering fatigue is one of the main symptoms. You won't feel like doing much other than lounging in bed or on the couch. Consider it a good excuse to take a needed break from the daily stresses of life. And if you absolutely must continue to work, at least get to bed earlier than usual and try to go into the office a little later in the morning.

Take aspirin, acetaminophen, or ibuprofen—if you must. "One of the characteristic symptoms of influenza is a high fever that ranges anywhere from 102 to 106 degrees Fahrenheit," says Kielhofner. "Headaches are also seen almost universally with influenza," she adds. Lowering the fever will help to prevent dehydration and will cut down on the severe, shaking chills associated with fever. On the other hand, since a fever may actually help your body fight the influenza bug (see "Influenza Myths"), you may want to try to let the fever run its course if you can. "The aspirin- and ibuprofen-containing drugs tend to work better against the aches and pains, while the acetaminophen works best on the fever," says Bell. But both doctors warn that people who have a history of gastrointestinal problems and/or ulcer disease should avoid taking aspirin and ibuprofen, because these medications have been shown to further complicate these conditions. And Glezen adds that individuals aged 21 and under should avoid taking aspirin during the flu season because the combination of aspirin and the flu in this age group has been associated with Reye's syndrome, an often-fatal illness characterized by sudden, severe deterioration of brain and liver function.

◆◆◆ Influenza Myths ◆◆◆

Despite evidence to the contrary, there are a few myths about the flu that continue to prevail. One myth has to do with what people often refer to as the "24-hour flu." This is an illness characterized by the sudden onset of vomiting and diarrhea, accompanied by a general feeling of malaise. It can be quite intense in the first few hours but tends to subside completely after 24 hours. While this illness is indeed caused by a viral agent, it is not caused by the influenza virus, and so therefore is not a form of the flu at all, according to Evan T. Bell, M.D. The correct term for this type of upset is "gastroenteritis," which indicates an infection of the gastrointestinal tract.

Another common myth about influenza is that being cold or chilled makes us more susceptible to it (as well as to the common cold). According to W. Paul Glezen, M.D., several scientific studies on humans have shown that those exposed to severe temperatures for several hours fare no worse as far as becoming ill than those who are kept warm and dry. The myth is perpetuated because severe chills are one of the first symptoms of the flu, leading people to believe that they somehow "caught a chill" that led to the illness.

An additional myth is the belief that using medicine to keep the fever down helps us to get over the illness. "Experimental studies on the flu in animals show that more of the virus is excreted over a longer period of time when the body temperature is lowered with medication," says Glezen. "So while such treatments may make you feel better, they don't necessarily help you get over the virus."

Drink, drink, drink. This doesn't mean alcoholic beverages, of course. But drinking plenty of any other nonalcoholic, decaffeinated liquid (caffeine acts as a diuretic, which actually increases fluid loss) will help to keep you hydrated and will also keep any mucous secretions you have more liquid. "Clear broth that is salty and warm tends to agree with people when they have the flu and are experiencing a general loss of appetite," says Glezen. Juices are also good for keeping some nutrients coming in when you're not eating much else.

Humidify your home in winter. "Influenza viruses survive better when the humidity is low, which explains why they tend to show up more during the winter, when we use artificial heat to warm our homes," says Glezen. Humidifying your home in the winter not only helps to prevent the spread of flu, it also makes you feel better once you have it. "When you are really sick, a little extra humidity in the form of a warm- or cool-mist humidifier works wonders," he adds.

Suppress a dry cough. For a dry, hacking cough that's keeping you from getting the rest you need, you can reach for over-the-counter relief. "Cough remedies containing dextromethorphan are best for a dry cough," says Kielhofner.

Encourage a "productive" cough. A cough that brings up mucus, on the other hand, is considered productive and should not be suppressed with cough medicines. Drinking fluids will help bring the mucus of a productive cough up and will ease the cough a little as well, according to Glezen. ◆

Should You Get a Flu Shot?

Anyone who wants to reduce their chance of getting the flu should consider being vaccinated against the flu. However, it is especially important for the following groups of individuals to get a flu shot, according to Evan T. Bell, M.D., and Marcia Kielhofner, M.D.:

• *Individuals with chronic heart and lung disease. The flu virus can aggravate these conditions to the point of causing serious complications and even death.*

• *People over the age of 65, especially if living in a nursing home or chronic-care facility. Viruses spread more rapidly in such environments. What's more, the flu virus attacks the already weakened immune systems of elderly people, which can lead to pneumonia and even death.*

• *People with other chronic diseases, such as asthma, diabetes, kidney disease, or cancer. Any time the body is fighting one disease, getting another illness can cause serious problems.*

• *Children who take aspirin regularly for problems such as chronic arthritis. Again, Reye's syndrome may be triggered by the flu virus in children who are on aspirin therapy.*

• *Health-care providers. While catching the flu may not seriously endanger these individuals, it can be deadly to the patients they are treating.*

• *Pregnant women who fall into any of the high-risk groups mentioned. The vaccine must be given after the first trimester of the pregnancy to prevent the possibility of harming the fetus.*

◆ FLUID RETENTION ◆

29 Ways to Stop Swelling

Nearly everyone has experienced some form of fluid retention at one point or another—whether as swelling from a bumped shin or ankle sprain or as a bloated feeling following a very salty meal or preceding the monthly menstrual period. Anyone who has had to stand or sit for hours on end knows that inactivity can cause a temporary swelling in the legs. Ironically, overexertion can also result in swelling. Typing nonstop or weeding a garden—any activity in which the same movements are performed over and over—can be the culprit. Fluid retention can also be an indicator of a deeper problem, such as a heart, blood vessel, or kidney disorder.

"Swelling is the body's first obvious response to injury, and if it's not treated, it can lead to joint stiffness, which compromises function and delays healing," says Pamela Kirby, O.T.R./L., C.H.T., an occupational therapist and certified hand therapist at The Hand Center in Greensboro, North Carolina. That's why it's important to take steps to bring down swelling from an injury as soon as possible.

The following are some tips for bringing down minor swelling and for keeping excess fluid from accumulating in the first place. However, if you suspect that swelling is the result of a sprain or fracture, if swelling persists for more than a few days, if it is more pronounced in one extremity than another, or if it encompasses the whole body, see your doctor.

Bag some ice. Applying an ice pack can help bring down swelling caused by a sprain or strain. Ice cubes placed in a sandwich bag that has a zipper-type seal make an effective ice pack, says Kirby. You can also use a bag of frozen peas or frozen unpopped popcorn. Specially made hot/cold packs can be effective, too. For rheumatoid arthritis, alternating hot and cold treatments on a swollen joint may help, says Kirby.

Keep it dry. "Wet compresses can be too harsh on the skin," says Kirby. "So use a dry barrier between the ice pack and you." She suggests a napkin, a cloth or paper towel, or a cotton T-shirt. Dry compresses also seem to allow the ice to affect deeper body tissues than damp barriers, she notes.

Go above your heart. By elevating your hand or foot, you're allowing gravity to help drain the fluid and draw the swelling out. Raising the extremity above the level of your heart is even more beneficial. "When your hand swells, sit up and elevate it, so your thumb's about even with your nose," advises Kirby. Prop up your arm or leg on a couple of pillows or on the back of a couch.

Don't get wrapped up in bandages. "Elastic wraps don't apply a consistent pressure," says Kirby. "Since the amount of pressure applied can't be controlled, many people invariably make them too tight, which, ironically, can cause more swelling above or below the wrap." If you think you need the support of an elastic bandage, consult your physician, who may recommend a variety with a more consistent pressure. If you suffer from arthritis, you can help minimize swelling with department-store stretch gloves. You can also ask your doctor about special gloves for this purpose.

Support your legs. For minor swelling that results from being on your feet all day, over-the-counter support hose may help. There are also stockings specially made to apply more pressure to the lower leg to help keep fluids from collecting. A doctor prescribes the stockings, which are available in various lengths and degrees of compression. Prescription stockings can help pregnant women who suffer swelling, says Claudia Holland, M.D., assistant clinical professor of obstetrics and gynecology at Columbia–Presbyterian Medical Center in New York.

Walk and walk some more. When it comes to swelling in the legs, "it's very important to keep the legs moving," says Robert C. Schlant, M.D., professor of medicine (cardiology) at Emory University School of Medicine in Atlanta. Whether you are at your desk or on a plane, get up periodically and stretch your legs. "Simply taking a walk around your desk can help," he says. Better yet, put on a pair of sneakers, and take a walk during your lunch break or during a layover at the airport. Besides helping the leg muscles pump blood and other fluids back toward the heart, walking and other aerobic activities can help build the heart and leg muscles, making them more efficient. If you find that exercise itself causes swelling in your hands, wear a pair of stretch gloves while working out, suggests Kirby.

Flex your legs. For people who are limited in their activity, due to arthritis, for instance, flexing is the next best thing to walking. While sitting, flex your knee and ankle joints up 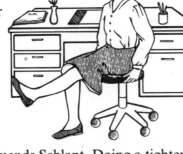 and down, recommends Schlant. Doing a tighten-and-release routine on the thigh and calf muscles can also help.

Take a break. Since repetitive motion is one cause of swelling in the hands and wrists, make sure you take breaks to give them a rest. For more information on repetitive motion injuries, see the section entitled CARPAL TUNNEL SYN-DROME.

Don't cross your legs. This can restrict blood flow through the veins in the thighs, which in turn can aggravate swelling in the lower legs.

Massage the swelling. Gentle massage will help increase circulation to the tender injury site, says Kirby. For hand injuries, gently bend the joints to prevent stiffness.

Don't pull on the puffiness. "Some people think that if they jam their finger, they should pull on it to stop the swelling," says Kirby. "What they don't realize is that they can actually cause more injury to the area because their pulling can tear the ligaments and tendons, creating a bigger problem than they originally had."

Get some over-the-counter help. Aspirin and ibuprofen can be an aid in controlling the inflammation that sometimes accompanies swelling, as is the case with rheumatoid arthritis and sprains and strains. (Acetaminophen, on the other hand, is not an anti-inflammatory medication, although it can help to relieve pain.)

Consider your medications. Some prescription drugs, including certain blood pressure medications (such as reserpine and nifedipine) and hormonal regulators (such as birth control pills), can cause fluid retention, says Allan D. Marks, M.D., associate professor of medicine and director of the Hypertension Clinic at Temple University Health Sciences Center in Philadelphia.

Avoid constricting clothing. Tight garments, such as belts, garters, and girdles, should be avoided because they can apply too much pressure on the upper thighs and waist, says Schlant. This pressure can restrict the removal of fluids and cause edema (swelling) in the lower legs.

Adjust your jewelry. Wristwatches, rings, and bracelets (for the wrist or ankle) that are worn too tight can aggravate, and in some cases even cause, swelling, says Missy Donnell, O.T.R., C.H.T., an occupational therapist at The Hand Clinic in Austin, Texas.

Put Your Foot Down on Swelling

Ill-fitting footwear and hosiery can cause, as well as aggravate, swelling. The following tips can help you choose shoes and socks that fit properly, according to Glenn B. Gastwirth, D.P.M., deputy executive director at the American Podiatric Medical Association in Bethesda, Maryland.

Buy shoes later in the day. Your feet can swell by as much as half a shoe size over the course of a day. If the pair you buy is too small, swelling can occur or become more pronounced.

Measure your foot while standing. This will give you the most accurate measurements of the length and width of your foot so you don't buy the wrong size.

Opt for lace-up shoes. Slip-on styles are usually not too forgiving when it comes to swollen feet. With lace-up shoes, you can always loosen the laces to allow your feet more room.

Go with a flat or low heel. A flat or low heel allows the foot to move more naturally when walking, with the sole flexing from heel to toe. Higher heels are more likely to restrict this movement. Swelling can result because the leg muscles, which help keep the lower circulatory system moving, are not pumping as efficiently as they could be with a proper stride.

Boot uncomfortable boots. Many boots weren't made for walking. Styles that constrict the calf or have very high heels will also aggravate swelling and restrict proper stride.

Wear a style that suits your feet. As is the case with clothing, some styles are fashioned to fit certain shapes better than others. Shoes with shallow toe boxes, for instance, aren't good for people with thicker digits, and very pointy shoes will never feel comfortable to someone with broad feet.

Buy natural. Shoes made from leather, suede, and canvas keep the feet cool and dry by allowing them to "breathe." On the other hand, rubber and vinyl are nonporous and will trap moisture. The result: excessive heat and humidity, which can aggravate swelling.

Choose socks that let your feet breathe. Some studies have shown that socks made of certain acrylic fibers tend to pull moisture away from the feet. (Nylon, however, tends to generate heat and absorb moisture like a sponge.) On the other hand, some doctors stand by the traditional natural fibers—cotton and wool—as being best for keeping the feet cool and dry. Try a pair of each, and see which type works best for your feet. If you find that your feet perspire heavily no matter what type of socks you wear, you may need to change your socks two or three times a day.

Don't assume socks will fit. Though their packages may say it, one size does not fit all. Socks are made based solely on shoe size, with no consideration for the fact that some people have thicker ankles or calves. If you get the socks home, and they feel like a vise on your legs, don't wear them. Elastic banding that is too tight can restrict circulation and lead to or aggravate swelling.

Don't use your hands as tools. Instead of putting extra stress on your hands to carry out tasks, use tools made for the job, advises Kirby. For instance, don't use the heel of your hand as a hammer. Arthritis sufferers should adapt the tools of their everyday tasks for ease of use. A toothbrush or hairbrush with a built-up handle, for example, can take the stress off the hands. (For more tips, see ARTHRITIS.)

Take the pressure off your palms. When you lift something, don't hold it from the bottom with your palms flat; instead, hold it at the sides, recommends Kirby. The reason: When the palms meet great resistance straight on, the wrists take the brunt of the load, which can lead to injury and swelling.

Maintain the proper weight. "Overweight people have more of a chance of developing edema," says Schlant. They are also more likely to be affected by heat and humidity, which can aggravate swelling, says William F. Ruschhaupt, M.D., a staff physician in the Department of Vascular Medicine at the Cleveland Clinic Foundation in Ohio.

Shake the salt habit. Sodium causes the body to retain fluid. But keeping the shaker off the table isn't the only way to cut back on salt. Avoid heavily salted snacks; opt for no-salt potato chips, pretzels, and popcorn instead. Processed foods can be high in sodium, so check labels. Virtually salt-free: Fresh and frozen fruits and vegetables, whether eaten raw or steamed. If you cook them, do not add salt to the water.

Try to stay calm, cool, and collected. While stress doesn't have a direct effect on edema, some doctors believe it can have an indirect one. "Stress can leave you lethargic and sedentary, leading to inactivity, which can aggravate swelling," explains Ruschhaupt. ◆

◆ FOOD POISONING ◆

8 Coping Tips

As anyone who's had a bad case of food poisoning can testify, it is an experience so thoroughly awful that you wouldn't wish it upon your worst enemy. Not only does everything you've eaten for the last 24 hours seem to want to escape out of both ends of your body simultaneously, but the cramps and pain you experience can make you want to crawl into a hole and die.

The good news is that food poisoning is rarely life-threatening. In most cases, it will pass within 24 hours, leaving you as good as new. The bad news is that once it's started, there's no real way to put the brakes on it until it has run its course.

The following tips, however, may help minimize your discomfort and shorten the duration of your symptoms.

Replace your body's fluids. If your stomach will tolerate it, be sure to keep taking liquids, especially if you have diarrhea, says Zachary T. Bloomgarden, M.D., an internist and assistant clinical professor of medicine at Mount Sinai School of Medicine in New York. "Sometimes people feel that if they drink more, they'll throw up more or have more diarrhea," he says. "However, these illnesses require acute hydration. Even if you do have a little more diarrhea, you'll still be ahead of the game if you've been drinking more. Also, you feel worse if you are dehydrated." He recommends gelatin, decaffeinated soda, decaffeinated tea with sugar, or water.

Avoid rich or spicy foods. When your stomach is feeling irritated, eating fatty or highly seasoned foods may send you right back to the toilet bowl, says John C. Johnson, M.D., past president of the American College of Emergency Physicians and director of the Emergency Department of Porter Memorial Hospital in Valparaiso, Indiana. If you feel hungry, it's probably best to stick with clear liquids, plain toast, mashed potatoes, bananas, or other bland foods.

> ## ◆◆ Hello, Doctor? ◆◆
>
> *In rare instances, food poisoning may be downright dangerous. It's time to head for the doctor or the emergency room if you are experiencing severe cramps, you are weak or dizzy, or you can't keep anything at all down, says John C. Johnson, M.D. Ditto if you have a fever of over 102, if you faint, if the symptoms persist longer than 48 hours, or if you see any blood in your stool or vomitus, says David Posner, M.D. Other symptoms that signal an emergency are paralysis, double vision, breathlessness, or weakness in a limb, Posner says.*

Go with the flow—literally. If you've been poisoned by contaminated food and your stomach is reacting by having diarrhea or vomiting, you can trust your body's impulses, according to Johnson. "Don't run out and buy antidiarrheal medications," he says. "If there's something in your system, you may feel better sooner if you let it out. The same goes for vomiting—wait a while before you take anything orally. Your stomach doesn't want anything more down there. If you give it a chance to rest, it will usually take care of itself."

Be careful with pain medications. Some people make the mistake of taking prescription or over-the-counter pain medications to reduce the discomfort of intestinal cramps, says Johnson. "The side effect of many of these drugs is to irritate the stomach or gastrointestinal tract," he says. The one exception is acetaminophen, says David Posner, M.D., a gastroenterologist and assistant professor of medicine at the University of Maryland School of Medicine in Baltimore. Drugs containing aspirin or ibuprofen are definitely out when your stomach is irritated.

Try a hot-water bottle. One thing that may help cramps is a hot-water bottle placed on the stomach, according to Posner. "Make sure it's not too hot to the touch," he cautions.

Treat it like the stomach flu. Just like with the stomach flu, there's really not a whole lot you can do, except to be good to yourself and wait it out, says Bloomgarden. Cancel your appointments, rest, take it easy, and take solace in the fact that it's guaranteed to pass, most likely within 24 hours.

Replace your potassium. Vomiting and diarrhea may lead to a depletion in your body's supply of potassium, which may leave you feeling even worse, according to Johnson. Twenty-four hours after your symptoms started (and hopefully when you're feeling a bit better), a sports drink or a banana "may perk you up," he says.

Report it to the health department. If you were the only person affected by food that may have been contaminated, reporting your condition may not be necessary, according to Posner. However, if you were one of a group of people who ate at a restaurant or other food establishment and more than one of you became ill, tell the restaurant, your physician, or your local health department, he says. "If it turns out to be an infection, such as dysentery, the health department may want to track it down," he adds. ◆

Prevention Is the Best Medicine

The best way to treat food poisoning is to avoid getting it in the first place. Although you can't control the conditions in the restaurants you patronize, you can take several precautions in your own home, say John C. Johnson, M.D., and David Posner, M.D.

"Mixed foods, such as potato salads, creamy coleslaws, and other foods containing dairy products, are likely to breed bacteria, especially if they are not kept well refrigerated or if they get warm and are later refrigerated," Johnson says. Summer picnics are notorious for such conditions, he adds.

Another problem arises at holiday times when people tend to thaw and stuff turkeys or roasts hours before guests arrive, leaving them out of the refrigerator for long periods of time, according to Johnson.

"Make sure that perishables are kept cold," Posner says. "Cook chicken, pork, and beef very thoroughly, and wash hands and utensils in very hot water and soap after using them to cut meat."

◆ FOOT ACHES ◆

22 Ways to Ease the Agony

Our poor, overworked feet. In a single day, they absorb about 1,000 pounds of force as they carry us from place to place. And we mistreat them terribly—we stand on them for hours; we walk on hard, unyielding surfaces; and we cram them into shoes that may be fashionable, but are often very far from comfortable. So it's really no wonder that four out of five adults eventually suffer from foot problems.

Foot pain is so common, podiatrist Andrew Schink, D.P.M., past president of the Oregon Podiatric Medical Association and podiatrist in private practice in Eugene, quips, "At parties, I've stopped telling people what I do for a living."

While certainly not as glamorous as the heart or the brain, the feet are amazing pieces of engineering, perfectly designed to give years of service—if you treat them right. Each foot has 26 bones—together the feet have almost one-quarter of the bones in the entire body. Thirty-three joints make the feet flexible and 19 muscles control movement of foot parts. Tendons stretch tautly between muscles and bones, moving parts of the feet as the muscles contract. Two arches in the midfoot and forefoot, constructed like small bridges, support each foot and provide a springy, elastic structure to absorb shock. Numerous nerve endings in the feet make them sensitive (and ticklish). And the whole structure is held together by more than 100 ligaments.

As incredible as our feet may be, few of us ever think about them until they hurt. And when they do hurt, it's difficult to think of anything else. Fortunately, if your dogs are barking, there are several things you can do to soothe and pamper your tired, aching, overworked feet. There are also some simple steps you can take to prevent serious foot problems from developing in the first place. Here are some suggestions:

Take a load off. Much of the foot pain we experience comes from tired muscles. "The leg has four basic muscle groups that move the foot up, down, and from side to side," explains Schink. "After a period of time, the foot flattens out because the muscles get overly fatigued from trying to hold up the foot."

If you have to stand a great deal, take breaks to take the weight off your feet. The same advice applies if you do a lot of walking. Whenever you can, elevate your feet at a 45-degree angle to your body, and relax for 10 to 15 minutes. Elevating your feet will move blood away from the feet and help reduce swelling.

Give them a soak. Put two tablespoons of Epsom salts (available without a prescription at your local drugstore) into a basin of comfortably warm water and give your aching feet a relaxing bath for 15 minutes, says Schink. Then, pat your feet dry with a soft towel, and moisturize them with your favorite cream or lotion.

Alternate hot and cold. Sit on the edge of the bathtub and alternately run cold water then (comfortably) hot water (for one minute each) on the feet; end with cold water. If you are diabetic, however, do not try this without your doctor's approval.

Give them the squeeze. There's nothing quite as relaxing as a foot massage. Have a partner massage your feet with massage oil, baby oil, or moisturizing lotion. Or treat yourself by massaging your own feet. First, apply oil, and condition the foot with medium-light strokes, using your thumbs and fingers. Next, starting with the ball of the foot, work across and down the entire foot using the thumbs to make small, circular motions. Use the thumbs to make long, deep strokes along the arch of the foot, moving in the direction of the toes. Gently squeeze, rotate, and pull each toe. End by cupping the foot between both hands and gently squeezing up and down the length of each foot.

Ice 'em. A cool way to refresh your feet after a long, hard day is to ice them down with a washcloth filled with ice. It'll make them feel wonderful and decrease swelling.

Exercise your feet. Like any part of the body, the feet stay healthiest if they're kept strong and flexible with regular exercise. Walking in shoes that provide good support and cushioning is excellent exercise for the feet.

Feet also benefit from specific foot exercises. Michael Martindale, L.P.T., a physical therapist at the Sports Medicine Center at Portland Adventist Medical Center in Oregon who specializes in athletic injuries, suggests the following:
• **Golf-Ball Roll:** With your shoe off, place your foot on top of a golf ball, and roll (don't stand) on the ball using only the weight of the foot.
• **Spill the Beans:** Scatter beans or marbles on the floor, and pick them up with your toes.
• **Circle and Stretch:** Sit in a chair with your feet out in front of you, and make four or five small circles in both directions with your feet. Next, stretch your toes out as far as you can; then stretch them up toward you. Repeat six times.

Trim your toenails. Ingrown toenails may be inherited, but improper nail trimming can make the problem worse. Trim the nails straight across and only to the end of the toe, then file the corners to remove sharp edges that might cut the skin (see INGROWN TOENAILS).

Maintain ideal weight. Being overweight puts excess strain on your feet, as well as on all of the other weight-bearing joints of the body.

Buy shoes that fit. Too often, people buy shoes that don't fit their feet. They opt for fashion rather than fit or comfort. "I could make almost any foot problem feel better with the right pair of shoes," says Schink.

He says to look for shoes that:
• Have plenty of room in the toe area (toe box).
• Don't slip. The foot should not slide around in the shoe.
• Are wide enough. Your foot shouldn't bulge over the edges of the shoe.
• Fit in the store. Don't buy shoes that are too small for your feet believing that you'll "stretch them out" with wearing.

Know your feet. Different types of feet require different kinds of shoes, according to Martyn Shorten, Ph.D., former director of NIKE's Sports Research Laboratory. "High-arched feet tend to be rigid and need shoes that provide good cushioning and absorb shock," he says. "Flat feet have lots of flexibility so they need shoes that can control excess motion."

To find out what kind of foot you have, wet your bare feet and stand on a concrete floor or piece of paper. If you have high arches, the outline of your foot will appear very narrow and curved like a half-moon. If the outline looks like a slab, you're probably flat-footed.

Wear the right shoe for the activity. "The wrong shoe can cause injuries such as tendinitis in the knees, chronic foot pain, heel spurs, and stress fractures," says Kathleen Galligan, D.C., a chiropractor in Lake Oswego, Oregon, who specializes in sports injuries.

She says each activity has its own set of repetitive movements that require special support and cushioning. You wouldn't play basketball in a pair of heels. Likewise, don't rely on that old pair of sneakers if you're going climbing or hiking. Spend the extra money to buy shoes that are specific for the activity you're doing. The investment could save you and your feet a good deal of discomfort.

Replace worn shoes. It's tough to give up those old favorite shoes, but often we wear shoes long after they've lost their ability to support and cushion the foot. "Shoes are often worn out before you can see the wear," says Galligan.

She advises paying attention to the worn-out-shoe messages from your body. "If your feet hurt, your legs feel tired, your knees are sore, or your hips hurt, it's definitely time to buy a new pair of shoes." ◆

◆◆◆ High-Heel Hell ◆◆◆

Remember your grandmother's feet? Chances are good they were misshapen with corns, bunions, calluses, and curled toes. Chances are equally good your grandfather had long, well-formed feet. A genetic difference? No, it's probably high-heel hell, the purgatory women's feet are put through by high-heeled shoes.

"The body can tolerate a heel up to about an inch," says Kathleen Galligan, D.C., who frequently sees the results of high-heeled shoes in her chiropractic practice. "But over an inch rocks all your weight onto the ball of your foot. It causes the Achilles tendon to shorten and the pelvis to shift forward."

The result of this precarious sliding forward can cause all kinds of structural problems, including back pain and foot pain. Podiatrists often see women for "forefoot shock"—pain, fatigue, and a wobbly gait caused by the body's weight being centered on the ball of the foot.

Sometimes, we just can't get around the convention of wearing high-heeled shoes at work or social gatherings. But here are a few ideas to help you minimize the strain on your feet.

• Wear the lowest heel you can find.

• If you must wear high-heeled shoes, wear lower-heeled or flat shoes to and from work and during lunch and breaks.

• Look for shoes that are more rounded in the toe area; avoid pointy shoes that pinch the toes.

• Buy shoes that are large enough to accommodate added padding or an arch support. A half insole can help keep your foot in place when you wear heeled shoes. Experiment and see what works for you.

• Buy the thickest heel possible for the greatest stability.

◆ FOOT ODOR ◆

13 Steps to Sweeter-Smelling Feet

If removing your footwear at the end of the day calls to mind the scent of a postgame locker room, you may be suffering from what is scientifically known as bromhidrosis—sweaty, smelly feet.

While neither painful nor contagious, foot odor causes unmitigated social suffering to those who are burdened with it. Under normal conditions, each of your feet produces half a pint of sweat by means of some 20,000 sweat glands. In most people, this perspiration evaporates. In people with bromhidrosis, however, more sweat is produced, and it doesn't evaporate as easily. The result: odoriferous feet.

If you suffer from this problem, don't worry. You don't have to stand for it anymore. Simply follow these suggestions for keeping your feet drier and sweeter smelling.

Wash well. Those sweat glands on the soles of your feet produce perspiration composed of water, sodium chloride, fat, minerals, and various acids that are end products of your body's metabolism. In the presence of certain bacteria, these sweaty secretions break down, generating a foul smell. Obviously, washing away the bacteria will short-circuit this process. "Washing your feet often with a deodorant soap and drying very carefully can *temporarily* make your feet smell sweet," says Joseph C. D'Amico, D.P.M., a podiatrist in private practice in New York.

Wash wisely. How often should you wash your feet? Enough to remove the offending bacteria but not so often that you remove all the protective oils from your skin. For strong foot odor, you may need to bathe your feet several times a day. However, if you notice that your feet are becoming scaly and cracked, cut back on the number of washings.

Soak the sweat out of them. Suzanne M. Levine, D.P.M., a podiatrist in private practice in New York, suggests the following treatment for sweaty feet. First, alternate footbaths of hot and cold water to help decrease blood flow to your feet and reduce perspiration. Next, dip your feet into another footbath containing ice cubes and lemon juice. Finally, rub your feet with alcohol. In hot weather, when your feet tend to perspire more, this form of treatment should be repeated daily. If you have diabetes or any other condition that causes decreased circulation, do not try this treatment at all.

Salt your tootsies. For extra-sweaty feet, try adding half a cup of kosher salt (it has larger crystals than ordinary table salt) to a quart of water and soaking your feet in the solution. After soaking, don't rinse your feet; just dry them thoroughly.

Treat them like underarms. "The key to controlling foot odor is to use either an antiperspirant or a deodorant right on your feet," advises Levine. Foot deodorants, like underarm deodorants, contain antibacterial agents that can kill bacteria. They won't stop the sweat, but they will eliminate the odor that ensues when sweat meets bacteria. Antiperspirants, on the other hand, stop the sweat and the smell at the same time.

Take a powder. Spray or put on foot-deodorant powder. Be sure it contains aluminum chloride hexahydrate, advises Levine.

Sock 'em away. "Clean feet need clean coverings," notes Mary Papadopoulos, D.P.M., a podiatrist in private practice in Alexandria, Virginia. Wear socks that let your feet breathe. (Some experts advise cotton or wool, others suggest acrylic; try different fabrics until you find the one that seems to keep your feet driest.) If possible, change your socks at least once during the day, and don't wear the same pair two days in a row. Contrary to conventional wisdom, white socks are not sterile and do contain dye, so they are not necessarily preferable to colored socks.

Shoe it away. "Stay away from solid-rubber or synthetically lined shoes, because they don't allow your feet to breathe easily, allowing odor-producing bacteria to flourish," says Levine.

Wash your sneakers. Some shoes—such as sneakers and other canvas footwear—should go right in the washing machine, says D'Amico. Let them air dry rather than throwing them in the dryer.

Let your shoes breathe. Try airing out your shoes between wearings, too. If you can, alternate shoes on a daily basis so that you don't wear the same pair two days in a row. Loosen the laces and pull up the tongue on the pair you're not wearing, and let them dry out in the sunshine.

Sprinkle your shoes. Sprinkle the inside of your shoes with cornstarch to help absorb moisture and keep your feet drier.

Eat wisely. "Eating certain strong foods, such as onions, garlic, scallions, peppers, and even curry, can cause strong foot odor," says D'Amico. The odoriferous products pass through the blood-stream and eventually concentrate in the perspiration. While this effect is not restricted to foot perspiration, it certainly won't help a case of smelly feet.

Keep calm. Stress and anxiety increase production of sweat, giving those nasty little bacteria even more to feed on. "A level of stress so high that it produces foot odor should be dealt with right away, because other parts of the body are probably feeling the toll, as well," says Levine. ◆

◆ FROSTBITE ◆

25 Ways to Deal with Jack Frost

For fans of winter sports, there's nothing more exhilarating than crisp, cold air and a blanket of snow for skiing, snowmobiling, sledding, or just plain horsing around. But the nip in the air can have an unforgiving bite if you're not dressed properly to ward off the elements. Indeed, you may not realize how cold it actually is outside—until frostbite develops.

Frostbite occurs when the fluids in the skin tissues begin to freeze, or crystalize, restricting blood flow to the affected area. Most cases of frostbite occur on the hands, feet, toes, nose, and ears. The reason is that as the body temperature drops in reaction to prolonged exposure to cold, the heart attempts to protect vital organs by increasing circulation to the torso at the expense of the extremities.

While it is wise to have any suspected case of frostbite checked out by a doctor, you need to take steps right away to rewarm and protect the affected areas. The tips that follow can help you care for frostbitten skin and help you protect yourself from Jack Frost's bite in the future.

TREATING FROZEN SKIN

Here's what to do—and what *not* to do—if you suspect that you are developing frostbite:

Watch for the warning signs. The sooner you notice the symptoms of frostbite, and the faster you take measures to rewarm the areas, the better the outlook for recovery. The skin may first start to tingle, as ice crystals begin forming in the tissues. Then, pain develops, accompanied by redness, burning, itching, and swelling. If exposure to cold continues, numbness sets in, the pain decreases, and the skin becomes whiter and waxy looking. At this stage, immediate action is necessary to prevent gangrene, or death of skin tissue.

Warm up the right way. If you become frostbitten, don't run to the nearest radiator, hot stove, or roaring fire. "The numb extremity may not sense the intense heat, and you may burn the delicate, damaged tissues," says Roger Thurmond, M.D., a dermatologist in private practice in Fairbanks, Alaska. For the same reason, do not use a heat lamp, hot-water bottle, or heating pad to warm up. Submerging the affected extremity in a sink or basin full of warm water (104 degrees Fahrenheit to no more than 110 degrees Fahrenheit) is the safest way to treat the frostbite. Once your fingers or toes are warmed up, very gently wiggle them to increase the circulation to the area. For frostbitten ears or a frostbitten nose, moving to "a heated room should be enough to warm them up," says Thurmond. If not, gently apply warm compresses to the affected area; do not rub the delicate tissue.

Warm up rapidly. Experts have found that rewarming the frostbitten area as quickly as possible "promotes faster healing, reduces tissue loss, and helps prevent complications, such as gangrene—and even loss of a limb," says Jerome Z. Litt, M.D., an assistant clinical professor of dermatology at Case Western Reserve University School of Medicine in Cleveland. Rapid rewarming may initially cause more pain, redness, and swelling, and result in bigger blisters. The payoff: Mild to moderate frostbite should heal in a week or two.

Don't thaw and then refreeze. Thawing and then refreezing a frostbitten area can cause even more damage, so if you cannot keep the injured area warm, it may be best to postpone rewarming until you are safely out of the cold.

Stay as warm and dry as possible. Even if your clothes are dry, they may be cold enough to keep you from warming up. Clothing that is wet depletes heat even more and should be removed. However, if you are out in the cold with no chance of getting to a warm place quickly, your better bet may be to just add layers of warmth to what you already have on.

Huddle with a buddy. A friend's body heat will help warm you up.

Drink plenty of fluids. Sipping warm or tepid fluids may make you feel better and, more importantly, will keep you from getting dehydrated, which can make your frostbite worse. (Becoming dehydrated also makes you more susceptible to frostbite in the first place.) Do not, however, eat snow. And stay away from alcoholic beverages, which actually encourage fluid loss.

Elevate the affected area. This minimizes edema, or swelling, of the affected area. It's important to do this because swelling can interfere with proper circulation, which is necessary for proper healing.

Don't use snow. "That's just old folklore," says Litt. "Rubbing frostbite with snow or ice will break down the skin cells and possibly lead to gangrene."

Don't rub or massage the frostbitten area. This will also cause further damage to the skin, says Litt.

Keep off your feet. If possible, don't walk on your frostbitten toes. As with any frostbitten area, they need to be immobilized for proper healing.

Keep your toes or fingers apart. Use sterile gauze to separate the affected digits. "This helps to immobilize the delicate tissues, which may be apt to stick together as they blister and heal," says Thurmond.

Try this solution for blisters. During the thawing process, blisters may develop and persist for weeks. If this occurs, mix Burow's solution (available without a prescription in packets and tablets at pharmacies) and warm water (between 104 degrees and 110 degrees Fahrenheit) according to the package directions, and apply the solution to the blisters with wet compresses for 15 to 20 minutes every two to three hours until the blisters have begun to dry up, says Litt.

PREVENTING FROSTBITE

With a little advance planning and preparation, you can protect your skin and keep frostbite from developing in the first place. Here's how:

Wear fabrics specially made for cold or wet weather. "The ideal outerwear traps a lot of air between you and the elements," says Litt. "Loosely woven bulky wool and acrylics are good choices," he says. Litt and other experts also recommend clothing made with Thinsulate, Hollofil, Gore-Tex, or other "high-tech" materials, which can help keep you both warm and dry.

Keep your head covered. You can lose a significant amount of body heat from the neck up, says Litt. This is due to the disproportionately large amount of blood circulating there. "That's why it's true when they say that if your feet are cold, you should put a hat on," says Philip Gormley, W.E.M.T., operations director of Wilderness Medical Associates in Bryant Pond, Maine. He suggests wearing a wool hat and scarf and earmuffs in order to help keep your whole body warm.

Layer, layer, layer. Gormley suggests polypropylene liners on the hands and feet, followed by down mittens and wool socks, respectively. Jonti Fox, former associate program director of the Colorado Outward Bound School in Denver, recommends wearing a lightweight shirt, then a heavier-weight one over it, covered by a chinchilla jacket, and, finally, a water-resistant windbreaker. Boots with separate, removable inner liners of felt or Gore-Tex are also recommended. Experts agree that clothing and footwear should not be tight. Too-tight cuffs and boots, for instance, can decrease circulation to the extremities. "The best-fitting boots will allow you just enough room to move your toes, even if you have an extra pair of socks on," says Fox.

Put sandwich bags in your boots. The bags act as a barrier to keep your feet dry if your boots should get wet, says Gormley.

Give your hands a spin. If your fingers start to tingle, whirl your hands round and round at the wrist. "The centrifugal force you create should help get more blood circulating to the chilled fingers," says Thurmond.

Eat right and get plenty of rest. Poor nutrition and fatigue can exacerbate the problem by lowering your resistance and hindering circulation, making you more prone to frostbite. For strenuous outdoor activities, Fox recommends foods with complex carbohydrates and fats, such as pasta and nuts, for long-term energy, and simple sugars, such as candy, for quick energy boosts.

Avoid alcohol. Alcohol can impair your awareness of how cold you are. Alcohol is also a diuretic, which can contribute to dehydration.

Do not smoke. Some people light up when they're cold thinking it's going to make them warmer. The truth is that smoking constricts the blood vessels and decreases circulation to the extremities, which is why smokers are at higher risk for frostbite.

Be aware that medicines play a role. "Prescription drugs, such as tranquilizers, and over-the-counter medications, such as sleeping aids and antihistamines, can also impair your judgment as to how cold you've become," says Litt. There are many drugs that can act in this way; check the label or ask your pharmacist to find out if any medication you are taking could have this effect.

Don't touch metal. Coming in contact with metal in the cold can cause instantaneous frostbite, causing you to stick right to it. If this should happen, pour warm water (again, at about 104 degrees to 110 degrees Fahrenheit) over the injury site to loosen it.

If stranded on a wintry day, stay with your car. This is your best bet, unless, of course, you are in immediate danger or you can seek help very nearby. "Leaving the car to brave the elements will deplete your energy and dehydrate you," says Thurmond. This predisposes you to frostbite and hypothermia (see "Hypothermia: The Deep Freeze"). You also run the risk of getting lost.

◆◆ Hypothermia: ◆◆ The Deep Freeze

When the temperature within the body drops from its average 98.6 degrees Fahrenheit to below 95 degrees Fahrenheit, hypothermia can occur. The symptoms of hypothermia include shivering, numbness, drowsiness, muscle weakness, and disorientation, often marked by "mumbling and stumbling," says Philip Gormley, W.E.M.T. In severe cases, the victim may become unconscious. Hypothermia is an emergency that requires immediate medical attention. In the meantime, the victim should be covered with extra blankets or other wraps and, if conscious, given sips of a warm, nonalcoholic beverage. If the victim is unconscious, do not attempt to administer fluids.

Furthermore, rescue crews can more easily spot a vehicle than a person in distress. So stay put.

Always keep emergency supplies in the car. In addition to a first-aid kit and tools for repairing minor problems such as flat tires, these supplies should include protection for you. Stuff a box with a blanket or two, an extra pair of gloves, a hat, boots, earmuffs, a sweater for everyone who will be traveling, candles, and matches. Hot packs used by hunters may also come in handy. ◆

◆ GENITAL HERPES ◆

17 Home-Care Hints

Suspect that you may have genital herpes? Know that you have it but want more information? Read on.

Genital herpes is a viral infection marked by sores that look like fever blisters on the genital area. There's a reason they resemble fever blisters, too. Both genital herpes and fever blisters are caused by the herpes simplex virus. There are two strains of herpes simplex virus—Type I and Type II. The Type I virus usually causes fever blisters, also called cold sores, on the mouth, face, and lips, although it can also cause sores in the genital area. The Type II virus, on the other hand, most often causes sores in and around the genital area.

Herpes is a "contact virus." In other words, you can only get it from skin-to-skin contact with someone who is infected. Herpes is passed from partner to partner through oral or genital sex. Infected persons can pass the virus on to a partner when the virus is in an active state (when sores are apparent) or a preactive state (marked by itching or tingling in the area where sores generally appear). However, in some cases, the virus can be passed before the infected person knows he or she is shedding the virus.

The bad news is that once you contract herpes, it cannot be eradicated. "Once the herpes virus enters the body through mucous membranes in the genital area or mouth, these tiny organisms travel up the nerve endings to the base of the spine," says Sadja Greenwood, M.D., assistant clinical professor in the Department of Obstetrics, Gynecology, and Reproductive Sciences at the University of California at San Francisco. Once established, the virus stays in the body permanently, feeding on cell nutrients. It may remain dormant, causing no symptoms, or it may recur at any time.

The first episode of herpes, before the body has built up defenses, is usually most intense and occurs a couple of days to two weeks after exposure to an infected partner. The first signs are itching, tingling, and a burning sensation or minor rash. Then, small, red sores develop. In women, the sores can occur in and around the genital area and, in some cases, on the buttocks, anus, navel, and thighs. In men, the sores usually appear on the shaft and head of the penis, although they can also develop on the testicles, in the area around the penis, and on the buttocks, anus, and thighs.

If you develop a sore or rash in the genital area, you need to see a doctor for correct diagnosis and treatment. Doctors don't have a cure for herpes, but prescription medications can help relieve the symptoms and, in some cases, shorten the duration of an outbreak. You can, however, take steps at home to ease your herpes symptoms, lessen the number of recurrences, and prevent the virus from spreading.

Keep a herpes diary. Such a log can help you identify the things that trigger your herpes recurrences, such as certain foods, stress, drugs, trauma, and menstruation, says Anne Simons, M.D., a family practitioner in the San Francisco Department of Public Health. "Ask yourself: 'What occurred just before my outbreak? Did I change my diet? Was I under any unusual stress? Did I use recreational, over-the-counter, or prescription drugs?' If you can identify and avoid your triggers, you may be able to avoid painful outbreaks," she says.

Ice it. At the first sign of symptoms (tingling, burning, itching), apply ice to reduce pain and swelling, says Amanda Clark, M.D., assistant professor of obstetrics and gynecology at Oregon Health Sciences University in Portland. Place crushed ice cubes in a plastic bag (a bag of frozen peas or frozen unpopped popcorn also works), and wrap it in a cloth that is the thickness of a sheet (a terry-cloth towel is too thick to transmit the cold effectively). Place it directly on the area. Keep it in place for 10 to 15 minutes at a time. Reapply several times throughout the day.

Dry it out. External drying remedies like baking soda and cornstarch may lessen the itching, says Greenwood. You can also try using a hand-held hair dryer on a cool setting to help dry out the sores.

Wear baggy pants. Tight-fitting underwear, nylons, or pants can irritate the genital area and stimulate a herpes outbreak, says Susan Woodruff, B.S.N.,

childbirth and parenting education coordinator at Tuality Community Hospital in Hillsboro, Oregon. They can also increase discomfort when sores are present. She advises opting for comfortable, baggy shorts and slacks.

Tea for one, please. "The tannic acid in black tea is very soothing to genital tissues," says Clark. "Place cold, wet tea bags right on the sores."

Cool it with Burow's. Simons recommends applying cool compresses soaked in Burow's solution (available without a prescription in pharmacies) to

---

◆◆◆ Hello, Doctor? ◆◆◆

While home remedies for herpes can help ease the discomfort, decrease recurrence, and prevent the spread of the virus, it is important to see your physician for proper diagnosis whenever you develop any rash or sores in the genital area. You may think you have herpes, but you may have another, more serious sexually transmitted disease (STD) such as syphilis that can be life-threatening if left untreated.

Here's a brief outline of what you can expect when you visit the doctor for genital herpes. First, the doctor will do a visual exam of your genital area. If you have active lesions, the doctor may be able to identify them, but the diagnosis should be confirmed by a lab test.

Herpes can be identified in three ways: the Tzanck test (cytological smear); a viral culture; or a blood test. If you have active sores, your doctor may opt for taking a smear from the sores for cytologic examination under a microscope. If your symptoms have just appeared, your doctor may take a cell sample and grow the virus in a culture medium. However, the most effective way to find out if you've ever had a herpes infection is with a blood test, which measures virus antibodies in the

blood. This test requires two blood samples, one sample during the initial attack and another sample one to four weeks later.

Medical treatment for herpes isn't perfect. It doesn't cure the condition but only reduces the frequency and length of outbreaks. The oral antiviral drug acyclovir may shorten the initial herpes attack by a few days; unfortunately, the drug's effectiveness often decreases over time. "If it's the first outbreak of herpes," says Amanda Clark, M.D., "taking oral acyclovir might shorten a three-week outbreak to ten days."

Oral acyclovir decreases the number and severity of outbreaks if taken continuously. (In rare cases in which herpes requires hospitalization, acyclovir may be given intravenously and orally.) Oral acyclovir is also less effective in recurrent attacks and can have numerous side effects, including nausea, vomiting, diarrhea, joint pain, rash, and fever. "If you're going on a trip or something special and you need to prevent an outbreak," says Clark, "oral acyclovir is effective."

Most doctors believe acyclovir is relatively safe. However, if you've taken this drug for a year or more, talk with your doctor about reassessing its effectiveness.

the sores four to six times a day. Follow package directions for preparing the Burow's solution.

Take a hot bath. Sitting for five to ten minutes in a hot "sitz" bath (a bathtub filled with three to four inches of water) three or four times a day sometimes inactivates the sores and speeds healing by drying out the sores, says Woodruff. "The warm water brings circulation to the area, which seems to have a positive effect," she says.

Take a nonprescription pain reliever. Over-the-counter analgesics like acetaminophen, ibuprofen, or aspirin can reduce pain, says Greenwood. Take two tablets every four hours as needed for pain.

Wear cotton underwear. Avoid synthetic fabrics that can trap heat and moisture in the genital area. Choose cotton underwear that "breathes."

Avoid arginine. Although the link between food and herpes remains fuzzy, some experts believe that the herpes simplex virus is stimulated by arginine, a substance found in foods like chocolate and peanuts. Experiment for yourself. If you find your herpes is affected by arginine-containing foods, avoid them, says Greenwood.

Keep dry. Keep the genital area as dry as possible. After a bath or shower, *pat* (don't rub) the area dry with a soft, dry towel. Use a different towel to dry the rest of your body to avoid spreading the virus to other parts of the body, and never share your towels with others. If the area is too tender to towel dry, try using a hand-held hair dryer on the cool setting, says Simons.

Don't use ointments. Viruses, including the herpes virus, like environments that are moist. Avoid using petrolatum or antibiotic ointments on your sores; these products may prevent drying and slow healing.

Hands off. Keep in mind that herpes is a *contact* virus. You get it and pass it from skin-to-skin

◆◆◆ Herpes and ◆◆◆ Pregnancy

While not life-threatening in adults, herpes is very serious in newborns, according to Sadja Greenwood, M.D. "Mortality rates in babies born with herpes are as high as 65 percent," she warns. "Survivors may suffer brain damage."

Women who contract their first herpes infection near the time of delivery are at greatest risk for infecting the baby during delivery. Women who have previous histories of herpes and become pregnant may also transmit the virus to their newborn during delivery. Greenwood offers this advice for women concerned about infecting their newborns with the herpes virus:

• Have your physician screen you regularly with vaginal and cervical cultures (to determine if you have active virus).

• Women who have an active lesion at the time of delivery should discuss with their doctor the option of a cesarean section to protect the baby from infection.

contact. If you have herpes sores and touch them, you can spread the virus to other parts of your body, such as your eyes or mouth. Avoid directly touching any active herpes sore.

Relax. While mind-body science is still in its infancy, and researchers aren't sure exactly why stress affects herpes, the experience of many women indicates that herpes sores tend to erupt when one feels run-down or overly stressed. Hence the association between colds and cold sores. To minimize any possible effect from stress, try to get plenty of rest and, if necessary, try some form of stress-reduction technique, such as regular aerobic exercise or progressive relaxation, says Greenwood.

Practice safe sex. If you or your partner have active sores or feel sores coming on, avoid sexual contact, advises Greenwood. (A condom *may* prevent herpes spread from an infected man, but protection isn't always 100 percent. Condoms won't halt virus transmission from an infected woman.) Talk with your sex partners honestly about your sexual histories. Use a condom with all new partners.

Maintain good general health. The body's immune system is better able to fight off the advances of the herpes virus and other organisms if you're in good health. Keep the machinery running at full power by eating a well-balanced, low-fat diet and exercising regularly. Avoid immune-lowering activities like cigarette smoking and using drugs and alcohol.

Get support. Stress promotes herpes and herpes tends to cause stress. It seems like a vicious cycle. How do you break it? Get support by joining a herpes support group in your area. Many people feel embarrassment, guilt, and frustration about their herpes. Talking with others who share your problem can be healing. They may not only help you overcome your negative feelings about herpes, they may offer coping tips and strategies that they've developed through experience—strategies that may, in turn, help you. To find a herpes support group in your area, call the American Social Health Association at 919-361-8400, or write to them at P.O. Box 13827, Triangle Park, North Carolina 27709. The American Social Health Association also publishes an excellent newsletter, *The Helper,* for herpes sufferers. ◆

◆ GINGIVITIS ◆

16 Hints for Healthier Gums

You're brushing your teeth, and when you rinse and spit, you see a little blood. No big deal, you think to yourself. It happens all the time. Well, it's time to think again—and get to a dentist—because that bit of blood may be a much bigger deal than you think. It may be a sign of gingivitis, the first stage of gum disease. According to the American Dental Association (ADA), gum disease—not dental caries, or "cavities"—is the leading cause of tooth loss among adults.

Gingivitis is inflammation, swelling, and bleeding of the gum tissue caused by the bacteria that naturally coat everyone's teeth. The bacteria form a sticky, whitish film on the teeth called plaque. If plaque isn't thoroughly removed every day, the bacteria produce toxins that irritate the gums and make them red, swollen, and likely to bleed easily. Eventually, the toxins destroy gum tissue, causing it to separate from the tooth and form pockets. The pockets hold more bacteria and detach even further. This is periodontitis, an irreversible stage of gum disease that can destroy the bone and soft tissue that support the teeth.

If you have gingivitis, you're not alone. According to the ADA and the American Academy of Periodontology, three out of four adults have gingivitis. Most gingivitis results from poor oral hygiene—not brushing and flossing correctly or often enough and not having teeth professionally cleaned on a regular basis. Ronald Wismer, D.M.D., a dentist in private practice in Beaverton, Oregon, who routinely sees gingivitis among his patients, says other factors may increase the risk of developing gingivitis. "Stress is a big factor in gingivitis," he says. "Hormonal imbalances like pregnancy, menstruation, and the changing hormones of adolescence can increase gingivitis. Some diseases like diabetes and drugs like Dilantin [phenytoin] can cause a gingivitis flare-up. Even habitually breathing through the mouth, which tends to dry out the gums and cause an overgrowth of gum tissue, can increase your risk of developing gingivitis."

For most of us, it's lack of good oral hygiene that's the problem. Good oral hygiene is also a major part of the solution. "The clinical definition of gingivitis is that it involves only the gums," explains Sandra Hazard, D.M.D., managing dentist for Willamette Dental Group, Inc., in Oregon, "so it's entirely reversible. If you can get things cleaned up, the damage can be taken care of."

If you suspect that you have gingivitis, you need to see a dentist, because only a dentist can diagnose gum disease. If you have been diagnosed with gingivitis, the following tips, used in addition to your dentist's advice and treatments, can help you improve your oral-hygiene habits and keep gum disease from stealing your smile.

Use the "three-three" rule. Whenever possible, brush your teeth three times a day for at least three minutes each time. The ADA says that most people spend less than one minute *per day* on dental hygiene. Ken Waddell, D.M.D., a dentist in private practice in Tigard, Oregon, understands why people don't brush and floss more. "Undoubtedly, brushing and flossing are the two most boring activities on earth, so we don't devote enough time to them," he says. "But to do it right, you've got to brush for at least three minutes each time." (For more information on proper brushing technique, see TARTAR AND PLAQUE.)

Try brushing dry. Waddell says you can take some of the boredom out of dental hygiene by "dry" brushing—or brushing without toothpaste—while doing other activities such as watching television.

Be consistent. "Find a routine and stick with it," suggests Waddell. "Start at one spot in the mouth each time and work around the mouth the same way each time. It'll help you be consistent and prevent missing tooth surfaces."

Lighten up. One of the biggest mistakes people make when they brush is pushing too hard with the toothbrush, says Waddell. Try the following experiment. Apply the bristles of your toothbrush to the back of your hand. Push as hard as you normally would for toothbrushing, and try to move the brush around. Then apply only a tiny amount of pressure and move the brush. You'll find that the hard pressure doesn't allow the tips of the bristles—the part of the brush that cleans the teeth—to move.

In addition, Waddell says to avoid a "traveling" stroke. Instead of moving the brush up and down and traveling rapidly over several teeth, brush a couple of teeth at a time, holding the brush in one place.

Use a softie. Often, people choose toothbrushes that have bristles that are too stiff. "Stiff bristles can actually injure the gums and create gingivitis," says Jack W. Clinton, D.M.D., associate dean of Patient Services at Oregon Health Sciences University School of Dentistry in Portland. "The softer the bristles, the less you have to worry about technique."

Brush your tongue and palate. In addition to brushing your teeth, Waddell advises brushing your tongue and the roof of your mouth to cut down on the amount of bacteria present and to increase circulation in the tissue.

Electrify 'em. Okay, so you hate to brush. It's awkward and boring, or maybe it's too difficult because you don't have as much dexterity as you used to. Try one of the new "rotary" electric toothbrushes. "I advise anyone I see who has a gum disorder to use an electric toothbrush," says Waddell. But, he warns, not all electric toothbrushes are created equal. Ask your dentist for a recommendation.

Floss, and floss again. "No matter how good a toothbrusher you are, you aren't going to get your

---

◆◆ Hello, Doctor? ◆◆

Regular dental checkups and cleanings are essential to your oral health. If you notice any of the following symptoms between your dental visits, call your dentist.

- *You have persistent bad breath.*
- *There is pus between the teeth and gums.*
- *Your "bite," the way your teeth fit together, has changed.*
- *You have loose or separating teeth.*
- *Your gums consistently bleed.*
- *The gums at the gumline appear rolled instead of flat.*
- *Your partial dentures fit differently than they used to.*

---

toothbrush bristles in between your teeth," says Hazard. "That's why flossing becomes important." You might want to try a waxed floss (it may be easier to move between the teeth without getting hung up). Whenever possible, floss at least twice a day, advises Wismer. (For more information on proper flossing technique, see TARTAR AND PLAQUE.)

Irrigate it. While water irrigation devices like the Waterpik don't take the place of flossing, they do clean debris out from pocket areas and from between the teeth and they massage the gums, says Hazard.

Use tartar-control toothpaste. Tartar is a hardened material that often contains bacterial debris and sometimes even plaque. "Tartar-control toothpastes help control some of the mineralization of plaque," says Hazard. "Look for products that have the American Dental Association Seal of Acceptance or Recognition, which means they've been put through a testing process and their claims have been proven."

Brush with baking soda. Once or twice a week, brush your teeth with baking soda. "Baking soda is a good abrasive, but not too abrasive so that it damages the enamel," says Hazard. "It cleans the teeth well and makes the gums feel terrific." Make a paste with a little baking soda and water, and brush thoroughly, especially around the gum line. Not only will the baking soda scrub off the plaque, it also neutralizes acidic bacterial wastes, deodorizes, and polishes your teeth.

Rinse it. Despite what many of the television advertisements seem to say, only one over-the-counter dental rinse, Listerine, has the acceptance of the ADA's Council on Dental Therapeutics for reducing plaque. Ask your dentist if he or she thinks adding Listerine to your dental arsenal would be helpful for you. Hazard warns, however, that no mouth rinse will take the place of thorough brushing and flossing.

Bring on the salt water. Clinton recommends rinsing the mouth with a warm saltwater solution (half a teaspoon of salt to four ounces of warm water). Swish it around in your mouth for 30 seconds and spit (don't swallow). "The salt water is very soothing to the inflamed tissue and gets rid of some of the bacteria," says Clinton.

Swish. If you can't brush right after eating, at least rinse your mouth out thoroughly with water, advises Clinton. "Even plain water can flush out debris and help prevent the inflammation of gingivitis," he says.

Eat a balanced diet for overall good health. According to some researchers, a poor diet may cause gum diease to progress more rapidly or may increase the severity of the condition. So be sure to choose a wide variety of foods from the basic food groups—fruits and vegetables, breads and cereals, meat and dairy products—to make sure you are giving your body all of the nutrients it needs for good health.

Schedule regular dental appointments. Having your teeth professionally cleaned and checked on a regular basis is essential for preventing and treating gum disease. It is especially important since you can have gum disease—or a recurrence of it—without noticing any symptoms. Talk to your dentist about how often you should schedule appointments. Then be sure to keep those appointments. ◆

◆ GOUT ◆

6 Ways to Tame the Pain

Last night, you fell into bed, exhausted from the day . . . you drifted into a peaceful sleep . . . and then it happened. You awoke to an excruciating pain in your big toe. When you turned on the light and took a look, you found that your big toe was red, swollen, and hot to the touch. No matter what you tried, the pain didn't subside.

When you finally made it in to your doctor's office, she took some blood tests and made her diagnosis. "You have gout," she said. But when you reached into your memory bank to pull out what you knew about the disease, all you could think of was reading about it in history books. Well, here's a short refresher course.

"Gout was formally introduced in the Thirteenth century, but was described by Hippocrates long before that," says Don Stewart, M.D., chairman of the family practice department at Overlake Hospital and Medical Center in Bellevue, Washington.

"The classic symptom is pain in the joint at the base of the big toe," he continues. But gout can affect any other joint of the feet and hands, as well as the knees, shoulders, and elbows. "Sometimes you'll even get a fever and chills because the joint gets so swollen and inflamed," he adds. Gout comes on very suddenly, produces severe pain, and usually lasts three to five days if untreated. But Stewart warns that it can recur and last a lot longer than that. Many patients describe gnawing pain accompanied by a feeling of pressure and tightening in the area. "The pain is like that of a dislocation, yet the parts feel as if cold water were being poured over them," says Denise Kraft, M.D., F.A.A.F.P., a family practitioner in private practice in Bellevue, Washington.

There are several conditions that can result in gout, but the primary cause is an abnormally high level of uric acid in the blood, either from the body's producing too much or from the body's not excreting it properly. Uric acid is a waste product of cell activity. When the level of uric acid in the blood increases, sodium urate crystals may form. "The crystal deposition in itself is not symptomatic," says Peter A. Simkin, M.D., a rheumatologist and professor of medicine in the Department of Medicine at the University of Washington in Seattle. "It's when those crystals deposit in a joint and cause arthritis that you start to see the classic symptoms of gout."

High blood pressure and obesity are also contributing factors, says Kraft. Stewart adds that diseases involving the breakdown of tissue—including cancer, lymphoma, psoriasis, and anemia—can cause high levels of uric acid in the blood and result in an attack of gout.

"Gout is overwhelmingly a problem in men rather than women because women are more efficient in the way they excrete uric acid in the kidneys," says Simkin. Stewart clarifies this further. "Gout is classically a disease of middle-aged men who are fat and who drink too much," he says. But frequently it affects perfectly healthy individuals as well. "Severe dehydration can also bring on an attack of gout," says Kraft.

"Gout itself isn't necessarily dangerous, but the underlying causes for it are," warns Stewart. Gout, therefore, requires diagnosis and treatment by a doctor. Once you've seen your physician, however, there are a few things you should do on your own.

Don't put any weight on the joint. This usually means staying off of your feet as much as possible until the episode subsides, according to Stewart. Any pressure you put on the joint will increase the pain and possibly damage the area further. "This is a serious condition because it can go on to cause a lot of major joint damage and destruction," warns Stewart.

Keep the joint elevated. "This again will reduce some of the pain and keep the blood from rushing to the area, which can cause additional inflammation," says Stewart.

Immobilize the joint. "This could be achieved by lying still or by actually building a splint for the joint," says Kraft. The less you move the joint, the better it will feel.

Take ibuprofen. "This will help to reduce some of the swelling and decrease some of the pain associated with that swelling," says Kraft. Both ibuprofen and aspirin are anti-inflammatories, but Stewart warns against taking aspirin to relieve the symptoms. "Aspirin in low levels can actually exacerbate the problem," he says.

Avoid icing or heating the area. "Heat may feel good on the area, but it also increases circulation to the area and brings in more white blood cells, which can make it more irritated," says Kraft. Simkin adds that icing the joint can cause more crystals to form.

Wear comfortable shoes. "Many people like to wear stylish shoes with narrow, pointed toes. But any shoe that forces the big toe inward can make the problem of gout worse," says Simkin. ◆

Preventing Attacks of Gout

If you have a tendency toward attacks of gout, there are a few things that you can do to help ward off these attacks. Taking any medications prescribed by your doctor is the first step. The following measures can also help, whether used in conjunction with prescribed medication or, if no medication has been prescribed, on their own.

Maintain desirable weight. *Since obesity is a contributing factor, Denise Kraft, M.D., F.A.A.F.P., and Peter A. Simkin, M.D., recommend getting down to a healthy weight. "This should not be done with a crash diet that promotes rapid weight loss," warns Simkin. "Dietary reduction should be achieved with a balanced-calorie diet and should promote gradual weight loss," he continues. Kraft specifically recommends a moderate-protein, low-fat diet. Talk to your doctor or to a nutritionist if you need help in setting up such a diet plan.*

Avoid alcohol. *"Beer, wine, and ale are especially bad, as they can precipitate attacks of gout," says Kraft. "Alcohol is a problem because it causes urate retention," adds Simkin.*

Avoid nonprescription water pills and other diuretics. *"These things tend to keep you from properly excreting uric acid, which enables it to build up in your system and cause gout attacks," says Don Stewart, M.D. If you have been prescribed a diuretic for another condition, such as high blood pressure, be sure the doctor knows that you have a tendency toward attacks of gout.*

Drink eight six-ounce glasses of fluid a day. *"In addition to causing gout, high serum urate levels can also cause kidney stones. Keeping your fluid intake up tends to reduce the amount of crystallization and lessen your chance of developing stones," says Kraft.*

Wear comfortable, well-fitting shoes. *"In addition to relieving some of the pain of an attack of gout, wearing comfortable shoes can also help to prevent these attacks," says Simkin.*

Check out your diet . . . maybe. *One treatment for gout that was recommended in the past was to stay on a low-purine diet. "On theoretical grounds, avoiding the high-purine foods makes all the sense in the world. The problem is, going from a regular diet to a diet free of purines in general makes only a modest change in the serum urate levels of patients," says Simkin. "Purine is largely found in the organ meats," adds Stewart. Anchovies, sardines, legumes, and poultry are also high in purines. If you are willing to try a low-purine diet, go ahead. It won't hurt you. But don't expect it to help much either.*

◆ GRINDING TEETH ◆

11 Ways to Conquer the Daily Grind

Everybody handles excess stress differently. Some people develop an ulcer, some people develop high blood pressure, and some people grind or clench their teeth.

Stress, it's now believed, is the major cause of grinding and clenching, say dental researchers. In the past, a malocclusion (the way your teeth fit together) got the blame, and dentists would grind the teeth down, trying to readjust the bite.

In a small percentage of cases, sleep patterns are responsible, says Daniel M. Laskin, D.D.S., M.S., professor and chairman of the Department of Oral and Maxillofacial Surgery and director of the TMJ and Facial Pain Research Center at the Medical College of Virginia in Richmond. The reasons children grind remain unclear.

The problem with bruxism, as the habit of grinding and clenching is called, is the wear and tear on your teeth. "It can wear away tooth enamel, causing decay and sensitive teeth," says Laskin. Expensive dental work can get destroyed in the process, too. "And, you can get aching jaw muscles, which may be confused with pain in the joint and the symptoms of temporomandibular [jaw] joint disorder [TMJ]," Laskin adds. (See TMJ.)

Prolonged grinding may damage the jaw joint enough to cause osteoarthritis, says John D. Rugh, Ph.D., professor in the Department of Orthodontics and director of research for the Dental School at the University of Texas Health Science Center at San Antonio. And it can increase bone loss in periodontal (gum) disease, although it does not actually cause gum disease.

You may inherit the tendency to grind, says Rugh. Three times as many women as men brux, says Thomas F. Truhe, D.D.S., codirector of the Princeton Dental Resource Center in New Jersey. Bruxism is most common in those between 20 and 40 years of age.

Ironically, the regular grinder may do less harm than the intermittent grinder—sort of like the weekend athlete who's not in shape for intense activity. The regular grinder can wear down teeth, but his or her muscles get stronger from the habit, says Laskin.

Clenching may do more harm than grinding, adds Laskin. "Your jaws are constructed for bruxing, or chewing, but clenching loads the joint isometrically and can end up causing degenerative changes in the joint."

People who grind are usually aware of their habit, too, says Laskin. They wake up with a stiff or tired jaw, or their spouse hears the noise during the night. Clenchers, on the other hand, may be ignorant of their problem. "If you notice the pain gets worse as the day goes on, then you're doing something in the daytime," says Laskin.

Here's what you can do to try to stop bruxing and to cope with discomfort until you do:

Wear a night guard. Your dentist can make a plastic or acrylic appliance for you to wear at night. It will redistribute the forces from grinding and protect your teeth from damage. "It's a little like banging your head against the wall and putting a pillow between your head and the wall so it doesn't hurt anymore," says Rugh. Opinions are divided as to whether it will actually keep you from grinding. Your dentist will want to see you regularly to check for any tooth movement or cavities that might result from wearing such an appliance. Keep in mind, however, that in order for the night guard to do any good, you must remember to put it in.

Keep your lips sealed, but your teeth apart. Your teeth should be touching only when you're chewing or swallowing. Drop your jaw and feel the muscles relax—then try to maintain that feeling.

Take a warm bath before bedtime. You may temporarily relax your jaw muscles, although they may not stay that way, says Laskin.

Stress Thermometer

When he was a young dentist in the military, Thomas F. Truhe, D.D.S., says he would see more evidence of tooth grinding and clenching among women whose husbands were at sea.

"Use your bruxism as an indicator that you're pushing yourself too hard—it's like taking your stress temperature," says John D. Rugh, Ph.D. Remind yourself to slow down and take it easy.

Exercise. Your body, not your jaw, that is. A walk or other mild exercise may help relieve some of the tension and stress that's causing bruxism, says Rugh.

Remind yourself. If you're a daytime clencher, you can put a red dot on your phone, stickers on your wristwatch, or even a string on your finger to remind you to keep your jaw relaxed, says Rugh.

Relieve stress. "Change jobs, get a divorce, get married, move the kids out, but if you can relieve stress, you can relieve the bruxism," says Rugh.

"Don't forget that good things as well as bad things can cause stress," says Laskin. "I've had patients say they don't have any stress, then they go on to say they've got a wonderful husband, two kids, a great job, they're active in the PTA, they do this and that, and it's all good, but it's overload." (See "Stress Thermometer.")

Learn coping skills. See a psychologist or psychiatrist. Take an assertiveness training course. Practice techniques such as progressive relaxation or guided imagery or self-hypnosis. Listen to relaxation tapes. In other words, find something that helps you to better handle the stress in your life.

Take a mild analgesic. Ibuprofen, for example, can dull the pain and help relax stiff muscles.

Apply heat. Warm, moist heat is best. The simplest method: Soak a washcloth in hot water, wring it out, and hold it up to your jaw. You can use a heating pad, although moist heat will penetrate better. A hot shower's nice, too. "Think of these muscles like the baseball pitcher treats the sore muscles in his pitching arm," suggests Truhe.

Massage. It works for the rest of your body, so try a gentle massage to your jaw muscles.

Give your jaw muscles a break. Avoid the steak, the hard-crusted bread, and the popcorn for a while. "Your muscles aren't able to tolerate that much activity," says Laskin. Chewing gum's a no-no, too, if your jaw muscles ache. ◆

◆ HAIR LOSS ◆

6 Ways to Fight It

A clump of hair in the shower drain or scattered on the pillowcase can alarm anyone. For many folks, their mane is their crowning glory. When they're having a "good hair day," it adds extra zip to their step. So anytime it looks like they may be losing their locks, they're not happy.

In reality, it's normal to shed between 50 and 100 hairs a day. That's generally not a problem, since the typical head of hair has about 100,000 hairs. It's simply part of the shedding phase that all hair goes through. Hair first goes through a growth stage, which lasts anywhere from months to years. "Women with very long hair have long growing phases. It's not an acquired trait; either you have it or you don't," says Alvin Solomon, M.D., associate professor of dermatology and pathology at Emory University School of Medicine in Atlanta. Hair then moves into a resting phase for about three months. Finally, the shedding phase occurs, and the whole cycle starts over again with a new hair.

By far, the most common cause of hair loss for both men and women is pattern balding. In men, this hereditary condition affects the front and/or top of the head. "All men undergo this to some degree," says Douglas Altchek, M.D., assistant clinical professor of dermatology at Mount Sinai School of Medicine in New York. Pattern hair loss in women isn't generally as severe as it is in men, and it's more diffuse, with the thinnest patches of hair usually at the top of the head. Still, the number of women with pattern balding is "much more than most people think," says Solomon. While there is no cure for pattern balding, there are treatments available (see "Help for Pattern Balding").

Hair loss does occur for other reasons, some of which you can have control over if you know about them. In most of these instances, the hair loss is temporary, although you may have to wait six to eight months after the precipitating cause has been removed before you see the growth begin again. The following tips can help you prevent some of the other situations that can cause hair loss:

Stay healthy. Easier said than done sometimes, but a whole host of diseases may have the unfortunate result of causing hair loss. "These diseases may have the effect of shortening or interrupting the growth phase of the hair cycle," says Marty Sawaya, M.D., Ph.D., assistant professor of dermatology and biochemistry at the State University of New York at Brooklyn. Illnesses as diverse as measles, thyroid disease, lupus, pneumonia, anemia, diabetes, syphilis, polycystic ovaries, and tumors on the adrenal gland may all produce hair loss.

Watch your medications. "Literally hundreds of different medications can cause hair loss," says Solomon. Chemotherapeutic drugs (medications used in the treatment of cancer) certainly affect the hair, but the list of offenders also includes some birth control pills, high blood pressure medications, certain types of steroids, diuretics, antidepressants, and even aspirin when taken chronically. Whether you will be affected by your medication in this way depends on your own sensitivity. Check with your doctor to see if the medications you are taking are associated with hair loss and whether there are alternative medications available, suggests Altchek. However, do not stop taking any prescription medication without first talking to your doctor about it.

Eat a balanced diet. People who eat a very-low-protein or iron-deficient diet run the risk of shedding more than normal amounts of hair. This can happen, for instance, when someone eats a poor diet or tries crash dieting. This holds true especially for women. "We don't understand it fully, but some investigators have been finding that in women, iron and iron metabolism have an effect on the hair cycle," says Sawaya. On the other hand, going overboard with certain vitamins can harm hair, too. Taking Vitamin A or D in excess can cause hair loss. "People who are taking the so-called megavitamin regime should be very careful," warns Altchek.

Keep calm. Severe stress or a traumatic event like a death in the family can bring about heavy shedding of the hair. But moderate stress can leave its mark on your mane as well. "Gradual hair loss or thinning of the hair can be brought on by constant, low-grade stress," says Altchek. Try to find a way to cope with stress and minimize its effects on your health—and your hair. Do whatever works for you, whether it's exercising, practicing meditation or some form of relaxation technique, or making time for a hobby.

Don't overprocess or overstyle your hair. We do many things to our hair to make it look beautiful, but some of them may not be good for our tresses. Cornrowing, tight braiding, bleaching, teasing, chemically straightening, and using hot rollers or hot combs can all cause hair breakage. "The rule of thumb here is the less you do to your scalp, the better," advises Altchek. Whoever told women to brush their hair 100 times a night gave them "the worst possible advice," he says. If you can't forgo the styling and processing altogether, at least try to space them out a bit and give your hair a break from these treatments whenever possible.

Check out your supplements. Selenium supplements taken in excess and foreign herbs that contain heavy metals can cause hair loss. If you are taking any such supplement and notice hair loss, discontinue the supplement and see your doctor to be sure that the supplement has not caused other complications that may not be as readily apparent as the hair loss. ◆

Help for Pattern Balding

Unfortunately, for the millions who suffer from hereditary pattern balding, there aren't any "miracle remedies," says Douglas Altchek, M.D. The Food and Drug Administration has banned as ineffective any nonprescription hair cream or lotion that claims to grow hair or prevent baldness. They also state that there's no evidence that any vitamin or food supplement retards baldness or grows hair.

There are medical treatments, however, to help restore lost or thinning hair. The prescription drug minoxidil, sold under the brand name Rogaine, is currently the only medication on the market for treating hair loss. It grows hair in about 20 to 25 percent of those who use it. Minoxidil is a clear solution that you apply to your scalp twice daily. The medication generally has to be used for at least four months before any signs of new growth occur (if new growth occurs at all), and it has to be continued for as long as you want to retain the new hair. In other words, once you stop using minoxidil, you will most likely lose the new hair. Researchers are developing new drugs that may be combined with minoxidil to give an enhanced effect, says Marty Sawaya, M.D., Ph.D. If you would like to know more about minoxidil, contact your doctor.

Your other option is a hair transplant. Often, a hair transplant can be done in a doctor's office under local anesthesia. These procedures are usually quite successful.

◆ HANGOVERS ◆

8 Tips to Get You Back on Your Feet

Ah, the morning after. There's nothing in the world quite like it, except, perhaps, being flattened by a steamroller and living through it.

Although they are the most revered of self-inflicted ailments, hangovers are not well understood. Many physicians believe that they arise from two phenomena—a slight swelling of the brain and dehydration.

The mechanism causing the swelling of the brain is not clear, but it may be a selective effect of alcohol, according to Joseph A. Lieberman III, M.D., M.P.H., chairman of the Department of Family and Community Medicine at the Medical Center of Delaware in Wilmington. The dehydration occurs because alcohol acts as a diuretic, causing you to urinate more frequently.

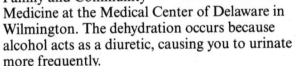

Whatever the exact reasons that you're feeling so bad, the bottom line is that you do. The tips that follow are the doctor's prescription for some relief.

Replace your fluids. Since much of the discomfort of a hangover comes from the dehydration your body experiences, drinking lots of liquids may make you feel better, according to Lieberman. "Rehydrate yourself with something that is not offensive to your stomach," he says. "The alcohol tends to make the mucous membranes of the stomach and small intestines sensitive and irritated. Acidic fluids, like orange juice, may make it worse." Some tried-and-trues are water and mildly carbonated sodas. Skip the Bloody Mary mix.

Treat it early. Hangovers are one ailment where the treatment may be more effective if it precedes the symptoms, according to E. M. Hecht, M.D., a New York-based general practitioner. Also, "with any pain syndrome, it's best to treat it in its earliest stages," he says. He recommends drinking plenty of fluids before going to bed, and, if you suspect that you'll be waking with a headache, taking a dose of acetaminophen.

Stick with clear liquids. Until you feel that you've really recovered, it's probably best to avoid food, especially foods that are spicy or highly seasoned, says Lieberman. He recommends sticking with liquids until you feel you are able to tolerate something solid.

Eat a banana. "Some people believe you need to replace potassium because of what you may lose with the frequent urination that you experience when you drink alcohol," Hecht says. If your stomach can handle it, eating a few bananas may help you feel better more quickly, he explains.

Take two acetaminophen. Nonaspirin pain relievers, especially acetaminophen, are probably the best cures for a hangover-induced headache, says Lieberman. Although aspirin will probably also work for pain, it can aggravate an already irritated stomach, he says.

Skip the hair of the dog. Some people swear that a morning drink of whatever you drank last night will cure a hangover. However, doctors don't tend to agree with this "hair-of-the-dog-that-bit-you" philosophy. "It will dehydrate you further. Don't do it," says Gary H. Goldman, M.D., an assistant attending physician at The New York Hospital–Cornell Medical Center in New York.

"Drinking the next day will only re-create the problem," says James E. Bridges, M.D., a family physician in Fremont, Nebraska.

Common sense says that the logic of this remedy seems to be lacking. After all, if you hit your thumb with a hammer, would you hit it again to stop it from hurting?

Treat it like an illness. 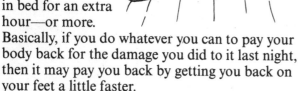 Cancel your appointments for the day. Call in sick to work, if you can. Draw the shades. Take the telephone off the hook. Stay in bed for an extra hour—or more. Basically, if you do whatever you can to pay your body back for the damage you did to it last night, then it may pay you back by getting you back on your feet a little faster.

Take it easy on your tummy. "Eat sick foods, such as toast, soup, or tea, if you can hold anything down," suggests Goldman. Try nibbling rather than sitting down to a full meal. Let your stomach be your guide as you go through the recuperation process. ◆

◆◆◆ Rules of Prevention ◆◆◆

By following a few simple guidelines, you may be able to avoid ever getting a hangover in the first place, according to Joseph A. Lieberman III, M.D., M.P.H.

Although the most obvious prophylaxis is abstaining from alcohol altogether, you may also prevent a hangover by slowing the pace of your partying. "Try to delay the absorption of alcohol into your system," Lieberman says. "Don't drink on an empty stomach. You'll be protecting yourself as long as you have something in there to compete with absorption of alcohol." He suggests having something to eat within two hours of drinking or snacking while you drink. Another good rule of thumb is to drink no more than one alcoholic drink (a 6-ounce glass of wine, a 12-ounce beer, or an ounce of hard liquor) per hour.

You might also try staying away from red wine to help prevent that morning-after headache. All

alcohol, but especially red wine, contains high amounts of an amino acid called tyramine, according to E. M. Hecht, M.D. Tyramine has been associated with headaches (migraine patients are often told to avoid alcohol). If red wine seems to bother you, try switching to another type of drink.

Drinking fluids before you go to bed may also be helpful in warding off the dehydration that contributes to the development of a hangover, says Hecht. Some proponents of this theory suggest drinking one glass of water for every alcoholic drink you consumed.

The worst kind of hangover is the kind that can come from drinking and driving. This kind of hangover can land you, an innocent third party, and/or those you love in the hospital or the cemetery. The best prescription for preventing this type of a morning after is simple: Don't drink and drive.

◆ HEADACHES ◆

16 Ways to Keep the Pain at Bay

Headaches. We've all had them. From the morning-after-celebrating-too-much headache to the tough-day-at-the-office headache to the you-might-as-well-kill-me-now-because-I'm-going-to-die-anyway headache. Sometimes, an aspirin or other analgesic may ease the pain; at other times, nothing short of waiting it out seems to help.

If you suffer from frequent, severe headaches that put you out of commission several times a month, you need to seek medical attention. Likewise, if your headaches are associated with physical exertion, changes in vision, or weakness, numbness, or paralysis of the limbs, skip the urge to self-treat and see a doctor. If you're already seeing a physician and aren't getting relief, think about getting a referral to a headache specialist or headache clinic.

However, if you are prone to occasional headache pain, read on. The tips that follow can help you feel a lot better—fast.

Don't overdo the pain pills. Although an occasional dose of an over-the-counter analgesic may help alleviate your headache for a few hours, taking these drugs too often may actually worsen the pain, according to Sabiha Ali, M.D., a neurologist at the Houston Headache Clinic in Texas. "These drugs are OK in limited quantities," she says, "but if you need to take more than two doses a day, you should see a doctor."

Lie down. Lying down and closing your eyes for half an hour or more may be one of the best treatments for a bad headache. For some types of headaches, such as migraines, sleep is the only thing that seems to interrupt the pain cycle. "The most important thing is to recognize that the faster the patient with a severe headache stops what they're doing and goes to bed and rests, the faster the headache will go away," says James R. Couch, Jr., M.D., Ph.D., professor and chairman of the

Headache Resources

The following associations provide support and information for headache sufferers:

The American Council for Headache Education (ACHE). *ACHE provides patient information and referrals to headache specialists. The organization also sends out free informational pamphlets about headache treatment. In the future, ACHE plans to set up patient-support groups around the country. You can contact ACHE at 1-800-255-ACHE.*

The National Headache Foundation. *This organization sends out free headache information to patients and publishes a headache newsletter. You can contact the Foundation at 1-800-843-2256.*

Department of Neurology at the University of Oklahoma Health Sciences Center in Oklahoma City. "You need to recognize when the big headache is coming. That's the time to give up and go to bed."

Don't let the sun shine in. Especially if your symptoms resemble those of a migraine (such as severe pain on one side of the head, nausea, blurred vision, and extreme sensitivity to light), resting in a darkened room may alleviate the pain. Bright light may also cause headaches, according to Seymour Diamond, M.D., founder of Diamond Headache Clinic in Chicago. "Sometimes, looking at a computer screen may bring on a headache," he says. "Tinted glasses may help."

Use a cold compress. A washcloth dipped in ice-cold water and placed over the eyes or an ice pack placed on the site of the pain are other good ways of relieving a headache, says Fred D. Sheftell, M.D., director and founder of The New England Center for Headache in Stamford, Connecticut. "Other good solutions are the 'headache hat,' which is an ice pack that surrounds the head, and the ice pillow, which is a frozen gel pack that is inserted into a special pillow," he says. (These special ice packs can be found in some pharmacies; if you don't see them at yours, ask your pharmacist about ordering them.) Using ice as soon as possible after the onset of the headache will relieve the pain within 20 minutes for most people, Sheftell adds.

Try heat. If ice feels uncomfortable to you, or if it doesn't help your headache, try placing a warm washcloth over your eyes or on the site of the pain, Ali says. She recommends leaving the compress on for half an hour, rewarming it as necessary.

Think pleasant thoughts. Many headaches are brought on or worsened by stress and tension, according to Couch. Learning to handle life's difficulties in a calm way may keep the volume down on a bad headache, he says. "Turn off all thoughts of unpleasant, crisis-provoking things," he says. "Think about pleasant things. Just for the moment, try to forget about the confrontation with the boss or the coworker. Try to relax while you work out a strategy to cope with the problem."

Check for tension. Along with the preceding tip, Sheftell recommends that patients periodically check their body for tension throughout the day. "If you notice that you get these headaches frequently, check the body for signs of tension," he says. "Are your jaws set very tightly? Are you scrunching your forehead? You want to check

◆◆◆ Dr. Diamond's ◆◆◆ Antiheadache Diet

At Diamond Headache Clinic in Chicago, patients are advised to eat a diet low in tyramine, an amino acid that is known to promote headaches, nausea, and high blood pressure in certain individuals. People who take certain antidepressant drugs called monoamine oxidase (MAO) inhibitors are especially prone to accumulating high amounts of tyramine. The following diet keeps tyramine levels to a minimum.

Beverages
Foods allowed: Decaffeinated coffee, fruit juices, club soda, noncola sodas. Caffeine sources to be limited to no more than two cups per day.

Foods to avoid: Caffeine (does not contain tyramine, but aggravates headache symptoms): coffee, tea, colas in excess of two cups per day. Hot cocoa, all alcoholic beverages.

Dairy
Foods allowed: Milk: homogenized, low-fat, or skim. Cheese: American, cottage, farmer, ricotta, cream cheese. Yogurt: limit to one-half cup per day.

Foods to avoid: Cultured dairy, such as buttermilk, sour cream, chocolate milk. Cheese: blue, boursault, brick, Brie types, Camembert types, cheddar, Swiss, Gouda, Roquefort, Stilton, mozzarella, Parmesan, provolone, Romano, Emmentaler.

Meat, Fish, Poultry
Foods allowed: Fresh or frozen turkey, chicken, fish, beef, lamb, veal, pork, eggs (limit three per week), tuna fish.

Foods to avoid: Aged, canned, cured, or processed meats; canned or aged ham; pickled herring; salted, dried fish; chicken liver; aged game; hot dogs; fermented sausages (no nitrates or nitrites allowed), including bologna, salami, pepperoni, summer sausage; any meat prepared with meat tenderizer, soy sauce, or yeast extracts (it's not the yeast itself that's a problem, but yeast contains an enzyme that alters an amino acid to become tyramine).

Breads and Cereals

Foods allowed: Commercial breads: white, whole wheat, rye, French, Italian, English muffins, melba toast, crackers, bagels. All hot and dry cereals: cream of wheat, oatmeal, cornflakes, puffed wheat, rice, bran, etc.

Foods to avoid: Hot, fresh, homemade yeast breads; breads and crackers containing cheese; fresh yeast coffee cake, doughnuts, sourdough breads; any breads or cereals containing chocolate or nuts.

Starches

Foods allowed: Potatoes, sweet potatoes, rice, macaroni, spaghetti, noodles.

Vegetables, Legumes, and Seeds

Foods allowed: Asparagus, string beans, beets, carrots, spinach, pumpkin, tomatoes, squash, corn, zucchini, broccoli, green lettuce. All except those listed in the next paragraph.

Foods to avoid: Pole, broad, lima, or Italian beans; lentils; snow peas; fava, navy, or pinto beans; pea pods; sauerkraut; garbanzo beans; onions (except as a condiment); olives; pickles; peanuts; sunflower, sesame, or pumpkin seeds.

Fruit

Foods allowed: Prunes, apples, cherries, apricots, peaches, pears. Citrus fruits and juices: Limit to one-half cup per day of orange, grapefruit, tangerine, pineapple, lemon, or lime.

Foods to avoid: Avocados, bananas (one-half allowed per day), figs, raisins, papaya, passion fruit, red plums.

Soups

Foods allowed: Cream soups made from list of allowed foods, homemade broths.

Foods to avoid: Canned soups, bouillon cubes, soup bases with autolyzed yeast or monosodium glutamate (MSG)—read labels.

Desserts

Foods allowed: Fruits listed above, sherbets, ice cream, cakes and cookies made without chocolate or yeast, gelatin.

Foods to avoid: Chocolate-flavored ice cream, pudding, cookies, or cakes; mincemeat pies.

Sweets

Foods allowed: Sugar, jelly, jam, honey, hard candy.

Foods to avoid: Chocolate candies, chocolate syrup, carob.

Miscellaneous

Foods allowed: Salt (in moderation), lemon juices, butter or margarine, cooking oils, whipped cream; white vinegar and commercial salad dressing in small amounts.

Foods to avoid: Pizza, cheese sauce, soy sauce, monosodium glutamate (MSG) in excessive amounts, yeast, yeast extracts, Brewer's yeast, meat tenderizers, seasoning salt, macaroni and cheese, beef stroganoff, cheese blintzes, lasagna, frozen dinners, and any pickled, preserved, or marinated foods.

to see if your fists are clenched. Also, when you stop at a red light, are your hands gripping the wheel very tightly?" If the answer to any of the questions is yes—stop, relax, and take a deep breath or two (don't go beyond a couple of deep breaths, though; otherwise, you may begin to hyperventilate).

Quit smoking. Smoking may bring on or worsen a headache, Couch says, especially if you suffer from cluster headaches—extremely painful headaches that last from 5 to 20 minutes and come in groups.

Don't drink. Alcohol, aside from its notorious morning-after effect, may also bring on migraines and cluster headaches, according to Diamond. Alcoholic beverages contain tyramine, an amino acid that may stimulate headaches (see "Dr. Diamond's Antiheadache Diet" for other foods and beverages that contain tyramine).

Start a program of regular exercise. Regular exercise helps to release the physical and emotional tension that may lead to headaches, according to Ali. She recommends walking or jogging. These and other aerobic activities, she says, help to boost the body's production of endorphins (natural pain-relieving substances).

Cut down on caffeine. "Caffeine can increase muscle tension and your anxiety level," Sheftell says. "It also creates difficulties in sleeping, which can cause headaches." Another problem is that many people drink several cups of coffee a day during their work week but cut their consumption on weekends. This can lead to weekend caffeine-withdrawal headaches, according to Sheftell. "My advice to those people is for them to slowly decaffeinate themselves," he says. "Decrease your caffeine intake by one-half cup per week. I suggest that people who are prone to headaches cut down to the equivalent of one cup of caffeinated coffee per day," says Sheftell. One five-ounce cup of drip

coffee contains about 150 milligrams of caffeine. A five-ounce cup of tea brewed for three to five minutes may contain 20 to 50 milligrams of caffeine. And cola drinks contain about 35 to 45 milligrams of caffeine per 12-ounce serving. Sheftell also recommends checking the caffeine content of any over-the-counter drugs in your medicine cabinet.

Fight the nausea first. Some headaches may be accompanied by nausea, which can make you feel even worse. What's more, the gastric juices produced by stomach upset may hinder the absorption of certain over-the-counter and prescription analgesics, which may make these drugs less effective at relieving the pain of your headache. So, by first taking care of the nausea, the pain of the headache may be easier to treat, says Sheftell. He says that many of his patients have found that drinking peach juice, apricot nectar, or flat cola has helped alleviate nausea. Over-the-counter antinauseants such as Emetrol and Dramamine may also be useful.

Rise and retire at the same time every day. Going to bed and getting up at the same time every day also helps prevent headaches, according to Diamond. "Changes in body chemistry that occur when you oversleep can precipitate migraines or other headaches," he says.

Keep a headache diary. If you get frequent headaches, try to tease out the factors that seem to be responsible, says Sheftell. "Pick up patterns. Figure out a way to record headaches and rate them on a zero-to-three scale of intensity: no headache, mild headache, moderate to severe headache, incapacitating headache. Start to look at what foods you are eating. Women should begin tracking their periods, as well as their use of hormone-replacement medications or oral contraceptives. You can show this calendar to your doctor." ◆

Recipes for Relaxation

In addition to being given an antityramine diet (see "Dr. Diamond's Antiheadache Diet"), patients at Diamond Headache Clinic in Chicago are instructed in relaxation techniques. The following is a typical relaxation exercise. The exercise can be memorized, or the written instructions can be recorded on a cassette tape. The entire exercise, which relaxes the facial area, neck, shoulders, and upper back, takes about five minutes. Before you begin, make sure you won't be disturbed—close the door and take the phone off the hook.

1. Settle back quietly and comfortably into a favorite chair or sofa. Allow your muscles to become loose and heavy.

2. Wrinkle up your forehead, hold it, then smooth it out, picturing the entire forehead becoming smoother as the relaxation increases.

3. Frown, creasing your eyebrows tightly, feeling the tension. Let go of the tension, smoothing out your forehead once more.

4. Close your eyes more and more tightly. Feel the tension as you hold them shut. Relax your eyes until they are closed gently and comfortably.

5. Clench your jaws and teeth together. Feel the tension build, then let go and relax, letting the lips part slightly. Allow yourself to feel relief in the relaxation.

6. Press your tongue hard against the roof of your mouth. Again, feel the tension, then relax.

7. Purse your lips together more and more tightly, then relax. Notice the contrast between tension and relaxation. Feel the relaxation all over your face, forehead and scalp, eyes, jaws, lips, and tongue.

8. Press your head back against your chair, concentrating on the tension in the neck. Roll your head to the right and feel the tension shift. Repeat to the left. Straighten your head and bring it forward, pressing chin to chest. Finally, allow your head to return to a comfortable position.

9. Shrug your shoulders up to your ears, holding the tension, then drop. Repeat the shrug, then move the shoulders forward and backward, feeling the tension in your shoulders and upper back. Drop the shoulders and relax.

10. Allow the relaxation to spread deep into the shoulders, into your back. Relax your neck and throat. Relax your jaws and face. Allow the relaxation to take over and grow deeper and deeper. When you are ready, slowly open your eyes.

Fred D. Sheftell, M.D., recommends the following relaxation exercise to his headache patients:

Lie down and relax your muscles. Place your hand on your stomach and take a deep breath. As you inhale to the count of five, feel your stomach rise. Allow yourself to slowly exhale to the count of five, letting your stomach fall. Imagine that you are breathing in relaxation and breathing out tension. As you breathe, visualize the muscles in your head and neck as if they were scrunched up, tense. Then, picture them becoming relaxed and smooth, parallel to one another. Continue the deep breathing for five minutes, then slowly open your eyes.

♦ HEARTBURN ♦

21 Ways to Beat the Burn

Heartburn. The word evokes a frightening picture: Your heart on fire, sizzling and smoking, without a fire fighter in sight. Fortunately, the word is a misnomer. It's not your heart that's on fire, it's your esophagus. But heartburn is easier to say than "esophagusburn."

The "burn" part, however, they got right. Your esophagus, the food tube that carries what you swallow down to your stomach, can literally be burned by the acids released by your stomach. Those acids are industrial-strength stuff and are meant to stay where the tough stomach lining can handle them.

Unfortunately, we can experience something called reflux. That's when some of the stomach contents, including the acid, slip back up through the esophageal sphincter, the valve that's supposed to prevent the stomach's contents from reversing course.

David M. Taylor, M.D., a gastroenterologist and assistant professor of medicine at Emory University in Atlanta and at the Medical College of Georgia in Augusta, puts it plainly: "If it goes south, that's good; if it goes north, you're in trouble."

Reflux causes an uncomfortable burning sensation between the stomach and the neck. Most people feel the discomfort right below the breastbone.

The easy way to avoid a simple case of heartburn? Moderation. Heartburn is generally the result of eating too much too fast. But if it's too late for moderation, here are some ways to put out that fire and keep it from flaring up again.

Take an antacid. Over-the-counter antacids in tablet or liquid form can help cool the burn. Take a dose about every six hours as needed, says Nalin M. Patel, M.D., a gastroenterologist in private practice and clinical instructor at the University of Illinois at Urbana-Champaign. Don't overdo it, though, because too much antacid can cause constipation or diarrhea.

♦♦♦ Is It Really ♦♦♦ Heartburn?

If symptoms don't subside, you may have something other than a simple case of heartburn.

"Persistent heartburn can be a sign of significant disease," warns David M. Taylor, M.D. "They [persistent-heartburn sufferers] can have hiatal hernia or esophagitis [inflammation of the esophagus], they can have an ulcer in their stomach, they can have an ulcer in the duodenum [part of the small intestine], and in an older person, they can even have cancer. And sometimes heartburn can mimic coronary disease, and they can have heart trouble."

The best advice: If symptoms persist, see your doctor.

Don't forget your bedtime dose. Even if you forget to take an antacid during the day, try to remember to take one at bedtime to protect yourself from the pooling of stomach acids. 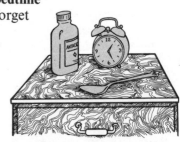 "Nighttime damage is probably the worst that will occur, because you're bathing your esophagus in acid, and you're much more prone to burn it," says Douglas C. Walta, M.D., a gastroenterologist in private practice in Portland, Oregon. Try keeping a bottle of antacid on your nightstand so that you remember to take your nightly dose.

Keep your head up. Another way to protect your esophagus while you sleep is to elevate the head of your bed. That way, you'll be sleeping on a slope, and gravity will work for you in keeping your stomach contents where they belong. Put wooden blocks or bricks under the legs at the head of your bed in order to bring it up about six inches, advises Patel.

Have a glass of milk. Milk can sometimes cut the acid and decrease heartburn, says Taylor.

Get rid of your waterbed. "People with waterbeds who have reflux have to get rid of their waterbeds," says Walta. "They don't like to hear that." The problem with a waterbed is that your body basically lies flat on the water-filled mattress. You can't effectively elevate your chest and so can't keep your stomach contents from heading north.

Say no to the couch. Tempting as it may look, the couch is not your friend after eating a meal. People who lie down with a full stomach are asking for trouble. "Stay upright for one hour after meals," says Patel.

Don't eat before bed. Heading from the dinner table to bed is a no-no for heartburn sufferers. In fact, doctors recommend warding off sleepy time for two to three hours after a meal. And by that, they mean staying upright for that amount of time. "You should stay upright until the gastric contents are emptied," says Walta.

Pass on seconds. "If you overeat, it's kind of like a balloon," says Walta. "If you blow it up real tense, it's more likely to empty quickly if you release the valve." A stomach, ballooned by too much food and drink, may partly empty in the wrong direction.

Loosen your belt. "Avoid tight clothing around the waist," says Patel. "This tends to increase acid backing up into the esophagus."

Lose the fat. If you're fat on the outside, you can be sure you're fat on the inside, too, says Walta.

Heimlich Maneuver Won't Help This

Heartburn can become very serious, says Douglas C. Walta, M.D. The acid reflux of heartburn can sometimes burn the lining of the esophagus so badly that scar tissue will build up. The resulting strictures can cause food to get stuck in the esophagus.

A person with a piece of food stuck in his or her esophagus can still breathe and talk, says Walta. "It doesn't interfere with breathing, but if it totally occludes, all of a sudden you can't swallow your saliva."

The Heimlich maneuver, used for dislodging an object that is obstructing the airway, is not the appropriate treatment in this case. Usually, a doctor must use a special instrument that is inserted into the esophagus to dislodge the food. So if it feels as if you have food stuck in your esophagus or if you are having trouble swallowing your saliva, see a doctor.

"The fat competes for space with your stomach." Fat pressing against the stomach can cause the contents to reflux.

Don't blame the baby. For the same reason that fat can impede normal digestion—competition for space—pregnancy can cause heartburn. That's all the more reason expectant mothers should watch what they eat and give up that nonsense about eating for two. Remember, pregnant or not, you only have one stomach. Be sure to discuss with your doctor any questions you may have about proper diet and weight gain during pregnancy.

Get in shape. "Couch potatoes have heartburn," states Taylor. "You almost never have heartburn when you exercise." Even mild exercise done on a regular basis, such as a daily walk around the neighborhood, may help ease digestive woes. However, avoid working out strenuously immediately after a meal; wait a couple of hours.

Watch your diet. "A high-carbohydrate, low-fat, high-bulk diet is the best thing," says Taylor. Fried foods and fatty foods should be avoided, he says, because they take longer to digest. Highly spiced foods sometimes contribute to heartburn as well.

Don't smoke. Nicotine from cigarette smoke irritates the valve between the stomach and the esophagus, as well as the stomach lining, so smokers tend to get more heartburn.

Be careful of coffee. It may not be the caffeine that's the problem. The oils contained in both regular *and* decaffeinated coffee may play a role in heartburn. Try cutting your coffee intake to see if your heartburn troubles subside.

Be wary of peppermint. For some people, peppermint seems to cause heartburn. Try skipping the after-dinner mints and see if it helps.

Hold the pepper. For people with heartburn problems, using pepper is not such a hot idea, says Kimra Warren, R.D., a registered dietitian at St. Vincent Hospital and Medical Center in Portland, Oregon. Sprinkling or grinding pepper, whether red or black, onto your food may be contributing to your heartburn troubles, so try going easy on it.

Take it easy. "A big contributor to heartburn is stress," says Taylor. Stress can create increased acid secretion and can cause the esophageal sphincter to malfunction.

Don't crack open a cold one. Alcohol can relax the sphincter, notes Taylor. It can irritate the stomach, too, which can lead to reflux.

Slow down on soda. Carbonated beverages and soda pop can contribute to heartburn woes. "Carbonation causes stomach distention due to gas, and that causes acid rolling back up into the esophagus," Patel explains.

Check your painkiller. If you're about to pop a couple of aspirin in your mouth, think again. Aspirin, ibuprofen, and products that contain them can burn the esophagus as well as the stomach, warns Walta. Opt for acetaminophen instead. ◆

◆ HEART PALPITATIONS ◆

7 Ways to Control Them

In the language of romance, a racing, thumping heart is a sure sign that you're in love. In the language of medicine, those same symptoms indicate that your heart's rhythm is out of whack. One common—and altogether normal—alteration is a speeding up of the heart rate during exercise or during an intense emotional experience. All of the body's cells and tissues demand more oxygen-rich blood at such times, and the heart accommodates by accelerating the delivery process. In spite of a rapid heartbeat, the normal rhythm stays steady: Once you have stopped exercising, the heartbeat will slow to what is called the "resting heartbeat"—72 regular beats a minute is the average, although an individual's resting rate may be as low as 40 (during sleep or in athletes) or as high as 100.

Another common disturbance in heart rhythm is called a premature beat—or extrasystole. In this situation, a beat, which originates in the upper or lower chamber of the heart, happens a little earlier than anticipated. It may be followed by an unnervingly long pause, in which you sense a little flutter in the neck and chest and a sudden empty feeling in the stomach. Then there is the noticeable thump of another heartbeat, whereupon the symptoms disappear as quickly as they started. (Such extra beats may also occur without noticeable symptoms.)

Everyone has experienced at least one episode of premature heartbeat. Sometimes, the sensation is so vague and fleeting that the event may pass unnoticed. Such episodes may be more noticeable when you are at rest and your attention is not otherwise occupied. If you are trying to fall asleep, the sensation may prevent you from doing so. Premature beats occur in normal hearts as well as in those that have been damaged by some form of heart disease. While they are bothersome, they are not usually serious. (If you experience irregular

Runaway Heartbeats

Several types of prescription and nonprescription drugs have a stimulant effect, which can cause a rapid or pounding heartbeat as well as other symptoms. If you are taking any of the following types of medications and have experienced heart palpitations, there is probably a link. Don't stop taking a prescription medication on your own, however; call your doctor or mention it during your next regular visit.

- *Monoamine oxidase (MAO) inhibitors (antidepressant medications)*

- *Appetite suppressants (amphetamine and nonamphetamine types)*

- *Asthma medications (sympathomimetics and theophyllines)*

- *Cough/cold medications (oral, nasal drops, spray, and inhalers containing nasal decongestants)*

- *Attention deficit disorder medications*

- *Narcolepsy medications*

- *Thyroid medications*

heartbeats on a regular basis or if they are associated with pain, breathlessness, dizziness, and/or nausea, see "Heartbreakers.") Still, there are some steps you can take that may help keep your heartbeat steadier.

◆◆ Heartbreakers ◆◆

"While occasional palpitations—especially when the episodes can be traced to a specific reason, such as exercise or excitement—are no cause for concern, some heart-rhythm disturbances are extremely worrisome and should be brought to the immediate attention of a doctor," says Jonathan S. Steinberg, M.D.

Which palpitations warrant medical attention? The answer depends on what else is going on. If the symptoms come on out of the blue, if they happen repeatedly in a very short time span, and if the heartbeat is very rapid, very intense, and long lasting or if the sensations are accompanied by lightheadedness or fainting, you should contact your doctor.

If three or more premature beats occur, the condition is called a tachycardia, which can originate in any one of the heart's four chambers. Abnormal heart rhythms can also result from conduction abnormalities that slow the heart down or even cause the heart to stop sending out signals altogether. Any of these situations are potentially dangerous and should be carefully evaluated. The doctor may recommend that you wear a portable heart monitor, which records the heart's electrical activity, for 24 hours or more in order to detect and evaluate the abnormality. Other specialized tests may also be performed.

Consider your caffeine intake. Caffeine is a nervous-system stimulant that is present in coffee, tea, and cola-type soft drinks as well as in chocolate. In small amounts, caffeine may "rev" you up and even keep you from falling asleep at your desk. In large doses or in sensitive individuals, however, it may cause palpitations and other unpleasant side effects. "Since caffeine is habit forming, it may be difficult to wean yourself away from the different caffeine-containing products you use in the course of a day, but the positive result will be worth it," says Jonathan S. Steinberg, M.D., director of the Arrhythmia Service at St. Luke's–Roosevelt Hospital Center in New York.

How much caffeine is too much? "Keep your caffeine intake below 500 milligrams a day," advises Steinberg. A five-ounce cup of drip coffee contains about 150 milligrams of caffeine. A five-ounce cup of tea brewed for three to five minutes contains 20 to 50 milligrams of caffeine. Cola drinks generally contain about 35 to 45 milligrams per 12-ounce can. As you tally up your caffeine intake, keep in mind that cough and cold products, menstrual-discomfort products, and pain medications may contain appreciable amounts of the stimulant; check the labels.

Nix the nicotine. In addition to the havoc nicotine wreaks on other parts of the body, it also speeds up the heart rate and can cause it to become irregular. So, if you have not stopped smoking yet, don't wait a minute more!

Ease up. One of the most common causes of palpitations is anxiety. "Worry and tension may actually cause the heart rate to increase," notes Lynda E. Rosenfeld, M.D., associate professor of medicine and pediatrics at Yale University School of Medicine in New Haven, Connecticut. "What's more, anxious individuals may have a heightened awareness of body functions, such as heartbeat, even if those functions are normal."

Turn in earlier. If you have been trying to get by on too little sleep, your palpitations may be your heart's way of telling you to slow down. "During a long night's sleep, your body's demand for oxygen-rich blood is reduced so that your heart can relax just a little in its never-ending pumping job. After a few nights of uninterrupted sleep, you may find that your palpitation problem has resolved," says Steinberg.

Check your iron. Palpitations may reflect a case of severe iron-deficiency anemia. A major function of your blood is to transport oxygen —via red blood cells —to every part of your body. When you are deficient in red blood cells or in iron, which is the mineral in red blood cells that carries the oxygen, the tissues in your body become undernourished. Consequently, your heart beats faster, trying to send more of the iron-poor blood to the organs in

an effort to make up for in quantity what is lacking in quality. "If you are severely anemic, you may also be feeling extremely fatigued in general and be noticing that your skin—especially on the palms of your hands—is pale," notes Arnold J. Greenspon, M.D., clinical professor of medicine and director of the Cardiac Electrophysiology Laboratory at Thomas Jefferson University Hospital in Philadelphia. "While eating iron-rich foods, such as green, leafy vegetables, can help, the best way to get a diagnosis and a treatment is to see your doctor." Once your anemia has been diagnosed and corrected, your heart palpitations should abate, as well.

Dump the diet pills. If you are trying to lose weight with over-the-counter diet pills, you may be losing a steady heart rate in addition to pounds. The active ingredient in these products—phenyl-propanolamine, or PPA—should not be used by people with heart-rhythm problems. "Drugstore aids for weight loss tend to lose their effectiveness in a very short time," notes Greenspon. "Thus, you take more and more of them—with a further increase in heart rate." (Diet pills are not the only drugs that can cause heart palpitations, however; see "Runaway Heartbeats.") ◆

◆ HEAT EXHAUSTION ◆

21 Ways to Regulate Your Thermostat

Sometimes, it's just too darn hot. Extreme heat, especially when coupled with exertion, can put a terrible strain on the body. Occasionally, it's enough to make the hypothalamus go haywire and send the body's temperature-control system into turmoil.

The hypothalamus is a cherry-sized part of the brain that serves as the body's thermostat. Thanks to the hypothalamus, the body switches on its temperature regulators, such as sweating and shivering, to protect us from extreme heat or cold. When the hypothalamus is not able to produce the desired responses to keep the body from overheating, however, the result can be heat illness.

There is a progression of symptoms associated with heat illness. It may start with heat cramps in the thighs and buttocks, then move on to a headache and dizziness. In extreme cases, there may be vomiting, disorientation, a dangerous drop in blood pressure, and even death.

Symptoms of heat exhaustion—headache, nausea, profuse sweating, fatigue, feeling faint—are considered middle range. In other words, you're not doing too well, but you're not as bad off as someone with heatstroke, which is considered the most severe and the most life-threatening of the heat illnesses.

Still, heat exhaustion is nothing to take lightly. "It's the first step on the road to having heatstroke," says Ronald Shelton, M.S., a certified athletic trainer in Rockford, Illinois. "If you get heatstroke, the hypothalamus shuts down. That's when you have somebody going into shock."

Here's what to do to keep out of danger:

Preload with water. James Rogers, M.D., an adolescent and sports medicine physician at Virginia Mason Medical Center and clinical associate professor of pediatrics at the University of Washington School of Medicine, both in Seattle, recommends drinking a full pint of water before beginning an activity in the sun. "Preloading gives you a better ability to sweat," he says.

Don't wait for thirst. Waiting until you feel thirsty is courting danger, says Shelton. "Once the body's thirst mechanism kicks in, it's already too late." Drink plenty of water before, during, and after the activity, whether or not you feel thirsty. Nina L. Turner, Ph.D., a research physiologist at the National Institute for Occupational Safety and Health (NIOSH), recommends drinking five to eight ounces of water every 15 to 20 minutes during the activity, or as long as you're sweating profusely.

Weigh yourself. Turner says it's easy to believe you've satisfied your need for water when your body actually is still dehydrated. One way to make sure you replace the water your body lost through sweat is to weigh yourself before and after an event. Any difference in weight represents lost water—water that needs to be replaced.

Make it cool, not cold. While you may be craving an icy cold drink of water, you're better off opting for one that's just cool. "If it's really cold, that inhibits gastric emptying of the fluid," says Turner. In other words, your body won't be able to use the water as quickly to fulfill its needs, including maintaining blood volume.

Go the distance with a sports drink. If you're planning to participate in an endurance or long-distance athletic event, like a marathon or long-distance bicycle race, a sports drink such as Gatorade may be a better choice than plain water. Such drinks contain some calories and some potassium and sodium. You'll need to dilute it with water, however, to make it easier to digest. "If it's a commercially available drink, it should be diluted, the more diluted the better," says Turner. "Certain components of commercial drinks cause inhibition of gastric emptying." In diluted form, these drinks are preferable to water for events lasting two hours or more, says Rogers.

Take frequent breaks. If you have to work or perform in the heat, avoid serious problems by taking frequent breaks—preferably including a cool drink—in a cool spot.

Don't play hero. Athletes or workers who are exerting themselves in the heat should never attempt to "run through" or "work through" the early symptoms of heat illness. "If people tend to exercise through that, then the body will go into something closer to heatstroke," says Shelton, "and that's a medical emergency." If you're participating in an athletic event, marching in a band, or working in the heat, take a break if you feel symptoms. "If you get to the point where you're dizzy and you're nauseated and feeling faint, you should be withdrawn from the event," says Rogers.

Don't be fooled. The symptoms of heat exhaustion sometimes can fool a victim into believing that it's a case of the flu. If your flulike symptoms of nausea, headache, and weakness coincide with overexposure to heat, it's probably not the flu at all. Get out of the heat and start replacing fluids.

Step into the shade. Moving out of direct sunlight or into a cooler environment, such as an air-conditioned building, may bring relief by lowering the body's core temperature, says Turner.

Get horizontal. If you start to experience symptoms of heat illness, lie down with your feet elevated. If possible, do so in a cool place.

Use ice with caution. Early symptoms of heat illness, such as muscle cramps, may be helped by

◆◆ The Galloping ◆◆ Symptoms of Heat Illness

Things can go from bad to worse quickly with heat illnesses. Once a person progresses toward symptoms of heatstroke, the situation becomes a matter of life and death. Medical attention must be sought immediately. Until help arrives, the victim should be kept cool through fanning and sponging with cold water.

During heatstroke, the body's heat-regulating mechanism, the hypothalamus, ceases to function. The core temperature of the body rises to a dangerous level. Blood pressure drops, and coma may occur. Death may follow if medical treatment does not begin immediately.

There is no way of guessing at what point a case of heat exhaustion will escalate to a potentially fatal condition. "Each case of heat exhaustion should be viewed as having the potential to progress to heatstroke," says Nina L. Turner, Ph.D.

Even the earliest symptoms of heat illness cannot be taken lightly. These symptoms have a tendency to gallop into more critical conditions without a moment's notice. So from the first sign of heat illness, get out of the heat and take care of yourself—before it's too late.

applying ice to the muscles. Putting ice bags across the major muscles helps cool the body's core temperature, as well, says Shelton. But he warns that too rapid cooling could worsen a person's condition and may even contribute to shock.

Fan yourself. Air blowing against skin helps dissipate heat, says Shelton. Turn on a fan or fan yourself with a newspaper, paper plate, or whatever's handy. This is only effective, however, if the air is relatively cool. It's not much help to blow hot air on someone with a heat illness.

Wear cool duds. The type of fabric and the fit of your clothing can be a factor in how heat affects you. Loose, cotton clothing is the best choice on a hot day. "Cotton is an airy fabric that breathes and allows the body to dissipate heat better," says Shelton.

Lighten up. Wear light-colored clothing, says Shelton. Darker colors absorb heat.

Don't strip. Going shirtless may look cooler, but you'll end up hotter than if you were wearing a light, loose-fitting top. Wearing a shirt helps wick away perspiration and heat from your skin. "If you didn't wear any shirt at all, your body couldn't get rid of the heat as efficiently," says Rogers.

Just say no. Say no to alcohol, particularly before having to exert yourself in the heat. "You're usually dehydrated after moderate alcohol consumption," says Turner. "Dehydration is a predisposing factor for heat exhaustion."

Avoid salt pills. Because some sodium is lost in perspiration, it used to be common practice to give salt tablets to athletes and other individuals who

were exerting themselves in the heat. However, this practice is, for the most part, not a good idea. That's because when you're very warm and sweating, you lose a lot of water, but only small amounts of salt. "Salt pills don't replenish any of the water loss, and you probably lose a liter per hour during vigorous exercise." If you gulp down salt tablets, you can actually increase your blood-sodium level, causing more discomfort. "You can easily make up the amount of salt lost in sweat by putting salt on your food," says Rogers.

Acclimatize. If you know you're going to be working or performing athletically in the heat, try to get your body used to the conditions so it will be able to produce sweat more efficiently. "If you are a triathlete and you want to do the Hawaii Ironman, you would do well to go two or three weeks before the event to train," says Rogers, who is a triathlete himself.

Lose weight. Obese people are more susceptible to heat illnesses. "The bigger you are, the more heat you'll produce," says Rogers.

Know your medications. Several common medications, including propranolol, may mask signs of heat exhaustion or make you more susceptible to it. Ask your doctor or pharmacist whether any medication you may be taking could have this effect and what precautions you can take.

Protect your children. Children are prone to heat illness because they do not sweat as efficiently as adults do, says Rogers. They should, therefore, limit their play in the sun and drink plenty of water. Children are particularly at risk if they're already dehydrated from a recent illness that included vomiting and/or diarrhea. ◆

◆ HEMORRHOIDS ◆

14 Ways to End the Torment

When was the last time you heard a party conversation turn to the subject of hemorrhoids? The condition is rarely discussed, even between close friends and relatives, although Americans spend $150 million a year on remedies that promise relief.

Hemorrhoids are swollen and stretched-out veins that line the anal canal and lower rectum. Internal hemorrhoids may either bulge into the anal canal or protrude out through the anus, in which case they are called "prolapsed." External hemorrhoids occur under the surface of the skin at the anal opening. Regardless of type, hemorrhoids cause cruel distress: They hurt, burn, itch, irritate the anal area, and, very often, bleed.

About one-half to three-fourths of all Americans will develop hemorrhoids at some time in their lives. The following factors contribute to them, and some can be avoided.

• **Gravity.** Humans stand upright, which causes a downward pressure on all veins in the body, including those in the anal canal and rectum.

• **Genes.** If one parent has hemorrhoids, it is more likely that his or her child will develop them in adult life; if both parents have hemorrhoids, it is an almost certain outcome.

• **Age.** While hemorrhoids usually begin to develop when an individual is twenty years old or even earlier, symptoms usually do not appear until the thirties and beyond.

• **Constipation.** Difficulty in passing fecal matter creates pressure and possible injury to veins in the anal canal and rectum.

• **Low-fiber diet.** Highly refined foods (white flour products, sugar, foods high in fat and protein and low in complex carbohydrate) result in a fiber-deficient diet, with resulting constipation and hemorrhoids.

• **Obesity.** Added pounds put more pressure on veins. What's more, overweight individuals may be more likely to favor refined foods and a sedentary lifestyle.

• **Laxatives.** Improper use of these products is a major cause of constipation and, as such, it may also be considered a prime factor in the development of hemorrhoids.

• **Pregnancy.** As the fetus grows, it puts additional pressure on the rectal area. Pregnancy-related hemorrhoids usually retract after the baby is born, unless they were present beforehand.

• **Sexual practices.** Anal intercourse also puts pressure on veins in the anal canal.

• **Prolonged sitting.** Without some form of exercise, the heart muscle works more slowly in returning blood in the body's veins to the heart.

• **Prolonged standing.** The pull of gravity continues unabated on the body's veins in individuals who are on their feet all day.

Fortunately, most cases of hemorrhoids respond to basic self-care methods, so you may never have to tell a soul about them. (If you notice blood, see "Could It Be Something Else?") Here are the most effective steps you can take to soothe your achy bottom and keep hemorrhoids from flaring.

Rough up your diet.
"People who consume large amounts of food 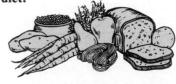 containing fiber—or what grandmothers used to call 'roughage'— rarely have problems with hemorrhoids," says Thomas J. Stahl, M.D., assistant professor of general surgery at Georgetown University Medical Center in Washington, D.C. Fiber passes through the human digestive tract untouched by digestive enzymes. As it travels, it has the capacity to absorb many times its weight in water; by the time it reaches the colon in combination with digestive waste, it produces a stool that is bulky, heavy, and soft—all factors that make it easier to eliminate. "Straining to have a bowel movement day after day because of

◆◆◆ Could It Be ◆◆◆ Something Else?

"Often people attribute symptoms to hemorrhoids when other conditions are to blame," notes Norton Rosensweig, M.D. Itching may be the result of poor anal hygiene, perianal warts, intestinal worms, medication allergies, psoriasis, other forms of dermatitis or local infection, or too much coffee. Pain can result from fissures—small cracks in the skin around the anus.

Erroneously attributing bleeding to hemorrhoids can be a serious mistake. Bleeding can be a symptom of colorectal cancer, which kills 60,000 people every year. "Rectal bleeding must be followed up promptly," cautions Rosensweig. While bright-red bleeding usually heralds hemorrhoids, don't try to make a diagnosis yourself. If you notice blood, see your doctor.

constipation is probably the main cause of hemorrhoids," says Norton Rosensweig, M.D., associate clinical professor of medicine at Columbia University College of Physicians and Surgeons in New York. According to medical experts, adding fiber to the diet is the only treatment necessary for about half of all hemorrhoid cases (see "An Apple a Day").

Drink up. Be sure to drink lots of water to keep the digestive process moving right along. A minimum of eight large glasses of water or other fluid a day is recommended, says Gayle Randall, M.D., assistant professor of medicine in the Department of Medicine at the University of California Los Angeles School of Medicine. And remember, fruits and vegetables, which are important sources of dietary fiber, come packaged in their own water.

Avoid sweat and strain. Don't try to move your bowels unless you feel the urge to do so. And don't spend any more time on the toilet than it takes to defecate without straining. "You should not try to catch up on yesterday's reading while sitting on the toilet," advises Rosensweig. Once your bowels have moved, don't strain to produce more.

Heed the call of nature. On the other hand, don't wait too long before responding to the urge to eliminate. The longer the stool stays in the lower portion of the digestive tract, the more chance there is for moisture to be lost, making the stool hard and dry. "The frenzied pace many people follow today can lead to elimination always getting low priority," says Stahl.

Try a different position. It has been suggested that squatting is a more natural position than sitting for moving one's bowels; unfortunately, Western toilets are not designed to make this possible for most people. "Try putting your feet on a small footstool to raise your knees closer to your chest," advises Randall.

Soften it. Sometimes, eating more fiber-packed food and increasing water intake aren't enough to solve a severe constipation problem. In this case, you might want to ask your doctor to recommend a laxative known as a stool softener (such as Colace or Correctol) or one that contains a natural bulking agent (such as Metamucil and Effer-Syllium). Experts agree, however, that the safest and best way to add fiber to the diet is through foods. Don't—repeat don't—use laxatives that act on the muscles of the colon and rectum; prolonged use of these products can cause permanent malfunction of the bowel in addition to severe irritation of the anal area. Avoid mineral oil, as well, since it can interfere with the absorption of some essential nutrients such as vitamin A. "Ordinary laxatives are short-term solutions that lead to long-term problems," says Rosensweig.

Take a walk. Regular exercise helps your digestive system work more efficiently. No need for strenuous aerobics, however; a lengthy walk at a brisk pace will do quite nicely.

Keep it clean. Keep your rectal area clean at all times. Residual fecal matter can irritate the skin, but so can vigorous rubbing with dry toilet paper. Randall's suggested solution: "Gently rinse the area with plain water while sitting on the toilet. Then pat the area dry and dust with powder, preferably nontalc and unperfumed." More convenient, but also more expensive, are premoistened wipes designed for anal care. These

Those Over-the-Counter "Shrinks"

Drugstore remedies for hemorrhoidal discomfort usually achieve part of what they promise: temporary relief of pain and itching. Claims that they can shrink hemorrhoids or reduce inflamed tissue, however, don't hold up when put to the test, say the experts.

Over-the-counter aids are available in three forms: cleansers, suppositories, and creams and ointments. The cleansers, although effective, are more costly than ordinary warm water, which works very well. Suppositories may be of little use, according to some experts, because they may slip up into the upper rectum, bypassing the area they are meant to soothe. Ointments are greasy and tend to retain moisture, which can lead to increased irritation. Creams, especially hydrocortisone creams, are effective; however, their prolonged use may lead to dependency and can also cause thinning of the skin.

Furthermore, while some drugstore remedies may feel good, they may cause more harm than good in the long run. Some of these products should not be used by individuals with certain medical conditions, such as heart disease or diabetes, so you'll need to check the label of any product you are considering. In addition, many preparations contain a number of ingredients, including anesthetics, astringents, counterirritants, and skin protectants, which may cause an allergic reaction in some persons that is far worse than the discomfort of the hemorrhoids themselves.

The Food and Drug Administration has also made some specific rulings about products marketed for hemorrhoidal use.

• Boric acid is no longer allowed. While it's safe enough for ordinary skin, it is toxic if absorbed by the mucous membranes.

• Painkilling ingredients are out, too, because rectal nerves don't sense pain and, therefore, such ingredients are unnecessary.

• Lanolin alcohols, cod liver oil, and Peruvian balsam are banned as ineffective rather than unsafe.

• Product labels must say "If your condition worsens or does not improve in seven days, consult your doctor."

• Product labels claiming to shrink tissue must also caution: "Do not use this product if you have heart disease, high blood pressure, thyroid disease, diabetes, or difficulty in urinating due to an enlarged prostate gland unless directed by a doctor."

Keep in mind that, according to the experts, using petroleum jelly or zinc oxide ointment or powder may be as beneficial as any "hemorrhoid preparation" you can buy.

◆ An Apple a Day ◆

One of the most important moves toward healing hemorrhoids is a change in diet. "By all means, increase your intake of fiber-rich foods—but do it gradually," advises Norton Rosensweig, M.D. Too rapid an increase can cause gas, abdominal cramps, or diarrhea. As it is, you can expect some increase in intestinal gas at first, but this will subside in a week or two as your system and the bacteria that inhabit your colon adjust to your new diet.

Here are some foods that can increase the fiber content of your diet when eaten regularly:

Vegetables	**Grains**
Carrots	Wheat, whole
Brussels sprouts	Rye, whole
Eggplant	Rice, brown
Cabbage	Corn, milled
Corn	Oatmeal,
Green beans	unprocessed
Lettuce	Oats, rolled
	Bran,
Fruits	unprocessed
Apples	miller's
Oranges	
Pears	**Legumes**
Figs	Lima beans
Prunes	Soy beans
Apricots	Kidney beans
Raisins	Lentils
	Chick peas

wipes, however, may cause irritation in some people, says Randall. If you want to try them, they are available without a prescription at pharmacies and drugstores.

Rinse well. Soap residue can also irritate the anal area. "Be sure to rinse the anal area completely after a bath or shower," says Randall.

Skip the soap. If you find that, even with thorough rinsing, soap still irritates the anal area, look for a special perianal cleansing lotion in your drugstore. Follow the package directions.

Soften your seat. If your job demands that you sit all day, try sitting on a donut-shaped cushion—an inexpensive device that takes the pressure off the sensitive area. "But it's still important to get up and walk around whenever possible," says Stahl.

Sitz around. Sit in six inches of warm water on your donut cushion or a towel twisted into a circle big enough to support your bottom. "Taken three or four times daily, a half-hour sitz bath will soothe inflamed tissues and relax muscle spasms," says Randall.

Take the heat. Even if you can't manage a full-scale sitz bath, applying a washcloth moistened with warm water can soothe the painful area.

Slim down. If you are overweight, you'll be doing your bottom a favor by getting your weight closer to the desirable range. Of course, you'll be doing the rest of your body good, too. ◆

◆ HICCUPS ◆

13 Techniques Worth a Try

"It's a reflex similar to your leg jerking when a doctor hits a hammer to your knee." So says George Triadafilopoulos, M.D., a gastroenterologist and associate professor of medicine at the University of California at Davis, in describing hiccups. Hiccups result when the vagus nerve or one of its branches, which run from the brain to the abdomen, is irritated. And the vagus lets you know by tweaking the phrenic nerve, which leads to the diaphragm, the muscle below the lungs that helps you breathe. The diaphragm then spasms, causing the "hic."

Experts say hiccups are most often a reaction to common digestive disturbances. And luckily, they're usually more a nuisance than anything else. But what about the times when we seem to hiccup for no apparent reason? No one knows for sure why these seemingly innocuous bouts occur. What experts do know is that even infants hiccup, and the reflex continues, about three to five times a year, throughout life.

The home remedies used to stop a hiccuping bout are believed to work on two principles. Some basically rely on overstimulating the vagus nerve. "Nerves deal with a number of different sensations, from temperature to taste," Triadafilopoulos explains. "When one sensation is more overwhelming than another, the vagus nerve tells the brain that there's something more important to deal with. The brain then shuts off the hiccup response." Other methods, which interfere with breathing, increase the amount of carbon dioxide in the blood, probably causing the body to become more concerned with getting rid of the carbon dioxide than making hiccups. Here are some tried-and-true remedies from both "camps."

Play "hear no evil." Some doctors recommend that you put your fingers in your ears—and not because they don't want you to hear yourself hiccup. It seems that branches of the vagus nerve also reach into the auditory system, and by stimulating the nerve endings there, the vagus nerve goes into action. "The pressure you create in the ears," says Triadafilopoulos, "is similar to the gag reflex caused when you put a finger in the back of your mouth." Of course, other doctors insist that you should never put anything smaller than your elbow in your ear in order to avoid irritating or damaging the ear canal. So if you do decide to try this hiccup reliever, be gentle, and don't stick your fingers too far into your ears.

Get scared silly. Having someone surprise you may be the one method that overwhelms the vagus nerve more than anything else. "It's similar to the method an adult uses to quiet a child who's crying endlessly. Out of frustration, a parent may yell at the child to stop, and sure enough, the child will stop, almost as if on cue," says Triadafilopoulos. Scaring the vagus may shut it up.

Drink water. Swallowing water interrupts the hiccuping cycle, which can quiet the nerves. Gargling with water may also have the same hiccup-stopping effect.

Sweeten the hiccups. Mary Poppins sang that a spoonful of sugar helps the medicine go down. But does it help hiccups? Many experts think so. "The nerve endings in the mouth become overloaded with the sweet sensation," Triadafilopoulos explains. Have a teaspoonful of sugar, and if you can, place the sugar on the back of the tongue, where "sour" is tasted. This way, the sugar overload will pack the most punch.

Pull on your tongue. Sticking out your tongue and yanking on it may stop hiccups, says Howard Goldin, M.D., clinical professor of medicine at The New York Hospital–Cornell Medical Center in New York.

◆ When You Can't ◆ Stop the Hiccups

Though thankfully rare, "chronic or consistent hiccups can be a sign of a more serious problem," says George Triadafilopoulos, M.D. He estimates the number of causes at as many as 100. Among the medical reasons: infection; renal (kidney) failure; liver disease; cancer, including lung cancer, nervous system or abdominal problems, such as ulcers; and even heart attacks. Virtually anything that affects the head, chest, or abdomen can be implicated, reports the National Heart, Lung, and Blood Institute in Bethesda, Maryland.

"Normally, people get hiccups about three to five times a year," says Howard Goldin, M.D. A common bout usually lasts no more than an hour, and the hiccups occur at a rhythmic interval of about every 30 seconds. It's time to worry if the hiccups continue with frequency for more than an hour or as many as 12 hours plus, with no relief from home remedies. And "hiccups that keep you awake at night should be diagnosed," says Allan Burke, M.D.

In some cases, a physician will prescribe antacids or a sedative to help calm the digestive system. And in instances of severe, nonstop hiccuping, surgery may be performed to cut the phrenic nerve's link to the diaphragm in order to stop the spasms.

Tickle it away. Tickling the soft palate of the roof of your mouth with a cotton swab may do the trick. Or, if you're the type who enjoys getting tickled, it may be more fun to have someone find your ticklish spots.

Hold your breath. Hold your nose and close your mouth—like when you jump in a pool.

Bag those hiccups. Breathing into a paper bag is believed to work on the same principle as breath-holding. They increase the amount of carbon dioxide in the bloodstream, and the body becomes preoccupied with getting rid of it.

Take an antacid. "One or two tablets should help, especially if you take the kind that contains magnesium," says Allan Burke, M.D., assistant professor of clinical neurology at Northwestern University School of Medicine in Chicago. Magnesium tends to decrease the irritation and quiet the nerves, he says.

Eat more slowly. "People who eat too fast tend not to chew well, which can cause hiccups," says Triadafilopoulos. And besides that, you swallow more than the meal. "Air gets entrapped between pieces of food," he explains. Chew deliberately and take smaller sips of drinks.

Don't pig out. Overloading the stomach with food is another cause of hiccups. Triadafilopoulos has a theory as to why some digestive disturbances trigger a bout: "If you're eating too much or too fast, hiccups may be the body's way of stopping you from continuing to binge, which gives the digestive system a chance to catch up and recover."

Avoid spicy foods. Some spices can irritate the lining of the esophagus (the food pipe) and stomach. At the same time, they can also cause acid from the stomach to leak into the esophagus. The extra acid can bring on a bout.

Drink only in moderation. Like spices, alcoholic beverages can cause a simultaneous irritation of the esophagus and the stomach. And with time, excessive drinking can damage the lining of the food pipe. But long-time alcoholism isn't the only cause. Parties, like the kind some college students attend, where people are sometimes dared to consume a lot of alcohol as quickly as possible, can lead to what is called acute ingestion. The digestive system not only becomes irritated by the alcohol, but big gulps of it cause the esophagus to expand rapidly, resulting in hiccups. ◆

◆ HIGH BLOOD ◆ CHOLESTEROL

21 Heart-Healthy Ways to Lower It

Heart attacks are the leading cause of death in the United States. In 1989 alone, says the American Heart Association (AHA), heart attacks claimed the lives of 497,850 American men and women.

What causes a heart attack? In most cases, an attack occurs when the blood supply to part of the heart muscle is severely reduced or stopped, according to the AHA. This stoppage is caused when one of the arteries that supply blood to the heart is obstructed, usually by the fatty plaques that characterize atherosclerosis, a result of coronary-artery disease.

Although it's not clear where the plaques come from in each individual case, the most common causes are a blood cholesterol level that's too high, a hereditary tendency to develop atherosclerosis, and increasing age (55 percent of all heart attack victims are 65 or older, 45 percent are under 65 years of age, and 5 percent are under 40). Other factors that contribute to the likelihood that heart disease will develop are cigarette smoking, high blood pressure, and male sex (although after menopause, a woman's risk rises to almost equal that of a man), according to the AHA.

You can't change your age, your gender, or your genes, but you can make positive lifestyle changes that can sharply reduce your risk of developing heart disease. Getting your blood cholesterol down to a level that's considered low risk (see "Low, Borderline, High—What Do the Numbers Mean?") is an important first step. The following tips are designed to help you take that step.

Adopt a new lifestyle. Making a commitment to lowering blood cholesterol and improving your heart health requires a change of mind-set, not a temporary fad diet, according to Henry Blackburn, M.D., Mayo Professor of Public Health and a professor of medicine at the University of Minnesota in Minneapolis. "You need to adopt a healthy lifestyle, a familywide lifestyle," he says. "Even if one member of your family has a low risk of developing heart disease, that doesn't mean his or her risk will stay low. Our risk rises as we get older, and it takes a lifetime to establish good habits." Lifetime good habits also mean avoiding "yo-yo" dieting—losing weight and gaining it back repeatedly. Yo-yo dieting has been shown to cause cholesterol levels to rise.

Know it's never too early to act. Although much of the emphasis on heart disease risk is placed on people with a total blood cholesterol level over 240, the numbers can be a bit misleading, says William P. Castelli, M.D., director of the Framingham Heart Study in Massachusetts, the oldest and largest heart disease study in the United States. "Most heart attacks occur in people with a total cholesterol level between 150 and 250," he says. "Many doctors don't understand that. That group up at the top, the highest-risk group (with cholesterol levels above 240), only produces about 20 percent of the heart attacks." Even if you're in a low or borderline group, you still need to pay attention to your lifestyle habits, he advises.

Ignore the magic bullets. This week it's rice bran, last week it was oat bran and fish oil. All were touted as the solution to your cholesterol problem. While it's the American way to search for shortcuts, such an approach just doesn't cut it when you're dealing with your health, according to Basil M. Rifkind, M.D., F.C.R.P., chief of the Lipid Metabolism and Atherogenesis Branch at the National Heart, Lung, and Blood Institute in Bethesda, Maryland. "We are very cautionary about these magic-bullet remedies," he says. "If someone's cholesterol is high, we know that it comes about by eating a bunch of foods that are

The American Heart Association Diet

The following are the dietary guidelines put forth by the American Heart Association. They are designed to prevent heart attacks, stroke, and other manifestations of cardiovascular disease from occurring in healthy adults.

1. Total fat intake should be less than 30 percent of daily calories.

2. Saturated fat intake should be less than ten percent of daily calories.

3. Polyunsaturated fat intake should not exceed ten percent of daily calories.

4. Cholesterol intake should not exceed 300 milligrams per day.

5. Carbohydrate intake should constitute 50 percent or more of daily calories, with an emphasis on complex carbohydrates.

6. Protein intake should provide the remainder of the calories.

7. Sodium intake should not exceed three grams (3,000 milligrams) per day.

8. Alcohol consumption should not exceed one to two ounces of ethanol per day. Two ounces of 100-proof whisky, 8 ounces of wine, and 24 ounces of beer each contain 1 ounce of ethanol.

9. Total calories should be sufficient to maintain the individual's recommended body weight, as defined by the Metropolitan Tables of Height and Weight (Metropolitan Life Insurance Company, New York, 1959).

10. A wide variety of foods should be consumed.

higher than the optimum in fat and cholesterol. We need to address the source of the problem, instead of paying attention to garlic, fiber, or fish oil."

Stay away from saturated fats. Many people make the mistake of believing that if their blood cholesterol level is high that it's because they ate too many foods containing cholesterol. Not exactly true, says W. Virgil Brown, M.D., past president of the AHA and professor of medicine and director of the Division of Arteriosclerosis and Lipid Metabolism at Emory University School of Medicine in Atlanta. The number-one cause of high serum cholesterol is eating too much saturated fat, the kind of fat that is found in full-fat dairy products and animal fat, he says. Another culprit is partially hydrogenated vegetable oil, which contains *trans* fatty acids, substances that increase the cholesterol-raising properties of a fat. The best rule of thumb is to stick with fats that are as liquid as possible at room temperature, according to Brown. "For example," he says, "if you are going to use margarine, use the most-liquid kinds, such as the tubs or squeeze bottles."

Read your meat. The small orange labels stuck to packages of meat at the grocery store aren't advertisements or promotions; they're actually grades of meat, says Castelli. "Prime," "Choice," and "Select" are official U.S. Department of Agriculture shorthand for "fatty," "less fatty," and "lean," he explains. "Prime is about 40 percent to 45 percent fat by weight, Choice is from 30 percent to 40 percent fat, and Select, or diet lean, is from 15 percent to 20 percent fat," he says. You could have a hamburger made from Select ground beef for breakfast, lunch, and dinner and still not exceed your daily saturated fat limit, he adds.

Learn to count grams of fat. The AHA's dietary guidelines outline the percentages of daily calories that should come from fat (see "The American Heart Association Diet"). However, since most package labels show grams of fat, not percentages, it can be difficult to figure out exactly what you're eating, Castelli says. Instead, he recommends counting grams of fat. How many grams of fat, and how many grams of saturated fat, can you have each day? Multiply your total number of calories per day by .30, then divide by 9 to find the number of grams of total fat allowed. (You divide by 9 because each gram of fat provides 9 calories.) Multiply your total number of calories per day by .10 and divide by 9 to find the number of grams of saturated fat allowed each day.

"If you're on a 2,000-calorie-per-day diet, you should eat no more than 22 grams of saturated fat a day," Castelli says. "The average American eats twice as much."

What can you eat for 22 grams of fat? One serving of Choice beef contains from 12 to 15 grams of fat, whereas a serving of Select contains 4 to 10. One tablespoon of butter is just under seven grams, while many brands of low-fat margarine contain only one gram per tablespoon. Whole milk has a whopping five grams per cup; skim milk just one. You add it up. After all, if you choose the lower-fat versions of each item, maybe you'll have enough saturated fat calories left in your daily budget to indulge in some low-fat frozen yogurt, a cup of which may contain as little as two grams of saturated fat.

Go to the extreme. Although the AHA recommends deriving 30 percent or fewer of your daily calories from fat, some heart specialists believe it's not only safer, but better, to go even lower than that. (The average American derives about 37 percent to 40 percent of his or her calories from fat.) "It's quite appropriate for a person with a high degree of risk for heart disease to go to these sort of extremes," says Blackburn. "That means reducing fats way down. You can go down even to five percent of your calories from fat without hurting yourself. We've examined populations in Japan who consume 9 percent to 12 percent of their calories from fat and they are perfectly healthy and have very low cholesterol. It's worth the effort."

Eat as much like a vegetarian as possible. Dietary cholesterol is found only in animal products;

animal products also tend to be higher in fat (skim-milk products are exceptions), especially saturated fat. Foods derived from plant sources, on the other hand, contain no cholesterol and tend to be lower in fat. The fats they do contain tend to be polyunsaturated and monounsaturated, which are healthier than the saturated kind, says Peter F. Cohn, M.D., chief of cardiology at the State University of New York at Stony Brook. (The exceptions are coconut oil, palm oil, palm kernel oil, and partially hydrogenated oils, which contain higher amounts of saturated fatty acids.) You'll be doing your arteries a favor if you increase your intake of vegetable proteins, such as beans, whole grains, and tofu, and keep servings of high-fat animal products to a minimum.

Increase your carbohydrate intake. Adding extra servings of complex carbohydrates into your diet will fill you up and make you feel more satisfied, leaving less room for fatty meats and desserts, says Cohn. Complex carbohydrates include fruits, vegetables, pasta, whole grains, and rice.

Grill it. Grilling, broiling, and steaming are heart-smart ways to cook food, says Brown. Unlike frying, they require no added fat.

Skin a (dead) chicken. The skin of chicken (and turkey, too, for that matter), is an absolute "no-no" for people who are watching their fat intake, according to Cohn. The skin contains high amounts of saturated fat, he says.

Skip the pastry. One hidden source of saturated fat is pastry—donuts, Danishes, piecrust, éclairs, and so on, says Brown. These confections are often made with shortening or butter—two things that should be limited by people who are working to

Low, Borderline, High—What Do the Numbers Mean?

According to the American Heart Association (AHA), total levels of blood cholesterol under 200 milligrams per deciliter represent a low risk for coronary heart disease. Levels between 200 and 240 are considered to be borderline risk, and over 240 is considered dangerously high risk.

While total levels of blood cholesterol are considered important, other factors come into play, as well. For example, if someone has a borderline-high total cholesterol level, but has very low levels of HDL, the "good" cholesterol, he or she may still have a high risk of heart disease. In general, doctors worry about the ratio of LDL (the "bad" cholesterol) to HDL.

A desirable HDL level is over 50, according to W. Virgil Brown, M.D. For LDL, a level below 130 is desirable, 130 to 160 is borderline high, and over 160 represents a high risk of heart disease, he says. Although these numbers aren't absolute (for example, levels of triglycerides, another fatty acid, also enter into the big picture), they do represent a fairly good predictor of heart disease risk, according to Brown. "We know that, on average, for every one percent increase in total blood cholesterol, there is a two to three percent increase in heart disease rates," he says. "For a person with a total cholesterol of 220, their risk is ten percent higher than a person with a total cholesterol of 200. A person with a level of 250 has a 50 percent higher risk than the person with 200."

reduce their saturated fat intake. Stick with whole-grain bread and rolls, and read labels to be sure you know what's in the package, he suggests.

Eat fish. Fish oil, as a cholesterol reducer, has gotten a lot of play in the media in the past few years. And it is true that the slimy stuff contains high levels of omega-3 fatty acids, substances that have been associated with lower cholesterol levels, according to Blackburn. However, the greatest benefit has been achieved in people who frequently substitute their intake of higher-fat meats with fish. Also, fish oil itself tends to be high in fat, Blackburn says. His advice is to add more servings of fish into the diet (as substitutes for some of the meat dishes) and reap the oil's benefits naturally.

Go easy on yolks. You can have all the eggs you like, as long as you leave the yolks behind. Egg yolks are more than 50 percent fat and also contain high amounts of cholesterol. Egg yolks may also be hidden inside processed foods, so be sure to read labels carefully. The AHA recommends limiting egg yolks to no more than three per week, including those found in processed foods or used in cooking.

Eat smaller meat portions. One way to cut down on saturated fat without giving up steaks is to keep your portions small, says Brown. "Reduce the size of the meat portions, even chicken, to about three ounces per serving," he advises. "Try to have a vegetarian lunch. Then you can have six ounces at dinner." A three-ounce serving is about the size of a deck of cards, Brown says.

Give up organ meats. Like eggs, organ meats are something best left behind as a memory of foods gone by, says Brown. Although rich in iron and protein, these meats are also tremendously high in fat and cholesterol. And remember—pâté is made from liver, so it, too, should be restricted.

Increase your fiber intake. Soluble fiber, the kind found in fruits and brans, has been shown to be effective in lowering cholesterol levels, says Brown. However, to exert this effect, it must be consumed in high amounts; a bowl of oatmeal a day probably won't make much difference. "You have to eat about a quarter pound of oatmeal per day to get ten grams of soluble fiber a day, the amount that can lower cholesterol," he says. He recommends a daily one-teaspoon dose of a psyllium-husk powder, such as Metamucil, which provides a lot more bang for your buck. "For the person whose cholesterol is still borderline high after changing their diet, psyllium may give them another eight percent to ten percent reduction in their LDL," he says. And no need to go overboard, either. More than ten grams a day won't make much more of a difference, he says. It's also prudent to increase your fiber intake gradually in order to give your system time to adjust.

Eat like the rest of the world. "Four billion of the 5.3 billion people on this earth eat 15 grams of saturated fat or less each day," says Castelli. "Where do they live? Asia, Africa, and Latin America. They are the four billion people that never get atherosclerosis. We want our 250 million people to eat like those 4 billion. If we accomplished this, we could get rid of heart attacks, stroke, and other manifestations of cardiovascular disease. We could live five years longer, which isn't much. However, we wouldn't have heart attacks in our 40s, 50s, 60s, 70s, or 80s. That is the vision for America."

Quit smoking. Most of us are aware that smoking can cause lung cancer and raise the risk of heart attack, but few people know that smoking can actually affect your cholesterol levels, says Brown. "When you stop smoking, your HDL levels rise significantly," he explains. "A two-pack-a-day smoker who quits may have an eight-point rise in their HDL cholesterol."

Add exercise to your daily routine. Studies have shown that regular aerobic exercise can boost levels of HDL, says Brown. "Exercise can be very useful in reducing body weight, which can help cholesterol levels," he says. "When you engage in even modest amounts of exercise, your triglycerides come down, your LDL comes down, and your

---

◆◆◆ Heart-Smart ◆◆◆ Glossary

The following are definitions of terms commonly used in discussions of cholesterol and cardiovascular health:

LDL: *Low-density lipoprotein, the "bad" cholesterol often implicated in the development of atherosclerosis*

HDL: *High-density lipoprotein, the "good" cholesterol thought to protect against atherosclerosis*

Triglycerides: *Another type of fatty acid found in the blood that doctors measure when they evaluate heart-disease risk*

HDL goes up after several months." He recommends 30 to 45 minutes of moderate exercise, such as walking, five days per week. It is important to accelerate your heart rate and keep it up for at least 20 minutes, he says. However, he adds, it is not necessary to do your exercise all at once. Try parking your car a quarter mile from work and walk it twice a day. Take the stairs instead of the elevator. It all adds up.

Know it's never too late. Even if you've had a heart attack or have other evidence of heart disease, changing your lifestyle can still dramatically reduce your risk of a recurrence, says Rifkind. In the past, heart specialists thought that lifestyle changes couldn't make much of a difference for people who already had heart disease. They now believe differently. "We want the cholesterol to be much lower in these people than in their healthy counterparts," he says. "For these people, the target levels of total serum [blood] cholesterol are between 160 and 170." ◆

◆ HIGH BLOOD PRESSURE ◆

13 Ways to Reduce It

At last count, 62,770,000 Americans had or were being treated for high blood pressure, according to the American Heart Association (AHA). That's almost one-quarter of our country's population. Every year, 31,630 of these individuals die as a direct result of the condition, the AHA says. An additional 147,470 deaths every year occur from stroke (a blood clot that travels to the brain), making it the number-one fatality related to high blood pressure. Another 2,980,000 Americans have had a stroke and lived. Many of these people are now severely disabled and unable to care for themselves.

High blood pressure, or hypertension, is defined as having blood pressure (the force that is created by the heart as it pumps blood into the arteries and through the circulatory system) equal to or higher than 160 systolic (the top number) over 95 diastolic (the bottom number), according to William P. Castelli, M.D., director of the Framingham Heart Study in Framingham, Massachusetts, the oldest and largest heart-disease study in the United States. Between 140 and 159 systolic over 90 to 94 diastolic is considered "borderline" high. Below these numbers is considered normal.

In addition to strokes, high blood pressure can cause blindness, kidney failure, and a swelling of the heart that may lead to heart failure.

Who's at risk for high blood pressure? People with a family history of the condition, blacks (they have an almost one-third greater chance of having high blood pressure compared to whites), overweight individuals, and aging individuals. Also at risk are women who are pregnant or who are taking oral contraceptives.

The good news is that, together with your doctor, you can control hypertension. It won't be easy—you'll have to change the way you think and act. You may have to take medication for the rest of your life. You'll definitely have to cut out some bad habits and begin some new, more healthful

ones. However, your efforts are likely to pay off in a longer, healthier life. Here's to your health!

Join the club. It may sound trivial, but the first step toward controlling your blood pressure is actually accepting that you've got a problem to begin with, says David B. Carmichael, M.D., medical director of the Cardiovascular Institute at Scripps Memorial Hospital in La Jolla, California. "People must accept the fact that they've got hypertension," he says. "The worst person in the world is an aggressive 40-year-old male who comes in feeling fine and is told he has hypertension and will have to monitor his blood pressure. They often just won't believe it. In fact, if I ask myself what type of patient has left my practice over the years, I would say it has been the hypertensives." Carmichael likens this type of acceptance to joining a fraternal lodge. "You've got to do certain things: go to the doctor, take your medications faithfully, modify your diet, report bizarre symptoms. You have got to join the club."

Lose weight. "At all levels of blood pressure, increased weight contributes to the degree of blood pressure elevation," says Robert A. Phillips, M.D., Ph.D., director of the Hypertension Section and associate director of the Cardiovascular Training Program in the Division of Cardiology at Mount Sinai Medical Center in New York. "Weight loss lowers blood pressure—not in everybody, but in many people. It's worth a try." Phillips explains that for each pound of excess body weight that is lost, blood pressure may drop by two points. "It's always a good thing to do, even if you are severely hypertensive," he says. "If you are mildly hypertensive, that weight loss may enable you to stay off of medication." Even a modest amount of weight loss is better than none at all, according to Castelli. "The most common problem in hypertension is borderline hypertension—between 140 and 159 systolic and 90 to 94 diastolic," says

Castelli. "That level of blood pressure increases the risk of stroke three times. And yet, virtually all of those people would be cured with a ten-pound weight loss."

Invest in a home blood pressure monitor. If you have been diagnosed as hypertensive, or if your doctor wanted more blood pressure readings before making a definitive diagnosis, he or she may have prescribed 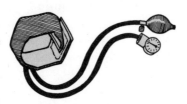 you a home blood pressure monitor. At-home monitoring has several benefits—first and foremost, warning you if your pressure becomes dangerously high, so you can get medical attention early. Second, a monitor can save you money, because it will save you trips to the doctor. "This is now very common," says Carmichael. "It is also easy to do. If the patient is afraid to use the monitor [some people become panicky if they find their pressure is high], another person, such as a spouse, can do it for them. The blood pressure should be checked at close to the same time of day, under the same conditions." Carmichael says that most insurance companies will cover the purchase of such devices if prescribed by a physician.

Start an exercise program. Along with helping with weight loss, exercise confers additional benefits for those with high blood pressure, says Phillips. "For people who are severely hypertensive, they shouldn't exercise until their blood pressure is controlled," he says, "but people with mild hypertension can exercise aerobically for 20 to 30 minutes, three times per week, and will benefit with a reduction in blood pressure by about eight points that will last at least half a day." It's best to check with your doctor before beginning any exercise program, especially if you have been sedentary. The types of exercise that are most likely to benefit your blood pressure are walking, jogging, stair-climbing, aerobic dance, swimming, bicycling, tennis, skating, skiing, or anything else that

elevates your pulse and sustains the elevation for at least 20 minutes. Nonaerobic exercise, such as weight lifting, push-ups, and chin-ups, may actually be dangerous for hypertensives. These types of exercise should not be done without the explicit consent of your doctor.

Take your blood pressure medicine. The biggest danger with hypertension, Carmichael says, is that it is usually asymptomatic until its final stages, where it becomes fatal. That's why the condition is often labeled "the silent killer." Unlike people who have other chronic illnesses, such as diabetes, you'll probably feel just fine if you don't take your medicine. However, inside your body, the disease will continue to progress, damaging the arteries in your eyes, destroying your kidneys, causing your heart to swell, and so on. Another problem that can occur when you stop taking your blood pressure medicine is a rebound phenomenon, where the blood pressure rises to a higher level than it was before you started taking the medication. The moral of the story? "If you're starting and stopping taking your medication, you haven't joined the club," says Carmichael.

Cultivate a taste for less-salty foods. "There is no question that salt in the diet has a relationship with blood pressure," says Jeffrey A. Cutler, M.D., a hypertension specialist and chief of the Prevention and Demonstration Research Branch of the National Heart, Lung, and Blood Institute in Bethesda, Maryland. "We Americans take in far more salt than we need. We've become accustomed to the taste. However, the fact is that our taste sense is adaptable. People who lower the salt in their diets, after a period of time, have been shown to taste something as salty at a much lower level of salt than before." The average American takes in about eight to ten grams of salt a day, Cutler says. However, studies have shown that by cutting that amount down by a third, blood pressure can be significantly reduced, he says. Ideally, he says, people should cut down to six grams per day as a short-term goal, and to about four-and-a-half grams per day as a long-term goal.

Read labels. So how do you know how much salt you're eating? As far as table salt goes, one teaspoon contains over two grams—almost half of the recommended daily amount. Also, says Cutler, the average American adult takes in somewhere between one-and-a-half to two extra teaspoons of salt a day without knowing it. These insidious salt sources are frozen entrées, canned vegetables, even antacid medications. To avoid this extra salt, read labels. Many labels will express the amount of sodium in milligrams (1,000 milligrams is equivalent to 1 gram). To calculate the amount of sodium chloride, or salt, multiply the amount of sodium by two-and-a-half, Cutler says.

Say no to a second round. Restriction of alcohol consumption to one drink (1.5 ounces of hard liquor, 4 ounces of wine, or 12 ounces of beer) per day does not appear to increase the risk of high blood pressure, but consuming two or three drinks per day is associated with an elevated risk of hypertension, according to Phillips.

Eat a banana. One substance (other than prescription medication) that has been proven to reduce blood pressure is potassium, says Cutler. However, it may be difficult to increase your intake of potassium enough to lower blood pressure, he adds. While supplements may help, they are not recommended without the permission of a doctor, since they may be hazardous in individuals with certain medical conditions. "The average person needs three to four servings of potassium-rich fruits and vegetables per day," he says. "It would probably benefit your blood pressure in a detectable way if you could double that number of servings. A little more may be a little better, and a lot more may be a lot better." Potassium-rich foods include bananas, raisins, currants, milk, yogurt, and orange juice.

Drink your milk. Some studies have shown that extra calcium added to the diet may have a modest effect on blood pressure, says Phillips. Although the effect may not be significant, there's certainly

---

◆◆◆ Pregnancy and ◆◆◆ Hypertension

If you have been diagnosed as having high blood pressure and you become pregnant, you should see your doctor as soon as possible to discuss ways to control your condition during pregnancy.

During pregnancy, your blood volume triples, placing a great deal of additional strain upon the heart. Perhaps because of this increase in blood volume, many women who never had a problem with blood pressure become hypertensive, a condition called pregnancy-induced hypertension.

The problems of hypertension in pregnancy are twofold: First, the condition is extremely dangerous, posing a risk of stroke, preeclampsia (a condition that causes sudden weight gain, extreme water retention, blurred vision, and other symptoms), stillbirth, premature delivery, and low

birth weight. Second, blood pressure may be difficult to control without medication, and many medications may pose a danger to the developing fetus.

However, several studies have shown that extra calcium has a definite blood-pressure-lowering effect in pregnant women, according to Johns Hopkins researcher John T. Repke, Ph.D. Repke's findings show that pregnant women may need to take between one-and-one-half and two times the recommended daily allowance of calcium to keep their blood pressure at safe levels. However, he cautions that pregnant women should check with their doctors before taking supplements or exceeding the recommended amount of any nutrient.

The recommended daily allowance for calcium during pregnancy is 1,200 milligrams per day, the amount contained in about eight servings of low-fat milk, yogurt, or broccoli.

no harm in adding a few extra glasses of skim milk, low-fat yogurt, or leafy green vegetables to the daily diet, he says.

Add polyunsaturated oils to your diet. Most people know that by substituting polyunsaturated oils for saturated fats in their diets they can reduce their level of blood cholesterol. However, what most people don't know is that polyunsaturates can also reduce blood pressure, according to James A. Hearn, M.D., an assistant professor of medicine at the University of Alabama at Birmingham. "Switching to canola and safflower oils in cooking can cut your blood pressure by ten points," he says.

Quit smoking—now. Cigarette smoking is the number-one taboo for hypertensives, says Phillips. Not only does the nicotine in the smoke cause blood pressure to rise, but it dramatically raises your risk of stroke, he says. According to the AHA, cigarette smoking can thicken the blood and increase its propensity to clot. Blood clots in the arteries leading to the heart can cause a heart attack, while blood clots in the artery leading to the brain may cause a stroke, according to the AHA. The good news is, you get an immediate benefit by giving up the habit right now. "Two years after you quit smoking, your risk of developing coronary artery disease has dropped to the same level as someone who never smoked," Phillips says. In contrast, it can take much longer for a person's risk of lung cancer to drop to that level. Your doctor can be a great source of help to you in quitting smoking. He or she may prescribe nicotine gum or skin patches to reduce withdrawal discomfort. Your local Heart Association may also be able to provide you with resources.

Learn to relax. Many people misunderstand the term hypertension, believing it to mean a condition where the patient is overly tense. This isn't true. The term is defined solely by blood pressure levels. However, many hypertensives are the consummate "Type A" personality—aggressive, workaholic, hostile, frustrated, or angry, says Carmichael. For these people, some form of relaxation, be it prayer, yoga, biofeedback, or just resting, may be an

---

◆◆◆ Symptoms of ◆◆◆ a Stroke

If you are experiencing any of the following stroke symptoms, call your doctor or an ambulance at once. Waiting too long or not recognizing the signs could mean the difference between life and death. If you experience any of these symptoms and then feel better within 24 hours, you may have had a transient ischemic attack, or TIA. A TIA is a warning sign that a full-blown stroke is on its way. Again—call your doctor at once.

• *Sudden weakness or numbness of the face, arm, or leg on one side of the body*

• *Sudden dimness or loss of vision, particularly in only one eye*

• *Loss of speech, or trouble talking or understanding speech*

• *Sudden, severe headaches with no apparent cause*

• *Unexplained dizziness, unsteadiness, or sudden falls, especially along with any of the previous symptoms*

(Source: "1992 Heart and Stroke Facts," by the American Heart Association.)

---

important component of treatment, he says. "People need to recognize their personality traits and do their best to change," he says. Some chronically stressed-out individuals release a lot of adrenaline into their systems. That rush of hormone can constrict the arterioles (tiny blood vessels), causing them to go into spasm. It is difficult for the heart to push blood through constricted arterioles. The effect? Higher blood pressure, says Carmichael. ◆

• HIVES •

14 Methods for Relieving Them

Just about anything can make you break out in hives: Foods such as peanuts or strawberries, drugs such as penicillin or aspirin, vitamin supplements, heat, cold, sunlight, exercise, fever, stress, and even scratching or rubbing the skin are among some of the possibilities.

Some substances actually cause an allergic reaction that results in hives, while others have absolutely nothing at all to do with allergies. Strawberries, for example, contain a chemical that can cause cells in your body to release histamine, a chemical also produced in allergies, which allows blood plasma to leak into the skin and form the hives, explains Philip C. Anderson, M.D., chairman of dermatology at the University of Missouri–Columbia School of Medicine.

And sometimes only a tiny amount of the culprit is needed to set off a reaction. "You can be sensitive to fish and order something completely different in a restaurant. But it's cooked in a pan that was previously used to fry fish, and you break out in hives," explains Larry Borish, M.D., staff physician at National Jewish Center for Immunology and Respiratory Medicine in Denver.

Don't confuse hives with other skin eruptions. Hives (or urticaria) occur when blood plasma leaks into the skin, causing "wheals" or swollen areas. They can be as small as a pencil eraser or as large as a dinner plate, and they usually last only a few hours. But new hives may form continuously. And as they form, they often itch.

An attack of hives generally lasts a short time, often just a few days. (Some people, however, may be plagued with recurrent outbreaks or with hives that persist for years.) Here are some tips for relief.

Top Triggers of Hives

According to the American Academy of Dermatology, here are the most common foods that cause hives*:

Peanuts
Eggs
Nuts
Beans
Chocolate
Strawberries
Tomatoes
Seasonings such as mustard, ketchup, mayonnaise, and spices
Fresh fruits, especially citrus
Corn
Fish
Pork

The drugs most likely to cause hives are*:

Aspirin (check the labels on over-the-counter drugs, which may contain aspirin)
Penicillin
Sulfa drugs
Tetracyclines
Codeine

*This is not an all-inclusive list.

Take an oral antihistamine. The most recommended remedy is over-the-counter Benadryl but it may cause drowsiness. "That may not be so bad, since hives are generally worse at night, and the itch is more annoying then," says Borish.

Don't scratch. "It's said that with hives, a million scratches are never enough and one is too many," says Borish. Scratching can increase local inflammation and even cause more hives.

Wear gloves to bed. If you think you'll scratch in your sleep, gloves will help prevent damage.

Wrap up the affected area. Wrap an elastic bandage around the area with hives or cover it with clothing so you can't reach it with your fingernails.

Use a milk compress. Wet a cloth with cold milk and lay it on the affected area for 10 to 15 minutes at a time. "Don't freeze the skin," warns Judy Jordan, M.D., a dermatologist in San Antonio and a spokesperson for the American Academy of Dermatology. "Just cool it."

Chill the itch. Hold an ice pack or ice cubes in a thin towel on the skin for five minutes at a time, three to four times a day.

Take a bath. Put half a box of baking soda or one cup of oatmeal in the water first, says Jordan.

Try cortisone. A one percent cortisone preparation, available without a prescription, may help.

Try to ferret out the cause. "In the overwhelming number of patients, there's no explanation found," says Borish. "We only find the cause 20 to 30 percent of the time." Do remember that hives generally show up within half an hour of eating. "You don't get hives the next day from something you ate the night before," he says.

Avoid the trigger. This one's pretty obvious, but if you know that cold sets off hives, don't put your hands in the freezer. In fact, jumping into cold water could be life-threatening, points out Borish. And there's no question, he says, that if you're prone to hives, stress will trigger them.

Treat the underlying infection. If hives turn into a chronic problem, they may be due to an infection. "You can have a tooth or yeast infection and not be aware of it," points out Jordan. Consider these possibilities and have them checked out.

◆◆ Hello, Doctor? ◆◆

Many episodes of hives are short-lived inconveniences that go away on their own in a day or two. But sometimes hives become a long-term problem or indicate a more serious condition. See your doctor or visit the emergency room if you:

- *Have a lot of swelling around your face and throat*

- *Feel nauseated or dizzy*

- *Have trouble breathing*

- *Have a fever*

- *Are losing weight or suffering from malaise*

- *Have hives that persist for four to six weeks*

In some cases, diseases like thyroid disorders, hepatitis, lupus, or even some cancers can have hives as a symptom. Don't ignore hives that won't go away. "If you're sick otherwise and you're suffering from hives, you need to see the doctor," says Philip C. Anderson, M.D. "Hives could signal a serious internal disease in that case."

Relieve the pressure. Hives often form where clothing is tight, such as under bra straps or waistbands.

Use a moisturizer. If dry skin contributes to the itch, apply a moisturizer to relieve it.

Don't make the problem worse. Nonprescription anti-itch lotions or creams can cause allergic reactions. If you react to topical Benadryl and topical products ending in "-caine," you'll be in worse shape after using them. Calamine lotion, that old standby for so many itches, doesn't do much for hives either. ◆

HYPERVENTILATION

12 Ways to Catch a Breath

Shortness of breath, dizziness, blurred vision, numbness, heart palpitations, chest pain. Sounds serious. What is it?

More often than not, these frightening symptoms are part of a non-life-threatening condition called hyperventilation.

The problem with hyperventilation is that it's brought on by anxiety and certain breathing habits; then, after some or all of those scary symptoms kick in, it's heightened by the additional anxiety caused by the symptoms. Mounting anxiety causes a release of adrenaline in large quantities. Your body instinctively experiences the "fight or flight" response, a defense mechanism we humans share with animals. The heart rate quickens and blood is routed to the large muscles, in order to ease our "escape."

Hyperventilation occurs as a result of over-breathing. When frightened or anxious, people tend to blow off too much carbon dioxide. When carbon dioxide levels in the blood fall, blood vessels constrict in the brain and elsewhere in the body. Due to the "fight or flight" response, blood flow to the brain is already diminished. This cumulative reduction in blood to the brain causes dizziness, tingling, and/or numbness. Occasionally, people will hyperventilate to the point of passing out. Before that happens, try out these tips:

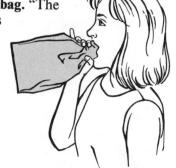

Breathe into a paper bag. "The theory behind that is the carbon dioxide will build up in the bag, and you'll rebreathe it," explains Michael B. Heller, M.D., F.A.C.E.P., an associate professor of medicine in the Division of Emergency Medicine at the University of Pittsburgh School of Medicine. Normal levels of carbon dioxide in the blood will then be restored.

◆◆ Don't Do This ◆◆ on Purpose

Voluntary hyperventilation is commonly done by some divers, especially "free divers," those who don't use air tanks, in order to prolong their dives.

But diving instructors adamantly counsel against it, says scuba instructor Andy Marshall.

"Most of the world-champion free divers have blacked out every once in a while, and there have been some deaths," says Marshall.

He says divers would exhale deeply several times before diving and deliberately blow off carbon dioxide. With less carbon dioxide in their blood, their brains failed to respond to the need for air, and they could stay underwater longer.

"You're just fooling yourself into thinking you have enough oxygen in your body, and you don't," says Marshall.

Don't try this with a plastic bag. It may seem obvious to you, but somebody out there might try it. It won't work, and you'll probably be worse off for even trying. Breathing into a plastic bag can cause suffocation.

Seek reassurance. In the grips of hyperventilation, it's hard to believe that you're really not suffering from a serious illness. Hearing it from someone else helps. "In terms of treatment, the most important thing is reassurance that the symptoms have a basis in anxiety, that they're not imagining these symptoms," says John H. Phillips, M.D., Lassen Professor of Cardiovascular Medicine at Tulane University School of Medicine in New Orleans. "We assure them of the absence of physical disease."

Find a friend. If at all possible, don't go through a hyperventilation episode alone. "Sometimes a friend can talk to them and have them breathe more slowly and deeply, rather than rapidly and shallowly," says Heller. "Sometimes that's enough."

Concentrate on something else. If you force yourself to think about something other than the panic you're experiencing, you may be able to trick yourself into feeling calm. Visualize a tropical beach, a snowy mountaintop, or some other scene that you perceive as tranquil.

Start exercising regularly. Exercise tends to build self-confidence while helping the body produce natural tranquilizers called endorphins, says Phillips. Stress reduction may cut down on incidents of hyperventilation.

Know thyself. Learn more about how your body responds to stress by doing biofeedback, suggests Heller.

Evaluate your stressors. "Sit down and write down all your sources of stress and then look at them," says Phillips. Figure out what things you can eliminate or modify. Find ways to live with the things you can't change.

Follow a schedule. With regular meals and regular sleep, your stress level will probably be reduced, and you'll be less likely to have hyperventilation episodes, says Phillips.

Reduce stimulants. Are you drinking a lot of coffee? What medications are you taking? Phillips says caffeine, diet pills, aspirin in large doses, and decongestants can aggravate anxiety and hyperventilation.

◆◆ Hello, Doctor? ◆◆

Hyperventilation is a disease of healthy people. If you're not young to middle-aged and in general good health, but you think you are experiencing the symptoms of hyperventilation, give up the guesswork and see a doctor.

"Generally, in younger people, the diagnosis (of hyperventilation) is fairly easy, but when you get into middle and older age, we have an intermingling of physical disease," says John H. Phillips, M.D.

People with hyperventilation have normal chest X rays and may have normal electrocardiograms (a method of testing electrical activity in the heart to detect abnormalities), says Phillips.

But if there truly is a physical basis for some of hyperventilation's typical symptoms, the person is sick indeed. For example, one of the anxiety-based symptoms is shortness of breath at rest. If it's not anxiety based, however, it spells trouble. "For a person to be short of breath at rest, if it's on the basis of physical disease, you have to have lost well over 50 percent of your lung function, or you have to have lost 30 to 40 percent of your heart function, or it has to be a severe anemia, with a 50 percent decrease in what your blood count should be," says Phillips.

Take a pill. Some people find that an over-the-counter oral antihistamine like Benadryl will relieve their symptoms, says Heller. Some antihistamines have a sedative effect and may calm your anxiety; check the label. While this may help in the short run, however, you still need to look into and modify the causes of your anxiety.

Have some milk. Drinking milk also seems to have a calming effect, Heller notes. ◆

◆ IMPOTENCE ◆

17 Ways to Improve Your Sex Life

Impotence. The word somehow sounds like failure, weakness. If you feel that you are impotent, you may also feel that you have somehow lost part of your dignity, your masculinity, your wholeness.

There are many degrees of erectile difficulties. Some men may be able to achieve an erection, but are not able to maintain it. Others become erect, but not extremely rigid. Still others only have problems when they are with a new partner or with a long-time partner. And of course, there are those who cannot achieve an erection at all.

Do not despair. You may be suffering from a physical or emotional problem (or both) for which there are definite solutions. If your problem is of an emotional nature, the following tips may help. If your erectile problems arise from a medical condition (see "Could It Be a Medical Problem?"), there are now many new surgeries and therapies that can help restore your sexual health.

Whatever the nature of your problem, remember that almost every man has difficulties with erection at some point in his life. You are not abnormal, nor are you alone. There is no need to suffer in silence. Don't let embarrassment keep you from sexual health and happiness.

Remove the performance demand. It's not unusual for a man to have an occasional episode of impotence, after drinking alcohol or after a particularly stressful day, for example. However, if he places too much emphasis on the incident and harbors fear that it may happen again, the anxiety itself may become a cause of erectile difficulties, says Michael E. Geisser, Ph.D., an assistant professor in the Department of Clinical and Health Psychology at the University of Florida in Gainesville. "Some men engage in thinking that distracts them or takes away from their sexual performance," he says. "Generally, we teach them behavioral exercises that take the performance demand out of the situation and relieve the anxiety

about having to get an erection." One strategy that sex therapists often use is to have couples abstain from intercourse altogether, telling them instead to engage in cuddling and nonsexual touch. Gradually, over a period of weeks or months, depending on the couple, the partners work toward more sexual touching, then intercourse. The idea is to make sex a less-threatening experience, Geisser says.

Break out of a rut. "One problem in people's sex lives is that they get into certain ruts and routines and they don't have much novelty," says William O'Donohue, Ph.D., an assistant professor of psychology at Northern Illinois University in De Kalb. "For example, they always have sex at 11:00 at night with the lights off, with the same foreplay, and so on. Their sex lives are relatively invariant. Soon, their partner becomes about as exciting to them as a flounder." His recommendations? Incorporate some variety—go to a hotel or a different setting. Vary the routine. Buy your wife some new lingerie. In short, spice up your sex life.

Learn to relax. Stress, arising either from performance anxiety or from other life situations, can also be a culprit in erectile problems, according to Geisser. Regardless of the cause, it's difficult to enjoy yourself when you've got too much on your mind. "Relaxation exercises are helpful," Geisser says. He recommends deep breathing or progressive muscle relaxation, where the person consciously tenses and relaxes each part of the body in sequence. "In and of itself, as a treatment for impotence, relaxation is not effective," Geisser says, "but it may be a good first step for someone trying to improve their own functioning."

Express your feelings. Marital or relationship difficulties are notorious contributors to sexual problems, according to Raul C. Schiavi, M.D., professor of psychiatry and director of the Human

Sexuality Program at Mount Sinai School of Medicine in New York. Anger, resentment, and hurt feelings often spill into the couple's sex life, turning the bedroom into a battlefield. This situation is especially likely to develop if partners are noncommunicative, therapists agree. "You need to verbalize your feelings," Schiavi says. "Not in terms of accusations, such as 'you did this,' or, 'you did that,' but more like 'I felt upset or hurt when you said that.'" In other words, use "I" statements, and keep the focus on your feelings, instead of on your partner's actions. Doing a thorough housecleaning of the relationship, instead of storing up emotional debris, may very well clear the way for a healthier sexual union.

Talk about sex. Sometimes, erectile problems can come right down to not feeling aroused. In these cases, sex therapists often work to help patients communicate more openly about their sexual relationship, according to Geisser. "This can be an embarrassing area, one that people don't talk about," he says. "Not talking contributes to the problem. We encourage people to communicate about what they like in sexual situations, so they can get more pleasure and stimulation out of it." Again, to avoid defensiveness and hurt feelings, "I" statements are key, Geisser says. Choose to make assertive, rather than aggressive, statements.

Don't drink before sex. Drinking alcohol or being drunk can significantly impair your sexual functioning, says Schiavi. His advice is simple—sex and booze don't mix.

Remember your successful experiences. If performance anxiety has undermined your confidence, thinking about positive sexual relationships or experiences you have had in the past may help boost your self-esteem, says Geisser. It may also convince you that you can have a fulfilling sex life in the future. "We have patients think about past successful sexual experiences, to try to shift the focus from worrying about the current situation and to help them experience it in a more pleasurable fashion," Geisser says.

◆◆◆ Could It Be a ◆◆◆ Medical Problem?

The word "impotence" can be a little vague, since it refers simply to erectile failure and does not address the source of the problem. However, the causes of erectile difficulties can range from diseases (such as diabetes) to guilt about sex. So how do you tell the difference between a physical or a psychological cause?

"Both factors contribute a great deal," says Raul C. Schiavi, M.D. "Even if the patient has a clear physical factor, there are always psychological factors contributing to the problem." The most common diseases that cause impotence are diabetes, cardiovascular disease, Parkinson's, multiple sclerosis, and epilepsy. In younger men, accidents, such as a gunshot to the spinal cord, car crashes, and skiing wipeouts, are often responsible. Other problems can include hormonal imbalances, says Schiavi. Lastly, there are several prescription drugs that can impair erectile function. Among the most common in this category are blood pressure medications and antidepressants. Of course, alcohol, marijuana, and cocaine can also keep you from achieving an erection.

If you have a sexual problem and have one of the illnesses listed above or have just started taking a prescription medication, contact your physician, Schiavi recommends.

Likewise, if you have doubts about whether your problem is physical or emotional, see your doctor.

Involve your partner. Although erectile difficulties originate with the man, they are a couples' problem and have couples solutions, according to Kenneth R. Fineman, Ph.D., a clinical psychologist and associate clinical professor of medical psychology at the University of California at Irvine School of Medicine.

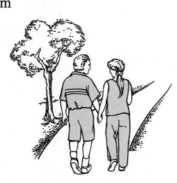

If the problem is not a medical one, there are many strategies that can help. However, your chances for improvement are much better if your sexual partner is involved in the solution, Fineman says. "If you are in a committed relationship, you need to develop a strategy to get your partner in there. Convince her that she is the most logical solution to the problem."

Know that you are not abnormal. It can never be stated enough: Having problems with erection does not mean that you are physiologically or psychologically abnormal in any way. It is not your fault. "People tend to feel guilty about their sexual problems," says Geisser. "Men often feel that, to a certain extent, they have lost their masculinity. It may bring on a significant decline in self-esteem. But the truth is, most men, for one reason or another, experience erectile failure. Even if periodic failure occurs, try not to get too upset about it. Oftentimes, people really come down hard on themselves or have a partner that gets very distressed and feels that it is because they're unattractive or unwanted. Getting too upset can lead to performance anxiety. Do your best to be open and understanding about the problem."

Read, then talk. Many of the sex therapists interviewed for this section said that they were often surprised by their patients' lack of knowledge about the sex act itself. There is a

◆◆◆ Prevention Tips ◆◆◆

Several types of medical conditions and injuries can make you impotent—permanently, according to Irwin Goldstein, M.D., a professor of urology at Boston University School of Medicine and codirector of the New England Male Reproductive Center at University Hospital in Boston. Here is his advice on preventing the most common physical causes of impotence:

Quit smoking. *Studies conducted at Boston University School of Medicine have shown that smoking is associated with blockages in the penile arteries, obstructing the blood flow that is necessary for an erection. The findings aren't really a surprise, since previous studies have linked smoking to blockages in the arteries of the heart, according to Goldstein. "Impotence is similar to vascular diseases, such as arteriosclerosis," he says.*

"It is the manifestation to the penis of those types of disorders. The smart person would say: Don't smoke, exercise, don't eat high-fat foods. In short, be smart about your cardiovascular health. That will impact on your potency and your sexual health." Quitting smoking won't reverse existing damage, but it can help prevent it from worsening.

Protect your crotch from injury. *One very common cause of impotence, especially in young men, is an injury to the crotch area. Often, these injuries (and the impotence they cause) do not heal of their own accord and must be treated with surgery. "People who bicycle should be very protective of the crossbar," says Goldstein. "Other activities that require caution include karate, horseback riding, rodeo riding, and anything else that may cause injury to the crotch." If you believe that your erectile difficulties were caused by such an accident, you should see a doctor.*

plethora of helpful written resources out there—books that can help you and your mate solve your problems and work toward a more mutually satisfying sex life, says Fineman. "Read the various manuals, the ones that are appropriate, not X-rated material," he says. "Then dialogue about it. One person says 'I think that's silly,' and the other might say, 'Well, why not? I'd like to try that.' Read books about sex, even if you don't choose to go on to try the exercises."

Develop coping strategies. Just as penis size isn't the measure of sexual prowess, neither is the rigidity of the penis, says Schiavi. "In a study of 100 healthy, aging couples, there was a decrease in sexual drive as age progressed," he says. "There was also a decrease in the rigidity of the penis and in the frequency of intercourse. However, couples who developed coping strategies to bypass these difficulties, by assisting insertion manually or by developing alternative ways of reaching orgasm, still rated themselves as sexually and maritally satisfied." The moral of the story is: Creativity pays off.

Skip the aphrodisiacs. Spanish fly and other so-called aphrodisiacs are usually little more than placebos—sugar pills that do nothing but boost your confidence, says Geisser. In fact, he adds, no drug has ever been shown to boost sexual performance with any degree of reliability. What's more, Spanish fly can be very dangerous to use and can even be fatal.

Employ fantasy. Many men with erectile problems engage in "spectatoring," or constantly observing their own sexual performance, says Schiavi. This takes the individual out of the moment and leads to being overly critical, he says. "We try to set up a situation where the attention is focused someplace else—on experiencing pleasure as one is being caressed or on experiencing the pleasure of caressing someone else. We also may advise the use of fantasy—focusing on a sexual fantasy that may involve the partner. This helps to minimize spectatoring and enhance sexual arousal."

Try masturbation. Performance anxiety is just that—anxiety over performing. But sex between loving partners was never meant to be an off-Broadway production. Don't forget that while it's important to please your partner, you're also there to please yourself. Masturbation—bringing yourself to orgasm while you are alone—may be helpful by reteaching you how to achieve your own pleasure (as long as it's not overdone). The next step is to bring that ability into a sexual situation with your partner—changing the focus from performance to mutually pleasurable interaction, says Fineman.

Don't be afraid to seek help. When you've tried everything, to no avail, it's time to seek medical attention, says Geisser. Studies have shown that therapy can significantly improve a couple's sex life. Where you go is up to you, but do your homework and shop around. Many states have certifications in sex therapy. Licensed psychologists will also be able to help you (and may be better regulated, according to Geisser). Get referrals if you can. The most important thing is to find a certified or licensed professional who has helped others with problems similar to your own. ◆

◆ INCONTINENCE ◆

20 Steps to Greater Security

Have you stopped taking an aerobics class because you're afraid you might have an "accident"? Do you worry when it's time to take a long car trip on highways with few roadside rest areas? Do you dread sneezing, coughing, even laughing, because you're not sure if you'll stay dry?

Rest assured, you're not alone. Help for Incontinent People (HIP), a not-for-profit organization in Union, South Carolina, estimates that at least 12 million, and perhaps as many as 20 million, people in the United States and Canada suffer with urinary incontinence, oftentimes in silence. Indeed, it's a problem that's only been recognized relatively recently in America as a treatable condition and not merely an unavoidable symptom of old age. As a matter of fact, other cultures in times past seemed to have been much more aware of the problem. The ancient Egyptians developed products for incontinence, and in Great Britain around the turn of the century, it was perfectly acceptable for a woman to hold what was called a "slipper" under her dress to relieve herself during a long church service.

The loss of bladder control is not a disease but a symptom with any of a host of causes. It can affect anyone at any age—from children to the elderly, both women and men. Women, however, are three times more likely than men to be incontinent, due in part to the physical stresses of childbearing and a decrease in estrogen after menopause. The cause of incontinence may be as minor as an infection triggered by a cold or the use of certain prescription or over-the-counter medications. Incontinence may also be the result of sagging pelvic-floor muscles. This set of muscles located at the bottom of the pelvis supports the lower internal organs and helps them maintain their shape and proper function. Childbirth and certain types of surgery, such as a hysterectomy in a woman (removal of the uterus) or a prostatectomy in a man (removal of the prostate gland), can cause these pelvic-floor muscles to become deficient. (See

"Exercises for Incontinence" for help in toning up and strengthening the pelvic-floor muscles.)

Incontinence reveals itself in a number of ways, and one person can suffer from more than one form of it. Stress incontinence occurs from rigorous or spontaneous activity, like playing tennis or sneezing. Urge incontinence is marked by a sudden need to go but possibly not making it to the bathroom in time. Overflow incontinence is a full bladder that begins to dribble. And reflex incontinence is marked by an unawareness of the need to urinate (caused by an enlarged prostate gland, for example), which results in leakage. Here are ways to cope:

Keep a diary. "This is very helpful in establishing symptom patterns," says Katherine Jeter, Ed.D, E.T., executive director of HIP. By maintaining a voiding diary, or uro-log, you'll have a record of when you urinated and the circumstances causing it. The diary should include: the time of day of urination or leakage; the type and amount of fluid intake that preceded it; the amount voided in ounces (pharmacies carry measuring devices that fit right inside the toilet bowl); the amount of leakage (small, medium, or large); the activity engaged in when leakage occurred; and whether or not an urge to urinate was present. Keeping such a diary for at least four days, if not a full week, before you see a doctor can help him or her to determine what type of incontinence you have and the course of treatment. When you see a doctor, take along a list or the actual bottles of any prescription or over-the-counter medicines you have been taking, because some medications can cause incontinence.

Watch what you drink. Experts are not entirely sure why some beverages seem to irritate the bladder lining and, as a result, cause bladder leakage. But you may want to eliminate certain substances from your diet or at least decrease your intake of them to see if your urine control improves. The caffeine in coffee, for instance, may irritate the bladder, and the ingredients that give coffee its distinct aroma (also found in decaffeinated varieties) can be irritating, too. Tea, another favorite breakfast drink, is not only a diuretic, which means it pulls more water from the kidneys as it passes through, but also a bladder irritant. (HIP recommends substituting hot grain beverages, found in your grocer's coffee and tea aisle.) Citrus fruits and juices, such as grapefruit and tomato, can be a problem. Carbonated sodas may be irritating, too, according to HIP (you might be able to tolerate seltzer water, which is not as highly carbonated as sodas). And, finally, alcoholic beverages should be avoided. Your safest bet: water, perhaps with a twist of lemon for flavor (a few drops of lemon should not be enough citrus to cause or aggravate an incontinence problem).

Try these juices. Grape juice, cranberry juice, cherry juice, and apple juice are not irritating to the bladder and may, in fact, control the odor of your urine. And surprisingly, orange juice is not an irritant, because it is metabolized by the body into a more alkaline, or less acidic, fluid before it reaches the bladder, says Jeter.

Keep drinking. "Too often, people who suffer with incontinence limit their fluid intake, believing that the less they take in, the less they'll urinate. But dehydration can occur," warns Thelma Wells, Ph.D., R.N., F.A.A.N., F.R.C.N., a professor of nursing at the University of Rochester School of Nursing in Rochester, New York. Dehydration can lead to constipation, which in turn can irritate nearby nerves that will trigger the bladder to void. The result: incontinence. Instead of cutting back on how much you drink, schedule the time that you drink. Having liquids at set intervals during the day will keep your bladder from becoming too empty or too full. "The bladder becomes irritated if its fluid level is too low or too high," explains Wells. A normal bladder holds about two cups of fluid; problem bladders may hold as little as half a cup or as much as a quart and a half. If you find

yourself constantly waking up in the middle of the night to go to the bathroom, you might try to taper off your fluid intake between dinner and bedtime, says Wells. Experts suggest an average total fluid intake of six to ten 8-ounce cups a day.

Watch what you eat. Again, experts are not sure why certain foods aggravate the bladder, but you may want to try cutting back on the following foods to see if it helps: hot spices and the foods they're used in, such as curry powder and chili; tomato-based foods; sugars, such as honey and corn syrup; and chocolate.

Try a recipe for success.
If you are constipated, adding fiber to your diet may relieve your constipation, and in turn, your incontinence. Here's an easy-to-make-snack recipe from HIP that may help. Combine one cup of applesauce, one cup of oat bran, and a quarter cup of prune juice. Store the mixture in your refrigerator, or freeze premeasured servings in sectioned ice-cube trays. Begin with two tablespoons every evening, followed by a six- to eight-ounce glass of water or juice (one of the acceptable varieties mentioned previously). After seven to ten days, increase this to three tablespoons. Then, at the end of the second or third week, increase your intake to four tablespoons. You should begin to see an improvement in your bowel habits in about two weeks. The extra fiber may cause increased gas or bloating, but this should decrease after a few weeks. Be sure to keep up your daily fluid intake in addition to using this fiber recipe.

Lose weight. Obesity can cause muscles to sag, including the pelvic-floor muscles, which aid in proper voiding.

Do not smoke. Here's another reason to give up the habit. Nicotine can irritate the bladder, and for heavy smokers, coughing can contribute to stress incontinence.

Buy yourself some insurance. There are numerous products on the market today that will absorb any accidents, whether urine or a bowel movement, and at the same time, protect your clothing or bedding from wetness. Specially made disposable and reusable briefs, diapers, liners, inserts, and linen protectors can add a measure of confidence. For some people, sanitary napkins or panty liners may be an acceptable alternative that provides enough protection. And a new product may be on the market soon. "Within the next year or two, urethral plugs, which can block the flow of urine during everyday activities, will be available in the United States," says Peter K. Sand, M.D., associate professor of obstetrics and gynecology at Northwestern University School of Medicine and director of the Evanston Continence Center at Evanston Hospital in Evanston, Illinois. These plugs, now in use in Europe, can be inserted by the user and later removed by means of an attached string.

Be confident on the road. External collecting devices that are specially designed for use by females or males can make traveling a little more comfortable. These on-the-go urinals, which are also convenient for bedside use, are available at medical-supply stores and pharmacies and through medical-specialty mail order.

Exercises for Incontinence

The pelvic floor is a set of muscles at the bottom of the pelvis that supports the lower internal organs, such as the bladder and uterus, and controls the sphincter muscles, which are the muscles that control the urethra and rectum. When you stop and start your urine stream, you're working these muscles. When this set of muscles becomes weak, incontinence may occur. Since these muscles can be controlled voluntarily, exercises may help strengthen them and in turn help control leakage, especially in cases of stress incontinence. This is true only if the exercises are done properly, however.

Here are a few simple exercises recommended by Help for Incontinent People (HIP) that should be done on a daily basis for best results. If you need additional instruction, HIP can provide manuals and tapes, or you can consult your doctor. In addition, your doctor may recommend exercises of increasing difficulty, depending on your specific case.

1. Lie on your back with your knees bent and feet slightly apart. Contract all the openings in the pelvic floor—the rectum, urethra, and, in women, the vagina, too. To help you isolate the muscles, first squeeze as if trying to keep from passing gas. Then (for women) contract the vagina as if trying not to lose a tampon. Then, proceed forward as if trying to stop urinating. Hold the tension while slowly counting to three. Then slowly release the tension. Repeat five to ten times. You should feel a "lift" inside you. Be sure to breathe smoothly and comfortably and do not tense your stomach, thigh, or buttocks muscles; otherwise, you may be exercising the wrong muscles. Check your abdomen with your hand to make sure the stomach area is relaxed.

2. Repeat the first exercise while using a low stool to support the lower part of your legs. Raising your legs will help further relax the pelvic-floor muscles for the exercise.

3. Third, repeat the first exercise while kneeling on the floor with your elbows resting on a cushion. In this position, the stomach muscles are completely relaxed. If you are unable to kneel, roll up a blanket and place it under your groin while you lie on your stomach.

Go before you go. Empty your bladder before you take a trip of an hour or more, whether you have the urge to go or not.

Then go again. After voiding, stand up and sit down again. Then lean forward, which will compress the abdomen and put pressure on the bladder, to help empty the bladder completely, suggests Wells.

Wear clothes that are easy to remove. Women's clothing, in particular, can pose a problem. Jumpsuits or unitards can slow you down when you're in a hurry to go because these one-piece outfits must be removed from the top down. Skip such suits or look for ones with a snapped opening at the crotch for quick-and-easy removal. Carry extra clothing with you so that you can change if an accident occurs. If your clothes happen to become stained with urine, soak them for three hours in a mixture of one gallon of water and one cup of dishwashing detergent.

Weight for results. Resistive exercise—when force is exerted against a weight—can be applied to the sphincter muscles of the urethra and rectum, which are important to regaining continence, says Wells. Cones that are about the size of a tampon and that come in varying weights are designed for use in the vagina (women) or rectum (men). When a cone is inserted, the sphincter muscles must contract in order to hold the weight and not let it drop. "Over a few months and with progressive use of the varying weights, the pelvic-floor muscles should get stronger," says Jeter. These weight sets are available from physicians, who can guide your use of the cones, or from medical-supply stores. Be sure to carefully read and follow the accompanying instructions on proper use for best results. Start by holding in the lightest weight for 15 minutes, two times a day. Once successful at that weight, try the next heaviest weight for the same amount of time. Some versions of these cones come with an electronic biofeedback system, called a perineometer, which reports on the amount of pressure you're applying to the inserted cone.

Take control of your muscles every day. To prevent leakage, contract the pelvic-floor muscles when coughing or sneezing or when carrying or lifting something. Do so by standing close to the object to be lifted with your feet slightly apart, one foot just in front of the other. Then, bend your knees but keep your back straight. Lean forward slightly as you contract, or tighten, your pelvic muscles. Then lift the object.

Be wary of exercise gimmicks. Carefully investigate any exercise contraption that claims to help decrease incontinence. A company may promote the fact that its gadget will tone the pelvic-floor muscles, but the device may actually exercise an unrelated muscle group, if it does anything at all. An exerciser for use between the thighs, for instance, will not strengthen the pelvic-floor muscles. If you're not sure if a certain exerciser will benefit your incontinence problem, don't waste your time or money. Check first with your health-care provider.

Make a phone call. Call 1-800-BLADDER, a toll-free number sponsored by HIP, for details on how to receive a free packet of information on services and products for incontinent people. ◆

◆ INFERTILITY ◆

14 Tips to Help You Get Pregnant

OK, so you want to have a baby. Your chances of succeeding are excellent: About 85 percent of all couples who try to conceive will do so within one year. (After one year, couples are considered infertile.) Twenty to 22 percent will get pregnant within the first month of trying.

There are some obvious rules to this game. The first is that you and your partner need to have sexual intercourse, with the penis in the vagina. The penis must ejaculate inside the vagina, depositing sperm near the cervix, the mouth of the uterus. In addition, intercourse must occur at or around the time of ovulation.

There are also a lot of misconceptions and old wives' tales surrounding this issue. For example, it is not necessary for the woman to achieve orgasm in order for conception to occur, according to Paul A. Bergh, M.D., an assistant professor of obstetrics and gynecology in the Division of Reproductive Endocrinology at Mount Sinai Medical Center in New York. Bergh explains that the fallopian tubes, the tubes that carry the egg from the ovary to the uterus, actually draw the sperm inside, coaxing them to unite with the egg. This occurs with or without orgasm, he says.

The following tips will help increase your chances of getting pregnant. Also refer to "When and Why to Seek Help" for a list of conditions that should prompt you to see a doctor *before* your year of trying is over. Good luck!

Get a physical. Before spending a year trying to get pregnant, it's a good idea to have a thorough physical examination, according to Sanford M. Markham, M.D., an assistant professor of obstetrics and gynecology at Georgetown University Medical Center in Washington, D.C. "Make sure that there aren't any physical problems, such as masses or cysts in the pelvic area," he says. "Your doctor should also treat any low-grade vaginal infections that you might have. He or she should also check for sexually transmitted diseases." Other conditions that can interfere with pregnancy are ovarian cysts, fibroids, and endometriosis, an inflammation of the lining of the uterus, Markham says.

Have sex around the time of ovulation. The woman's egg is capable of being fertilized for only 24 hours after it is released from the ovary, according to Richard J. Paulson, M.D., an associate professor of obstetrics and gynecology and director of the In Vitro Fertilization Program at the University of Southern California School of Medicine in Los Angeles. The man's sperm can live for between 48 and 72 hours in the woman's reproductive tract. Since sperm and egg must come together for an embryo to be created, a couple must try to have sex at least every 72 hours around the time of ovulation (see "Methods of Ovulation Prediction") in order to hit the mark, Paulson says. "Every 48 hours is even better," he says. However, he adds, the man should not ejaculate more frequently than once in 48 hours, since that may bring his sperm count down too low for fertilization.

Men should ejaculate every two to three days. Along with the advice to have sex no more often than once every 48 hours, men should also try to ejaculate at least once every two to three days throughout the month, says Bergh. Men need to keep ejaculating to keep up their sperm supply, he adds.

◆ INGROWN TOENAILS ◆

13 Ways to Curb Them

Here's the good news: "Ingrown toenails can be simply solved with a minimum of pain and discomfort," says Donald Skwor, D.P.M., a podiatrist in Memphis and past president of the American Podiatric Medical Association.

Now for the bad news: A simple nail infection, if not treated properly, can swiftly lead to further complications. When a sharp edge of a toenail grows into the skin folds at its edge, it will result in pain and discomfort, especially if the wound gets infected.

Diabetics and people with vascular disease in particular should get immediate medical treatment for ingrown toenails (see "Hello, Doctor?"). People without circulatory problems, however, can usually take care of an ingrown toenail themselves, if they follow these tips from the experts.

Go soak your toe. To relieve the soreness, soak your foot in warm, not hot, water. Put a tablespoon or two of Epsom salts in a basin of warm water, suggests Raymond Merkin, D.P.M., a podiatrist in Rockville, Maryland. Soak your toe for five to ten minutes, once or twice a day.

Try a different solution. Rock G. Positano, D.P.M., M.Sc., codirector of the Foot and Ankle Orthopedic Institute at the Hospital for Special Surgery in New York, is a fan of something called Domeboro solution. It's an antibacterial, anti-inflammatory soak that's available without a prescription. Positano recommends nightly soaks of 20 to 30 minutes. Soaking in this solution should help bring down inflammation so that the nail can grow out naturally.

Apply ointment. Spread a topical antibiotic dressing, such as Neosporin, on the wound to prevent infection, says Merkin.

Don't play surgeon. You're not helping matters by performing bathroom surgery on your toe. First of all, the implements in your medicine cabinet are

---

◆ Too Much Nail, ◆ Too Little Toe

Raymond Merkin, D.P.M., likens this situation to when a child's teeth grow in and the need for braces is suddenly very obvious. There seem to be too many teeth for the kid's mouth.

Sometimes, a similar thing can happen with toenails. The growth pattern may change for some reason. The nail seems to be growing wider than before. The result may be a persistent problem with ingrown toenails.

Merkin says a podiatrist can solve the problem with minor surgery using a local anesthetic. "Treatment is to try to permanently narrow the nail by removing part of the side nail border and some of the root of the nail—the matrix, a group of cells that line the base of the toenail. By removing some of the matrix cells, that corner that digs down into the skin is eliminated." If you have persistent ingrown toenails, see a podiatrist.

---

probably chock full of bacteria. Secondly, you could hurt yourself. "The first thing to do is *not do* bathroom surgery," says Positano, "especially with a dirty instrument. You're many times introducing bacteria or foreign bodies." If the nail has grown in so deeply that it is causing serious infection, see a podiatrist.

Go straight. No more curved toenails! Get in the habit of cutting them straight across. "You can file the corners if they're sharp," says Merkin.

◆◆ Hello, Doctor? ◆◆

If you are diabetic or have vascular disease or any other condition that affects circulation, don't even think of trying to treat a nail infection yourself. Furthermore, you shouldn't even be doing your own foot care.

"If someone is a diabetic, they shouldn't be cutting their own nails, period," says Rock G. Positano, D.P.M., M.Sc. "They should be going to a health-care professional who's trained in nail care."

Because diabetics have poor circulation in their extremities, any foot wound or infection takes longer to heal. Without proper treatment, an injury could worsen quickly and bring other complications.

"A simple nail infection can be absolutely catastrophic," Positano warns. "It has led to half a foot being amputated."

The reduced circulation also affects the foot's sensitivity to pain, which can delay detection of a minor injury. For this reason, diabetics and others with poor circulation need to examine their feet daily and should not hesitate to call their doctor at the first sign of foot injury.

Don't cut too short. When we stand up, pressure pushes the skin up in front of the toenail. "As the nail grows forward, it imbeds into the skin. So it's best to cut the nail to the end of the skin, rather than below the end of the toe," says Merkin.

Step into a different shoe. An ingrown toenail may be nature's way of telling you to go shopping. It's time for some new shoes, ones that don't pinch your toes. If you're a woman, avoid high heels. Try a lower heel (about one inch high) to relieve the pressure on your toes, suggests Skwor. Men and women should shop for shoes with a roomier toe.

Get some sandals, too. If the weather allows, wear open-toed sandals to allow your ailing toe to breathe. Positano describes the space inside socks and shoes as "a very hostile environment" for feet, one that's dark, damp, and hot. Healing will be speedier in the open air.

Watch where you walk. Now that you're padding around in sandals, Positano wants you to be careful where you walk in them. "Don't walk in the city streets," he cautions. There is too much bacteria that could enter your hurt toe. Wear your sandals around your home, but choose shoes with closed toes for urban excursions.

Guard your toes. Even while wearing shoes, you can hurt your toes pretty badly by dropping something on your foot. "If you drop something on your toe that causes you to lose your toenail, the nail may grow in when it grows back," says Skwor. If dropping things is a problem for you, wear steel-toed shoes, he advises.

Don't stub. Stubbing your toe can result in an injury that affects the nail. Skwor notes, "That can cause your nail to grow in a thickened manner or cause it to grow in."

Ignore old wives. There's an old wives' tale that by cutting a "V" in the top center of the nail, pressure will be relieved. That doesn't make sense, says Skwor, because the nail grows from the base of the toe. Another tale he has heard concerns rubbing coal oil into the affected area. "They say it helps," says Skwor, but he can't imagine why.

Pass on some pedicures. If you intend to have a pedicure, be sure the person who is performing it does not use metallic instruments to remove dead skin, says Positano. Pumice stones are OK. ◆

◆ INSOMNIA ◆

21 Ways to Sleep Tight

You know the story: It's 5:00 A.M., and the first traces of dawn have begun to appear in the nighttime sky. You've been awake since 2:00 A.M. and are beginning to feel hopeless about ever getting back to sleep. How will you function at work tomorrow (today)? How will you cope with your presentation at the board meeting? How will you keep yourself from yawning through that dinner with your boss? How will you make it through another day after yet another night without sleep?

Insomnia is the most common sleep disorder in North America and in Europe. A whopping one-third of the U.S. population cannot sleep well enough to function well during the day. One-half of those people have only one or two bad nights a week. The other half spend countless sleepless nights tossing and turning, staring at the alarm clock, and feeling miserable. They also spend countless days exhausted.

Insomnia is also one of the least-understood sleep disorders. German Nino-Murcia, M.D., founder and medical director of the Sleep Medicine and Neuroscience Institute in Palo Alto, California, talks about the frustration he feels at not being able to help more patients who suffer from sleepless nights. "Ten years ago, when I was the director of Stanford University's Sleep Disorders Center, I couldn't do a thing for a quarter of the insomniacs I saw," he says. "Twenty-five percent, after treatment, said they weren't sleeping any more than before they first sought help."

Luckily, after many years of study, sleep experts have come up with many tried-and-true strategies for putting an end to insomnia. The results of their work appear in the tips that follow. Try them out, and see what works for you. If nothing has helped after six months—if you're still struggling to get a decent night's sleep—consult your doctor for a referral to a sleep clinic near you, or call the National Sleep Foundation at 213-288-0466 for a referral to a sleep specialist.

Make it as nonpunishing as possible. The worst thing that an insomniac can do is to lie in bed tossing and turning, says Peter Hauri, Ph.D., a professor of psychology and director of the Mayo Clinic Insomnia Program in Rochester, Minnesota. Hauri, one of the country's leading authorities on insomnia, is coauthor of the book *No More Sleepless Nights*. "Pass your time reading in bed or watching television, rather than lying in bed frustrated," he says. "This goes for everyone. If you are lying in bed, even if you are not sleeping, your body will still get the same amount of recovery as if you had slept. Although your brain doesn't get any recovery, you'll still be better off than if you spend the time watching the clock, tossing and turning. Hide the clock; put it out of view. You'll only watch it getting later and later and get more and more tense."

Don't nap. "Napping tends to make matters worse for the chronic insomniac," says Karl Doghramji, M.D., director of the Sleep Disorders Center at Jefferson Medical College of Thomas Jefferson University in Philadelphia. The concept is similar to the reason you shouldn't stay in bed late the morning after you had trouble sleeping: you'll have more trouble getting to sleep the next night, thereby compounding your insomnia. It's best to let yourself get good and sleepy so that it will be easier to get to sleep the next night.

Change your interpretation of the problem. Several misconceptions about sleep can make people overly concerned about their insomnia and can actually keep them awake, says Nino-Murcia. One example is when people wake up out of what seems like a deep sleep and feel wide awake. They think that because they feel so alert that they will never be able to get back to sleep. However, says Nino-Murcia, this is not the case. "What happens is that if insomnia wakes you from your REM stage [REM stands for Rapid Eye Movements, the stage of sleep in which you dream], you will be very alert. However, all you have to do is wait for 30 minutes and you will easily fall back to sleep." The key is to understand that your awakening is natural and that you just have to wait it out, he says. Another instance of mistaken perception is that when people wake, they often have the feeling that they were never asleep at all. But most people sleep much longer than they think, according to Nino-Murcia.

Try earplugs. Sometimes, insomnia is caused by being awakened repeatedly by loud noises. Often, the sleeper is not aware of what awakened him or her, according to Doghramji. "The classic case is a person who lives near an airport," he says. He suggests minimizing ambient noise as much as possible and, failing that, investing in a good pair of earplugs.

Try a sleeping pill. You're not admitting defeat by asking your doctor for a prescription sleeping pill or trying an over-the-counter remedy, says J. Christian Gillin, M.D., a professor of psychiatry at the University of California at San Diego and an adjunct professor in the Department of Psychology at San Diego State University. However, prescription pills should not be used for more than a month at a time, says Gillin. They should also not be used for insomnia at high altitudes, since that type of insomnia may be caused by trouble breathing and a lack of oxygen. Taking sleeping pills at high altitudes may slow your breathing rate even further and may be dangerous. (If you often suffer insomnia at high altitudes, ask your doctor for a prescription drug called Diamox, says Gillin. It may make sleep easier.)

Some doctors don't endorse over-the-counter sleeping pills, however, since they can cause side effects such as drying out your mucous membranes (they often have antihistamines as ingredients) and can make you drowsy the next day. Of course, if you are pregnant, are nursing a baby, or have a serious medical problem, you should consult your doctor before taking any drugs. Sleep medications may also worsen snoring and sleep apnea, a dangerous condition in which breathing is labored during sleep.

Never take sleeping pills throughout the night. If you do choose to take medication to help you fall asleep, make sure you only take your dose before you go to bed, says Nino-Murcia. If you take the medication when you wake in the middle of the night, it won't have a chance to wear off before morning, and you're likely to end up being sleepy during the day, he says.

Get a comfortable bed. Sleep may also be disturbed because the individual is uncomfortable in his or her bed, says Doghramji. In this case, the sleeper will probably be unaware of why he or she was awakened. "Soft beds are usually better for sleeping than firm ones are," he says.

Don't drink alcohol. Although alcohol can make you feel drowsy and may actually put you to sleep, it has the unpleasant side effect of waking you up later on in the night, says Gillin. "After drinking alcohol, people often wake up in the middle of the night because of headaches, a full bladder, or gastric upset," he says. In addition, once alcohol's sedative effect wears off, there's a rebound effect that actually makes the individual more likely to have trouble falling back to sleep. So skip the nightcap for a better night's sleep.

Cut down on caffeine. We all know that too much coffee, tea, or soda with caffeine can impede the ability to go to sleep at night. But how much is too much? Hauri recommends no more than two cups of coffee or other caffeine-containing beverage in the morning and none after noon.

Don't switch beds or move to the couch. It is important to associate your bed, and only your bed, with sleep, according to Doghramji. "We are all creatures of habit," he says. "Regularity has to be enforced to facilitate sleep. Even animals tend to sleep in the same place every night."

Try to maintain a normal schedule. Perhaps the most important rule for people with insomnia is to keep a strict sleep-wake schedule, even on weekends, sleep specialists agree. "Many insomniacs become so desperate that they'll go to sleep any time that they can," says Gillin. If you can't sleep one night, simply get up at your usual time the next morning and don't take any naps. Chances are, you'll be ready for a sound sleep by the next night, he says.

Confine work to the office. For the same reason that you shouldn't switch beds or move to the couch every night, you shouldn't do work in bed, says Doghramji. It's important to associate your bed with sleep, not with unpleasant things, like work. Relaxing activities, like reading a novel or watching television, are OK bedtime activities. It's also OK to have sex in bed.

Take a hot bath. A hot bath taken two hours before bedtime is a wonderful way to relax your body and make it ready for sleep, says Hauri. For most people, taking a bath closer to bedtime may be stimulating and may delay sleep (of course, there are always exceptions, he says, so be your own guide). Hauri recommends making the water very hot, like a hot tub, and staying in it for at least 20 minutes. Do not bathe in very hot water, however, if you are pregnant or have any significant health problems; ask your doctor if you are unsure.

Establish a bedtime relaxation ritual. When parents bathe their children or read to them every night before bedtime, they are reinforcing a signal that it's time to settle down and get ready for sleep. Establishing such a ritual may also be helpful for adults, says Doghramji. "Learn how to relax," he says. "You can try systematic muscle-tension-and-

How Much Sleep Do You Need?

The word of the day is that adults need eight hours of sleep per night. But is that the case for everyone?

Sleep researchers answer with a resounding "no."

Peter Hauri, Ph.D., in the book No More Sleepless Nights, *says that while different individuals have very different sleep needs, the amount remains amazingly constant for each person. He tells the story of a 70-year-old nurse who slept only one hour each night, took no naps during the day, and said that she never felt tired. In fact, she said she didn't understand why other people wasted so much time in bed. She had averaged the same amount of sleep each night since she was a child.*

Other people may need 9, 10 or even 11 hours of sleep per night. There is no "norm."

"Studies demonstrate that people perform just as well cognitively if they are sleep deprived," says German Nino-Murcia, M.D. "What happens is that people start to demonstrate intellectual problems when they are worried about how little they sleep. If you think you will be impaired, you will be. If you sleep for 90 minutes and when you wake up I tell you that you have slept for eight hours, you will feel great. But if you sleep for eight hours and I wake you up and tell you that you have only slept for 45 minutes, you will feel exhausted."

relaxation exercises: Tense all of your muscles, one at a time, then let go. Buy a tape of ocean or bird sounds. There are plenty of things available. Most insomniacs have a problem with not being able to relax prior to bedtime. They worry about the insomnia." Doghramji recommends doing a relaxation exercise of some sort every night before you retire.

Drink hot milk. Try drinking warm milk or a malted-milk drink before bed. Even if it doesn't help make you drowsy, it can be comforting and certainly can't do any harm (unless you are allergic to milk or are lactose intolerant).

Cut down on the time you spend in bed. "Drastically curtail your time in bed," says Hauri. "About 90 percent of people I talk to stay in bed too long. The farther you spread your sleep out, the thinner it gets. If you stay in bed ten hours and you only need seven hours of sleep, you'll sleep ten hours, but it won't be very high-quality sleep. In the morning, you'll be more tired than if you only had slept for seven hours. Stay in bed two hours less than you do now. Try it for a week and see if it makes you sleep sounder and increases the restorative value of your sleep."

Evaluate your medications. Certain prescription medications, such as those for asthma and thyroid problems, may cause insomnia, says Gillin. Check with your doctor if you suspect that one of your medications is causing your insomnia.

Be your own sleep scientist. There is no one formula for perfect sleep, says Hauri. Different things work for different people. The important thing is to give everything a fair and persistent trial (for at least a week or two, not just one night) and see what works best for you. "Think back to 10 or 15 years ago when you were not an insomniac," Hauri says. "How much did you sleep then? What helped you sleep?" He recommends keeping a sleep log, a notebook of what works and what doesn't work for you.

Never try to go to sleep. Sounds counterintuitive, right? Well, it's not. Falling asleep is something that requires the opposite of effort. Effort is work, and work keeps you awake. "The harder you try to go to sleep, the harder it will be to go to sleep," Gillin says. Instead, simply lie still, relax, and let sleep come.

Stay cool. For high-quality sleep to occur, the internal body temperature should be a few degrees cooler than it is during the day, says Hauri. However, many insomniacs lack the proper internal controls to regulate their body temperature. That's why a hot bath helps—after raising the body's temperature, it drops it back down within a couple of hours. Exercise, done at least six hours before bedtime, has the same effect, Hauri says. Keeping the bedroom cooler than the rest of the house may also be helpful.

Eat a sandwich. Although you may have been told that eating before you go to bed may give you nightmares, the reverse is true, according to Hauri. Going to bed on a full stomach may actually help you sleep, he says. That may be part of the reason why folks are always nodding off after a big holiday dinner. ◆

IRRITABLE BOWEL SYNDROME

15 Tactics for Taming It

Like an unannounced visitor who stops by when you're just about to go out, or the annoying caller who won't let you off the phone, irritable bowel syndrome, or IBS, comes calling whenever and wherever it likes. In fact, as many as half the people who visit a doctor complaining of digestive problems probably have IBS, according to the National Institutes of Health in Bethesda, Maryland.

As its name suggests, the symptoms of IBS are indeed irritating but can also be painful, as constipation hits one moment and diarrhea the next, sometimes coupled with bloating and cramping. What can be just as irritating is someone who tells you that "it's all in your head." Nothing could be further from the truth. No cause or cure for IBS, also known as spastic colon, has been found, but what health-care specialists do know is that there are ways to fend off this abominable abdominal beast.

Keep a diary. This is important in helping you and your doctor to determine what the cause of your discomfort may be or what factors may aggravate it. For about two weeks, keep a record of what you've eaten, the kind of mood you're in, the stress you're experiencing, and how your tummy feels. (Women should also record the dates of their menstrual period, since some women suffer more acutely from IBS around the time of their period.) "The diary has a lot of benefits," says Douglas A. Drossman, M.D., professor of medicine and psychiatry in the Division of Digestive Diseases at the University of North Carolina at Chapel Hill. "Most importantly, virtually all of the factors involved in IBS are modifiable." By writing down your stresses, for instance, you may be able to pinpoint their causes and, as a result, take necessary action to change a stressful circum-stance. And you may be able to cut back on or eliminate certain foods that may aggravate your symptoms (see "Is Your Diet to Blame?").

Learn how to relax. "For 34 percent of IBS sufferers, stress exacerbates the symptoms," reports William Whitehead, Ph.D., professor of medical psychology at Johns Hopkins University School of Medicine in Baltimore. As a matter of fact, some sufferers have their most serious bouts of IBS soon after a stressful situation. The first step in learning how to relax is to simply be aware of when your muscles have tensed up, so you can detense them.

In order to do this, you can try progressive muscle relaxation, suggests Barbara Greene, a clinical psychology doctoral candidate at the State University of New York at Albany. In this technique, you tense and then relax each muscle group throughout the body. "This way," Greene explains, "you'll realize what your muscles feel like when they're truly relaxed, and you'll become more aware of when they're not."

While this technique can be helpful to some, your best bet is to try different methods of relaxation and see what suits you. Something as simple as a hobby or reading may do the trick.

Be ready to roll with the punches. Too often, people see the world in black and white instead of shades of gray. "They are slow to compromise or negotiate and expect absolute perfection from themselves and others," says Greene. And a negative attitude can have a negative effect on the digestive system. Indeed, people who have a healthy outlook on life may stay healthier and not suffer so severely from IBS. So IBS sufferers can help themselves by confronting and understanding their fears and concerns. A professional counselor may also be of help.

Picture yourself in stress-free surroundings.
"Mental imagery can also have a positive effect,"
says Greene. Close your eyes and dream up a
relaxing scene. You may find that relaxation tapes
or tapes of soothing sounds or music can help you
visualize relaxing scenes.

Add exercise to your routine. "Exercise increases
peristalsis motility," says Whitehead, which
basically means it helps the digestive system work
properly. Exercise also aids in mental health by
giving an IBS sufferer "something else to focus on
besides discomfort," says Suzanne Rose, M.D.,

assistant professor of medicine at the University of
Pittsburgh Medical Center. The feel-good effect of
exercise is also tied in to the release of endorphins,
hormones that help control pain, says Drossman.
"But don't overdo it," he cautions, "because too
much exercise can cause diarrhea." Long-distance
runners, for instance, have been known to suffer
from it.

Take a deep breath when stressed. This is the
quickest, easiest way to release the tension from
your body when you can't run off to exercise or
take time off to relax. Breathe deeply and slowly,

◆ Is Your Diet to Blame? ◆

*While no single food has been found to cause
irritable bowel syndrome (IBS), some foods may
aggravate the condition. Not all IBS sufferers are
adversely affected by the same foods, however.
Here's a list of the kinds of foods that may be
contributing to your symptoms. Test the suspects
by eliminating only one type at a time from your
diet to see if you feel better, and record the results
in your diary.*

*Dairy products. Some IBS sufferers also have a
lactose intolerance (see LACTOSE
INTOLERANCE). This means they can't digest
lactose, the sugar in milk and other dairy products.
(Yogurt and hard cheeses don't seem to cause any
symptoms because their bacterial content converts
much of the lactose to lactic acid before they're
consumed.) To find out if you are indeed lactose
intolerant, a physician can do a simple breath test
on you to check. If you are, lactase enzyme is
available in tablet form and even in some food
products to help alleviate the symptoms. Whole-
milk dairy products also contain fat, which may be*

*an irritant. Opt instead for products made with
low-fat or skim milk.*

*Gas producers. The last thing an IBS sufferer needs
is more gas. Among the offenders: onions, beans,
broccoli, brussels sprouts, cabbage, red and green
peppers, and carbonated beverages.*

*Spicy foods. Forgo the spices in your dishes and see
if that makes a difference.*

*Wheat products. Those who find that foods
containing wheat are a problem should consult their
physician as to how to maintain or increase their
fiber intake without using wheat.*

*Citrus fruits. Of all the types of fruit, citrus
varieties, such as oranges and tangerines, seem to
be the most-common offenders.*

*Sugar. Some IBS sufferers have what's known as
fructose, or sugar, intolerance.*

*Chocolate. It not only contains caffeine but high
amounts of sugar and fat.*

*Sugarless gum and candy. Specifically, those made
with sorbitol can aggravate IBS symptoms because
the artificial sweetener is not digestible.*

allowing your chest to rise and fall slowly and purposefully, suggests Greene.

Eat more slowly. If you gobble down your food, you're more likely to swallow air, which can cause gas. Chewing gum can also have the same effect.

Eat several smaller meals. Large meals can overload the digestive system, causing cramping and diarrhea, according to the National Institutes of Health. Smaller, more frequent meals over the course of the day are easier for the body to handle.

Increase your fiber intake. Fiber, well known as an aid in relieving constipation, may alleviate some IBS symptoms as well. "But increase your fiber intake gradually," cautions Whitehead. As the body adjusts to the added fiber, it's common to experience bloating, which should dissipate after the first two to four weeks, says Rose. "The important thing is to stick with an increased-fiber diet." And be sure to drink plenty of fluids, especially water, she adds. Fresh fruits and vegetables and whole-grain breads and cereals are all good sources of fiber.

Cut down on caffeine. Found in coffee, tea, and caffeinated sodas, caffeine can stimulate the intestines, says Gary R. Lichtenstein, M.D., assistant professor of medicine at the University of Pennsylvania School of Medicine in Philadelphia. "Caffeine is also known to cause heartburn and abdominal cramping," says Rose.

Trim the fat in your diet. "Fatty foods are very hard to digest," says Lichtenstein. These include fatty meats, butter, and oils.

Watch your use of laxatives. "Overuse of laxatives containing stimulants can damage the bowels," says Lichtenstein. However, magnesium-based laxatives are relatively safe to use (except by those with kidney problems). Check labels.

Cut back on alcohol. "In large quantities, alcohol can cause diarrhea," says Drossman.

Don't smoke. It may have an effect on the motility, or movement, of the digestive system, says Rose.

Set up a self-help group. Often, people with IBS feel as if they're suffering alone. To help sufferers help themselves and each other, support groups have begun all over the country. If you'd like to start one in your area, here's how to get information on setting up, publicizing, and managing a group. Write to the Intestinal Disease Foundation, Inc., Attn: HR, 1323 Forbes Avenue, Suite 200, Pittsburgh, Pennsylvania 15219. ◆

◆ KIDNEY STONES ◆

11 Ways to Avoid Them

According to an old fairy tale, a single tiny pea placed beneath 20 mattresses and 20 featherbeds was enough to keep the true princess awake throughout the night. In real life, a tiny pea-sized stone, lodged in one or the other of your kidneys, is enough to keep you not only awake all night but crying out in pain and gritting your teeth until you can get to a doctor for relief.

Until recently, there were only two unpleasant alternatives for a stone sufferer: waiting to let the stone slowly pass through the urinary tract or undergoing major surgery to remove it. Today, a new treatment called lithotripsy, in which kidney stones are destroyed by shock waves, has brightened the outlook for those unlucky enough to be stone formers.

Scientists really don't know why kidney stones form. Kidney stones tend to run in families, so individuals with a close relative who has been through a stone episode should be careful. Most first-time victims are between 30 and 40 years old and are otherwise in very good health. Men are four times more likely than women to get kidney stones, the theory being that female hormones may prevent kidney stones from forming.

Despite the improvements in treating kidney stones, it's definitely preferable to avoid having them in the first place. If you have been through a bout with a stone in the past or think that you might be a candidate for developing a stone, you should do your best to beat the odds, which say that if you get kidney stones once, you run a 10 percent risk of developing more within a year and an 80 percent chance of developing a new stone within 15 years. Here's how to fight those odds:

Drink more than your fill. Increasing fluid intake should be the first step (and may be the only step needed) to keep free of kidney stones. One hundred ounces—that's at least 12 eight-ounce glasses a day—is the minimum. "Any fluid qualifies, including water, juice, soda, even tea and coffee," says Glenn M. Preminger, M.D., associate professor of urology/internal medicine at The University of Texas Southwestern Medical Center at Dallas. The only restriction, says Preminger, is avoiding tea for persons with high urinary oxalate and avoiding too much milk because of the calcium it contains.

Check it out. Sometimes, it's not easy to keep track of your daily water intake. That's why measuring your urine *output* may be a better indication of fluid intake. "I advise my patients to make sure they are urinating 1,200 to 1,500 cubic centimeters, or 40 to 45 ounces worth," says Michael Wechsler, M.D., assistant professor of clinical urology at Columbia–Presbyterian Medical Center in New York. Anything below 1,000 cubic centimeters a day is too little, he adds.

Keep the lid on dairy products. By far the most common kidney stones are those formed by calcium: calcium oxalate or calcium phosphate. "Some individuals who are prone to calcium-type stone formation should try to limit their calcium intake," says Demetrius H. Bagley, M.D., professor of urology and professor of radiology at Jefferson Medical College of Thomas Jefferson University in Philadelphia. If you have been dosing up on calcium supplements in hopes of strengthening your bones, you may actually be increasing your risk of stone formation. Dairy products are the greatest dietary source of calcium. Limit butter and cheese first; these are also high in the kind of fat that your heart will be better off without.

Don't oversoothe your tummy. Some over-the-counter antacids are calcium based. Check the label, and if the word "calcium" appears there, select another type of stomach medication.

Eat less meat. Individuals who form uric-acid stones are usually found to eat diets high in animal

◆◆◆ A "Berry" ◆◆◆ Good Idea?

One folk remedy that has long proved effective without anyone knowing why is the use of cranberry juice to treat urinary tract infections. The effectiveness was always explained by the juice's power to render urine highly acidic and, therefore, inhospitable to bacteria. Why other juices that have the same acidifying effect on urine did not seem to help urinary tract infections was always a mystery until researchers found that (in female mice, anyway) cranberry juice actually diminishes the ability of bacteria to adhere to the bladder lining.

Does it follow, therefore, that cranberry juice has the same protective benefits against kidney stones? There's no scientific proof, says Michael Wechsler, M.D., but if you like the taste of cranberry juice, drink up—it will add to your fluid intake.

protein, which can accelerate formation of uric acid and calcium in the urine. "People who are prone to kidney stones should cut back on animal proteins," says Wechsler.

Go easy on the oxalates. Eating large quantities of fruits and vegetables gives you lots of vitamins and minerals; however, some of these foods can also give you oxalates, which you may need to go easy on if you have a tendency toward kidney-stone formation. "In people with normal gastrointestinal function, oxalates may not be harmful, but it's still a good idea to lay off rhubarb and spinach," says Preminger. Other oxalate-rich foods include: chocolate, tea, cola, parsley, peanuts, and citrus fruit.

Be "A" enriched. Vitamin A is necessary for the overall healthy state of your urinary tract. Foods rich in vitamin A include sweet potatoes, pumpkin, winter squash, broccoli, and carrots. The Recommended Daily Allowance (RDA) of vitamin A for healthy adults is 5,000 international units, which should be easily met through a varied, balanced diet. Don't rush out for vitamin A supplements; if you get too much, your body won't excrete the excess, which can be toxic.

"B" fortified. Scientists have found that Vitamin B_6 may actually lower the amount of oxalate in the blood, thereby reducing the risk of stone formation. Magnesium, too, has a negative effect on stone formation. Your doctor may suggest a daily supplement of B_6 and/or magnesium or a drug that combines the two. If you take vitamin B_6, don't take more than 25 milligrams a day.

"C" less. With news of the positive powers of vitamin C appearing regularly, people may be led to think of it as a wonder vitamin. However, vitamin C in very high doses—more than 3,000 milligrams daily—can be a potential problem for those with kidney-stone tendencies. That's because vitamin C is converted to oxalate in the body. "People prone to kidney stones should stay away from vitamin C supplements, although foods containing vitamin C aren't a problem," says Wechsler.

Move it. One of the many benefits of regular exercise is that it facilitates the passage of calcium out of the bloodstream and into the bones. The result: stronger bones and less risk of stone formation. According to Preminger, it's "one more excellent reason to exercise regularly."

Don't shake it. There's also a high correlation between kidney stones and salt intake. "Two grams a day is the reasonable intake," says Bagley. ◆

◆ KNEE PAIN ◆

21 Knee-Saving Strategies

We bend them, kneel on them, run and jump on them daily, yet few of us give them a second thought. Knees. They're one of the most complex—and most injury-prone—joints in your body. Why? Blame the knee's design. Unlike the more stable hip joint, which is a ball in a deeply cushioned pocket, the knee joint is more exposed—and more vulnerable.

Essentially, the knee is a rounded bone that rests on a relatively flat one. The thighbone (femur) ends in two rounded knobs (condyles), which sit on the relatively flat shinbone (tibia). The kneecap is a small, rounded bone that sits in a groove between the thighbone and the knobby ends and gives strength to the joint. As the knee bends and straightens, the kneecap slides up and down in the groove. A tendon attaches the kneecap to the thigh muscles above, and a ligament connects it to the shinbone below. The kneecap acts like a pulley, increasing the power of the muscles attached to it.

"The knee flexes and extends, but it has little lateral rotation," says board-certified foot surgeon Elliot Michael, D.P.M., director of the residency program for Podiatric Medicine at Holladay Park Hospital in Portland, Oregon. "The upper and lower leg bones act like long levers on the joint, increasing power and force. A small change in the levers is magnified many times over in the knee," says Michael.

This intricate design can cause problems, especially for the kneecap, which accounts for about 20 percent of all knee pain, say knee experts. Proper functioning of the knee and its kneecap doesn't depend on the alignment of the bones themselves, but on the alignment of the surrounding structures. Think about the kneecap as a puppet controlled by "strings"—muscles, tendons, and ligaments. As long as all of the strings pull in just the right way, the kneecap moves back and forth smoothly in its track. But if any string pulls too strongly or not hard enough, the kneecap is pulled out of its track and can no

longer glide easily against the thighbone, which can cause pain and may even damage the kneecap.

Because women have wider hips, the upper-leg bone of a woman enters the knee at a greater angle, which twists the knee. This makes women more vulnerable to certain types of kneecap injuries, such as chondromalacia, in which the smooth layer of cartilage that undercoats the thighbone becomes roughened or cracked, according to orthopedic surgeon Michael Baskin, M.D., an assistant clinical professor in the Department of Orthopedics at Oregon Health Sciences University in Portland.

If the large muscles in the thigh (quadriceps) are inflexible due to disuse or lack of stretching before exercise or if these muscles are overused, they can cause inflammation of the knee tendons (patellar tendinitis), sometimes called "jumper's knee." Muscle imbalances, in which one group of muscles is stronger than another and pulls harder, can cause knee problems, too.

While knee problems can result from trauma due to falls, automobile accidents, and athletic injuries or from diseases like arthritis, the vast majority of knee problems are caused from overstressing the knee, according to Michael. "When there isn't an acute injury, most knee pain comes from doing too much too soon or from putting the wrong type of force on the knee," he says. "Often, people who start a running program develop knee problems early on. They don't realize they're subjecting their knees to four to five times their body weight with every running step."

Physical therapist Ellen Nona Hoyven, P.T., owner and director of Ortho Sport Physical Therapy P.C. in Clackamas, Oregon, says most of the knee problems she sees are caused by deconditioned muscles. "People put a high demand on their knees and their muscles without the proper conditioning," she says. "Or they overuse their knees by doing only one type of activity over and over like kneeling, running, or climbing."

Of course, you can't always prevent injuries from occurring, and any serious knee injury should be evaluated and treated by a physician. However, if your knee problems are caused from overuse, disuse, or improper training, you can use the following strategies to keep your knees healthy and, if you do develop pain, to help ease the hurt and speed healing.

Stay trim. Being over normal weight stresses all the joints of the body, but those extra pounds are particularly tough on the knees. "Because of the way the knee is structured, every time you take a step, you're putting one-and-a-half times your body weight on your knee," says Michael. "If you run, you're putting up to five times your body weight on the knees."

Twenty, thirty, forty, or more pounds of extra weight can really stress the knees. For example, if you're only 20 pounds overweight and you jog, you're putting 100 pounds extra force on each knee with every step. "If you're overweight," says Baskin, "it can really add to knee pain. Being overweight means you're going to need greater muscle strength to prevent injuries."

Keep your weight within normal limits with a low-fat diet and regular exercise.

Look at your feet. There's an old saying: "When your knee hurts, look to your feet." Hoyven agrees. "When the feet hit the ground, everything changes," she says. "Think of the body much like a slinky. If one part of the skeleton is out of balance, it will throw off the other parts. When the feet are not supporting the body properly, it can cause problems all over the body, including the knees."

A common cause of knee problems is overpronation, or rolling inward of the foot. A certain amount of pronation is normal, but too much can cause knee problems. "When the foot pronates, it rotates inward and flattens out," explains Michael. "At the same time, it rotates the lower leg, which malaligns the knee. This malalignment can cause the kneecap to track abnormally and grind, causing pain."

You can correct overpronation with supportive shoes designed to prevent pronation or with orthotics, which are special shoe inserts. You can buy ready-made, over-the-counter orthotics or you can get custom-made ones from a podiatrist, orthopedist, chiropractor, or sports-medicine specialist.

Buy the right shoes. "The right shoe can prevent all kinds of knee problems," says Kathleen Galligan, D.C., who specializes in sports injuries in Lake Oswego, Oregon.

Wear the lowest heel possible. Galligan says the body can tolerate a heel of about one inch. Higher heels throw the body forward and stress the knees.

If you tend to pronate, buy a shoe that has antipronation devices. "You can buy athletic shoes that have higher-density materials on the inside of the shoe sole and cushioning material on the outside edge of the sole," says Michael. "The higher density material doesn't allow the shoe to 'give' on the inside and helps prevent pronation."

Michael says you should also look for shoes that have a stiff heel counter, the part of the shoe that cups the heel. "A stiffer heel counter will stabilize the heel and help prevent overpronation," he says.

Then replace them. Often, knee problems are simply caused from running shoes that are worn out, says Louisa Silva, M.D., who sees plenty of knee problems in her private practice in Salem, Oregon. "Even if the sole of your shoe looks fine, the structure of the shoe may be worn out," she says. "Then the shoe isn't giving your foot the support it needs." Shoe experts estimate that running shoes are good for 400 to 600 miles; walking shoes for 600 miles or more before they need to be replaced.

Check your alignment. If you're bowlegged or knock-kneed, you may be at greater risk for knee problems, according to Baskin. To check your alignment, stand with your ankles touching. If you're in alignment, both your ankle bones and your knees should touch. If your knees touch, but there's a large space between your ankles, you're knock-kneed. If your ankles touch, but there's space between your knees, you're bowlegged. "If you're out of alignment," says Baskin, "you may need to avoid certain activities, like running, that stress the knees. Substitute activities like swimming, biking, or working out on a cross-country ski machine."

Don't rely on over-the-counter braces. Often, you see people wearing knee braces or bandages they've purchased at the pharmacy. An over-the-counter knee brace may make you aware of the knee and remind you to avoid overtraining, but it doesn't really correct or prevent problems, says Michael Martindale, L.P.T., a physical therapist at the Sports Medicine Center at Portland Adventist Medical Center in Oregon who specializes in sports injuries. "Know that over-the-counter braces don't take the place of exercises you should be doing to strengthen your knees," says Baskin. He says if you do use a knee brace, opt for the one-piece neoprene or elastic braces rather than the elastic wraps, which make it difficult to apply

◆◆ Exercise Those Knees ◆◆

Often, muscle imbalances, in which one muscle or muscle group is stronger than another, cause knee problems. In other cases, lack of flexibility can contribute to knee pain or injury. "Knees need both strength and flexibility," says Michael Baskin, M.D. "People often concentrate on the quadriceps [muscles in the front of the thigh] and forget the hamstrings [muscles at the back of the thigh], but both need to be flexible and strong to prevent knee problems."

While rest is important when you injure your knees, too much rest can contribute to knee problems. "If you have knee pain, the tendency is to stop using it and to stop exercising," explains Chrissy Kane, L.P.T., a physical therapist in the Outpatient Physical Therapy Department at Providence Medical Center in Portland, Oregon. "Lack of use can cause the muscles around the knee to become weak and cause the knee to become unstable. Gentle exercises can break this cycle."

Exercises can correct imbalances, increase flexibility, and prevent many injuries. However, Baskin warns that not all exercises are healthy for the knees. He recommends that you avoid loading the knee with weight when it's in a fully flexed, 90-degree position (such as when sitting), especially if you have kneecap pain. "The only time you should have your knee at this 90-degree angle," he says, "is when you're getting up from a chair."

For strong, flexible knees, try performing these exercises regularly:

Hamstring stretch. *Lie on your back, raise your right leg, and hold the thigh up with your hands. Gently and slowly straighten the knee until you feel a stretch in the back of the thigh. Don't bounce. Hold the stretch for 10 to 20 seconds. Repeat three to five times on each leg.*

You can also perform this hamstring stretch in a standing position with your leg on a chair. Slowly lean forward, reaching down the shin until you feel a stretch in the back of the thigh. Hold for 10 to 20 seconds.

Quadriceps stretch. *Stand with your right hand on the back of a chair. With your left hand, pull your left heel toward your left buttock and point your left knee to the floor until you feel a stretch in front of the thigh. Hold for 10 to 20 seconds. Repeat using the right hand and right leg.*

If you can't reach your ankle, loop a towel around your foot to pull back the leg, or do the stretch lying on your stomach on a bed or the floor.

Calf stretch. *Stand two to three feet from a wall and lunge your right foot forward. Keep your left leg straight, with your heel on the floor and your toes pointed forward; keep your right leg slightly bent. Lean into the wall, with both hands on the wall supporting you, until you feel a stretch in the left calf. Hold for 10 to 20 seconds. Repeat with your left leg bent and your right leg straight.*

pressure evenly to the knee. Michael warns against becoming dependent upon a knee brace. "If you've got pain that is persistent enough to buy a knee brace, you need to see a doctor," he says.

Avoid "knee-busting" activities. Deep knee bends may feel healthful, but they're too hard on the knees. "Knee bends put way too much pressure on the knees," says Michael. "I tell people to take squats and deep knee bends out of their exercise routine and to avoid kneeling whenever possible, especially on hard surfaces."

Hip-extensor strengthener. This exercise strengthens the muscles in the back of the hip. Lie on your stomach, tighten the muscle at the front of your right thigh, then lift your right leg eight to ten inches from the floor, keeping the knee locked. Hold for five to ten seconds. Do ten repetitions. Repeat with the left leg.

Hip-abductor strengthener. This exercise strengthens the muscles at the outside of the thigh. Lie on your left side, tighten the muscle at the front of your right thigh, then lift your right leg eight to ten inches from the floor. Hold for five to ten seconds. Do ten repetitions. Repeat on opposite side.

Hip-adductor strengthener. This exercise strengthens the muscles at the inside of the thigh. Lie on your left side, with your head supported by your left hand and your right leg crossed over in front of your left leg. Tighten the muscle at the front of the left thigh, then lift the left leg eight to ten inches from the floor. Hold for five to ten seconds. Repeat ten times. Switch legs, and repeat ten times.

Quadriceps strengthener. Lie on your back with your right leg straight and your left leg bent at the knee. Tighten the muscle at the front of your right thigh, and lift your right leg five to ten inches from the floor, keeping the knee locked. Hold for 10 to 20 seconds. Repeat ten times. Switch legs, and repeat ten times.

Silva says one of the most common causes of knee pain among her patients is weight training. "People can literally wear out their knees by lifting too much weight and putting the knee through its full range of motion," she explains. "There are tremendous forces on the knee in the fully flexed position."

Silva's recommendations to weight lifters: Never fully flex the knee, and keep the amount of weight you ask the knees to lift to a minimum.

If you're gardening or doing some other activity that requires kneeling, Michael says to use foam kneeling pads and to give your knees frequent rest periods.

Don't "run through" knee pain. Many people, especially athletes, believe that it's best to "run through" knee pain. However, they may be doing more harm than good. "Pain is an indicator that something is wrong," says Martindale. "If you're having pain, you may have biomechanical problems like overpronation, or you may be overtraining, training incorrectly, or wearing the wrong footwear."

Michael agrees. "You don't have pain in your body if everything is right," he says. "The body is sending you a signal if it's hurting. Don't keep going. Stop stressing the part that hurts. The body heals itself with rest."

Change surfaces. Michael, who was a national collegiate running champion, says running on the wrong surface can cause knee problems. "Roads are 'canted,' or slanted from the center," Michael explains. "Runners who run only on one side of the road often overstress the knees." He recommends running or walking on the flattest part of the road. Switch sides of the road frequently if it is safe to do so.

Hard surfaces such as concrete or asphalt can increase the beating the knees take, too. Michael recommends running or walking on a soft surface, such as a forest pathway. Be careful of too-soft sand, however, which can stress the knees.

Running or walking downhill can cause knee problems as well. The natural tendency is to "brake" with the knees downhill, which can overstress them. Slow down and, whenever possible, traverse down hills. If you're already having knee problems, avoid training downhill.

Mix it up. Martindale says he's seen an increase in knee problems with activities like step aerobics. "Anytime you overstress the knee with too much squatting or stepping, the knee is vulnerable," he says.

Michael recommends "cross-training," or doing a variety of physical activities rather than just one or two. "Any repetitive routine strengthens specific muscles," he explains. "Cross-training helps balance out the imbalances caused by training only particular muscle groups. It helps counteract the stress and strain caused from repetitive activities."

He suggests combining running or walking with biking, swimming, dancing, aerobics, weight training, or any other activity you might enjoy. He says if you choose biking as one of your cross-training activities, be sure to raise the seat up so that the leg is almost fully extended on the downward stroke to prevent knee strain.

R.I.C.E. it. OK, despite all the good advice, you've overdone it and your knee hurts. Give it

R.I.C.E.—rest, ice, compression, and elevation. Take the weight off the knee. During the first 24 to 48 hours, use an ice pack (20 minutes on, 20 minutes off) to keep the swelling down. Wrap the knee (not too tightly) in an elastic bandage to reduce swelling, and keep the knee elevated.

Take anti-inflammatories. Aspirin or ibuprofen can reduce the pain, inflammation, and swelling, says Silva. Don't use anti-inflammatories, however, if you have an ulcer, a bleeding condition, or a sensitive stomach, warns Baskin. "The only thing worse than a sore knee," he says, "is a sore knee and a bleeding ulcer." Acetaminophen can help with the pain and may be easier on your stomach, but it won't do much for inflammation.

Avoid heat. Ice prevents fluid buildup, but heat can promote it, says Michael. For the first 48 to 72 hours after a knee injury, avoid hot tubs or hot packs.

Massage it. While massage won't affect the bony structures of the knee, it does increase circulation and can loosen tight hamstrings or other structures around the knee, says Martindale. If you've already developed knee pain, says Michael, see a professional massage therapist or physical therapist, not just a friend, for a professional massage. ◆

◆ LACTOSE ◆ INTOLERANCE

10 Ways to Manage It

Many folks relish the thought of downing a frosty-cold glass of milk, polishing off a bowl of creamy ice cream, or biting into a piping-hot slice of cheesy pizza. For close to 50 million Americans, though, the aftereffects of indulging in these dairy delights may force them to forgo such foods or suffer some decidedly unpleasant consequences.

The common condition these people share is lactose intolerance. That means they don't properly digest lactose, which is milk sugar found in all milk products. This problem is usually due to a shortage of the enzyme lactase, which normally breaks down milk sugar in the small intestine into simple parts that can be absorbed into the bloodstream. The end result of this lactase deficiency may be gas, stomach pains, bloating, and diarrhea. The severity of the symptoms varies from person to person.

Who is lactose intolerant? It's not an equal opportunity problem. It affects some ethnic groups much more than others. The National Institute of Diabetes & Digestive & Kidney Diseases estimates that 75 percent of African-American, Jewish, Native-American, and Mexican-American adults and 90 percent of Asian-American adults have this condition. Only about 10 to 15 percent of adult Caucasians are lactase deficient, says David Alpers, M.D., a professor of medicine and chief of the Gastroenterology Division at Washington University School of Medicine in St. Louis. Though you may not fall into any of these categories, keep in mind that as we get older, we all lose some of the ability to digest lactose in milk.

Some people figure out that they are lactose intolerant on their own; for others, it takes a trip to a doctor to pinpoint the problem. "Among the

◆◆ Hidden Sources ◆◆ of Lactose

Lactose lurks in many prepared foods. Bread, cereals, pancakes, chocolate, soups, puddings, salad dressings, sherbet, instant cocoa mix, candies, frozen dinners, cookie mixes, and hot dogs may all contain lactose. While the amounts of lactose may be small, people with low tolerance levels can be bothered. "People need to read every single label and be careful of what they eat," says author Jane Zukin. When perusing ingredient labels, it's not just milk that you have to watch for. Whey, curds, milk by-products, dry milk solids, nonfat dry milk powder, casein, galactose, skim milk powder, milk sugar, and whey protein concentrate are all buzzwords that indicate the presence of lactose.

black or Asian community, it's kind of folk wisdom that these people don't do well with milk, so they tend not to drink as much," says Alpers. On the other hand, he says, "There's also a significant number of people who are having symptoms from milk sugar and really have no idea of what the problem is."

If you suspect you may be lactose intolerant but you're not sure, it may be worth a visit to a physician to rule out other possible problems (see "Hello, Doctor?"). Once you know that you are indeed lactose intolerant, you may want to follow these helpful tips to ease your symptoms:

Determine your level of lactose intolerance. The degree of intolerance differs with each person. The easiest way to do this is first to get all lactose out of your system. "That means having no dairy food and no lactose for about three to four weeks," says Jane Zukin, author of *The Dairy-Free Cookbook* and editor of *The Newsletter for People with Lactose Intolerance and Milk Allergies*. Then start with very small quantities of milk or cheese. Monitor your symptoms to see how much or how little dairy food you can handle. Once you know your limits, management becomes a little easier.

Stick with small servings. While you may not be able to tolerate an eight-ounce glass of milk all at once, you may feel fine drinking a third of a cup in the morning, a third of a cup in the afternoon, and a third of a cup at night. "If you have 'x' amount of lactase enzyme in your body that can only digest 'x' amount of lactose, it will be easier if you take in less lactose over a longer period of time than if you overload," says Zukin.

Don't eat dairy foods alone. If you eat some cheese or drink a little milk, plan to do so with a meal or a snack. "Having more in your stomach to digest slows the digestive process and may ease your symptoms," says Zukin.

Color your milk chocolate. A study by researcher Chong Lee at the University of Rhode Island in Kingston found that 35 lactose-intolerant people digested more lactose when they drank milk with cocoa and sugar added than they did when they drank plain milk. They also experienced less bloating and fewer cramps. No one is sure why this is so, but Alpers says it may be because "chocolate delays the emptying of your stomach." A slower emptying rate may mean fewer symptoms.

Supplement your diet. Lactase-enzyme supplements can supply your body with some of what it lacks. They're sold in tablet or liquid form, without a prescription. The tablets are chewed with or right after you consume a dairy product; you add the drops directly to milk. "These work quite well for some people," says Zukin. You can also try lactose-reduced milk.

Try yogurt. "By and large, lactose intolerant people tolerate yogurt pretty well," says Alpers. This holds true, however, only for yogurt with active cultures, which you may have to buy in a health-food store. If you can tolerate yogurt, it's to your advantage to include it in your diet, because this creamy food is a great source of calcium.

Choose hard cheeses. If you find yourself drawn to the cheese aisle at your grocery store, pick hard, aged cheeses such as Swiss, cheddar, or Colby, advises Elyse Sosin, R.D., Supervisor of Clinical Nutrition at Mount Sinai Medical Center in New York. They contain less lactose than soft cheeses.

Avoid processed foods. Lactose is used in a lot of processed foods where you might not expect to find it (see "Hidden Sources of Lactose"). "It's best for people to stick to as much fresh food as possible, and skip the cans, frozen foods, and stuff that comes out of a box," says Zukin. One added benefit to this strategy: You'll be eating a healthier diet.

Get calcium from other foods. Lactose intolerant people, especially women and children, should make sure their calcium intake doesn't plunge. Green, leafy vegetables, such as collard greens, kale, turnip greens, and chinese cabbage (bok choy), as well as oysters, sardines, canned salmon with the bones, and tofu, provide lots of calcium. If your diet is calcium poor, you may want to take calcium supplements; talk to your doctor for a recommendation on proper dosage.

Watch out for medications. Lactose is used as a filler in more than 20 percent of prescription drugs (including many types of birth control pills) and in about 6 percent of over-the-counter medicines. This may not matter to someone who takes medication only occasionally, but Zukin says, "for the person who takes medication on a regular basis, this can be a problem." Complicating matters is the fact that lactose may not be listed under the inactive ingredients on the label. To find out if what you're taking contains lactose, Zukin advises first seeking help from your doctor. You might also check with your pharmacist or write directly to the drug manufacturer. ◆

◆◆ Hello, Doctor? ◆◆

If you're feeling digestive distress that you think may be lactose intolerance but you're not certain, try this simple test. Lay off all milk products for a few weeks and see if your gut gets better. If things don't improve, it may be time to check in with your doctor. Other glitches in the digestive system may be causing your problems. For instance, you may have irritable bowel syndrome, another common digestive disorder that can produce symptoms similar to lactose intolerance (see IRRITABLE BOWEL SYNDROME). "Another thing that lactose intolerance can be confused with is an intolerance to caffeine," says David Alpers, M.D. So play it safe and get an expert's opinion, especially if you notice a major change in bowel patterns.

◆ LARYNGITIS ◆

18 Ways to Tame a Hoarse Throat

Your voice sounds more like a frog croaking than a human talking. Chances are, you can figure out the cause—whether it was all the yelling you did at last night's hockey game or that cold you've had for the past couple of days.

Don't confuse laryngitis with a sore throat, though. "Some people say they've got laryngitis when what they really mean is their throat is sore," says Michael S. Benninger, M.D., vice-chairperson of the Department of Otolaryngology at Henry Ford Hospital in Detroit.

True laryngitis is the loss of the voice or hoarseness, and it's the result of inflammation (swelling) of the larynx, or voice box, and the voice folds, explains Gary Y. Shaw, M.D., associate professor of otolaryngology, head and neck surgery at the University of Kansas Medical Center in Kansas City.

The most common cause of temporary laryngitis is an upper-respiratory infection, usually viral, like the common cold. If the infection is bacterial, you may need to see a doctor to get antibiotic treatment.

The second most common cause of laryngitis is voice abuse or overuse. "If you screamed at the top of your lungs at the football game, you'll be hoarse afterward," says Shaw.

The symptoms of acute, or short-term laryngitis, can include pain in the throat or around the larynx, hoarseness, raspiness, the loss of range (noticed especially by singers), easy fatiguability, and a scratchy feeling in the throat. Constantly clearing your throat can be another symptom.

If you suffer from chronic laryngitis, smoking may be the culprit. The smoke increases the mass of the larynx, explains Benninger, lowering the pitch of the voice.

One surprising cause of laryngitis is gastro-esophageal reflux. That's a long name for what a lot of us think of as heartburn, except that only about half of its sufferers actually feel any "heartburn," so they're unaware that the acid-rich contents of their stomach are coming back up in their throats, especially during the night. "It's the principal player in laryngitis in the elderly," says Benninger. "People complain there's something sticking in their throat, and they think it's mucus from postnasal drip." Symptoms are worse in the morning. You may wake up with a bad taste in your mouth, do a lot of throat clearing, and have hoarseness that gets better as the day goes on, says Shaw. "And you often feel like there's something in your throat all the time." If you suspect this is causing your laryngitis, see your doctor (also see HEARTBURN).

If you're experiencing laryngitis, here's what you can do to soothe your voice:

Drink. Water, that is. Take frequent sips of water to stay hydrated and keep your throat moist. Or choose other fluids, like juices, says Sally Wenzel, M.D., assistant professor of medicine at the National Jewish Center for Immunology and Respiratory Medicine in Denver. She adds that warm drinks may feel more soothing than cold.

Sip noncaffeinated tea with lemon. You want to avoid caffeine because of its dehydrating effects, says Benninger. Make sure the tea isn't too hot or too cold. The lemon helps stimulate the flow of saliva.

Suck on lemon drops. Again, lemon gets those juices flowing.

Use artificial saliva. It may sound unpleasant, but you can buy over-the-counter products that help keep your mouth moist.

Speak softly. "Speak in a confidential tone, as if you're telling someone a secret," says Benninger.

Don't whisper. Whispering is actually more stressful than speaking in a softly modulated voice.

Limit conversation. "It's sort of like limiting the motion of your knee when it's skinned," says Shaw. "I tell patients to use their voices only if they're getting paid for it," adds Benninger.

Don't clear your throat. You're actually irritating the situation when you try to clear up things, setting up "a vicious cycle," says Benninger.

Stop smoking. Chalk up one more reason to avoid tobacco. If you can't kick the habit completely, at least go without while your throat is healing.

Avoid smokers. Even passive smoke irritates the larynx. If you live with a smoker, ask him or her to take their habit outside.

Forget recreational drugs. Marijuana and cocaine are extremely rough on the larynx, Benninger says.

Abstain from alcohol. Alcohol dehydrates you, which is the opposite of what your voice needs.

Cut out the caffeine. Like alcohol, the caffeine in coffee, tea, and colas dehydrates you.

Humidify the air. Indoor heating takes moisture out of winter air. Use a humidifier or portable steamer. If nothing else, breathe in the steam from a teapot or pan of boiling water, suggests Shaw.

Avoid dusty environments. The dust is irritating, and such places are often also dry, which compounds the problem.

Beware of certain drying drugs. Medications such as antihistamines and diuretics can dry your mouth and throat. You shouldn't stop diuretics (they're often prescribed for high blood pressure), but think twice about taking over-the-counter antihistamines. Talk to your doctor or pharmacist if you have any questions about any medications you may be taking.

◆◆ Hello, Doctor? ◆◆

Laryngitis is usually a temporary inconvenience without serious consequences. But sometimes, persistent hoarseness or voice loss is your body's way of telling you something is wrong. When should you see a doctor?

- *If pain is present*
- *If the hoarseness continues for more than 72 hours*
- *If you've got an upper-respiratory infection with a fever that lasts more than a couple of days*
- *If you have trouble breathing*
- *If you notice a permanent change in the pitch of your voice, especially if you are a smoker*
- *If you cough up blood*

The problem may be as minor as a bacterial infection that needs antibiotics. You could have polyps or nodules on your vocal folds that cause them to vibrate more slowly, changing the sound of your voice. Or you could have cancer of the larynx, which can be treated with radiation if caught early.

Gargle with salt water. Add one-half teaspoon salt to a cup of warm (about body temperature) water, advises Wenzel. You don't want it too salty, warns Benninger. "It's not like ocean water. And too much salt could cause more irritation."

Protect your voice. To help your voice heal and to prevent future attacks of laryngitis, learn how to take care of your voice. Staying well hydrated is the first step. Avoiding voice abuse is the next. And if you depend on your voice in your career, you may want to invest in voice training, suggests Benninger. ◆

◆ MENOPAUSE ◆

11 Tips for Coping with "the Change"

For most women, menopause, the cessation of the menstrual cycle, is fraught with rumor and misinformation. Stories of menopausal hot flashes, vaginal dryness, wrinkles, weight gain, depression, anxiety, thinning hair, and loss of sex drive may have you dreading "the change." Relax. Most of the stories you've heard probably aren't true.

Too often, women confuse natural aging changes with menopause. The few symptoms actually associated with the hormonal changes during menopause can usually be handled with a few minor lifestyle changes. Contrary to what most women have heard about menopause, it's a natural period of transition that gives rise to an exciting and challenging period in life.

Menopause is a period of four or five years, usually two years before the last menstrual period and two to three years after it. For most women, menopause occurs between the ages of 45 and 53, although some women experience it earlier and others go through it at a later age. A woman generally experiences menopause at about the same age as her mother did.

Menopause begins with changes in the menstrual cycle—shorter or longer periods, heavier or lighter bleeding, decreased or increased premenstrual symptoms—until the menstrual periods cease altogether. Women should keep track of their irregular bleeding so their physician can help them determine whether these changes are normal or whether they indicate some abnormal changes in the uterine lining.

Although there is much talk about menopausal "symptoms," the only symptoms that have been clearly demonstrated to be associated with the hormonal changes of menopause are hot flashes and vaginal dryness. Mood swings or depression aren't related to hormonal changes as much as they are to fatigue caused from sleep disturbances due to hot flashes, according to Amanda Clark, M.D., assistant professor of obstetrics and gynecology at Oregon Health Sciences University in Portland. "The hormonal fluctuations of menopause aren't believed to cause any major psychological depression," she says.

But menopause signals more than hormonal changes. It is the doorway to a new life. Postmenopausal women are free of the discomforts of menstruation, free of the need for contraceptives, and, in many cases, free of child-rearing responsibilities. For the first time, many women find they can concentrate on their own agendas and do the things *they* want to do.

Here are some tips about how to make the most of this exciting transition called menopause:

Dress for hot flashes. Eight in ten women experience periods of sudden, intense heat and accompanying sweating often called "flushes" or "hot flashes," according to Sadja Greenwood, M.D., an assistant clinical professor in the Department of Obstetrics, Gynecology, and Reproductive Sciences at the University of California at San Francisco. "Hot flashes are the body's response to lower-than-usual estrogen levels," says Greenwood. She recommends wearing loose clothing that is easily removed, such as cardigan sweaters.

Douse it. If you're at home or in a place where it's convenient, you can "spritz" your face with a spray of cool water from a squeeze bottle or you can blot your face with a cool washcloth or moist towelette.

Avoid caffeine and alcohol. If hot flashes seem to be triggered by caffeine and alcohol consumption, Greenwood advises women to avoid them completely. Try substituting noncaffeinated teas or decaffeinated coffee for caffeinated beverages. (Keep in mind that caffeine withdrawal may cause headaches and fatigue for several days.) Greenwood says excess caffeine also causes the kidneys to excrete more calcium, a factor in bone thinning in postmenopausal women.

Carry a personal fan. Many women find they can get relief from the sudden heat of hot flashes by using a small personal fan. Inexpensive wood and paper fans or battery-powered personal fans are small enough to be carried in a purse and can be used anywhere.

Take your time with lovemaking. Hormonal changes associated with menopause often cause a woman's vaginal mucous membranes to become thin and secrete less moisture. The result can be painful sexual intercourse. Some of this lack of moisture can be overcome by taking more time to make love, according to Lonnie Barbach, Ph.D., a nationally recognized sex expert and author of numerous books on the topic. Barbach also suggests exploring other ways of pleasuring one another in addition to intercourse.

Use creams or lubricants. If patient lovemaking doesn't produce enough lubrication for the woman, Clark suggests using lubricating jellies (available in pharmacies), plain vegetable oil, or unscented cold cream. "One of the best lubricants is a product called Astroglide, because it's most like natural secretions," she says. "Jellies like K-Y Jelly are good, but Vaseline tends to be messy and gummy."

Exercise regularly. Menopause has been erroneously linked with depression. Several studies have found that women between the ages of 45 and 55 have no increase in susceptibility to depression. Mood swings during this time may have more to do with a woman's changing role and her self-concept and the physical changes of aging she's experiencing. "For many women," says Clark, "menopause is a milestone, a negative milestone, in their lives. They find the idea of menopause

Calcium-Rich Foods

Calcium is important at any age, but it becomes even more important for menopausal women in order to prevent the bone thinning of osteoporosis. Include these calcium-rich foods in your diet to ensure you're getting enough of this important mineral.

Almonds
Brewer's yeast
Cheese
    (opt for nonfat or low-fat varieties)
Dandelion greens
Ice milk or ice cream
    (opt for lower-fat varieties)
Kelp
Mackerel, canned
Milk (opt for skim or low-fat)
Mustard greens
Oysters
Salmon, canned with bones
Sardines, canned with bones
Soybean curd (tofu)
Yogurt (opt for nonfat or low-fat)

depressing. We need to discard those old ideas." Regular, aerobic exercise such as brisk walking does much to increase the general health level, fight fatigue, and raise the spirits. Exercise also appears to slow changes like loss of strength that many believe to be age related, but are actually more associated with a sedentary lifestyle.

Regular, weight-bearing exercises such as walking or jogging can also help stave off the bone thinning of osteoporosis, a problem for many menopausal women. Clark says bones get stronger with regular exercise no matter what your age. "Any weight-bearing exercise is good," says Clark. "But it has to be a weight-bearing exercise, not like swimming, to increase bone density."

Get support. "Another term for menopause is 'climacteric,'" says Susan Woodruff, B.S.N., childbirth and parenting education coordinator at Tuality Community Hospital in Hillsboro, Oregon. "That word applies because it is a really big change. You're closing one chapter in your life and moving on. You may notice body changes—new aches, pains, wrinkles. Menopause is one of life's major change signals. It's helpful to talk to other women about these changes."

Woodruff recommends joining a menopause support group sponsored by a local hospital, community college, or professional group. Or you might want to form your own support group with friends who are experiencing menopause. "Menopause affects how you see yourself, your self-concept, because your roles in life are changing at this time," says Woodruff. "A support group of other women who understand can really help you see yourself as a strong person experiencing a natural life change."

Get plenty of calcium. "Everyone loses calcium as they get older," says Clark. "But in women, as estrogen levels decline, the rate of bone loss increases."

Sonja Connor, M.S., R.D., research associate professor in the School of Medicine at Oregon Health Sciences University in Portland, says, "At menopause, there's an outpouring of calcium in response to the lower estrogen levels. Unless you have really good stores of calcium already, during this time you're going to have an increased need for calcium."

Clark says postmenopausal women taking hormone replacement need 1,000 milligrams of elemental calcium daily; women not taking hormones need 1,500 milligrams of elemental calcium.

Dairy products are good sources of calcium, although you'll be doing yourself an even bigger favor if you choose those that are low in fat, such as skim milk, nonfat yogurt, and low-fat cheeses.

◆◆◆ Estrogen ◆◆◆ Replacement Therapy

Many physicians recommend that women take hormones to make up for the decrease in estrogen levels that occurs during menopause. Estrogen replacement therapy, or ERT (also called hormone replacement therapy or HRT), can reduce or eliminate the hot flashes and vaginal soreness and, in some women, decrease the risk of osteoporosis, says Sadja Greenwood, M.D.

However, ERT isn't without risk. Some studies have shown ERT may increase the risk of developing cancer of the breast and uterus. Amanda Clark, M.D., says studies have shown the increased risk of breast cancer is quite small and that the increased risk of uterine cancer from estrogen replacement can be eliminated by adding the hormone progestin.

Women who have had any of the following are generally not *recommended for ERT: cancer of the breast or uterus; ovarian cancer; clots in the legs, pelvis, or lungs; high blood pressure; diabetes; gallstones or gallbladder disease; or large uterine fibroids.*

Clark believes that, for most women, the benefits of hormone replacement therapy outweigh the risks. "Fourteen studies have shown that hormone replacement therapy helps prevent heart disease," she says. "Estrogen also helps maintain calcium uptake, which helps prevent osteoporosis."

Greenwood says women should thoroughly discuss the pros and cons of ERT with their physicians. If a woman opts for ERT, Greenwood says, she should take the lowest dose possible and be sure the doctor prescribes a combination of both estrogen and progestin to reduce the risk of uterine cancer.

For example, an eight-ounce glass of whole milk and an eight-ounce glass of skim milk contain the same amount of elemental calcium (350 milligrams), but the whole milk contains about 70 calories more from fat. To add to your calcium stores, eat a diet that is also rich in vegetables, fruits, and complex carbohydrates (see "Calcium-Rich Foods").

If your diet isn't calcium rich or if your stores of calcium are seriously depleted from a lifetime of poor eating habits, Clark suggests taking calcium supplements. Keep in mind that the number of milligrams of calcium listed on the label of a supplement may not reflect the amount of elemental calcium in the product. For example, it takes 1,200 milligrams of calcium carbonate to get 500 milligrams of elemental calcium. Ask your doctor or pharmacist for advice on choosing a calcium supplement.

Eat a balanced, low-fat diet. Women at menopause not only have an increased risk of osteoporosis, they may also be at risk for heart disease. "At menopause, women's levels of LDL, or so-called 'bad' cholesterol, go up," explains Connor. "Within about ten years, they have the same risk for heart disease as men."

Connor says diet can go a long way toward preventing serious health problems like osteoporosis, cancer, and heart disease in menopausal women. "Diets high in animal products and salt cause the body to excrete more calcium, which contributes to osteoporosis," she says. "Menopausal women should eat less animal protein and less salt. If they switch to more foods from the vegetable kingdom and more complex carbohydrates, they'll be getting less fat [high-fat diets are related to some cancers and heart disease], more calcium, and more of the anticancer elements like beta carotene."

Plan for menopause. "The problem," says Connor, "is that most women eat the typical American diet: 40 percent of calories from fat, 20 percent from sugar, and 5 percent from alcohol—essentially empty calories. That means they're getting nutrients from only 35 percent of their calories. On top of that, they don't do any regular exercise. When menopause comes, they need medical intervention in the form of hormone therapy just to catch up with what they've done to their bodies all these years."

Connor believes only a small percentage of women would need hormone therapy if they'd anticipate menopause by eating right and exercising regularly for at least 20 years before the onset of menopause. "Prevention is the best thing," she says. "A lifelong lifestyle of low-fat eating, not smoking, and exercising regularly will usually get you ready to face menopausal changes without any problems." And, of course, no matter what stage in life you're in, it's never too late to benefit from switching to a healthier lifestyle. ◆

◆ MENSTRUAL CRAMPS ◆

6 Ways to Tackle Them

◆◆ Hello, Doctor? ◆◆

All of these experts agree that if you notice your cramps getting more severe, or if you've never had menstrual cramps before and suddenly develop them, it is time to visit your doctor. "Women with primary menstrual cramps start having them when they first begin menstruating or within one to two years of the onset of menstruation," says Harold Zimmer, M.D. "So if you notice a significant change, you should be evaluated to see if there is some secondary cause for the cramps," he continues.

"Secondary cramps also tend to be pretty mean cramps that are often accompanied by nausea, vomiting, and even diarrhea," says Phyllis Frey, A.R.N.P. "They can also occur with backache and pain down the thighs."

The causes for secondary cramps could include endometriosis (the presence of endometrial tissue in places where it is not usually found), pelvic congestion, pelvic varicose veins, pelvic infection, or fibroids (benign tumors in the uterine wall). "Secondary cramps caused by fibroids tend to occur during actual ovulation, while those caused by endometriosis may be present throughout the month," says Zimmer. "With pelvic congestion or pelvic veins, the cramps tend to occur four or five days before the menstrual flow itself," he adds. While you may get some relief from secondary cramps with self-treatment, the underlying conditions that cause them really need to be treated by a physician. And Zimmer warns that exercising may actually worsen secondary cramps.

Three weeks out of each month you feel great. But then comes your period, and with it, those awful cramps. You try to ignore them and go about your daily business, but the pain and discomfort continue to divert your attention. For most women, menstrual cramps last no more than one or two days each month. But this can seem endless when you're trying to function normally. And the congestive, bloating-type symptoms that often accompany these cramps may only compound the problem.

"Primary menstrual cramps are hereditary," says Phyllis Frey, A.R.N.P., a nurse practitioner at Bellegrove OB-GYN, Inc., in Bellevue, Washington. "There is no specific cause determined. It just seems that during your period, your uterus cramps up and your sensitivity to that cramping is pretty acute," she explains.

"Sometimes, primary cramps will lessen after giving birth," says Harold Zimmer, M.D., an obstetrician and gynecologist in Bellevue, Washington. "We are not sure why this is, but it could be that the stretching out of the cervix during delivery reduces the pulling against it that can occur when the uterus contracts or cramps up," he adds.

"Secondary menstrual cramps, on the other hand, are caused by some underlying condition, such as pelvic infection, pelvic lesions, fibroids, endometriosis, bad pelvic congestion, or pelvic varicose veins," says Zimmer. "They are usually a little worse than primary cramps, depending on how significant the underlying condition is," he adds.

In either case, menstrual cramps are usually the result of a prostaglandin excess. Prostaglandin is a hormone produced by the uterine lining that mediates many processes within the body. It can bring on headaches, intestinal cramps, and labor, according to Zimmer. While secondary cramps are usually treated by curing the underlying condition, primary cramps are largely self-treatable with over-the-counter medications and some basic comfort measures. Here are some suggestions:

Take ibuprofen or aspirin. "These medications help to lower the level of prostaglandins, which can lessen or alleviate the cramps," says Zimmer. "These drugs also cost much less than those that a doctor would prescribe for cramps," adds Frey.

Hold a heating pad to the cramped area. 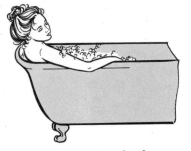 "The heat will relax the muscles and soften the pain of the cramping," says Frey. "It works best if you can lie down at the same time," she says.

Maintain a regular aerobic exercise program. "This doesn't mean you have to exercise through an episode of cramps. Keeping up a regular exercise or fitness program the rest of the month seems to make these episodes less intense when they do occur," says Frey. "Exercising also increases pelvic circulation, which helps to clear out the excess prostaglandins a little faster," adds Zimmer.

Take a hot bath. "Just as with a heating pad, a hot bath relaxes the muscles and increases circulation to the pelvic area," says Zimmer. It can also relieve some of the lower back pain that can accompany cramps.

Do some pelvic-tilt exercises. "Getting down on all fours, bringing the elbows to the ground, and rocking back and forth tends to help some women," says Zimmer. "It works especially well for women with a retroverted uterus [one that is more swollen and puts more pressure on the back]," he adds.

Talk to your doctor about birth control pills. "Birth control pills help to suppress ovulation, which lessens the severity of menstrual cramps," says Zimmer. "It is really not certain why they help so much," adds Frey. "It could be that by lessening the flow and length of a woman's period, the cramps are lessened as well," she continues. Birth control pills are not without side effects, however, and certain women should not use them, so be sure to discuss them thoroughly with your doctor. ◆

◆ MORNING SICKNESS ◆

13 Ways to Ease the Queasiness

The nausea and vomiting of early pregnancy were written about as early as 2000 B.C. Unfortunately, the ancient Egyptians didn't have a cure for the condition, either.

Some 50 to 70 percent of American women will suffer from nausea or vomiting, or both, during the first three months (also known as the first trimester) of their pregnancies. The severity and even occurrence vary not only from woman to woman, but from pregnancy to pregnancy in the same individual.

Some women never have even the slightest touch of queasiness. Some are ill in the morning and recover by lunch. And some stay sick all day for days on end, wondering why it's called "morning sickness" when it lasts 24 hours.

No one knows what causes morning sickness. It is less common among Eskimos and native African tribes than in Western civilizations. But today's doctors emphasize it's not psychological, as was once believed. "Morning sickness is not a psychological rejection of the pregnancy," says Donald R. Coustan, M.D., professor and chair of obstetrics-gynecology at Brown University School of Medicine and chief of obstetrics-gynecology at Women and Infants Hospital of Rhode Island in Providence. "It is not a symbolic attempt to vomit up the baby."

Since hormones run amok during early pregnancy, researchers theorize that these abnormal hormone levels contribute somehow to the existence of morning sickness. A suspected culprit is human chorionic gonadotropin (HCG), the hormone tested in home pregnancy kits, which hits an all-time high in those first months. But other hormones may play a role as well. High levels of progesterone, for example, result in smooth-muscle relaxation, slowing down the digestive process, says Cheryl Coleman, R.N., B.S.N., I.C.C.E., a childbirth educator at Hillcrest Medical Center in Tulsa, Oklahoma, and director of public relations for the International Childbirth Education Association.

◆ The Bright Side ◆

The good news about morning sickness? (You doubt that there's anything good to say about this subject?) Studies have shown that women who experience nausea and vomiting early in their pregnancies are more likely to deliver full-term, healthy babies.

Researchers in Colorado Springs, Colorado, and Albany, New York, studied 414 pregnant women. Nearly 90 percent said they had some of the symptoms of morning sickness. But these women were more likely to carry their pregnancies to full term and deliver a live baby than the women who had no morning sickness at all. On the other hand, don't panic if you don't experience morning sickness. Plenty of women sail through pregnancy without nausea and deliver healthy babies.

"There are a lot of changes going on in the pregnant woman's body," points out Kermit E. Krantz, M.D., university distinguished professor, professor of gynecology and obstetrics, and professor of anatomy at the University of Kansas Medical Center in Kansas City. "Your kidneys increase their activity by 100 percent. Your blood volume will increase by 50 percent."

If you're suffering from morning sickness, you probably don't care what causes it. You just want relief. Time will eventually take care of it; the condition usually subsides after the third month. (Scant words of comfort.) While you're waiting for the second trimester to arrive, however, here's what the experts suggest you try for relief:

Don't worry about crumbs in the sheets. Keep crackers by the bed. Eating a few low-sodium crackers as soon as you wake up—and before you get out of bed—is the first line of defense against morning sickness.

Graze. Eat frequent, small meals. You may want to eat five to six times a day. Sometimes, hunger pangs bring on the feelings of nausea. That's because acids in the stomach have nothing to digest when there's no food around.

Don't drink and eat at the same time. In other words, drink your fluids between meals, instead of during meals, to avoid too much bulk in the stomach, says Krantz.

Fill up on fluids. You need at least eight glasses a day, says Krantz. "Avoiding dehydration is most important, especially in the summertime."

Go for a liquid diet. You may find it easier on your tummy to emphasize liquids over solids, says Coustan. Get your nutrients from bouillon, juices, and other liquids.

Stick to bland foods. This isn't the time to try that new Thai restaurant. Spicy foods just don't cut it right now.

Choose complex carbohydrates. Pasta, bread, potatoes—the foods you think of as starches—are easier to digest and they're soothing, says Coleman.

Avoid fatty foods. Fats are harder to digest than carbohydrates or proteins, explains Coleman.

♦♦ Hello, Doctor? ♦♦

If morning sickness persists past the third month or you find yourself so ill that you're losing weight, see your physician. Watch out, too, for becoming dehydrated; you'll feel dizzy when you stand, or your urine output will be scanty and dark colored.

Don't sniff. Certain odors often trigger the feelings of nausea. "Pay attention to what these triggers are and avoid them," suggests Coustan. "Let someone else do the cooking if that bothers you, for example."

Avoid sudden moves. Don't change your posture quickly. "Don't sit up in bed too suddenly," advises Krantz. "Get up easily."

Take vitamin B₆. A number of physicians recommend this vitamin for morning sickness because of its ability to fight nausea. Talk to your doctor before trying a supplement, however, and be sure not to exceed 25 milligrams of the vitamin each day.

Take a hike. OK, go for a walk outside every day. "It's a positive thing you can do for yourself," says Coleman. "And the exercise and fresh air may make you feel better." Be sure to check with your doctor before trying anything more strenuous than a stroll, however.

Don't forget to brush. If you do succumb to vomiting, take good care of your teeth and brush afterwards. Otherwise, the frequent contact with the harsh acids in what you throw up can eat away at tooth enamel. ♦

◆ MOTION SICKNESS ◆

13 Ways to Still the Savage Beast

Oh that queasy sensation, when the world just won't stop swaying, bobbing, or just plain moving. No matter what the mode of movement—in the air, on the ground, or on the water—the result can be motion sickness. While many experts believe there may be a genetic tendency involved, they aren't exactly sure why some people get sick from riding in a car, boat, plane, or train. If you do, you're not alone. Motion sickness caused some pilots to drop out of training during World War II. And to this day, NASA astronauts are constantly combating this side effect brought on by weightlessness and space.

Motion sickness is believed to occur when the balancing system gets overloaded by the messages it's receiving from the eyes and inner ears. The brain responds to the conflicting messages by creating some of its own. "The first signs are usually sweating, hyperventilation, and light-headedness," says Michael S. Morris, M.D., an otolaryngologist and assistant professor at Georgetown University School of Medicine in Washington, D.C.

For some people, these reactions and the others associated with motion sickness, such as nausea, can be brought on merely by walking down the aisles in a supermarket or watching telephone poles whipping by a car window, says John Youngblood, M.D., associate professor at the University of Texas Health Science Center in San Antonio and president of the Austin Ear Clinic. And some people can get "motion" sickness from the sounds they hear, says Herbert Silverstein, M.D., president of the Ear Research Foundation and Florida Otologic Center in Sarasota.

No matter what the cause, once the symptoms set in, it's virtually impossible to stop motion sickness from running its course, says Silverstein. That's why it's important to try to prevent the symptoms before they have a chance to take hold. Here are some techniques you can try to keep motion sickness from setting in:

Look off into the distance. Not to daydream, but to focus on a steady point away from the rocky boat, plane, or car, to help you get your bearings. "Look as far to the horizon as you can," says Silverstein. This helps counteract the conflicting messages the brain is receiving from the topsy-turvy surroundings.

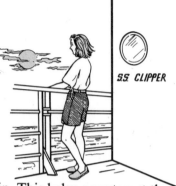

Stay on deck. If you're on a boat, going inside or below deck will only intensify the symptoms. Instead, stay on deck so you can look at the horizon to help your body cope.

Sit over the wing of the airplane. "The wing is the most stable part of the plane, since the plane's body pivots on it," says Youngblood. And if you can get a window seat in this midsection, all the better. Then you can look out and set your sights far from the plane if you should get queasy.

Face forward on the bus or train. This is so you can see the road ahead of you instead of concentrating on the busy movement taking place to the sides. And if you can, take a seat, because standing can also bring on motion sickness.

Volunteer to drive. Drivers are so busy watching the road that they're less apt to get carsick. If you haven't got a license, your next best bet is to "sit in the front seat so you can also anticipate the upcoming bumps and turns and, as a result, be less likely to get sick," says John W. House, M.D., associate clinical professor in the Department of Otolaryngology, Head and Neck Surgery at the University of Southern California at Los Angeles.

Eat a little or don't eat at all. About an hour before you leave, eat some plain crackers or a piece of bread or toast, some experts suggest. Others, such as Silverstein, recommend not eating at all before a trip to help keep your stomach calm and empty, in case you should start to get nauseated.

Avoid "heavy" foods and odors. For some unknown reason, the smell of spicy or greasy foods and strong odors can prompt motion sickness before or during a trip, reports the American Academy of Otolaryngology—Head and Neck Surgery in Alexandria, Virginia.

Say no to alcohol. Avoid alcoholic beverages before and during a trip. "Alcohol goes through the bloodstream and into the inner ear, stimulating it and making a case of motion sickness even worse," explains Silverstein.

Take it easy. After the first signs of illness, close your eyes and stay still until the queasy sensations pass, says Silverstein.

Stay calm, cool, and collected. "For anyone who's had motion sickness, just the thought of being in the same situation again can cause fear and anxiety, which can bring on a bout of motion sickness," says Silverstein. The same goes for those who are anxious about what they're about to do, like flying in a plane or riding in a boat. Try to stay as calm and relaxed as possible. Take a few deep breaths, close your eyes, and tell yourself that you will not get sick.

Leave your reading at home. Reading causes your eyes to move back and forth, so they are not fixed on a single point. At the same time, your body is sensing, and reacting to, the movement from your ride. The result: sensation overload and motion sickness. For the same reason, an action-packed movie on a plane may cause you to feel ill. On the other hand, "if the movie is not too visually demanding, it just may do the trick to help you relax, forget your fear, and prevent you from becoming sick," says Silverstein.

◆◆◆ Patch Up ◆◆◆ the Problem

Another option for preventing motion sickness is to use a transdermal (skin) patch. Available with a prescription from your doctor, the patch adheres to the skin behind the ear or on the neck or forehead and dispenses small amounts of scopolamine, a drug that suppresses the body's balancing mechanisms. In order to be effective, however, you must take care to use the patch properly. If you are prescribed patches, the first one must be applied at least 12 hours before departure. Do not dispense them to anyone else, warns John Youngblood, M.D. Children and the elderly, in particular, are more likely to be sensitive to the medication in the patch. Children, for example, can become hyperactive as a result of wearing the patch.

Try over-the-counter remedies. Antihistamines, such as Dramamine, Bonine, and Marezine, should be taken at least an hour before the trip for maximum effectiveness. "This gives the medication enough time to be absorbed into the bloodstream," says Youngblood. Always check the label for possible side effects, such as drowsiness or blurred vision, and take necessary precautions, such as not driving a car.

Stay away from others who are sick. The power of suggestion is very strong, especially if you have a tendency to get a bit "green" yourself. As callous as it may sound, let someone with a sturdier stomach tend to the sick; you should be looking at the horizon or at another steady point in the distance. ◆

◆ MUSCLE PAIN ◆

23 Steps to Relief

It was a pickup game of basketball with the guys. Nothing too serious. But a day and a half later, you can barely move. You're so stiff, it feels like you've aged 100 years nearly overnight. Every time you try to move, your muscles cry out, "Stop! It hurts!" What's going on?

Well, weekend jock, you've overdone it, and your body is letting you know. Overworking muscles causes the muscle fibers to actually break down, says sports-medicine expert and world-class runner Joan Ullyot, M.D., author of *Women's Running* and *Running Free*. "Ideally, you should be able to get into shape without getting stiff and sore," she says. "But most of us believe we have to overdo it so we feel like we've done something."

In addition to the tiny tears that occur in muscle fibers, the muscles swell slightly, and the accumulation of muscle breakdown products like enzymes contribute to the feeling of stiffness and soreness.

Another common source of muscle pain is a cramp, an acute spasm of the muscle that can send you to the ground clutching the offending muscle and howling in pain. Muscle cramps can be caused by anything that interferes with the mechanisms that cause muscles to contract and relax. "Muscle cramping means not enough blood is getting to the area," explains Ellen Nona Hoyven, P.T., physical therapist and owner and director of Ortho Sport Physical Therapy P.C. in Clackamas, Oregon. "The muscle objects with pain."

Knowing how muscles contract and relax can help you understand why muscle cramps occur and how to prevent them. To cause muscles to contract, the brain sends an electric "contract" message via nerves to muscles. When this signal reaches the muscle, the minerals sodium and calcium inside the muscle and potassium outside the muscle move and cause the signal to flow along the muscle, making it contract. For muscles to contract and relax properly, they need the right concentrations of minerals as well as adequate supplies of fat, sugar, and oxygen.

Michael Martindale, L.P.T., a physical therapist at the Sports Medicine Center of Portland Adventist Medical Center in Oregon, says, "A muscle goes into spasm because you've traumatized it somehow. Often, it's a sign the muscle has depleted its glycogen, its energy supply, and that there are too many waste products in the area. In response, the muscle goes into spasm. The spasms, in turn, decrease the blood flow, which causes pain. The pain then causes more spasm, which causes even more pain."

While muscle soreness and cramps aren't life threatening, they can be very bothersome. Here are some tips to ease the pain and prevent the problem from recurring.

Stop the activity pronto. If your muscle cramps up while you're exercising, STOP the activity. Don't try to "run through" a muscle cramp. "If you try to keep going while you have a cramp," says Ullyot, "you're likely to really injure the muscle by pulling or tearing it."

Give it a stretch and squeeze. When you get a cramp, stretch the cramped muscle with one hand while you gently knead and squeeze the center of the muscle (you can feel a knot) with the fingers of the other hand. "You want to stretch the cramped muscle in the opposite direction from the way it's contracted," explains Hoyven. "For example, if you have a cramp in the calf muscle, put your foot flat on the ground and lean forward. If you can't stand on your leg, sit on the ground and stretch the toes up toward the knee."

Walk it out. Once an acute cramp passes, don't start exercising heavily right away. Instead, walk for a few minutes to get the blood flowing back into the muscles.

Sip quinine tonic. Ullyot says many competitive swimmers drink quinine tonic water to prevent cramps. Quinine was once used to treat malarial cramping. While there may not be scientific studies to support drinking quinine tonic for muscle cramps, Ullyot says, "If it's a placebo, it's one that really seems to work." You might want to give it a try and see if it works for you.

Go bananas. Chrissy Kane, L.P.T., a physical therapist in the Outpatient Physical Therapy Department at Providence Medical Center in Portland, Oregon, says, "Sometimes a lack of potassium in the muscles can cause muscle cramps." If you're plagued by frequent cramping, Kane recommends that you eat a banana a day to increase your potassium intake and keep the cramps at bay.

Chill out. If you know you've overexercised, immediately take a cold shower or a cold bath to reduce the trauma to muscles, says Martindale. World-class Australian runner Jack Foster used to hose off his legs with cold water after a hard run. He told skeptics if it was good enough for race horses, it was good enough for him! Several Olympic runners are known for taking icy plunges after a tough workout, insisting that it prevents muscle soreness and stiffness. If an icy dip seems too much for you, Hoyven says ice packs work well, too. She recommends applying cold packs for 20 to 30 minutes at a time every hour. "Cold

Muscles that Go Cramp in the Night

You're sleeping peacefully when suddenly your leg is seized with a painful cramp. You're no longer sleeping and you're certainly no longer peaceful. What happened? You weren't even dreaming about exercise.

Cramps that occur during the night are usually due to a pinched nerve or an exaggeration of a normal muscle-tendon reflex. When you turn over in your sleep, nerves can get pinched, causing muscles to cramp. Other times, when you turn over, you contract muscles, and the tendons attached to the muscles stretch. The stretched tendon sends a message to the spinal cord, which, in turn, sends a message to the muscle, causing it to contract.

No matter what the cause of the cramping, the bottom line is that muscles that cramp at night have somehow gotten "stuck." The key is to short-circuit this cramping before it happens and disturbs your rest. Here's how:

Stretch before bed. Take a few minutes before retiring to stretch the muscles that are subject to cramping. Calves are often culprits of nighttime cramping. Try the "runner's stretch"—stand two to three feet from the wall and lean your chest against the wall, keeping your heels touching the floor. You should feel a stretch in your calves.

Be sure you get enough calcium. Nighttime cramps are often associated with a lack of calcium in the diet. Eat plenty of calcium-rich foods like broccoli, leafy greens, and low-fat dairy products. If cramping is still a problem, consider taking a calcium supplement.

Lighten the load. Sometimes, cramps in the legs and feet can be caused from a pile of heavy blankets. Toss off a few blankets and keep your muscles warm with an electric blanket set on warm.

Massage the muscle. If you develop a cramp despite using preventive tips, massage the cramped muscle with long strokes toward the heart. Sometimes a massage before you go to sleep can keep those muscles loose and free of cramps.

constricts the blood vessels and shunts blood away from the injured muscles, which reduces inflammation," she explains. "The cold numbs the surface skin and superficial structures in the area, which reduces pain. It also causes what we call a 'reflex inhibition' of the muscles, causing them to relax."

Avoid heat. Cold can reduce muscle trauma, but heat can increase muscle soreness and stiffness, says Hoyven, especially during the first 24 hours after overdoing it. "Heat may feel good," she says, "but it increases circulation to the area, causing blood vessels to dilate and fluid to accumulate. If you use it too long, it causes congestion in the area and more soreness and stiffness." If you absolutely can't resist using heat on those sore muscles, Hoyven suggests that you don't use it for more than 20 minutes every hour. Or, better yet, try contrast therapy—apply a hot pad for four minutes and an ice pack for one minute. After three or four days, when the swelling and soreness have subsided, Martindale says you can resume hot baths.

Take an anti-inflammatory. Aspirin and ibuprofen are great for reducing muscle inflammation, says Ullyot. Follow the directions on the label. If aspirin upsets your stomach, try the coated variety. Over-the-counter aspirin creams can also reduce pain and inflammation. They're greaseless and usually won't irritate the skin.

Do easy stretches. When you're feeling sore and stiff, the last thing you want to do is move, but it's the first thing you *should* do, says Martindale. "Studies have shown that light exercise the day after overexercising really helps," he says. "But take it really easy. Stretch gently and do only 20 minutes or so of easy walking."

Take a swim. Ullyot says one of the best remedies for sore muscles is swimming. "The cold water helps the muscle inflammation, and the stretching helps take out the kinks," she says.

Anticipate second-day soreness. You may feel a little stiff or sore a few hours after overexercising, but you'll probably feel even worse two days afterward. Don't panic. It's perfectly normal. "We call it delayed-onset muscle soreness," explains Martindale.

Drink plenty of fluids. One cause of acute cramps, especially when you're exercising during hot weather for an hour or longer, is dehydration. Be sure to drink plenty of fluids before, during, and after exercising. Ullyot recommends drinking at least half a cup of water every couple of miles.

Think twice about sports drinks. Ullyot says you really don't need them unless you're exercising for longer than an hour at a time. "Water is best absorbed by the body," she says. "For most people, drinking water is better than drinking sports drinks."

Martindale also says it's important to replace lost fluids if you've overexercised. So turn on the tap and drink up.

Pass the bouillon. If you know you're going to be exercising for longer than an hour in hot weather, Ullyot says you can prevent muscle cramps by drinking a cup of beef or chicken bouillon before exercising. "You can drink bouillon instead of sports drinks to replace the sodium you'll lose through sweating," she says.

Massage it. Gentle massage, done a day or two after a hard workout, can help ease sore, stiff muscles, says Ullyot. "Massage is wonderful for bringing circulation to the area," she says. However, if it is done too forcefully or too soon after the workout, massage can actually increase soreness and may even cause injury.

Avoid "hot" and "cold" creams. The pharmacy and supermarket shelves are loaded with topical "sports" creams designed to ease sore, stiff muscles. Unfortunately, they don't do much, according to Martindale. "Although those topical creams may feel good, physiologically they don't do anything," he explains. "They just cause a chemical reaction on the skin that gives the feeling of warm or cold, but they don't actually heat or cool the tissues." If you do use the topical sports creams, test a small patch of skin first to make sure you're not allergic, and never use these topicals with hot pads, because they can cause serious burns.

Wrap up. In cold weather, you can often prevent muscle cramping by keeping the muscles warm with adequate clothing. Layered clothing offers the best insulating value by trapping air between the layers. Some people like the compression and warmth offered by running tights.

Warm up your muscles. One way to prevent muscle cramping and injuries is to warm up muscles before exercise. Instead of stretching first, walk a little or bike slowly to "prewarm" the muscles. Then do a series of stretches appropriate for the exercise you're going to be doing. Even if you're only chopping wood or working in the garden, stretching before the activity will get your muscles ready for work and help prevent muscle cramping.

Learn your limits. The key to preventing muscle pain, soreness, and stiffness, says Martindale, is to learn your limits. "You don't have to overdo it to exercise," he says. "If you're feeling sore and stiff afterwards, you know you're doing too much. Take your time. Build up over several weeks. Learn what your body can and can't do, and pay attention to those limits." ◆

◆ NAUSEA AND VOMITING

9 Soothing Strategies

Perhaps it's the 24-hour flu bug, or maybe it was something you ate. Whatever the cause, now you're feeling queasy and sick.

The tips that follow are designed to reduce your discomfort and to help your symptoms go away as quickly as possible. If vomiting is violent or persists for more than 24 hours or if your vomit contains blood, see a physician without delay.

Evaluate the cause and treat the symptoms accordingly. Nausea and vomiting are two vague symptoms that can be caused by many illnesses, says Albert B. Knapp, M.D., an adjunct assistant attending physician at Lenox Hill Hospital in New York. If you suspect your symptoms are due to an ulcer, a headache, motion sickness, morning sickness, food poisoning, or a hangover, see the corresponding section in this book.

Stick to clear liquids. Your stomach probably doesn't need the added burden of digesting food, says Knapp. He recommends sticking to fluids until you feel a little better. "If you are vomiting, do not start fluids until the vomiting has stopped," he says. "Then start with warm fluids, since cold ones can irritate the stomach. The fluid should have sugar in it. The sugar helps absorption." Liquids are easier to digest and are necessary to prevent the dehydration that may occur from vomiting, according to Cornelius P. Dooley, M.D., a gastroenterologist in Santa Fe, New Mexico. He recommends diluted, noncitrus fruit juices.

Let it run its course. The best cure for the 24-hour stomach flu is bed rest mixed with a tincture of time, doctors agree. "You'll feel miserable, but you've got to let it run its course," says Dooley.

Don't drink alcohol. Alcohol can be very irritating to the stomach. The same goes for fatty foods, highly seasoned foods, caffeine, and cigarettes.

Stick to easy-to-digest foods. When you are ready to start eating again, start with soft foods, such as bread, unbuttered toast, steamed fish, or bananas, says Neville R. Pimstone, M.D., chief of hepatology in the Division of Gastroenterology at the University of California at Davis. "Avoid fats, and stick to a low-fiber diet," he says. What about chicken soup? "Chicken soup probably has too much fat," Pimstone says. Start with very small amounts of food and slowly build up to larger meals, says Steven C. Fiske, M.D., assistant clinical professor of medicine and gastroenterology at the University of Medicine and Dentistry of New Jersey in Newark.

Let it flow. The worst thing you can do for vomiting is to fight it, says Knapp. Trying to hold back the urge can actually cause tears in your esophagus.

Take Pepto-Bismol. Over-the-counter stomach medications that contain bismuth, such as Pepto-Bismol, may coat the stomach and relieve discomfort, says Pimstone. However, he advises against taking Alka-Seltzer, which contains aspirin and may irritate the stomach.

Try a cold compress. A cold compress on your head can be very comforting when you are vomiting, says Knapp.

Maintain your electrolyte balance. Along with replacing fluids, it is also important to maintain the balance of sodium and potassium (known as electrolytes) in your system, says Fiske. He recommends a sports drink, such as Gatorade, which is easy on the stomach and is designed to replace both fluids and electrolytes. ◆

◆ NECK PAIN ◆

16 Ways to Ease It

"This job is a pain in the neck." It may be more than just a saying. Tension on the job or at home, tasks that require a lot of leaning over, poor posture, and even a too-soft mattress can cause neck pain and stiffness. Of course, some neck pain is the result of injury or disease, but the vast majority of neck pain is due to simple muscle tension.

The neck, with its intricate structure and wide range of mobility, is particularly vulnerable to stress and strain. The head, which weighs between 10 and 20 pounds, is supported by a stack of 7 small bones called vertebrae and held in place by 32 complex muscles. Attached to and between the vertebrae are pads of fibrous cartilage called discs that act as cushions, or shock absorbers. Eight nerves and four major arteries that carry sensations (including pain) and blood between the head, shoulders, chest, and arms run through the neck. The delicate spinal cord runs through the center of the stack of vertebrae and is protected by it. Add to this complex structure the fact that the neck moves more than any other part of the body, and you've got a formula for trouble.

"When muscles become tense due to physical or emotional stresses," explains Michael Martindale, L.P.T., a physical therapist in the Sports Medicine Center at Portland Adventist Medical Center in Oregon, "the blood supply to the muscle shuts down, and the muscle feels pain."

It's a vicious cycle. Your muscles tense, decreasing blood supply and causing pain. Pain causes the muscles to tense further. Orthopedic surgeon Robert A. Berselli, M.D., who has been treating neck pain for more than 20 years, says breaking the tension-pain-tension cycle is a two-step process. "You have to relieve the emotional or physical pressure that's causing the muscle tension," he says. "Then you have to relieve the muscle spasms."

These tips can help you break the tension-pain cycle and learn new habits that will keep the tension from developing in the first place.

Take a load off. One of the simplest ways to relieve the pain is to lie down and give your muscles a chance to recover, says Martindale. Be sure not to use a thick pillow that crimps your neck.

Experiment. "Often, there's no scientific basis for what works," Berselli says. "What works for one person may not work for you. Experiment. Try different things until you find the combination of treatments that ease your pain."

Ice it. Ice effectively numbs pain and decreases inflammation, according to Mark Tager, M.D., coauthor of *Working Well* and president of Great Performance, Inc., a company in Beaverton, Oregon, that specializes in healthy workplaces. Put crushed ice in a plastic bag and cover the bag with a pillowcase (a terry towel is too thick to effectively transmit the cold). Apply to your painful neck for 15 minutes at a time.

Heat it up. After you've used ice to bring down any inflammation, you may find heat comforting. Use a wet towel or a hot water bottle, or stand in a hot shower. But don't keep it up for too long. Too much heat can aggravate symptoms and cause more pain.

Relax. "A lot of our muscle tension comes from emotional stress," says Martindale. "Learn to read the symptoms when you're holding your body tensely. Find out what makes you tense up. Recognize when you're in a stressful situation, and learn new ways to respond."

◆◆ Hello, Doctor? ◆◆

While most cases of simple muscle strain can be handled with home remedies, some types of neck pain should be checked by a doctor. Call the doctor if:

• Your pain is caused by an injury.

• Your neck pain is accompanied by fever, headache, and muscle aches.

• You have tingling or numbness in your arms or hands.

• You have visual disturbances.

• Your neck pain increases or persists for several days despite home treatments.

Martindale suggests developing stress-management skills through relaxation techniques, such as progressive relaxation or abdominal breathing. For progressive relaxation, find a quiet place where you won't be disturbed. Sit or lie down and close your eyes. Then, starting with your head and neck and working down the entire body, tense and then completely release muscles.

For abdominal breathing, sit quietly and take a deep breath all the way into your abdomen. Then exhale completely, gently sucking in your stomach. Breathe deeply like this for several minutes.

In addition to these two techniques, you may want to develop some of your own methods of relaxation. Do whatever works for you.

Use massage. Massage can help ease tense muscles and give temporary relief, and it may help you sleep better, says Martindale. First, take a hot bath or shower to relax the muscles. Then, have a partner use oil or lotion and rub your neck and shoulders using small circles with gentle pressure.

Next, have him or her rub your neck and shoulders using firm pressure and long, downward strokes. Don't forget the chest area. If you don't have a willing partner, try rubbing your own neck and chest area with oil or lotion for 10 or 15 minutes.

Take a nonprescription pain reliever. Over-the-counter pain relievers such as aspirin, ibuprofen, and acetaminophen can ease the pain. Asprin and ibuprofen can also reduce inflammation. "Aspirin is as good an anti-inflammatory as many more-expensive drugs, but without the side effects," says Berselli. "If your stomach is bothered by aspirin, try coated aspirin or acetaminophen."

Practice good posture. Posture has more to do with neck pain than people realize, according to Martindale. The head and spine balance in relation to gravity. When poor posture pulls the curve of the lower back forward, the upper back curves further backward to compensate. In response, the neck curves forward, in a strained position.

Berselli suggests improving your posture by using the "wall test." Stand with your back to a wall, heels several inches from the wall. Your buttocks and shoulders should touch the wall, and the back of your head should be close to the wall. Keep your chin level. Now, step away from the wall. Step back and check your position. Try to carry this posture throughout the day.

Stay trim. "Too much excess weight tends to exaggerate swayback in people," says Berselli. "This, in turn, causes the neck to compensate and become strained."

Strengthen stomach muscles. Just as poor posture and obesity can cause the neck to become overstrained, poor muscle tone in the stomach muscles forces the upper back to curve farther backward and the neck to curve forward. Tager suggests doing exercises like bent-knee sit-ups to strengthen abdominal muscles.

Do neck exercises. Two types of neck exercises can help ease and prevent neck pain: gentle range-of-motion exercises and isometric exercises. Berselli suggests applying moist heat to the neck before performing the exercises. Each exercise should be done five times per session, three sessions per day.

Range-of-motion exercises help stretch neck muscles. Sit erect and relaxed. Slowly turn your head to the right as far as you can, hold, and return it to the center. Repeat to the left. Then drop your chin down slowly toward your chest, hold, and relax. Bring your head back up. Now tilt your head toward your left shoulder, hold, and return to the center. Do the same on the right side. And finally, tilt your head backward so you're looking at the ceiling, hold, and then bring it back to the center.

Isometric exercises are performed against resistance *without moving your head.* Sitting erect and relaxed, press your forehead into your palm, and resist any motion. Then press your hand against the right side of your head. Push your head, trying to bring your ear to your shoulder, but resist any motion. Press both hands against the back of your head. Try to pull your head up, but resist the motion. And finally, press your hand against your temple, try to turn your chin to your shoulder, but resist the motion.

Stay in shape. "The stronger and more flexible your neck is, the more it will be able to resist injury," says Berselli. He recommends swimming as one of the best all-around exercises for strengthening the neck and back.

Work at eye level. If your neck discomfort comes on toward the end of the day, chances are good that your workstation or your work habits are causing the problem, says Berselli. People often get "desk neck" from looking down for long periods or from reaching up to work. If possible, always work at eye level. Change the height of your chair, desk, or computer screen; use an upright stand to hold reading material; and use a stepladder instead of reaching up, advises Martindale.

Take frequent breaks. Change positions often, especially if you have to be in a physically stressful position, says Tager. Get up and walk around at least once an hour.

Unlearn "neck-bashing" habits. Do you crimp the phone between your neck and shoulder? Do you shave with your head tilted back? Do you shampoo your hair in the sink? All of these habits can cause neck strain. Become aware of habits that strain your neck and replace them with neck-healthy ones.

Sleep on a firm mattress. If you wake in the morning with a stiff or sore neck, your mattress, pillow, or sleeping habits are probably the culprit. Use a firm mattress and keep your head level. Don't sleep on your stomach, since it forces your head up. Avoid pillows that are too thick, says Berselli. Try feather or crushed-foam pillows rather than those of solid foam rubber. ◆

◆ NIGHT TERRORS ◆

8 Tips to Calm Them

A 21-year-old man rages in his sleep like clockwork at the same time every night. He tosses and turns. "Get away!" he screams, jumping out of bed and clumsily knocking around his room. One night, after hearing suspicious noises, his mother opens the door to his room and finds him climbing out of the window of his second-story bedroom. Another morning, she finds him on the roof below his window, asleep. When she wakes him, she finds he has no memory of what has transpired.

The man is not psychotic, nor is he having nightmares. He suffers from night terrors, a sleep disorder known to affect somewhere between one percent and five percent of the population. Night terrors often begin in childhood or adolescence and taper off before adulthood (although they may continue in rare individuals).

A night terror may be as simple as the individual sitting up in bed, eyes bulging with fear, and screaming. It may be as dangerous as a child bolting through the glass of a closed window.

Night terrors occur, not because of a dream, but because the individual is stimulated into a state somewhere between sleeping and waking. He or she can neither waken fully nor return to sound sleep.

In children, night terrors often go away if they are allowed to run their course. In adults, they usually require treatment (see "Hello, Doctor?"). By following some simple steps, night terrors can often be kept to a minimum in both children and adults. The following guidelines are a good place to start. Night terrors do not represent any serious psychological or medical problems. Treated with understanding and care, they are likely to subside.

Maintain a regular sleep schedule. A strict schedule of sleeping and waking is the best insurance against night terrors for all individuals who suffer from them. In children, this advice is especially important, says Richard Ferber, M.D., director of the Center for Pediatric Sleep Disorders at Children's Hospital and assistant professor of neurology at Harvard Medical School in Boston. "If I ask parents 'How can you predict when your child will have a night terror?' the most common answer is 'When the child is overtired,' " he says.

Make the environment safe. If you or someone in your household experiences violent night terrors, it's wise to make the environment safe to protect the sleeper from injury, says Lee J. Brooks, M.D., assistant professor of pediatrics at Case Western Reserve University and director of the Sleep Disorders Center at Rainbow Babies and Children's Hospital, University Hospitals of Cleveland. For example, keep sharp objects out of the bedroom, put locks on the windows, and keep clutter off of the floor (to avoid tripping over things). Do not allow children with night terrors to sleep on the top bunk of a bunk bed. It may also be prudent to have the individual sleep on the first floor of the house, if possible. If the episodes seem excessively violent, it's best to consult medical help, Brooks says.

Avoid alcohol and drugs. Alcohol, which tends to make sleep less sound, may make susceptible individuals more likely to have night terrors, according to Brooks. Illicit drugs, such as marijuana, also alter the normal sleep patterns and may act as triggers, says Ernest L. Hartmann, M.D., a professor of psychiatry at Tufts University and director of the Sleep Disorders Center at Newton–Wellesley Hospital, both in Boston.

Limit fluids before retiring. Anything that disturbs a susceptible individual during sleep is likely to bring on a night terror. A nagging, full bladder is no exception. Brooks advises limiting fluids in the afternoon and evening to avoid this problem.

Don't try to wake the sleeper. Shaking or stimulating someone with a night terror is not advisable, since you will probably be unable to wake them and may make them more agitated or even violent, says Ferber. You may even be injured if the sleeper perceives your actions as an attack.

Stay calm and quiet. If you are witnessing the night terror, talk to the sleeper in calm and gentle tones and try to lead him or her back to bed, Ferber advises. If your efforts fail, simply give the sleeper some space and move objects out of the way to prevent injury.

Learn the triggers and avoid them. "Many parents report that children tend to have night terrors within the first two hours of sleep," says Mark Mahowald, M.D., president of the American Sleep Disorders Association and director of the Minnesota Regional Sleep Disorders Center at Hennepin County Medical Center in Minneapolis. "They know that sound or light stimulation may cause one to occur. Because of this, they won't close the child's bedroom door, cover the child, or turn lights off in the bedroom in the early part of the night."

Reduce stress. Stressful situations or events are among the most common causes of night terrors, according to Hartmann. "Sometimes, children have night terrors when their parents aren't getting along," he says. "Stress aggravates night terrors. Avoiding or reducing stress is important, although that's easy to say and hard to do." ◆

◆◆ Hello, Doctor? ◆◆

If night terrors are persistent or become particularly violent or worrisome, it may be time to seek professional help. Some sleep specialists will prescribe drugs, such as tranquilizers or antidepressants, to be taken in small doses before bed; others will advise counseling; and still others will suggest both. The important thing is not to avoid seeking help out of embarrassment or fear that the night terrors may be indicative of a serious psychological disorder. Help is available, and treatment may be highly effective. Also, since more serious disorders (such as epilepsy) may masquerade as night terrors, medical evaluation and treatment may prevent further problems from developing. You can ask your family physician for a referral to a sleep-disorders clinic in your area, or you can call the National Sleep Foundation at 310-288-0466 for a list of specialists.

◆ NOSEBLEEDS ◆

15 Ways to Get Out of the Red

You Should've Seen the Other Guy!

Any trauma to the nose—an errant snowball, a fight in the schoolyard, a fall—can make the nose bleed, possibly break, and almost always, swell. And it's more difficult to stop a swollen nose from bleeding, because you can't pinch the nostrils too well, and it's probably bleeding from far-back passages that you can't pinch anyway.

"Place gauze in each nostril to help stop the bleeding," recommends H. Christopher Moore III, M.D. "And don't lie down unless you absolutely have to. By sitting up, you'll keep your head above your heart, and by doing that, less blood will flow to the nose." Gauze is preferred to cotton because it won't shed particles in the nose.

Zeb Koran, R.N., C.E.N., C.C.R.N., suggests applying ice directly to the nose as quickly as possible to decrease the swelling and bruising.

Is the nose broken? "A nose doesn't have to be broken to swell," says Koran. "But if it is crooked or dimpled, you probably have a break."

On the other hand, "a fracture in the nose may be undetectable, especially if the nose is swollen," says James A. Stankiewicz, M.D. "You might not be able to tell until the swelling goes down." If you've taken a blow to the nose, it may be wise to have it checked by a physician.

"The nose is the most vascular area of the body," says H. Christopher Moore III, M.D., assistant professor of the Department of Otolaryngology/Head and Neck Surgery at the University of California at Irvine. This means that the nasal passages are packed with veins and capillaries, many lying just below the thin lining of the nostrils, practically waiting for the right conditions—very dry air, a picky finger, some dust or dirt—to get the blood flow started. Here's how to stop it:

Close your nose and open your mouth. Sit up, bend your head forward slightly, and pinch the soft part of the nose below the bony bridge, recommends Moore. At the same time, keep your mouth open to help you breathe. Having your head tilted forward keeps blood from going down the back of the throat, which can cause you to cough, choke, or spit up blood. "Only a slight tilt of the head is enough, because otherwise you're causing too much pressure in the head and nose," says Zeb Koran, R.N., C.E.N., C.C.R.N., director of Educational Services for the Emergency Nurses Association in Chicago. In addition, "you can monitor how much blood you're losing," says Moore. That's why the old wives' tale that says that lying down is best is not only old but untrue. "They were under the mistaken belief, I guess, that if you couldn't see the blood coming out that it must be stopping," says Moore. If the bleeding hasn't stopped after about 20 minutes, apply pressure for another 20 minutes or so. If the bleeding hasn't ceased at that point, go to the doctor or emergency room.

Make your nose cold. If your nosebleed is persistent, ice may stop the flow quicker. There are a few different ways to try the cold approach. "Studies have shown that sucking on ice can constrict the blood vessels," says James A. Stankiewicz, M.D., vice-chairman and professor of the Department of Otolaryngology—Head and Neck Surgery at Loyola University Medical School in Maywood, Illinois. Moore recommends a cold compress of ice wrapped in a towel or washcloth and placed on the forehead and bridge of the nose. He also says "a bag of frozen peas smashed up like a beanbag and wrapped up in a towel can be very effective." (Frozen, unpopped popcorn in a sealable plastic bag can also be wrapped in a thin towel and used as an ice pack.) Even after the nosebleed stops, a cold compress can help further constrict the blood vessels.

Spray the bleeding away. Over-the-counter nasal decongestant sprays may help stop a nosebleed. "Spray the nostrils every 10 to 15 minutes for about an hour to constrict the blood vessels," says Moore. If the bleeding does not stop after this time, stop using the spray and see a doctor.

Keep a child calm. Crying and sniffles will only prolong the bleeding.

Leave your nose alone. Resist the temptation to blow your nose, cough, sneeze, or sniffle after you've gotten the bleeding to stop. "If you do, you may dislodge the clot and start the bleeding all over again," says Koran. Also, try not to bend over for a while, as this creates pressure in the nasal passages. And if you must blow your nose, do it gently.

Moisturize. Dryness, especially the kind caused by forced-air heating in the winter, is one of the most common causes of nosebleed. "The elderly are particularly susceptible, since they are more likely to spend more time indoors in the winter," says Moore. To moisten the nose, Stankiewicz suggests applying a petroleum or water-based jelly just inside the front portion of the nostrils. He adds that the new over-the-counter saline sprays may be helpful, but they have yet to be studied by the American Academy of Otolaryngology—Head and Neck Surgery. Koran prefers a timeless remedy

for at-home relief: "Place pans of water on the radiators," she advises. She also suggests steaming up the bathroom during a shower for a blast of humidity.

Turn on a nebulizer. This type of humidifying unit "can deliver slightly warm or cool air in big droplets," says Moore. Humidifiers, which produce a cool mist, and vaporizers, which distribute warm air, can also help combat dryness in the home. Moore recommends cool mist as most effective in helping a dry nose. Some experts, including Moore, believe that these units should be filled only with distilled water to combat the growth of bacteria, which reportedly can irritate the nasal passages and the entire respiratory system. Other experts, however, say that tap water is fine, as long as the unit is cleaned frequently.

Avoid aspirin. Aspirin is an anticoagulant, or so-called "blood thinner," which can aggravate a sensitive nose and cause it to bleed. Prescription anticoagulants, often used in the treatment of blood clots, can do the same. However, if you are on a prescription anticoagulant, do not stop taking the medication before discussing it with your doctor.

Get enough vitamin C and zinc. Vitamin C, a component in the production of collagen, and zinc, helpful in the use of protein, are both important to the maintenance of body tissues, including the blood vessels. Be sure to eat a variety of foods in order to get enough of these nutrients. Good sources of vitamin C include citrus fruits and vegetables, including potatoes. Good sources of zinc include beef, liver, fish, whole-wheat products, brown rice, and popcorn.

Check your iron. "If you're prone to frequent nosebleeds, you may want to increase your iron intake," suggests Stankiewicz. He recommends seeing your doctor first for a blood count and analysis. Iron-rich foods include liver, most lean red meats, dark-meat poultry, spinach, and beans (such as kidney and lima).

◆◆ Hello, Doctor? ◆◆

Angiofibromas are benign (non-cancerous) tumors that, for an unknown reason, primarily afflict teenage males, says H. Christopher Moore III, M.D. These bumps lie in the back of the nasal passages and are difficult to diagnose. However, one symptom is frequent nose bleeding. If your teen has numerous nosebleeds with no identifiable cause, a visit to the doctor is in order.

Control your hypertension. People with hypertension, or high blood pressure, may also suffer from arteriosclerosis, or hardening of the arteries, which can make blood vessels stiff and noncompliant. Some experts believe that such vessels in the nose may be more prone to bleed. If you find yourself with frequent nosebleeds and no explanation, and hypertension runs in your family, see your doctor. Only your physician can diagnose high blood pressure and recommend the proper course of therapy to control it.

Don't smoke. Here's yet another reason not to puff. "Smoking can irritate and dry out the nasal passages," says Stankiewicz. Smoking is also a factor in hypertension.

Consider your hormones. Estrogen, especially in women, plays a part in the production of nasal mucus. The estrogen-level in women ebbs and flows during the menstrual cycle and all but disappears in postmenopausal women. "As we age, the mucous membranes begin to atrophy in both women and men," says Moore. This atrophy can make nosebleeds more likely. What can you do? Postmenopausal women can consider estrogen replacement therapy. Keeping the nasal passages moist can also help reduce the likelihood of nosebleeds.

Stop the picking. If you can't seem to keep your child from picking his or her nose, you may want to try this: "Tape a single layer of half-inch gauze over the nostrils," says Stankiewicz. "The child will be able to breathe but will not be able to get his finger through the gauze."

Teach your child to use tissues. "Children imitate what their parents do," says Koran. "So showing your child how to use tissues may keep him or her from picking." This, in turn, may help prevent nosebleeds. ◆

♦ OILY HAIR ♦

5 Tips for Cutting the Grease

You wash and style your hair every morning, but within a few short hours, it looks stringy and dirty. You, like millions of others, have oily hair.

A certain amount of oil secretion from oil glands on the scalp is healthy and necessary. Sebum, the natural oil produced by the oil glands, is secreted to protect your hair shafts from breaking. Oil also gives your hair luster and shine. But, let's face it, with oily hair, you've got too much of a good thing.

Oily hair is a second cousin to oily skin, according to Nelson Lee Novick, M.D., associate clinical professor of dermatology at the Mount Sinai School of Medicine in New York. "The oil is just coming up on a different part of the skin," he says. "It's usually a genetic problem. But at certain times, most people have oilier hair due to fluctuations in hormones."

Women often complain of oilier hair at the beginning and end of the menstrual cycle. Paul Contorer, M.D., chief of dermatology for Kaiser Permanente and clinical professor of dermatology at Oregon Health Sciences University in Portland, says that for many people, oily hair begins at puberty. "We often see teenagers with oily hair because the androgen hormones stimulate the sebaceous glands to produce more oil," he explains.

While you can't change your family background or your hormones, there is plenty you can do to get your oily locks under control.

Shampoo often. "People with oily hair can shampoo every day," says Contorer. "Keep in mind that hair is just dead protein. Washing often won't hurt it."

Use a "no-nonsense" shampoo. Often, shampoos have all kinds of additives and conditioners in them. People with oily hair need a good solvent-type shampoo, one that will cut the grease, says Contorer. "I tell my patients to add a couple of drops of Ivory Liquid to their shampoo," he says. If you don't like the idea of putting dish-washing liquid on your head, there are plenty of commercial shampoos that will cut through the excess oil, says Rose Dygart, owner of Le Rose Salon of Beauty in Lake Oswego, Oregon, and a cosmetologist and barber who has been teaching and practicing hair care for 35 years. "Look for a castile-type soap without conditioning additives," she advises. "Commercial products like Prell and Suave do a good job on oily hair." Dygart says normal hair needs a shampoo with a pH between 4.5 and 6.7, but oily hair requires a more alkaline product. Look for shampoos with a pH higher than 6.7, she says.

Rinse thoroughly. Whatever shampoo you use, be sure you rinse thoroughly. Soap residue will only collect dirt and oil more quickly, says Novick.

Forget conditioners. Conditioners coat the hair, something oily hair doesn't need, says Dygart. Apply a small amount of conditioner only to the ends if they've become dried out.

Try an acidic rinse. One way to decrease the oil is to rinse with diluted vinegar or lemon juice after shampooing. Dygart says to use two tablespoons of white vinegar to one cup of water or use the juice of one lemon (strained) to one cup of water. Rinse the mixture through your hair, then rinse your hair with warm water. ♦

◆ OILY SKIN ◆

10 Ways to Cope

You may welcome the shine from the sun, but, if you have oily skin, you probably dread the shine on your cheeks and forehead. Just as some people are born with dry skin, others are born with overly oily skin. "Oily skin is basically a genetic problem," says Margaret Robertson, M.D., a dermatologist in private practice in Lake Oswego, Oregon. "If your mother or father had oily skin, chances are good that you will, too."

Hormones also play a big part. "We often see people with oily skin who are in their teens or early 20s, people who are undergoing hormonal changes," says Nelson Lee Novick, M.D., associate clinical professor of dermatology at Mount Sinai School of Medicine in New York.

But oily skin doesn't just affect teenagers and young adults. Many women notice oily skin problems during pregnancy, around the time of their menstrual periods, or at menopause. Even some types of birth control pills can increase skin oiliness.

One of the biggest myths about oily skin is that it causes acne. "Acne is caused when oil becomes trapped below the skin's pores and becomes contaminated with bacteria," explains Novick. "When you have oily skin, the oil isn't blocked because it's coming to the skin's surface."

The good news about oily skin is that it keeps the skin younger-looking. Over time, people with oily skin tend to wrinkle less than people with dry or normal skin.

While you can't alter your genetics or completely control your hormones, there are plenty of things you can do to cope with your oily skin.

Keep your skin squeaky clean. As anyone with oily skin knows, the oilier the skin, the dirtier the skin looks and feels. To help combat this feeling, it's important to keep the skin clean. Vera Brown, skin expert to many of Hollywood's stars and author of *Vera Brown's Natural Beauty Book,* says oily-skinned people should wash the skin at least twice a day.

Dermatologist Paul Contorer, M.D., chief of dermatology at Kaiser Permanente and clinical professor of dermatology at Oregon Health Sciences University in Portland, recommends a detergent-type soap. "I tell my patients with oily skin to mix a couple of drops of dishwashing detergent like Ivory Liquid in with their regular soap," he says. "It's a great solvent for the oil."

Brown thinks detergent soaps are too harsh for even oily skin and recommends twice-daily cleansing with a glycerine soap instead. If you find detergent soap too irritating for your skin, try the glycerine variety.

Try aloe vera. Brown likes to follow a thorough facial cleansing with pure aloe vera gel (available in health-food stores). "The aloe vera helps absorb oil," she says, "and it helps cleanse the pores." She recommends dabbing the face two to three times a day with cool aloe vera gel (keep it in the refrigerator) and letting it dry.

Wipe with astringents. Contorer says that wiping the oily parts of the face with rubbing alcohol or a combination of alcohol and acetone (such as is found in Seba-Nil Liquid Cleanser) can help dry oiliness. "It's as good and less expensive than those astringents with perfumes in them," he says.

Frank Parker, M.D., professor and chairman of the Department of Dermatology at Oregon Health Sciences University in Portland, says oily-skinned people should wipe the face between washings with alcohol wipes. You can buy premoistened alcohol wipes in the cosmetic department of most stores. Novick recommends using alcohol, too, but he prefers the convenience of individually wrapped towelettes. "You can carry these with you and wipe the oil off every few hours," he says. "The alcohol acts as a degreaser."

Carry tissues. Novick says if you don't have towelettes, even paper facial tissues can help wipe away excess oils. You can also purchase special oil-absorbing tissues from cosmetics companies that are very effective in removing excess oil between cleansings, says Robertson.

Chill out with cold water rinses. Robertson advises splashing the face a couple of times a day with cold water. "The water is good for getting rid of excess oils, and I prefer it to adding more chemicals to the skin," she says.

Ban moisturizers. While people with dry skin are forever smearing on moisturizers, oily-skinned people shouldn't use them, says Robertson.

Brown agrees. "In all my years of dealing with skin care, I've never seen a moisturizer that's good for oily skin," she says. "Oily-skinned people should never go to bed with cream on their faces."

Novick suggests avoiding the application of oils, too. "Never put mineral oil or petroleum jelly on oily skin," he says. "Applying external oils to oily skin can clog the pores and cause acne."

Mist it. With all the cleansing and wiping, you might be concerned about overdrying the skin. But if you shouldn't use moisturizers, what should you do? Brown says to use a facial mist. "You can buy facial mists in health-food stores," she says. "They're mineral water with herbs and vitamins added. You just spray them onto the face. They add moisture without adding oil or chemicals."

Make a scrub. Brown says scrubs are excellent for removing excess surface oil. She recommends this almond-honey scrub: Mix a small amount of almond meal (ground almonds) with honey. Then *gently* massage the paste onto your skin with a hot washcloth. Rinse thoroughly. You can also make a scrub from oatmeal mixed with aloe vera, says Brown. Rub gently onto the skin, leave on for 15 minutes, then wash off thoroughly. If you suffer

◆◆ Hello, Doctor? ◆◆

In most cases, oily skin can be treated at home. However, you'll want to call a doctor if:

• *You develop acne.*

• *You notice any sudden change in your skin (if it suddenly goes from dry to oily, for example).*

from acne on your face, however, you should probably skip the scrub, since it can aggravate already-irritated skin.

Masque it. Masques applied to the face can reduce oiliness. Brown says you can purchase clay masques or mix Fuller's Earth (available at pharmacies) with a little water to make a paste. Apply to the face and leave on for about 20 minutes before rinsing off.

Use water-based cosmetics. Brown says oily-skinned people should stay away from cosmetics as much as possible. "Try and go without makeup as much as you can," she advises. When you do use makeup, Novick recommends water-based rather than oil-based types. "Go with the powder or gel blushers," he says. "And stay away from cream foundations that add oil." ◆

◆ OSTEOPOROSIS ◆

17 Ways to Combat Brittle Bones

Sometimes it may seem like a losing battle. We're responsible for giving the body all the calcium it needs. When we don't, it takes the bone-building mineral right from the reserves in the bones, "which leads to the breakdown of the bone structure," says Robert P. Heaney, M.D., John A. Creighton University Professor at Creighton University in Omaha, Nebraska.

Osteoporosis, or porous bones, affects many more women than men. There are a number of reasons why this is so. After puberty, males have more bone at most sites than females do, explains Conrad Johnston, M.D., chief of the Division of Endocrinology and Metabolism at Indiana University School of Medicine in Indianapolis. So at peak bone mass, men are at an advantage. What's more, while both men and women begin to lose bone mass as they age, this loss becomes accelerated in women at menopause, when estrogen levels drop. Bone loss in women eventually levels off to about one percent per year, says Johnston. Men begin to lose bone mass sometime around age 45 or 50, he says, but they lose only about half a percent per year. Why men lose bone mass is unclear.

The best prevention: building strong bones now to prevent fractures and other complications later. Here's how to win the war against brittle bones.

Make like Arnold Schwarzenegger. Well, not exactly. But weight lifting is a good way not only to build muscle but bone. "It stimulates the activation of new bone cells," says Richard C. Bozian, M.D., professor of medicine, assistant professor of biochemistry, and director of the Division of Nutrition at the University of Cincinnati. However, before beginning any weight-lifting program, consult your doctor. In general, always start with lighter weights and progress to heavier ones as you become stronger.

Use resistance to make your bones more resistant. "The skeleton is sensitive to mechanical load," says Johnston. Mechanical load is the amount of force you use against your skeleton, and certain activities that use the body's own weight as a force against gravity are the best way to "load up." The result: increased bone-cell production. You can actually see the results of loading in the significantly developed swinging arm of avid tennis and baseball players. "Exercise is one of the most positive things a woman can do to fight osteoporosis," asserts Bozian. While running is a top bone builder, some people find that it packs too much of a punch for their joints. Walking, besides being less stressful to the body, can be done by almost anyone, almost anywhere, without expensive equipment. And "the motion of walking helps the entire body," says Victor G. Ettinger, M.D., medical director of Bone Diagnostic Centres in Torrance and Long Beach, California. As for lower-impact activities, such as swimming and bicycling: "These are helpful, too," says Bozian. No matter which exercise you choose, Johnston recommends that it be performed one hour a day, three days a week for best results. Irony lies in the fact that those who exercise exhaustively, like professional athletes, can suffer from malnutrition. This can lead to a decrease in calcium intake. In women, it can also lead to amenorrhea, or no menstrual cycle, putting them at increased risk for osteoporosis.

Maintain a healthy weight. If you are underweight (say, more than ten percent lighter than the average weight for your age and height), you are at higher risk for a deficiency of calcium and other important vitamins and minerals, which can affect your bones' health. If you are overweight, you may have stronger bones than someone thinner; however, you also may be less active and less likely to follow an exercise routine, which is also important to keeping bones healthy.

Start drinking milk again. Mom was right when she made you drink milk at every meal. In addition to its calcium content, milk is fortified with vitamin D, and "vitamin D facilitates the absorption of calcium," says Bozian.

Get some sun. Rays of sunshine activate the vitamin D in the body. Studies have shown that women in Northern Europe and England, for instance, where the weather can be cold and dreary more often than not, have a higher rate of osteoporosis than women who are from warmer,

sunnier climates. That doesn't mean you should go out and bake yourself in the sun, however. Fifteen minutes of sun exposure on the hands, arms, and face each day may be all that you need and should not be enough to greatly increase your risk of skin cancer. (Sunscreen, by the way, blocks out the light rays that are responsible for activating vitamin D.) On the other hand, if you are at increased risk of getting skin cancer (because you are fair skinned, for example), your best bet may be to keep your skin protected from sunlight (see "Protect Yourself" in SUNBURN PAIN for tips on shielding your skin from the sun's damaging ultraviolet rays) and emphasize dietary sources of vitamin D, such as fortified milk, instead.

◆◆ How to Get Calcium ◆◆ Without Drinking Milk

For a variety of reasons, some people don't consume enough dairy products every day to get enough calcium. Dieters, for example, often shun dairy's high fat. Some individuals simply don't like the taste of milk and milk products. And yet others are lactose intolerant, which means their bodies have a hard time digesting dairy foods (see LACTOSE INTOLERANCE). Are these "dairy deserters" destined to a life of brittle bones? Not necessarily. There are many other sources of dietary calcium. To get the most calcium, eat foods in the raw; as foods are cooked, calcium can leach into the cooking water. Here are some nondairy, calcium-rich options:

Orange juice: *The calcium-fortified variety, that is. "This is a wonderful alternative for people who simply don't like milk, because it is fortified to the same extent," says Robert P. Heaney, M.D.*

Beans: *Kidney and pinto head the list, and for the adventurous, tofu (soybean curd) is calcium- and protein-rich.*

Broccoli: *Yet another good reason to munch a few stalks—preferably in the raw.*

Nuts: *Hazelnuts, Brazil nuts, and almonds are among the best choices.*

Fruit: *Figs and prunes are very high in calcium.*

Leafy greens: *Romaine lettuce, collards, and kale are good choices. The exception: spinach. "The calcium in spinach is not readily available to the body," explains Heaney.*

Salmon and sardines: *Salmon is also a good source of vitamin D.*

And for the lactose intolerant: More and more dairy products, made with easily digestible lactic acid, are on the market. Lactic acid tablets are also available. And, you shouldn't have a problem with these two dairy products:

Yogurt: *The lactose, or sugar, in yogurt, has already been broken down, so your digestive system won't have to do it. Substitute yogurt for sour cream in recipes.*

Hard cheeses: *The lactose breaks down during the aging process.*

Cut down on caffeine. "Caffeine stimulates the loss of calcium through the urine," says Bozian. One study found that drinking more than two cups of average brewed coffee or four cups of average brewed tea per day can increase calcium loss.

Pass up the salt shaker. Salt can also increase the amount of calcium lost through the urine. "The more sodium you excrete, the more calcium you excrete," says Rose Hust, osteoporosis coordinator at the Knoxville Orthopedic Clinic in Tennessee. High-sodium diets may also contribute to osteoporosis in a less direct way, she adds. If you take a diuretic to pull excess salt out of the body, it will also pull out calcium.

Don't worry about phosphorus. There has been some concern that consuming high levels of phosphorus can influence bone loss and risk of osteoporosis. The Food and Drug Administration addressed the issue, however, and found no evidence to substantiate this worry.

Be wise about protein. For healthy bones, protein is a double-edged sword. "Too much protein in the diet can increase calcium excretion," says Hust. However, protein is needed to help maintain a component of bone called collagen, which is made up of proteins. It's not so much a question of eating too much protein, but of not getting enough calcium to balance out the amount of protein in the diet. If you have an adequate calcium intake, you probably don't need to worry about getting too much protein. However, if you don't get much calcium in your diet, you'd be wise to avoid consuming an excess amount of protein.

Schedule your fiber intake. "Fiber can decrease calcium absorption by combining with calcium in the intestine, and at the same time, by increasing the rate at which food is passed through the intestinal tract," explains Hust. But don't eliminate fiber from your diet altogether. Just try to have calcium-rich foods or calcium supplements between—not during—fiber-rich meals.

◆ The Facts on Fluoride ◆

"Fluoride is the only substance we know that actually builds up bones," says Victor G. Ettinger, M.D. "But the problem is, we just don't know how much to give." While fluoride is a bone builder, it is generally believed that too much of it can actually make bones brittle. But even scientific studies have not yielded that same conclusion every time. "Some studies have found that fluoride had no effect on bone-fracture rate," says Conrad Johnston, M.D. "Others have shown a decrease in the amount of fractures suffered by patients." Inconclusive studies are one reason why "the use of fluoride therapeutically, especially in large doses, remains very controversial," Johnston adds.

Through similar tests, drugs containing fluoride have been studied but not approved by the U.S.

Food and Drug Administration (FDA). Others, like Didronel, are considered only experimental. Didronel was initially developed as a drug to help those with Paget's disease, a condition in which the bones thicken and soften. The drug was found to build bone, so it is used on a very limited basis to treat osteoporosis. A study, carried out by several medical centers and coordinated through Emory University in Atlanta, has shown a reduction in the rate of fractures in patients who have taken Didronel. However, the drug has been administered over a relatively short period of time and in relatively few patients. As typified by this study, the testing of fluoride drugs continues, so final recommendations about the use of fluoride in treating osteoporosis cannot yet be made by the medical community.

Make your own soup. When preparing stock from bones, add a small amount of vinegar to leach the calcium out of the bones. "The amount of calcium in a single pint of homemade soup is equal to the calcium found in a quart or more of milk," says Hust.

Say no to alcohol. Alcohol also interferes with the body's ability to absorb calcium.

Put out that cigarette. "Smoking has been shown to be associated with lower bone mass," says Johnston, since nicotine interferes with calcium absorption.

Check your medicines. Antacids that contain aluminum can interfere with calcium absorption. And some prescription drugs can increase the amount of calcium lost in the urine. For instance, diuretics, which are used to treat hypertension; tetracycline, an antibiotic often used to treat severe cases of acne; and high doses of cortisone drugs or steroids, such as those used to treat arthritis, are a few of the offenders.

Replace your estrogen in menopause. The hormone estrogen is vital to the maintenance of bone. When estrogen levels decrease after menopause, bone loss is "dramatically accelerated," says Ettinger. Estrogen replacement therapy can help slow that calcium drain. Estrogen replacement therapy is not for every woman, however, so be sure to discuss it thoroughly with your doctor.

Carefully consider calcium supplements. "Chances are, if you are a candidate for supplements, your diet is not only low in calcium but in other nutrients the body needs," says Heaney. "Your best bet is to primarily get calcium from the foods you eat." If your doctor recommends that you take a supplement, never exceed 2,500 milligrams per day; excessive calcium can lead to kidney stones. The supplement should be taken between meals with juice instead of water, says Hust. The reason: The vitamin C in fruit juices helps the body absorb calcium.

◆ For Dairy Lovers: ◆ How to Use Even More

• *Use milk instead of water to mix up hot cereals, hot chocolate, and soups.*

• *Substitute plain yogurt for half the mayonnaise in dressings.*

• *Top casseroles, omelets, toast, and baked potatoes with low-fat grated or shredded cheese.*

• *Add milk to coffee instead of adding fattening cream or nondairy creamer.*

• *Try low-fat and nonfat varieties of milk, cheese, sour cream, ice cream, and cottage cheese.*

Get the right amount of calcium. Women, especially, need different amounts of calcium at different times of their lives. The Recommended Daily Allowance (RDA) for females age 11 to 25—the big bone-building years—is 1,200 milligrams. After age 25, the RDA is 800 milligrams; however, the National Institutes of Health recommends 1,000 milligrams after age 25. The RDA for postmenopausal women is 1,500 milligrams, and for pregnant women, it's 2,000 milligrams daily. Men should increase their calcium intake as they age, from 800 milligrams to 1,000 milligrams a day. For both men and women, consuming close to 3,000 milligrams a day can be toxic, says Bozian, and can interfere with the absorption of the vital minerals copper and zinc. ◆

◆ POISON IVY, OAK, ◆
AND SUMAC

11 Prevention and Treatment Tips

The itching can drive you absolutely crazy. You try to ignore it, but you can't. All you want to do is scratch like a maniac. Getting a rash from poison ivy, oak, or sumac is maddening. It's almost enough to make you want to give up going outside ever again. Fortunately, you don't have to. You simply need to know how to take steps to avoid these foes and what to do to get relief if your preventive steps fail.

When you get a rash from poison ivy, oak, or sumac, you've had an allergic reaction to the oil, or sap, found inside the plant. This oil, which is clear to slightly yellow, is called urushiol. It oozes from any cut or crushed part of the leaves and stem, so just brushing a plant may not elicit a reaction. Oil content in the plants runs highest in the spring and summer, but cases are reported even in the winter, according to William Epstein, M.D., a professor of dermatology at the University of California at San Francisco.

Poison ivy, oak, and sumac are hardy weeds that can be found throughout the United States, except in Hawaii, Alaska, and some desert areas of Nevada, says Epstein. Poison ivy is found east of the Rockies, poison oak grows in the West and Southwest, and poison sumac thrives east of the Mississippi River. All three produce similar reactions, and if you're allergic to one, you'll probably react to the others as well.

Cases of poison ivy, oak, and sumac affect 10 to 50 million people in the United States each year, Epstein says. In fact, these plants constitute the single most common cause of allergic reactions. A lucky 10 to 15 percent of Americans are tolerant of these plants, but another 10 to 15 percent are quite sensitive to them. The rest of us fall somewhere in between, with varying levels of sensitivity.

What muddies the waters is that a person's sensitivity can change over time, even from season to season. You could be quite sensitive to poison ivy as a child and carry no allergy to the weed as an adult. "Some people will never get poison ivy, and others may get it at any age," says William Dvorine, M.D., chief of dermatology at St. Agnes Hospital in Baltimore. "It [a reaction to one of these plants] can appear early in childhood, or sometimes it can appear late in life," Dvorine says. So it's not safe to assume that you will always be immune if you are now. But on average, says Epstein, a person's sensitivity tends to decline with age.

Your level of sensitivity determines how bad a reaction you'll have. Once the oil touches the skin, it starts to penetrate in minutes. Within 12 to 48 hours, a red, itchy rash appears, followed by blisters that may weep and later get crusty. The area usually heals in about ten days. Among the very sensitive population, affected areas will quickly swell up, the rash can be severe and painful, and the reaction may take up to three weeks to clear up if left untreated. For those in this category, Epstein says it's important to see a doctor as soon as they realize they've been in contact with the plant.

Even for people who are not that sensitive, a rash from poison ivy, oak, or sumac is no fun. So here are some tips for preventing the problem in the first place and some simple ways to treat the rash if it does occur. (While the remedies often refer to poison ivy, the steps are generally appropriate for poison oak and poison sumac as well.)

Know the plant so you can avoid it. Find out what the plant looks like in your area, because

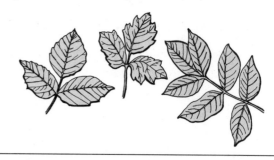

appearance will vary. "Poison oak in Northern California doesn't look like poison oak in Southern California," says Epstein. Typically, poison ivy is a vine or a low shrub with grayish white berries and smooth, pointed leaves usually in groups of three. The reddish leaves turn green in the summer and redden again by autumn, according to Charlie Nardozzi, an horticulturist with the National Gardening Association in Burlington, Vermont. Poison oak is a shrub or small tree with greenish white berries and oaklike leaves usually in groups of three. Poison sumac is a woody shrub found in swampy, boggy areas that has smooth-edged leaves and cream-colored berries. The leaves of poison sumac retain their reddish color and aren't grouped in threes. Spotting the plants isn't always easy. Poison ivy can mimic other plants, such as Virginia creeper, and can twine itself around English ivy. "I've tried to make myself an expert, yet I'm fooled all the time," says Hillard H. Pearlstein, M.D., assistant clinical professor of dermatology at Mount Sinai School of Medicine in New York. You'll decrease your chance of being exposed to one of these plants, however, if you become familiar with their typical appearance.

Cover up. Long pants, long-sleeved shirts, boots, and gloves provide a barrier between you and the plant's oil. This is especially important if you're sensitive and you know you're going to be in an area that might contain poison ivy. "My wife, who is a gardener, is exquisitely sensitive. She's learned to cover up or suffer the consequences," says Pearlstein.

Don't let your pets romp in wooded areas. If you get a rash from poison ivy but can't remember being near the plant, you may have your pet to thank. "A common way to get poison ivy is to pet a cat or dog that's run through the stuff," says Pearlstein. The oil gets on the animal's fur and can get transferred to you. Epstein also suggests that you be careful with gardening tools, bicycle tires, golf balls, and anything else you use outside that might come in contact with the oil. Once there, the oil can remain active for a long time, so you can get poison ivy again and again without touching the plant itself if you don't use care when handling these outdoor items and rinse them after each use.

Rinse your clothes outside. If you think you've had a close encounter with poison ivy, the oil may be all over your clothes. If you walk inside your home without rinsing your clothes, you may transfer the oil to rugs or furniture. Water deactivates the oil, so once your clothes are soaked, they're safe. Epstein also recommends rinsing camping, hunting, and fishing gear so you don't start off your next vacation with a case of poison ivy. Don't forget your shoes. "Many times, people will step on twigs or pieces of the vine and the oil will get on their shoes," says Dvorine. At night, if you take your shoes off by grabbing the sole or the heel, you may grab onto more than you bargained for and end up with a nasty case of poison ivy.

Head for water fast. This should be your first step if you suspect you've gotten into poison ivy. Whether it's a stream, lake, garden hose, or faucet, if you can get to water within five to ten minutes after contact with the plant, you may be able to wash the oil off before all of it sinks in. "The sooner you get wet, the better effect you're going to get," says Epstein.

Carry rubbing alcohol with you. The oil from poison ivy isn't absorbed into the skin all at once; it sinks in fairly gradually. If you move quickly enough, you may be able to use rubbing alcohol to extract some oil from the skin, suggests Epstein. If you think you've been exposed to the weed and you're heading back inside for the day, wash down the exposed areas with rubbing alcohol and then rinse well with water. Don't use a cloth wipe, Epstein cautions, because that may just pick up the oil and put it somewhere else. And don't use the alcohol near your eyes.

Cool off the itch. If preventive steps failed and you've got a rash, cool water may help ease the itch. "A cool bath or cool shower is wonderful," says Pearlstein. Placing ice-cold compresses on the rash may also provide relief.

Smooth on some calamine lotion. "People typically cover themselves with calamine lotion," says Pearlstein. "That's the time-honored solution." Indeed, calamine lotion can be mildly soothing and help to dry the rash. Apply it in a thin layer, however, so that the pores are not sealed.

Apply Burow's solution. This lesser-known product (sold without a prescription) can soothe and relieve mild rashes when put on compress-style. It's often sold under the name Domeboro, in a tablet or powder form that you mix with water (according to package directions). Ask your pharmacist if you're having trouble locating it.

Go soak yourself. Bathing in lukewarm water mixed with oatmeal or baking soda may help to dry oozing blisters and soothe irritated skin, says Epstein.

Try hydrocortisone creams. Sold without a prescription, these creams may offer some relief for mild rashes. Epstein says that for anything but the mildest cases, however, these over-the-counter creams are not strong enough to help. If you have a rash that is severe enough to take you to the doctor, he or she may prescribe more potent steroids. ◆

◆◆◆ Poison-Ivy Myths ◆◆◆

A number of widely held beliefs about poison ivy just simply aren't true. William Epstein, M.D., offers the real story on some long-standing myths:

Scratching poison ivy blisters will spread the rash. *The oil in the plant spreads the rash, not the fluid in the blisters. If you get the oil on your hands, for instance, and you touch different parts of your body, it will spread to them. This happens long before the blisters have even formed. It is true that you should avoid scratching the blisters, but only because your fingernails may have germs on them that could start an infection.*

The old saying "Leaves of three, let them be" always holds true. *This is usually the case for poison ivy and oak—but not every time. Leaflets may come in groups of five, seven, or even nine.*

You can catch poison ivy from someone else. *The rash can't travel from person to person through the blister fluid or any other way. Only the oil can be spread by contact.*

Dead poison-ivy plants can do you no harm. *This may seem logical, but it's not true. The oil from the leaves and stem can remain an active allergenic chemical for up to several years. "That's a very well-known syndrome now, because a lot of people are outdoors in the wintertime. They see sticks in the snow, collect them to make a fire, and it turns out they've picked up poison ivy," says Epstein.*

The juice from crushed plantain leaves will prevent a case of poison-ivy rash. *There's no scientific proof to back this claim, although hikers often try this as a preventive strategy.*

You can't be immunized against poison ivy. *You can, but Epstein doesn't recommend it. The procedure requires a great deal of time, effort, and commitment from both the patient and doctor, and there are side effects. If you're considering immunization, talk to an expert and get the facts. "The worst thing is to get started and then find out the treatment is worse than the allergy," says Epstein. In his opinion, immunization should only be used as a last resort.*

◆ POSTNASAL DRIP ◆

9 Ways to Slow the Flow

Hrmphh. Haack. Those sounds you make every morning to clear your throat could mean you're suffering from postnasal drip. That's a polite term for the feeling that there's an accumulation of mucus in the back of your throat. What you probably don't realize is that your sinuses normally produce one to two quarts of thin, clear mucus each day. "It's usually nonirritating and you don't notice it going from your nose to your throat," explains James A. Stankiewicz, M.D., professor and vice-chairman of the Department of Otolaryngology–Head and Neck Surgery at Loyola University Medical School in Maywood, Illinois. The mucus helps moisturize and cleanse the air you breathe and it keeps the tissues in your nose and sinuses lubricated so they can do a better job.

But when your nose runs amok and doubles up on production—or makes less, which ends up being thicker and stickier—the problems can start. "Sometimes patients think they're making too much mucus, when it's thicker because they notice it then," says Stankiewicz.

And sometimes you may not even notice the drip but may complain instead of a chronic sore throat, hoarseness, or the need to constantly clear your throat, says Gary Y. Shaw, M.D., associate professor of otolaryngology, head and neck surgery at the University of Kansas Medical Center in Kansas City. "If you control the postnasal drip, then these other symptoms improve."

What causes the sinuses to make this shift in production?

• **Allergies.** "That's one of the most common causes," points out Sally Wenzel, M.D., assistant professor of medicine at National Jewish Center for Immunology and Respiratory Medicine in Denver.

• **Colds.** A runny nose is probably the most noticeable symptom of a cold. Wait it out a week and you should start feeling better.

• **Obstructions.** Polyps, small tumorlike growths in the mucous membranes, or a deviated septum

---

◆ When the Cure ◆ Becomes the Problem

Over-the-counter nasal sprays offer temporary relief from a stuffy nose and clogged sinuses. But overuse of such products can leave you worse off than ever.

Sprays that contain phenylephrine hydrochloride, oxymetazoline hydrochloride, and xylometazoline hydrochloride have a rebound effect. They're vasoconstrictors; that is, they reduce inflammation or swelling of the nasal passages by preventing blood flow. But after using them for three or four days, constricted blood vessels rebel— they rebound and swell. So limit your use of such sprays to a few days at a time, recommend the experts.

(the partition that divides the nose into two sides) can block the flow of mucus or cause it to change by affecting the flow of air.

• **Sinus infection.** You'll probably need to see a physician for a prescription for antibiotics to clear up this one. If mucus is yellow or green and thick, you've probably got an infection.

• **Environment.** If you're exposed to a dry, dusty environment or to such irritants as cigarette smoke or pollutants, your mucous membranes will dry out and you'll end up with thicker, reduced amounts of mucus. Sometimes, switching from hot to cold temperatures suddenly, or vice versa, can turn on mucus-producing glands, says Shaw. "You go from hot, humid air outside in the summertime to dry, cool air indoors."

• **Pregnancy.** Stankiewicz suspects hormones are to blame.

• **Age.** The older you are, the less mucus your body makes. In addition, high blood pressure drugs and other medications may change mucus production, points out Stankiewicz.

If you're suffering from postnasal drip, here's how you can help clear up the problem:

Irrigate your nose and sinuses. It takes practice to get the hang of this, but some doctors swear by it. Take one cup of water at body temperature and add one-half teaspoon of salt and a pinch of baking soda. Use a nasal syringe and infect a bulbful of the saline solution into one nostril while you close off the back of your palate and throat. Tilt your head back, then forward, and then to the sides for about eight to ten seconds in each position. (You have four sinuses on each side, so you're trying to reach all of them.) Then forcibly blow out the solution. "It's not a pretty sight," Wenzel warns. Do three to four bulbfuls on each side. Be sure to keep your syringe clean; use rubbing alcohol and rinse with water after each use. If you don't have a bulb syringe, you can cup the salt solution in your hands and inhale. You can irrigate up to four to six times a day when you're suffering from problems, or twice a day "for maintenance," says Wenzel.

Use a saline spray. If you're a little squeamish about using a syringe, you can buy an over-the-counter saline nasal spray, such as Ayr, NaSal, or Ocean. Be sure you're getting a saline spray, however, and not a de-congestant nasal spray that can have a rebound effect after prolonged use. You can also "package" your own spray, according to Shaw's recipe: Bring one liter of water to boil, add one tablespoon of salt, boil, then let cool. Keep the solution in a closed container in the refrigerator and use it at room temperature in a spray bottle that provides a fine mist, or inhale it, cupped in your hands.

◆◆ Look to Your ◆◆ Stomach

Sometimes, what you're trying to clear out of your throat in the morning isn't mucus after all. It may be the contents of your stomach.

Gastroesophageal reflux, the medical name for heartburn, can result in the acid-rich contents of the stomach coming back up in the throat during the night. And it may not necessarily cause a burning sensation, the telltale sign of heartburn.

If you wake up with a bad taste in your mouth, do a lot of throat clearing, and have hoarseness that improves as the day goes on, your problem may not be postnasal drip at all, says Gary Y. Shaw, M.D.

Try elevating the head of your bed six to eight inches, avoiding meals or snacks within two hours of bedtime, and cutting out caffeine and alcohol, which relax the muscle that keeps the esophagus closed. You can also try over-the-counter antacids.

Other swallowing problems may also be to blame. The muscles used in the complicated process of swallowing become weaker with age. And you tend to swallow less frequently while sleeping. Plus stress can cause muscle spasms anywhere in the body—including in the throat.

Humidify the air. If you live in a dry climate or you're inside with artificially heated air during the winter, your sinuses can use some help. A home or room humidifier can help, as can placing open containers of water on the radiators in your home. "If you see a very light film of moisture on windows, then your indoor humidity is high enough," says Stankiewicz.

Drink fluids. In other words, keep your body well hydrated by drinking eight glasses of fluid a day. Don't rely totally on milk, coffee, or tea, and avoid alcoholic beverages. "Kids who drink a lot of milk aren't getting that much fluid," warns Stankiewicz. "Milk is more of a solid than a liquid." Caffeinated coffee, tea, and sodas—as well as alcohol—can actually have a diuretic effect and pull fluid from your system.

Avoid the allergens. That's the best—and probably most difficult—way to treat allergies, if they're responsible for your postnasal-drip woes. If you're allergic to cats, you can try to stay away from them. Allergies to ragweed pollen or house dust are harder (see ALLERGIES for suggestions).

Treat your allergies. You can also keep allergies under control with medications like antihistamines, decongestants, and prescription topical inhaled steroids. To fight drowsiness, a common side effect of nonprescription antihistamines, Stankiewicz recommends cutting an over-the-counter product in half and taking it every four to six hours instead of taking a whole one every eight hours. You could also try a combination antihistamine and decongestant, since the latter tends to be stimulating and may balance out the drowsiness caused by the antihistamine. If you find that an antihistamine quits working after a couple of months, try another one. "Your body becomes tolerant of one type and it won't be effective anymore," Stankiewicz says. Remember that antihistamines have a drying effect and tend to decrease and thicken mucous secretions.

> ## ◆◆ Hello, Doctor? ◆◆
>
> *If you suspect that you have a sinus infection, especially if your nasal mucus is thick and yellow or green, see your doctor. You may need a prescription for an antibiotic.*
>
> *In addition, if you have postnasal drip that just won't go away, you may want to have an ear, nose, and throat specialist (an otolaryngologist) examine you. He or she can determine if a mechanical problem, like polyps, is to blame.*

Take a decongestant. Over-the-counter products like Sudafed help the sinuses drain. Don't rely on decongestant nasal sprays, however; they can have a rebound effect (see "When the Cure Becomes the Problem"). And men over 60 who tend to suffer from urinary tract obstructions will have problems taking a decongestant, Shaw says.

Stay away from irritants. If you know that cigarette smoke triggers your sinuses, stay away from smoky areas. Ditto for anything else that causes trouble.

Gargle. It's no cure, but it may bring some relief for a sore throat, says Stankiewicz. Add one-half teaspoon of salt to a cup of warm water, says Wenzel. ◆

◆ PREMENSTRUAL ◆ SYNDROME

11 Ways to Ease the Discomforts

You've heard the joke before. A woman flies off the handle at work or at home and everyone around her chimes in with, "It must be that time of the month again."

The joke, of course, misses the point that women, at times, actually do get upset by their demanding husbands, whiny kids, and stressful jobs. For some women, however, the joke holds more truth than they'd like to believe. For these women, "that time of the month" really is a period of emotional imbalance, anger, depression, and anxiety. Situations that they normally cope well with suddenly become insurmountable. And the energy and health they enjoy most of the time give way to fatigue, achiness, and weight gain almost overnight.

These women have what is known as premenstrual syndrome, or PMS, a condition that has no known cause and no complete cure. But research into the topic has brought about several theories as to what may make some women more vulnerable to PMS.

"The two most widely held theories, neither of which has huge support, include an ovarian hormone imbalance of either estrogen or progesterone and a brain hormone change or deficiency," says Harold Zimmer, M.D., an obstetrician and gynecologist in private practice in Bellevue, Washington. Zimmer stresses that no single cause of PMS has ever been proven and that much of the research is contradictory.

Whatever the cause, the symptoms can include anxiety, irritability, mood swings, and anger; indeed, these symptoms occur in more than 80 percent of women who suffer from PMS. Other symptoms may include sugar cravings, fatigue, headaches, dizziness, shakiness, abdominal bloating, breast tenderness, and overall swelling. Much less common are depression, memory loss, and feelings of isolation. The symptoms, and their severity, vary from woman to woman.

"Symptoms are definitely cyclic, and that is one of the main criteria for diagnosing this condition. And the symptoms generally disappear with the onset of the woman's period," says Phyllis Frey, A.R.N.P., a nurse practitioner at Bellegrove OB-GYN, Inc., in Bellevue, Washington. "It's often the emotional symptoms that bring people in to the doctor," she adds.

As for what you can do to relieve the discomfort of PMS, there are several home remedies. And according to Zimmer, the home remedies probably work as well as, or better than, the medical remedies available. Here's what you can try:

Maintain a well-balanced diet. Include lots of fresh fruits and vegetables, starches, raw seeds and nuts, fish, poultry, and whole grains. "It is just sort of common sense dietary measures," says Zimmer.

Go easy on sugar. Your cravings for sugar may be strong during this time, but giving in to the sugar craving may make you feel even worse and can intensify your feelings of irritability and anxiety. To make fending off your sugar cravings a little easier, try keeping healthy snacks readily available and keeping sugary foods out of the house—or at least out of your reach. If you can't give up the sweets completely, try eating only small amounts at a time, and opt for things like fruits or apple juice that can help satisfy your sugar craving *and* provide nutrients.

Eat small, frequent meals. You don't want to go long periods without food because that can potentially intensify your premenstrual symptoms as well, says Zimmer.

Avoid alcohol. Both Zimmer and Frey stress that alcohol will only make you feel more depressed and fatigued. Alcohol also depletes the body's stores of B vitamins and minerals and disrupts carbohydrate metabolism. It also disrupts the liver's ability to metabolize hormones, which can lead to higher-than-normal estrogen levels. So if you need to be holding a beverage at that party, try a nonalcoholic cocktail, such as mineral water with a twist of lime or lemon or a dash of bitters.

Cut down on caffeinated beverages. These include coffee, tea, and colas. Caffeine can intensify anxiety, irritability, and mood swings. It may also increase breast tenderness. Try substituting water-processed decaffeinated coffee; grain-based coffee substitutes such as Pero, Postum, and Caffix; and ginger tea.

Cut the fat. Eating too much dietary fat can interfere with liver efficiency. And some beef contains small amounts of synthetic estrogens. Too much protein can also increase the body's demand for minerals. Opt for smaller servings of lean meats, fish or seafood, beans, peas, seeds, and nuts. Use more whole grains, rice, vegetables, and fruits to fill out your meals.

Put down the salt shaker. Table salt and high-sodium foods such as bouillon, commercial salad dressings, catsup, and hot dogs can worsen fluid retention, bloating, and breast tenderness.

Practice stress management. "Learning to control and reduce your level of stress has a great effect on reducing the symptoms of PMS," says Zimmer. Try joining a stress-management or stress-reduction program at your local hospital or community college; learning biofeedback techniques; meditating; exercising; or doing anything that helps you to relax and cope with stress.

Try not to plan big events during your PMS time. "I don't like to encourage my patients to plan their lives around their menstrual cycle, but if they have the option of planning a big social event at some time other than their PMS time, it would help them out to do so," says Zimmer. "The increased stress of the event will only make the PMS symptoms worse," he adds.

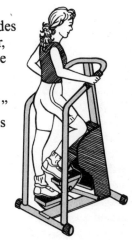

Exercise aerobically. "Besides being a great stress reducer, aerobic exercise triggers the release of endorphins (the natural brain opiates) and produces a 'runner's high,'" says Zimmer. "Good forms of aerobic exercise include running, stair-stepping, bicycling, or taking an aerobics class," he continues. "The social environment of a health club can also make you feel better by encouraging you to interact with other people," he adds. He also goes on to say that increasing the pelvic circulation can help to rid the body of some of the bloating associated with PMS. Try to exercise for 20 to 30 minutes at least three times a week. If you are too fatigued to exercise during the actual PMS period, don't. Doing so the rest of the month should help in itself.

Talk it over. Try to explain to your loved ones and close friends the reason for your erratic behavior. "One of the biggest stresses on a woman during this time is family. And it's not only the stress of feeling bad when she flies off the handle at someone, but also of having to apologize for her behavior later on," says Zimmer. He recommends enlisting the aid of your family and close friends by asking them to understand what the problem is and to realize that when you lash out at them you are not as in control as you would like to be. "If your child is really acting out and yelling at you for something during your PMS time, you might remind him that this is not the best time for him to be getting you angry. Hopefully, he'll see this as his cue to go outside and play," Zimmer explains. "You have to walk a fine line, though, and not begin using PMS as an excuse to be nasty to people," he adds.

If the emotional symptoms are causing problems in your relationships, consider getting some counseling from a mental-health professional. Ask your physician to refer you to someone. ◆

◆ PSORIASIS ◆

25 Coping Techniques

Psoriasis is a noncontagious, chronic skin condition that produces round, dry, scaly patches of different sizes covered with white, gray, or silvery white scales. If you suffer from this incurable disease, you're certainly not alone. According to the National Psoriasis Foundation, between three and four million Americans have the disease. Approximately 150,000 new cases are diagnosed every year.

Not only is psoriasis common, but it's also very mysterious because there seem to be few "absolutes" about it. Doctors aren't sure what causes it, although they believe it tends to run in families. However, you may have psoriasis and have no family history of the disease. It can appear at any age, but most often it strikes between the ages of 20 and 50. It's also been diagnosed in children and infants.

Psoriasis even behaves mysteriously. Sometimes, it can be very mild, with only a few patches. The next day, however, great patches of it may cover the body. Treatment is difficult because what works for one person may not work for another, and treatments that were effective often become ineffective or vice versa.

Doctors do know that whatever causes psoriasis somehow shifts production of replacement skin cells into overdrive. "Something is causing the upper layer of the skin to overgrow," explains Jon M. Hanifin, M.D., professor of dermatology at Oregon Health Sciences University in Portland. "Normally, it takes about 30 days for skin cells to migrate up to the surface. With psoriasis, it takes three to four days."

This speeded-up cell growth is what causes the scaly patches, called plaques. There are several types of psoriasis, but the plaque-forming type (called plaque psoriasis) is the most common. The plaques can appear anywhere on the body. However, they most commonly occur on the scalp and lower back and over the elbows, knees, and knuckles. When psoriasis affects the fingernails and toenails, it causes pitting and brownish discoloration and sometimes cracking and lifting of the nail.

While there currently isn't a cure for psoriasis, there are ways to make living with psoriasis easier. Follow these simple strategies:

Don't give up. Psoriasis isn't life threatening, but it can be terribly frustrating. Skin experts say a positive, never-say-die attitude can help people with psoriasis find relief. "At one time, the National Psoriasis Foundation conducted a survey and found that 75 percent of its members had given up trying to treat their psoriasis," says Hanifin. "Medicine is coming up with new treatments every day, and some old treatments that might not have worked in the past for you may work now."

Moisturize. "If the skin becomes too dry, it can crack and bleed. It also makes the skin susceptible to secondary infections," explains Diane Baker, M.D., a clinical professor of dermatology at Oregon Health Sciences University in Portland who serves as an advisor to the National Psoriasis Foundation. The solution is to never let your skin become dry, says Baker. Moisturizing also reduces inflammation, helps maintain flexibility (dried plaques can make moving certain parts of the body difficult), keeps the psoriasis from getting worse, and makes the scales less noticeable. The heaviest, or greasiest, moisturizers work best at locking water into the skin. Thick moisturizers like Eucerin, Aquaphor, and Neutrogena Norwegian Formula Hand Cream are all effective. But you can also use inexpensive cooking oils, lard, or petrolatum. "I tell my patients that Vaseline works as well as anything," says Mark Lebwohl, M.D., director of clinical dermatology at Mount Sinai School of Medicine in New York and medical advisor to the National Psoriasis Foundation. "It helps prevent drying and fissuring."

Get out in the sun. "A high proportion of people with psoriasis clear their lesions with exposure to sunlight," says Lebwohl. "I advise people to go to the seashore."

Although doctors aren't sure exactly what ultraviolet light does, it seems to slow skin cell replication. For many years, people have flocked to the Dead Sea to treat their psoriasis. "At 1,300 feet below sea level, the sunlight at the Dead Sea is like none other in the world," says Lebwohl. "Some people thought the psoriasis improvement might be due to the Dead Sea water, but they've tried taking the water to other places and it doesn't work. It's the sunlight."

While you may not be able to schedule your next vacation at the Dead Sea, you can take advantage of the healing effects of the sun. However, be careful not to burn, because this damages the skin. And Hanifin suggests "greasing up the scale with Vaseline or mineral oil before going in the sun."

Light up your life. Ultraviolet light B (UVB) therapy, also called phototherapy, can also be administered at home. According to the National Psoriasis Foundation, studies have shown 80 percent of psoriasis sufferers have good results with UVB light therapy. Home light units are similar to those used in a doctor's office. *Don't use a home UVB unit, however, without first talking with your physician.*

Be very careful to avoid burning, and have your skin checked regularly by a physician who can recognize skin cancer. When purchasing a UVB home unit, the National Psoriasis Foundation suggests these guidelines:
• Look for safety features like key switches or disabling switches that keep the machine from being used when the owner is not around.
• Make sure the unit has a reliable and accurate timer.
• Check to ensure there are safety guards or grids over the lamps.
• Look for equipment that is both stable and durable.
• Ask about replacement bulbs and their cost.

Take a soak. Showering, swimming, soaking in a tub, and applying wet compresses all can rehydrate very dry skin and help remove thick, scaly psoriasis without damaging the skin, says

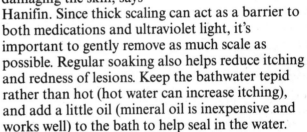

Hanifin. Since thick scaling can act as a barrier to both medications and ultraviolet light, it's important to gently remove as much scale as possible. Regular soaking also helps reduce itching and redness of lesions. Keep the bathwater tepid rather than hot (hot water can increase itching), and add a little oil (mineral oil is inexpensive and works well) to the bath to help seal in the water.

While soaking helps remove plaque scales, Lebwohl warns that it also removes the skin's oils, its natural protection against moisture loss. To prevent overdrying the skin, he recommends moisturizing with a heavy emollient immediately (within three minutes) after your soak.

Beat the tar out of it. Tar-containing shampoos, creams, and bath additives have been successful psoriasis treatments for many years. "Tar products are old standbys," says Hanifin. "There are effective over-the-counter lotions and tar shampoos like Baker's PNS that loosen scale."

Baker says tar-containing bath oils are especially helpful for psoriasis that is widespread on the body.

Bring on the salicylic acid. Lebwohl says over-the-counter salicylic acid shampoos and creams literally "eat scale."

Try over-the-counter cortisone. Hanifin says, "Cortisone creams can bring dramatic relief for psoriasis. They're especially helpful for psoriasis in body folds or on the face." Stronger, one percent cortisone creams are now available over the counter in pharmacies.

Pass the plastic wrap. Doctors have known for years that covering psoriasis lesions helps them go away. "Covering lesions also helps force medication into the skin and keeps moisture in the skin," explains Baker. You can use plastic wrap or you can buy over-the-counter patches (Actiderm). Apply the medication or moisturizer, and cover the area. Be careful, however, that the skin doesn't become too soggy and subject to secondary infection.

Choose soaps carefully. Harsh soaps can dry and irritate the skin and increase itching. Baker suggests using a mild, unscented soap. Many mild, "superfatted" soaps that contain moisturizers are available such as Basis, Alpha Keri, Purpose, Nivea Cream Bar, and Oilatum. You can also choose one of the many soap-free cleansers such as Lowilla Cake, Aveeno Cleansing Bar, and pHisoDerm Dry Skin Formula if your skin is dry and irritated. No matter what product you choose, Hanifin says to be sure to rinse off well to prevent drying and itching.

Pass the warm olive oil. If psoriasis scale is a problem on your scalp, Lebwohl suggests that you warm a little olive oil and gently massage it into the scale to help soften and remove it.

Wipe out the itch with antihistamines. Scratching can damage the skin, something you don't want to do with psoriasis, says Hanifin. He suggests trying over-the-counter antihistamines when the itch is more than you can handle.

◆ Kitchen Solutions ◆

Many anti-itch remedies can be made up right in your own kitchen. The National Psoriasis Foundation suggests the following do-it-yourself recipes:

• *Dissolve 1½ cups of baking soda in three gallons of water to use as an anti-itch compress.*

• *Add a handful of Epsom salts or Dead Sea salts to your bath water. You can also add a squirt of mineral oil or baby oil to the water with the salts.*

• *Put three tablespoons of boric acid (available in pharmacies) in 16 ounces of water and use as a compress.*

• *Add two teaspoons of olive oil to a large glass of milk and use it as a soothing bath oil.*

• *Add a cup of white vinegar to the bath to ease itching.*

Try fish oil. Recent research from the University of California at Davis and the University of Michigan at Ann Arbor suggests that large oral doses of fish-oil supplements may help control psoriasis. Doctors have long known that Greenland Eskimos, who eat large quantities of cold-water fish, rarely suffer from psoriasis. Some believe the Eskimos' consumption of fish-oil may be the reason. Participants in the fish-oil studies had to consume unusually large quantities of the oil to achieve positive results. Before you try fish oil yourself, talk with your physician.

Humidify. Dry indoor air is associated with dry skin, which is bad news for psoriasis sufferers. Hanifin suggests using room humidifiers to raise the humidity in your home or office. Even setting out pans of water on your radiators may help to increase indoor humidity somewhat.

Avoid injuring your skin. Robert Matheson, M.D., a dermatologist in private practice in Portland, Oregon, who frequently works with the National Psoriasis Foundation, says it's important to avoid injuring your skin. Even mild injuries like sunburn, scratches, and irritation from tight clothing can make psoriasis worse in some people. "Skin injuries often cause psoriasis to appear in the injury area," explains Matheson. "It's called the Koebner phenomena."

Use skin products carefully. Lebwohl says that the skin of people with psoriasis is more susceptible to irritating substances. He advises caution in using products, such as hair dyes and straighteners, that can irritate the skin. "Make sure your skin is in very good shape before you use these types of products," he says. "Don't use them if you have open wounds."

Treat infections pronto. Systemic infections like strep throat (streptococcal infections) can trigger psoriasis flares in some people. "If you suspect you have an infection like strep," says Matheson, "have it treated by a doctor right away."

Stay trim. For reasons doctors haven't been able to identify, psoriasis tends to be worse and harder to control among people who are obese, says Baker. While a weight cause-and-effect hasn't been established, it's a good idea to stay trim. If you're already overweight, try eating a low-fat diet and getting regular exercise to shed excess pounds.

Be careful with medications. Certain medications such as antimalarials, beta blockers (Inderal), lithium, and other drugs can worsen psoriasis in some people. Be sure your physician knows about your skin condition and discuss the possibility of reduced dosages or alternative medications.

Relax. Baker says stress is definitely a factor in psoriasis. "Stress can really make psoriasis flare up," she says. "Recognize that everybody's life has stress and learn to relax." ◆

◆ RESTLESS LEGS ◆ SYNDROME

14 Ways to Squelch the Squiggles

It's bad enough when you can't get to sleep and you just lie there, staring at the ceiling. But people who suffer from restless legs syndrome don't just lie there. They are seized by an uncontrollable urge to move their legs. Their legs actually twitch or jerk, while they experience the sensation of something squiggling under their skin. Consequently, restless legs syndrome can lead to problems associated with sleep deprivation, such as anxiety and depression.

Researchers say this is a condition still shrouded in much mystery. Although there seem to be connections with other conditions—such as heart, lung, and kidney disorders; circulatory problems; and arthritis—the culprit sometimes appears to be as simple as excessive caffeine consumption or too little exercise.

The following home remedies are designed to help you combat this problem. If you find that your legs are still twitching, however, it's time to get a medical evaluation.

Get up and walk. Walking around may be the only thing that helps, says Peter Hauri, Ph.D., professor of psychology and director of the Mayo Clinic's Insomnia Program in Rochester, Minnesota. A midnight stroll through the house may calm your legs enough to keep them still when you go back to bed.

Check out your caffeine consumption. "The first thing I'd ask is, 'Are you using too much caffeine or any other kind of stimulant that might be interfering with your falling asleep and jazzing your body up,'" says Richard B. Rosenbaum, M.D., a clinical associate professor of neurology at Oregon Health Sciences University in Portland. Coffee, tea, chocolate, sodas, and even over-the-counter medications may contain caffeine. Try cutting your consumption of caffeine-containing

---

Who Ya Gonna Call?

Doctors with some expertise in restless legs syndrome hail from a wide variety of medical specialties. Although neurology seems to be the logical category for this mysterious ailment, which was first identified about 50 years ago, some of the most informative studies on the syndrome have come from doctors who have chanced upon it while treating conditions that seem to be totally unrelated.

"There is no expertise in restless legs syndrome," states Myron M. LaBan, M.D. whose special interest is arthritis in the lower back and nerve irritability as they relate to restless legs syndrome.

So where do you turn for help when home remedies fail? Ask your doctor for a referral to a sleep-disorders specialist or to one of the hundreds of sleep-disorders clinics in the United States.

---

foods and medications (or substituting decaffeinated varieties) to see if your condition improves.

Try aspirin. It's typical of the mysterious nature of this ailment that some things work for some people but not for others. While some people may react unfavorably to the caffeine in aspirin products, other people find that taking a few aspirin before bed will help them avoid restless legs, says John H. Phillips, M.D., Lassen Professor of Cardiovascular Medicine at Tulane University School of Medicine in New Orleans.

Modify your medication. Some over-the-counter medications contain mild stimulants, warns Rosenbaum. "These might interfere with sleep and make the restless legs worse," he says. Examples are some cold medications and allergy pills. Ask your pharmacist if any medications you are taking contain stimulants.

Take a bath. Hauri says there may be many types of restless legs syndrome, but one type that may be related to circulatory problems probably would respond to a bath. "One might try a hot bath about an hour before going to bed," he says.

Change your temperature. A change from hot to cold, or cold to hot, may do the trick. Try putting a hot pad or hot pack on your legs for a short while. If that doesn't work, drape a cool towel over your legs, or dip your feet in cool water.

Pump iron into your diet. There are some indications that an iron deficiency may contribute to restless legs syndrome. Try eating more iron-rich foods, such as lean red meats, dark-meat poultry, spinach, and beans (such as kidney and lima).

Make a bedtime habit. Get into a regular routine that will help your mind and body prepare for bed. "Some people can help themselves get to sleep by developing a habit, like having a glass of milk before bedtime, or some sort of nighttime clue to their body that it's time to go to bed," says Rosenbaum.

Stick to a schedule. Getting to bed at about the same time each night and allowing for a full night's sleep may help avoid the fatigue that could be a contributing factor to restless legs syndrome.

Take a Benadryl. Phillips says some patients can combat their restless legs by taking one or two Benadryl pills before going to bed. Benadryl is an antihistamine that has a sedative effect.

Soothe your stress. Stress may not be the cause of restless legs syndrome, but "stress or anxiety or lack of sleep will aggravate it," says Myron M. LaBan, M.D., director of the Department of Physical Medicine and Rehabilitation at William Beaumont Hospital in Royal Oak, Michigan. Try to eliminate some of the stress in your life. Regular exercise and prudent diet and health habits may help.

Exercise your legs. "What I tell my patients is they should at least try a week of intense 20-minute or 30-minute leg exercises, which is bicycling or fast walking," says Hauri. Try exercising once a day for a week to see if it helps to calm your legs.

Stretch your legs. Rosenbaum tells his patients to do the same kind of stretches runners do before embarking on a run. But he tells them to do them right before they go to bed. "The best way to do that is to stand about a yard away from a wall and lean forward."

Wear socks to bed. Hauri notes that a lot of people who suffer from restless legs syndrome also seem to have cold feet. Although nobody has studied the connection, it might not hurt to bundle up your tootsies before bed. ◆

RINGING IN THE EARS

9 Sound Strategies to Quiet It

An ambulance with a shrieking siren races down the street and you put your hands over your ears until the sound subsides. A cat wails in the alleyway outside and you close the window to shut out the sound. Unfortunately, some people can't escape from annoying noise by simply covering their ears or shutting a window, because the sound is inside their heads. The sound may be a ringing, hissing, clicking, buzzing, or crackling. It may come and go, or it may be continuous.

The medical name for this sometimes tormenting condition is tinnitus, and medical researchers have made substantial headway into discovering why it happens. When vibrations from the outside world pass through tiny movable bones behind the eardrum, they reach a fluid-filled chamber deep in the inner ear. Within the chamber, thousands of tiny hair cells pick up the vibrations and send electrical impulses through the auditory nerve—or hearing nerve—to the brain. The brain translates these signals into sound that tells the hearer what is going on in the outside world. Sometimes, the hair cells can be damaged in such a way that they continuously send bursts of electricity to the auditory nerve even when there are no outside noises causing vibrations. In short, these hair cells are permanently turned on, making the brain believe that sound vibrations are entering the ear nonstop.

Among the many causes for hair-cell damage are excessive exposure to loud noise, earwax, middle-ear and inner-ear infection, a perforated eardrum, fluid accumulation, or stiffening of the middle-ear bones. Allergies, high or low blood pressure, a tumor, diabetes, thyroid problems, and injuries to the head and neck may all cause hair-cell damage. Degeneration of hair cells that occurs as a result of aging may also cause tinnitus.

Although tinnitus is not considered to be life threatening, it affects nearly 36 million people in the United States, and 7 million of them are so severely stricken that they cannot lead normal lives. Even at its worst, however, there are a number of measures a person can take to make the situation more bearable.

Stop the noise. As anyone who has been subjected to a blasting radio knows, the noise lingers on long after the melody ceases. "People seem to like listening to their portable audio cassette players at highest volume," notes Daniel Kuriloff, M.D., associate director of the Department of Otolaryngology–Head and Neck Surgery at St. Luke's–Roosevelt Hospital Center in New York. "If you do that daily and your ears continue to ring even after you have taken off your earphones, you are probably developing tinnitus, not to mention temporary or permanent hearing loss." Every additional exposure to loud noise damages the tiny hair cells in the inner ear even more, reducing the chance that damaged cells might heal or that the central nervous system might develop a tolerance level to block the noise out over time. People who attend loud rock concerts or who go hunting or target shooting may also be unwittingly damaging the tiny hair cells in their ears.

Check your blood pressure. Ringing sounds in the ears can often be traced to high blood pressure. "If your blood pressure is high enough to cause ringing in your ears, it is probably causing other damage to your body, as well," says John W. House, M.D., associate clinical professor in the Department of Otolaryngology, Head and Neck Surgery at the University of Southern California at Los Angeles. High blood pressure is a primary risk factor in heart disease, a far more serious condition than ringing in the ears.

Lick the salt habit. Sodium is not always problematic for tinnitus sufferers. If you have an inner-ear disorder such as Meniere's disease, however, you should cut out sodium. "Start with the obvious—limiting salty snacks, cooking with other seasonings in place of salt, and putting the salt shaker away," says Jack J. Wazen, M.D., associate professor of otolaryngology and director of otology and neurotology at Columbia University College of Physicians and Surgeons in New York. Be a careful label reader, too. Search out foods labeled "sodium free," which means that the item has less than five milligrams of sodium per serving.

Limit aspirin. Aspirin in high doses often causes reversible tinnitus for a day after it is taken. If aspirin is taken on a regular basis—say, for arthritis or chronic pain—the hair cells may suffer damage. Try to limit your intake of aspirin to see if your tinnitus improves; be sure to check labels on any over-the-counter medications you take, since many of them may contain aspirin. If you take aspirin for a chronic condition, talk to your doctor about alternate medications.

Avoid temporary "kicks." "Stimulants taken into the body can prod the hair cells into unnecessary action," says Kuriloff. Limit caffeine, which is found in coffee, tea, chocolate, and cola drinks, and eliminate tobacco and other addictive substances such as marijuana and cocaine.

Work it out. If poor circulation is the cause of ringing in your ears, a little exercise can go a long way toward improving the situation. "A brisk walk every day is the ideal goal," says Kuriloff.

Save time for rest. Becoming overly fatigued can lower your resistance to colds and flu, which can bring on swelling in the inner ear. "The human body needs periods of respite during the day," says House. "Being run-down leaves you susceptible to all kinds of adverse conditions in addition to ringing in the ears."

Don't worry. "As annoying and frustrating as tinnitus is, it's not life threatening," says Wazen. But the condition can be life impeding for people who constantly focus on the problem, searching in vain for cures and trying useless treatments.

◆◆ Hello, Doctor? ◆◆

Occasionally, tinnitus is related to a more serious medical condition, although treatment may not cure the ringing in the ears. Extremely high levels of triglycerides in your blood may bring on the condition. If the ringing is accompanied by slurred speech, numbness in the face or extremities, or a change in vision, it might be a stroke (in which case you should get medical attention immediately). Tinnitus is also a prime symptom of Meniere's disease, an inner-ear disorder marked by loss of equilibrium. Tinnitus may also be an early symptom of acoustic neuroma, a tumor of the ear nerve, which controls hearing and balance. So if there doesn't appear to be an obvious cause for your tinnitus, you'd be wise to set up an appointment for a medical checkup to determine if a more serious problem is causing the ringing.

Put on a mask. Ringing in the ears can often be countered by a competing sound, says Wazen. You can play background music at a low volume or turn your FM radio dial between two stations to create soft static. These outside sounds may be more pleasant—or at least more bearable—than the internal ones.

If you have more severe tinnitus, you might be able to mask the problem by wearing an electronic device that looks like a hearing aid and generates a competing but more pleasant sound. An audiologist can set the masking device to bring some measure of relief without interfering with conversational hearing. Maskers, however, seem to help only a few people. Wearing the device can be bothersome, so many people choose to use it only at night to help them fall asleep. ◆

◆ SCARRING ◆

6 Ways to Minimize It

Getting into a car accident, having an operation, or just cutting yourself is bad enough, but the scars you end up with can add insult to injury. Scars are nature's way of healing assaults to the skin, but most of us see them as imperfections. We accept them, but we don't often like them. Fortunately, if you know how to handle wounds as they heal and care for scars as they mature, you can make the best of a less-than-perfect situation.

First, it helps to understand the nature of a scar. "A scar is just a connection of collagen fibers that the body makes to repair a wound," says Stephen W. Perkins, M.D., a facial plastic surgeon in Indianapolis and a board member of the American Academy of Facial Plastic and Reconstructive Surgery. "The body basically glues the skin back together with a matrix of new collagen fibers."

Once the injury heals, the scar goes through several different stages. A typical scar usually looks red and irritated for the first few weeks, then it should gradually begin to improve. At the three- to six-week period, it may actually start appearing more red again, says Perkins. Don't worry, though—it's just a phase. The scar will "begin to soften and fade and get less red and pink," says Perkins. "Then, finally, it becomes pale or, hopefully, just blends into the normal skin color after six months to a year." Sometimes, it may take a year or two for a scar to develop a finished look.

In the meantime, here are some things you can do to give your scar the best chance of blending in.

Decide if you need to see a doctor should you cut yourself. Two major signs should send you to a doctor, according to Regan Thomas, M.D., director of the Facial Plastic Surgery Center and assistant clinical professor at Washington University School of Medicine, both in St. Louis. Get medical attention if a cut continues to bleed even after you've applied pressure to it to stop the flow. In addition, even if the bleeding has stopped, if the cut is gaping and the edges don't come together on their own, you'll probably end up with a better-looking scar if you get a doctor's help.

Carefully clean the wound. Once you've determined that your cut isn't serious, you'll need to cleanse it. It may sting a bit, but it's worth the effort. "Don't be afraid to wash with soap and water," says George Lefkovits, M.D., assistant professor of surgery at New York Medical College in Valhalla. You want to get any dirt and debris out and keep infection-causing bacteria away.

Use an antibiotic ointment. Applying a thin layer of antibiotic ointment (sold without a prescription) does two things. It helps counter potential infection, and "the moist barrier allows those cells that are trying to heal across the 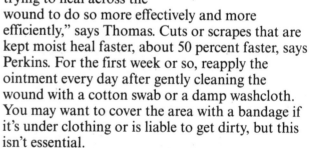 wound to do so more effectively and more efficiently," says Thomas. Cuts or scrapes that are kept moist heal faster, about 50 percent faster, says Perkins. For the first week or so, reapply the ointment every day after gently cleaning the wound with a cotton swab or a damp washcloth. You may want to cover the area with a bandage if it's under clothing or is liable to get dirty, but this isn't essential.

Keep new scars out of the sun. Once the injury has healed and a scar has begun to form, you should watch out for the sun's rays. You could end up with a scar that is darker or doesn't fade as well if you expose it to the sun. Lefkovits suggests that for the first three to six months, you keep the area covered, use a sunscreen on the scar, or simply keep the area out of the sun.

Try cosmetic coverups. After a wound has healed but while the scar is still young, you may want to camouflage the redness, especially if the scar is very visible. Special makeups designed to cover scars can do the trick. "Using these products can help the patient accept their scar while it's in the process of maturing better," says Perkins.

Massage your scar. Gently massaging a scar after the area is well healed but within the first six months of the injury can help. "What you do is help to break down the tough collagen fibers that are forming as part of the scar maturation," says Thomas. "In a practical sense, you're helping to stretch out and soften the scar." ◆

◆◆◆ What's Your ◆◆◆ Scar-ability?

All scars are not created equal. Many factors go into determining how well a wound will heal and to what extent scarring will occur. Here are some of the most important:

The type of injury. This affects the scar in a major way. There will be a great difference in the scar left by a clean, smooth surgical incision and a dirty, gaping wound with irregular edges, points out George Lefkovits, M.D.

The site of injury. "Certain areas of the body just heal better than other parts, no matter what you do," says Lefkovits. The face, for instance, usually heals better than the shoulder, back, chest, legs, or feet.

Proper nutrition. Eating an unbalanced diet may hinder healing. People with a deficiency of vitamins A, C, or B_{12} or of zinc can have impaired healing. Most of us easily get enough of these nutrients from the foods we eat. However, says Stephen W. Perkins, M.D., "people who are dieting or not absorbing their food well can give themselves a vitamin deficiency."

General health. Certain medical conditions, such as diabetes, anemia, heart disease, and lung disease, can interfere with healing, says Lefkovits.

Cigarette smoking. The wounds of heavy-duty smokers may not heal as well as those of nonsmokers. "Wound healing is interfered with by heavy nicotine intake because it shrinks the capillaries," says Perkins. The capillaries help to provide nourishment to the area that is healing. "We highly recommend against smoking during that healing period," he adds.

Medications. Taking certain medications can throw a curve at proper wound healing. Regan Thomas, M.D., notes that some of the cancer-fighting drugs can slow down wound healing. Chronic use of corticosteroids can get in the way of wound healing and even stretch scars that you've had for a long time, says Perkins.

Age. Older folks may have the edge here. While older people may heal a bit slower, they often end up with better-looking scars. The most common time for abnormal scarring to occur, says Lefkovits, is between the ages of 10 years and 30 or 40 years.

Racial background. Blacks, Hispanics, and Asians may have a slightly higher incidence of abnormal scarring, according to Lefkovits.

Skin texture. Oily skin may offer an advantage in the prevention of wrinkles, but it can be a drawback when it comes to scarring. According to Perkins, people with thick, oily skin tend to produce poorer-looking scars than those with thin, dry skin.

◆ SEASONAL AFFECTIVE DISORDER (SAD)

9 Ways to Stave Off the Sadness

Few people look forward to the gray days and long, dreary nights of winter. In fact, most people feel better in the summer, when the days are longer, sunnier, and warmer. We get out more, exercise harder, and eat less. But for some people, the transition from summer to winter is much more than a slight disappointment. It is nothing short of a nightmare.

For these individuals, the change in seasons signals a marked change in personality—from happy and relaxed to depressed and tense. Getting out of bed in the morning becomes a major effort, food (especially carbohydrates) becomes a major attraction, depression looms constantly, concentrating becomes all but impossible, and irritability runs rampant. Then, just when they think life isn't worth living anymore, spring comes along and they are suddenly back to their old selves again.

Until ten years ago, people suffering from this seasonal change in personality had no idea what was wrong with them. But then Norman E. Rosenthal, M.D., author of *Seasons of the Mind,* made the connection between the shorter, darker days of winter and the onset of seasonal depression. He and his colleagues began studying this phenomenon and gave it the name seasonal affective disorder (SAD).

As for what actually causes SAD, the experts aren't exactly sure. "Just what it is about the light deficiency that creates the low mood is the question. And while we don't have a final answer yet, we do have several theories," says David H. Avery, M.D., associate professor of psychiatry and behavioral sciences at the University of Washington School of Medicine, Harborview Medical Center, in Seattle. "One such theory suggests that there is a delay in the timing of the body clock in SAD patients that causes their temperature minimum to occur at 6:00 A.M. rather

than [at the normal time of] 3:00 A.M. As a result, they are attempting to wake up when physiologically it is the middle of the night," Avery says. "When we treat these people with bright light from 6:00 A.M. to 8:00 A.M., we not only improve their mood, we also see a shift in their temperature minimum to an earlier time. Using the light in the morning creates a phase advance," he adds.

Another theory is that the secretion of the hormone melatonin is responsible for the low mood and lack of energy. "It is known that the hibernation and reproductive cycles of animals are regulated by the secretion of melatonin. Melatonin is only secreted in the dark and is very light-sensitive," says Avery. "During the long summer days, melatonin secretion is markedly reduced because the nights are shorter. But during the long winter nights, melatonin secretion increases," he explains.

"Human melatonin production is also responsive to light, but it takes much more light to stop that production than it does in animals," says Raymond Lam, M.D., a psychiatrist in the Mood Disorders Program at the University of British Columbia in Vancouver.

"When melatonin is administered to normal individuals, it tends to lower their body temperature and cause drowsiness. So one initial thought about winter depression is that people who have it are secreting a lot of melatonin during the winter and not much during the summer," adds Avery. With this theory, the light therapy is thought to work because it shuts off the melatonin production.

Still, these and other theories have yet to be proven. And SAD can hit in varying degrees. In one study, 75 percent of the subjects had sought treatment for their depressions. "I have even had patients who have been hospitalized every winter," says Avery. Still, others say that they don't feel all that depressed; they simply have such low energy that they aren't able to accomplish the things they would like to accomplish.

For most people with SAD, it takes two or three days of bright sunshine to elicit a reversal of symptoms. And, consequently, a tipoff that you may have it is if you find great relief in your symptoms when traveling toward the equator.

Apparently, no one group is immune to the condition. "We see it in men and women of all ages and races and in all parts of the country," says Dan Oren, M.D., senior clinical investigator at the National Institute of Mental Health in Bethesda, Maryland. "But it does seem to occur in women more than in men, and specifically in women who are in their reproductive years," he adds.

So what can you do about SAD, short of taking a warm-weather vacation every few weeks during the winter months? According to these experts, the following strategies may help:

Getting Professional Help

If none of the remedies discussed here seems to work, it's time to seek the help of a professional. As for what type of professional, Dan Oren, M.D., offers the following advice: "I recommend a licensed health professional who has experience in the use of light therapy. This could be a psychiatrist, psychologist, social worker, doctor, or nurse," he says. But Raymond Lam, M.D., stresses that you should see your personal physician first to rule out any physiological cause for the depression, such as a thyroid disorder.

In addition to asking your doctor for a referral to a specialist in seasonal affective disorder (SAD), you can check the following sources to find a health practitioner in your area who has worked with patients who suffer from SAD:

• Your local medical school's department of psychiatry. "Call and ask if there is any kind of research program in your area for this disorder," advises Oren.

• Your local branch of the American Psychiatric Association. According to Oren, they may very well have a list of people who specialize in light therapy or may be able to get hold of one.

• The book Seasons of the Mind *by Norman E. Rosenthal, M.D. In addition to giving you a wealth of information about SAD, the book contains a listing of health professionals from all over the country who specialize in this area, according to David H. Avery, M.D.*

• The Society for Light Treatment and Biological Rhythms (SLTBR). While this is a nationwide professional society for experts in the field, its membership roster includes health professionals who are qualified to do light therapy, according to Oren. You can write to SLTBR at P.O. Box 478, Wilsonville, Oregon 97070, or call 503-694-2404.

• The National Organization for Seasonal Affective Disorder. "This national support group is very likely to be of help both in seeking treatment for and in coping with the condition," says Oren. You can write to them for information at P.O. Box 451, Vienna, Virginia 22180.

The treatments you would most likely receive from a professional include light-box therapy, dawn-simulator therapy, or tricyclic anti-depressants. "The data is very good that the bright-light-box therapy is an effective treatment for winter depression. But whether it returns patients completely to their summer selves is questionable," admits Avery.

"Light therapy is not magic, in that it doesn't work for everyone. But if you don't respond to light therapy, you almost always will respond to a conventional antidepressant medication," says Oren.

Soak up the morning light. Get as much natural light as possible between 6:00 A.M. and 8:00 A.M. "This could mean getting out and taking a morning walk every day," says Avery. "Sitting by a large window can help as well," he continues. "People who work at home or have an extremely short commute often get little or no natural light in the morning hours. And most people are not aware of the fact that the light in a home or brightly lit office is only one-tenth the intensity of natural light, even on a cloudy day," he adds.

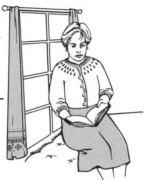

Eat foods containing the amino acid tryptophan. According to Avery, the carbohydrate craving common in people with this disorder is thought to be caused by decreased levels of the brain neurotransmitter serotonin. Since tryptophan is a precursor of serotonin, taking in more of this amino acid may increase the production of serotonin and help you to feel better. But he cautions that there is no data indicating that diet really helps. Foods that contain tryptophan include turkey, milk, and egg whites.

Avoid self-medication with alcohol or caffeine. "Using these drugs is a common way people deal with SAD," says Avery. But while caffeine may give you a brief lift, it can also cause anxiety, muscle tension, and gastrointestinal problems. Alcohol, on the other hand, is a depressant, which can further exacerbate depression.

◆ Summer Sadness ◆

While winter depression tends to be the most common type of seasonal affective disorder (SAD), some patients actually have the opposite problem; they experience depression during the warm, summer months. According to a study by Norman E. Rosenthal, M.D., and Thomas A. Wehr, M.D., these patients experience depression that begins between March and June and ends between August and October. The symptoms are similar to those found in the winter variety of SAD.

"For these people, it seems, the warm temperatures, rather than the light, are responsible for the mood shift," says Dan Oren, M.D. As with the winter SAD patients, several summer SAD patients note a relationship between latitude or climate and severity of illness. Improvement in the symptoms tends to occur when patients take summer vacations in the north, when they bathe in cold lakes in the summer, and when they are exposed to extreme amounts of air-conditioning during the warmer months.

Engage in regular aerobic exercise. While all of our experts admit that there haven't been any studies of the effects of exercise on SAD, they feel that it certainly can't hurt. "Intuitively, I think that exercise is good because it can get you outside in the morning light," says Avery. "Exercise also gives you a feeling of control," adds Oren. And Lam adds that when people start getting depressed, they start doing less and less, and this inertia builds up so that it gets easier to do less and less. Exercising, in his opinion, may prevent some of this inertia from setting in. But Avery admits that he has had SAD patients who were religious exercisers during the spring and summer and were not able to maintain their program during the winter because they were too tired.

Eat lunch outside. If you can't get out in the morning light, at least get out on your lunch break. "While morning light has been found to be most helpful in reducing the symptoms of SAD, any natural light you can get is better than nothing," says Oren. "Even the light from a cloudy day will do," he adds.

Maintain a regular schedule. "This will help synchronize your body clock," says Lam. "It's especially important to go to bed at the same time each night and wake up at the same time each morning," he adds.

Let the sun shine in. "Some people live in houses that are very dark anyway, so making a conscious effort to keep the blinds or curtains open as much as possible during the daylight hours can help," says Oren. "I've even had some patients who find that moving from a room that faces north to a room that faces east makes a tremendous difference in allowing them to get the morning sunlight," he adds.

Try a "dawn simulator." According to Oren, these low-level light boxes simulate dawn by coming on in your bedroom and getting brighter and brighter as the morning wears on. "Even people without SAD have been reported to feel much more energized after using these devices," he says. Avery cautions, however, that the best results may come from using these under the supervision of a qualified professional. "Light therapy is a fairly benign treatment, but it could be used incorrectly and fail to produce a good effect," admits Oren.

If possible, move to a sunnier climate. "This treatment comes up in my discussions with virtually every SAD patient, and it is a great treatment if you can do it. But for most people, family and career obligations make it difficult," says Oren. ◆

◆ SENSITIVE TEETH ◆

5 Tips to Keep You Smiling

You take a drink of iced tea, bite down on a candy bar, or slurp some hot soup and the electric stinging sensation in one or more of your teeth sends you flying out of your seat. You've got "sensitive teeth," a rather mild name for what can be a wildly uncomfortable condition.

So what's going on? Why do your teeth react to hot, cold, sweet, or sour, and sometimes even to pressure? Well, it could be many things, according to Jack W. Clinton, D.M.D., associate dean of patient services at Oregon Health Sciences University School of Dentistry in Portland. "The difficulty with sensitive teeth is there is a wide variety of problems that can cause the teeth to become sensitive," he says. "It can be as simple as a 'bruised' tooth from biting down too hard on something, to as complicated as necrotic, or dead, tooth pulp that requires root-canal work."

One or more teeth can become sensitive to pressure, even to mild chewing, when a tooth is "bruised" or traumatized from biting down too hard or from having a tooth worked on at the dentist's office. Often, teeth feel sensitive after they've been cleaned or filled. Sometimes this kind of sensitivity can take weeks or even months to go away. In other cases, people can cause tooth sensitivity by habitual tooth grinding or clamping the jaws tightly. This type of sensitivity to pressure isn't something to worry about if it happens once or twice and goes away in a day or two. The tooth or teeth simply need time to recover from the trauma. It's when the pressure sensitivity is persistent that you should suspect something like a break, crack, or decayed tooth and should see your dentist.

Sensitivity to temperature usually means teeth have been compromised in some way, says Clinton. Sometimes it means one or more teeth are hitting too soon or too hard and the "bite" must be readjusted by a dentist. "Teeth may be hard," explains Clinton, "but they move around. Bone is

◆◆ Hello, Doctor? ◆◆

While you can often self-treat generalized tooth sensitivity, see your dentist if:

• Your teeth are persistently sensitive to pressure.

• A single tooth is persistently sensitive. "This often indicates the pulp of the tooth is dead," explains Ronald Wismer, D.M.D.. "You need to see a dentist as soon as possible."

• Sensitivity doesn't decrease after two weeks of using desensitizing toothpaste.

• You have prolonged pain. "Any pain that lasts longer than one hour indicates you should see a dentist," says Sandra Hazard, D.M.D.

• The gums around a sensitive tooth change color.

• You have any obvious decay.

reabsorbed or, sometimes, habits like thumb sucking can move teeth around and change how the teeth come together."

By far, the most common cause of sensitivity to temperature and sweet or sour foods is exposed dentin, according to Sandra Hazard, D.M.D., managing dentist for Willamette Dental Group, Inc., in Oregon. Exposed dentin can be the result of dental decay, food or toothbrush abrasion, or gum recession. "Dentin is the material underneath the enamel and what the roots are made of," Hazard explains. "The dentin has microscopic nerve fibers that, when exposed, cause the sensitivity."

If you develop sensitivity in one or more teeth, first see your dentist to determine the cause. Then, if your sensitivity is caused by simple enamel abrasion or by normal gum recession, try these strategies for relief:

Bring on the desensitizing toothpaste. Unfortunately, widespread tooth sensitivity due to enamel abrasion or gum-line recession can't be treated with dental fillings. One of the best home remedies for overall sensitivity, says Hazard, are the desensitizing toothpastes available over the counter. "They contain a special ingredient that fills up the tubules in the dentin and decreases sensitivity," she says. In addition to brushing with desensitizing toothpaste, Ken Waddell, D.M.D., a dentist in private practice in Tigard, Oregon, suggests putting some of the toothpaste on your finger or on a cotton swab and spreading it over the sensitive spots before you go to bed. Spit, but don't rinse. "You should see considerable relief in two or three weeks," he says.

Try a fluoride rinse. Fluoride rinses, available without a prescription at your local pharmacy or in the dental section of grocery stores, can help decrease sensitivity, especially for people with decay problems, says Hazard. Use it once a day. Swish it around in your mouth, then spit it out.

Sometimes, people with sensitive teeth need a stronger fluoride rinse or gel than the ones available over the counter, says Ronald Wismer, D.M.D., a dentist in private practice in Beaverton, Oregon, who sees many patients with sensitive teeth. "If you've had a periodontal procedure like root planing to get rid of plaque," he says, "your dentist can apply a fluoride that can help decrease sensitivity."

Keep your teeth clean. It's particularly important to keep plaque, the white gummy substance that forms on teeth, off areas that are sensitive. "As plaque metabolizes, it produces acid, which irritates the teeth," explains Hazard. "It can cause sensitive teeth to react even more strongly when stimulated." Brush at least twice a day, preferably right after eating, and floss at least once a day.

Use a soft toothbrush. Often, people actually cause tooth sensitivity by brushing incorrectly with a hard-bristled brush. "Before I knew much about brushing, I brushed too hard with the wrong toothbrush and caused enamel abrasion on the right side of my mouth," admits Hazard.

When the gum line recedes (often as a natural part of the aging process), exposed dentin becomes even more vulnerable to toothbrush abrasion. "Enamel is very hard," says Wismer, "but dentin isn't and is much more subject to abrasion by things like brushing." Use a brush with the softest bristles you can find, and apply only a small amount of pressure when brushing. Avoid using a "scrubbing" action to clean the teeth.

Say enough to snuff. Chewing tobacco, also known as "dip" or "snuff," has become a popular habit, especially among many teenagers. They mistakenly believe it's less harmful than smoking cigarettes. However, in addition to causing mouth cancers, chewing tobacco causes the gums to recede, a major cause of gum sensitivity and decay. Habits like sucking on hard candy, while safer than snuff, can also cause enamel abrasion and tooth sensitivity. ◆

◆ SHAVING DISCOMFORT ◆

13 Ways to Nip the Nicks

You have probably seen those men who have little wads of toilet paper stuck to their face. In fact, you may be one of them. Therefore, you know perfectly well that those wads are not the latest fashion statement, designed to complement your tie or handkerchief. Those wads are there because you missed getting that most elusive of worldly things—the perfect shave.

You just missed it, too, didn't you? You missed it by a nick.

Nicks, scrapes, burns. It may sound like the inventory of an emergency ward, but most men encounter these discomforts on a regular basis in their own bathrooms.

So here are some tips on how to avoid turning your morning ritual into a nightmare and keep the toilet paper off your face. (Of course, women who shave their legs are not immune to these discomforts, either. So while this article is primarily geared toward men, the advice can help women get a softer, gentler shave as well.)

Be prepared. Proper preparation is the key to a good shave, says Gordon Scarbrough, owner of Moler Barber College in Portland, Oregon. That means moistening and softening your face before you even apply the soap. For the best results, do it with a warm, moist towel or washcloth held to your face. At the very least, splash warm tap water on your face. (Women should try soaking in the tub for a few minutes before shaving the legs.)

Follow the grain. Shave with the grain; that is, move the razor in the direction that the hair grows, advises Andrew Lazar, M.D., assistant professor of clinical dermatology at Northwestern University School of Medicine in Chicago. Generally, that means shaving down on the face and neck and up on the lower neck.

◆◆ Something for ◆◆ the Bearded Ones

We haven't forgotten you. Just because you're not shaving every day doesn't mean you don't have to take care of your face. Barber Gordon Scarbrough, who wears a beard himself, reminds bearded men that they should wash their face and beard daily. "The skin builds up on the chin just as dandruff would on the scalp if you don't wash it." He suggests shampooing your beard in the shower, at the same time you shampoo your hair. Otherwise, wash daily with facial soap.

Shave in the shower. It's the perfect place to shave, says Scarbrough, because the steam and hot water soften and moisten your skin and beard. Shaving your face as your final shower duty makes good sense for your skin.

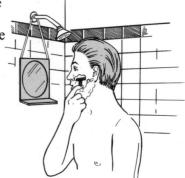

Cut up your credit cards. Well, at least don't use them as a measure of proper shaving. Joseph P. Bark, M.D., chairman of dermatology at St. Joseph Hospital in Lexington, Kentucky, says men have been trying to live up to an old shaving commercial that showed a credit card being rubbed against a shaved face. "If it made a lot of scraping sounds, you didn't pass the credit-card test," says Bark. He says to cash in that tired idea, and instead invest in the notion that shaving less closely will save you a lot of discomfort.

Stop playing doubles. "The bad actor in all this is the double-track razor," says Bark. He says the first blade pulls up the skin around hairs, then the second blade shaves off the nubbin of skin. "It's like using a nuclear weapon to mow your lawn," says Bark. Try a single-blade, disposable razor instead.

Froth your foam. Many men think that foam out of a can is moist enough to apply directly to dry skin. Wrong, says Scarbrough. You need added moisture, or it will almost be like shaving dry skin. Splash water on your face liberally before adding the foam.

Be sharp. A dull blade can scrape your skin, so don't try to get too many shaves out of one razor. Some men's beards are so coarse that a razor will be effective for only one shave, says Scarbrough.

Try an electric. Electric razors don't shave as closely as a double-track razor, so they may be less likely to irritate the skin, says Bark.

Use a quality aftershave. Cheaper brands are just plain alcohol, says Scarbrough. "They burn like sin and really don't do much." A good aftershave should refresh the skin, cleanse it of bacteria, plus heal it from the shaving. He looks for aloe vera or other natural healers as part of the ingredients.

Try a sunscreen. Bark recommends using a sunscreen as an aftershave. "Use a sunscreen as an aftershave every day of your life and you can look younger and not have skin cancer."

Heal thyself. While your face is healing from razor burn, use an over-the-counter hydrocortisone lotion as your aftershave, Bark suggests. It will speed the healing.

◆◆◆ Bumping Off ◆◆◆ Razor Bumps

Razor bumps, usually found on the neck and caused by ingrown hairs, are a common shaving problem encountered by curly haired men. The problem often can be solved by not shaving so close, and by shaving with the grain of the whiskers. For more tips on how to rid your face and neck of these painful, unsightly bumps, refer to INGROWN HAIR.

Quit shaving. If you need to be clean shaven on the job, how about giving up shaving for the weekend? Bark says growing just a quarter-inch beard will cure razor burn. "Guys lose their razor burn and razor bumps with even the slightest hair growth on their face," he says. Then, when it's time to shave again, don't shave too close.

Say styptic. Ask for it at the drugstore and keep it handy in the bathroom so you can use it when you nick yourself. You can get a styptic pencil or styptic powder. Dab it on the nick, press down momentarily with your finger, and the bleeding should stop. Alum contained in the pencil or powder draws the skin up to seal the wound, says Scarbrough. Rinse off any residue, and you're ready to face the world—without that snippet of toilet paper. ◆

◆ SHINGLES ◆

10 Ways to Handle the Pain

The chicken-pox virus never goes away. It continues to lurk in the nerve cells of your body years and years after you first suffer from this common childhood disease. You may not even remember having had chicken pox if yours was a mild case. But when the herpes zoster virus, as it's called, reappears in adults, it's known as shingles. The name comes from the Latin and French words for belt or girdle, because of the girdlelike outbreak of blisters on the trunk.

No one knows why the virus suddenly decides to attack. Some doctors think it occurs when the immune system is temporarily weakened. Shingles is more common in people over the age of 50, and older people are believed to have a lessened immune response. Injury or stress may be responsible. And anyone who's "immunosuppressed"—such as people who have had an organ transplant or those who have cancer or AIDS—is more prone to developing shingles.

Shingles often begins with pain or tingling. Then a red rash appears that's soon followed by blisters. The blisters may last anywhere from five days to possibly four weeks and then crust over and disappear. One important clue that you've got shingles: It will appear on only one side of the body. It's most common on the trunk, the buttocks, and the face.

It's after the blisters have healed that the real agony of shingles may be experienced. Called postherpetic neuralgia by the medical community, the sharp, shooting, piercing pain that can persist for years after an outbreak of shingles leaves victims in agony. The older you are, the more likely you are to experience lingering pain, but only about ten percent of all shingles patients will experience this.

Getting prompt treatment may reduce the odds that you'll suffer from pain after your bout with shingles. (And if it's any consolation, most people will only experience shingles once.)

◆◆◆ Your Eyes ◆◆◆ and Shingles

If the blisters from shingles appear close to the eye or occur on the tip or side of the nose, see a doctor immediately. Shingles can end up causing vision problems if it involves nerves around the eye.

If you suspect you have shingles, you need to get medical attention. If you are older; ill with another condition; or have shingles on your face (especially near your eyes, as it can lead to vision problems), leg, hand, or genital area, you need to see a doctor as soon as possible. "This isn't as urgent as a heart attack, but it's the next level," says Philip C. Anderson, M.D., chairman of dermatology at the University of Missouri–Columbia School of Medicine. Experts can't stress enough the importance of getting medical help immediately.

If the diagnosis is indeed shingles, you might want to ask your doctor about acyclovir. This antiviral drug, if given early in the course of shingles, may help prevent pain down the road.

Although the experts emphasize getting medical help, there are some things you can do to help relieve pain and itching during the early stage of shingles, when the blisters are present, and to cope with lingering discomfort once the blisters have cleared up.

Cool the pain. Cold packs can help relieve the pain from hot, blistered skin. Place a cold cloth on the blisters or wrap a towel around the affected area and pour ice water on it, suggests Anderson. Use for 20 minutes, then leave off for 20 minutes, and repeat until the pain decreases. Or try a cold milk compress, suggests Judy Jordan, M.D., a dermatologist in private practice in San Antonio and a spokesperson for the American Academy of Dermatology. Wrap a bag of frozen peas or frozen unpopped popcorn in a thin towel and place it on the affected area.

Stay in bed. Rest will help your body's defenses come to the rescue.

Take an anti-inflammatory drug. Ibuprofen helps reduce inflammation and is the first line of defense in fighting the pain. Aspirin may also be helpful. If you are allergic to ibuprofen and aspirin, you can take over-the-counter acetaminophen for the pain (although it won't do much for the inflammation). If these don't help, ask your doctor to prescribe something for the pain. Codeine or other mild narcotics can help reduce the pain in the early phase of shingles.

Rub on relief. Your doctor may recommend or prescribe a topical local anesthetic cream to be used on your blistered skin. Be leery of over-the-counter products that contain Benadryl or any ingredient ending in -caine, however; these can cause allergic reactions and may worsen the situation.

◆◆◆ The Pain Clinic ◆◆◆

After the blisters have healed, the pain may persist. It's unsettling; there's nothing on the surface of the skin to indicate it should hurt. But it does. And according to shingles sufferers, the pain can be excruciating.

Pain clinics, which have appeared around the country, offer numerous approaches for dealing with chronic pain such as that caused by shingles or other long-term conditions such as arthritis. "There are many different kinds of pain clinics, and they have many different orientations," explains Mitchell Max, M.D. Your best bet: Choose a clinic with a multidisciplinary, or team, approach.

No single approach, technique, or drug has yet been proven in studies to clearly reduce the pain after shingles. But if you've suffered for several months or years, you may be ready to try some different approaches. Once you've tried more conservative treatments like self-hypnosis,

antidepressants, or TENS, for example, you may decide to seek relief with extreme measures.

One such measure is a nerve block, in which a local anesthetic is injected into the nerve to block the pain. Although Max says evidence points to a reduction of pain in other conditions, nerve blocks haven't been shown effective yet in postshingles pain.

Another drastic measure is surgery in which the nerves carrying the pain are actually cut, says Max. But, he adds, the results have been disappointing. "It doesn't always remove the pain."

Max cautions against indulging in any drastic treatments during the first months following an outbreak of shingles. "Some of these techniques may be overkill this soon. Stay away from anything like nerve blocks or surgery that's irreversible. If you wait long enough, the pain after shingles often goes away on its own," he advises.

If you feel that you can't bear the pain any longer and are interested in trying a pain clinic, ask your doctor for a referral.

Don't pop the blisters. "It's a temptation for some patients," says Jordan. But it will only make matters worse.

Don't spread them. Although it won't bring relief to you, stay away from those at risk. Avoid people with any sort of immune problem, such as transplant patients, and children who haven't yet been exposed to chicken pox.

Consider a hot-pepper fix. Once the blisters have healed, but the pain persists, what options do you have? Apply hot peppers? Not exactly. But Zostrix, an over-the-counter cream containing capsaicin, derived from hot peppers, may help. Not everyone's impressed with it, however. "It may make the pain worse the first two or three days," says Jordan, "and none of my patients have been willing to tolerate that."

Try to relax. Learn self-hypnosis, imagery, or meditation or do whatever you can to relax. It certainly won't hurt you, and it may help you deal more effectively with the pain.

Try TENS. With this technique, a weak electrical current gives you a tingling feeling that may help block out the pain signal, explains Mitchell Max, M.D., chief of the Clinical Trials Unit at the National Institute of Dental Research/National Institutes of Health (NIDR/NIH) Pain Research Clinic in Bethesda, Maryland. You can purchase a TENS unit for home use; he says they should be priced below $100.

Consider an antidepressant. Some studies have shown that low doses of antidepressant medications help relieve postshingles pain, even in patients who are not suffering from depression. How? Antidepressants block the removal of a neurotransmitter called serotonin. If you have extra amounts of serotonin, it may keep pain signals from reaching the brain, so you don't feel the pain. Talk it over with your doctor to determine if an antidepressant may be of help to you in coping with postshingles pain. ◆

◆ SHINSPLINTS ◆

10 Ways to Say Goodbye to the Pain for Good

Perhaps you were in the middle of your morning run or your evening aerobics class and it came on like gangbusters: shooting pain starting in the front of your ankle and continuing up almost to your kneecap. Now, when you touch the area on either side of your shinbone, it feels sore and tender. Could it be shinsplints?

"'Shinsplints' is a garbage-basket term used to describe any kind of shin pain that comes from exercise," says Michael J. Henehan, D.O., director of the Sports Medicine Department at Stanford/San Jose Family Practice Residency Program in San Jose, California. "It is an injury that comes from overuse."

Most shin pain, although annoying, is minor and can be treated with the guidelines that follow. However, if the pain persists or recurs, see a doctor. You may be suffering from a stress fracture—a tiny chip or crack in the bone. Stress fractures won't go away on their own and, without treatment, may become serious.

Don't work through the pain. You won't earn points in athlete's heaven for trying to tough out the pain of shinsplints, says Henehan. At best, the pain won't get better and at worst, you'll be setting the stage for a more serious injury. "Stay off it until you're pain-free," Henehan says. "You can also cut back your mileage, if you're a runner, but you ought not to run at all, if the pain is severe."

Ice it. Ice is the treatment of choice for reducing the inflammation of any sports injury, and shinsplints is no exception, according to William E. Straw, M.D., a clinical associate professor of medicine at Stanford University School of Medicine in California and team physician for the San Francisco Giants. He recommends using water that's been frozen in a Styrofoam (or paper) cup; massage the area with the ice for ten minutes at a time, up to four times a day for a week or two. You can also try icing the area with a bag of frozen

Choosing a Sneaker

A good sneaker is an important investment for anyone who runs or does aerobics, doctors agree. Wearing shoes with worn-out or poorly cushioned insoles only paves the way for overuse injuries. When shopping for athletic shoes, look for a good fit (with at least a thumb's width of room at the toe and with the heel held firmly), good cushioning (especially in the forefoot, for an aerobics shoe) and extra-supportive material on the inside heel-edge of the sole, says Spencer White, director of research engineering at Reebok International Ltd. in Stoughton, Massachusetts.

Runners should replace their shoes approximately every 500 miles; aerobicizers every four to five months, White says.

vegetables, such as peas or corn kernels, suggests Jeffrey L. Tanji, M.D., an associate professor of family practice and director of the Sports Medicine Program at the University of California at Davis Medical Center.

Tape it. Taping up your shin with an Ace bandage or with a neoprene sleeve that fits over the lower leg may be comforting for shinsplints, says Henehan. "Compression seems to relieve the discomfort, perhaps by decreasing the amount of pull on the muscles."

Take two aspirin. Over-the-counter analgesics, such as aspirin and ibuprofen, are very effective in relieving the pain of shinsplints, according to Straw. These medications serve as anti-inflammatories, bringing down the swelling and inflammation that may come with these injuries. Acetaminophen may ease the pain but probably won't do much for inflammation. Women who are pregnant or nursing a baby, as well as aspirin-sensitive individuals, should check with their physicians before taking any medications.

Try an athletic insole. 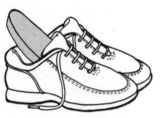 Since shinsplints often arises as a result of excessive pounding, a padded insole placed inside the shoe may help, according to Henehan. These insoles help soften the blow of your foot's landing on hard ground. You can purchase them at an athletic shoe store, sports supply store, or even some grocery stores. They range in price from about $7 to $20.

Tune in to your body. The biggest reason that people get overuse injuries is because they don't pay attention to the signals their bodies give them, says Tanji. "When you're running and you start to feel pain, you need to back off on the pace or the distance," he says.

Stay off the cement. Another way to lower the impact of your routine is to be sure you exercise on forgiving surfaces, according to Henehan. "For running, the best surface is a track where you have a material that is somewhat shock-absorbent," he says. "Crushed gravel and finely trimmed grass [without holes in the ground] are good choices. Asphalt is better than concrete. Also, rubberized, indoor track surfaces are good." If you do aerobics, stay away from cement floors, even carpeted ones, Henehan says. Suspended wood floors are best.

Cross train. One way to give rest to shinsplints without cutting out exercise altogether is to switch to another type of activity, according to Straw. "Stationary bicycling and swimming are good replacements for running or aerobics," he says. "You need to do something without the pounding."

Don't run on hills. Running up and down hills may contribute to shinsplints, says Tanji. He suggests avoiding hills until the pain goes away.

Prevent the injury from occurring in the first place. Warming up before exercise may help prevent injury, according to Frank Spano, M.D., an internist at Bridgeport Medical Group in Connecticut. "When you warm up, you increase your heart's supply of blood to your tissues," he says. "You also relax your muscles so that they don't start out so tight. This lowers the likelihood of injury." Spano recommends gentle stretching exercises and starting off slowly before building speed. Tanji tells his patients to do ankle circles before they run. ◆

◆ SIDE STITCH ◆

9 Ways to Stop It

You're running, biking, or walking briskly along when suddenly you're gripped with a sharp pain in your side. With each breath, the pain becomes more intense. You've developed a "side stitch," a sudden, sharp pain in the upper part of your diaphragm.

No one is actually sure what causes side stitch, according to fitness expert Covert Bailey, author of the best-sellers *Fit or Fat* and *The New Fit or Fat.* "No research has ever been able to demonstrate what's really going on with a side stitch," he says. "It remains one of the body's mysteries."

Most authorities believe a side stitch is a cramp in the diaphragm, the "breathing muscle," a large, flat, muscular membrane that separates the chest and abdominal organs and helps force air into and out of the lungs. Exactly why the diaphragm cramps, however, remains unclear. Some believe that exercise like running decreases blood flow to the diaphragm, causing it to go into spasm. Raising the knees to run contracts the belly muscles, which increases pressure inside the belly and presses on the diaphragm from below. During exercise, air tends to get into the lungs more easily than it gets out, so the lungs fill with air and press on the diaphragm from above. The dual pressure, says the theory, squeezes the diaphragm and shuts off its blood flow, resulting in cramping.

Another theory suggests that side-stitch pain results from gas trapped in the large intestine. Exercise, like running, speeds up intestinal contractions and pushes gas toward the end of the colon, or large intestine. If the colon is blocked by a hardened stool, cramping can result.

Some experts believe that, in some people, side stitch may be related to an intolerance to wheat or dairy products. People with such allergies, they say,

> ## ◆◆ Hello, Doctor? ◆◆
>
> *Sometimes, side stitch is mistaken for angina pectoris, a serious pain caused by lack of oxygen to the heart. See a doctor immediately if you have pain that:*
>
> • *Emanates from beneath the breastbone or from the neck or radiates down the left arm*
>
> • *Is accompanied by shortness of breath*
>
> • *And is brought on by emotional tension and/or physical exertion*

who exercise within 24 hours of eating these foods may develop cramping or even diarrhea. Others suggest side stitch can be brought on by any food in the stomach and exercising too soon after eating.

While the experts haggle about what causes side stitch, you can learn to prevent it and, if it does occur, make it stop quickly. Here's how:

Belly breathe. Competitive distance runner and sports medicine expert Joan Ullyot, M.D., author of *Women's Running* and *Running Free,* says most side stitches come from improper breathing. "Many people, especially beginning runners, don't breathe properly when they're exercising," she says. "They breathe too shallowly."

Michael Martindale, L.P.T., a physical therapist at the Sports Medicine Center at Portland Adventist Medical Center in Oregon, agrees. "People often learn to breathe using only their upper chest muscles rather than the diaphragm muscles," he explains. "During exercise, when they need more air, they breathe faster and even more shallowly."

Ullyot says the key to side-stitch prevention is deep belly breathing. To help people learn how to breathe, Ullyot has people lie on their back with a book on their abdomen. "I have them breathe in all the way into the belly," she says. "The book must move up when breathing in and down when exhaling."

Try the "grunt" exhale. Because it's much more difficult to empty the lungs than fill them during exercise, it's important to exhale all the way into your belly. Force air out while exhaling by pushing your abdomen out while making a grunting sound.

Slow down. Being out of condition and exercising too intensely causes you to breathe quickly—and more shallowly. Martindale suggests cutting back on the intensity of your activity. "Slow down," he says. "Build your endurance over several weeks."

Stop. Some people, particularly competitive runners, believe you should "run through" a side stitch. However, unless you're in a race, Ullyot says the best idea is to stop completely until the pain subsides.

Use the "one hour" rule. If you've eaten, wait at least an hour before exercising, says Ullyot. "Food in the stomach doesn't bother some people, but for others it can cause cramping," she says.

Massage it. "Anytime a muscle is denied blood, it will go into spasm and cause pain," says physical therapist Ellen Nona Hoyven, P.T., owner and director of Ortho Sport Physical Therapy P.C. in Clackamas, Oregon. "Massage increases circulation and relaxes muscles." If you develop a stitch, gently massage the area with your hands.

Use the "poke and blow" technique. One way to relieve diaphragm pressure is to reach deeply with your fingers into your belly just below your ribs on the right side. At the same time, purse your lips tightly and blow out as hard as you can, advises Martindale.

Practice running fast. One of the possible causes of side stitch is weak abdominal and diaphragm muscles. To increase endurance and strengthen the diaphragm, try running fast a couple of times a week.

Strengthen abdominal muscles. Strong abdominal muscles can help prevent side stitch. Try doing bent-leg partial sit-ups in which you raise the shoulders about six inches off the ground (it's less stressful to the back than full sit-ups). Or lie on your back and lift your straight legs a few inches off the ground and hold for 20 to 30 seconds at a time. ◆

◆ SINUSITIS ◆

5 Ways to Head It Off

Like it or not, your nose is an immeasurably valuable part of your anatomy. On the outside, it serves to hold your sunglasses in the vicinity of your eyes. On the inside, it incorporates an intricate system of narrow passages and hollow, air-containing spaces—connected to both your eyes and ears—that enable you to inhale air from the environment and process it along to your lungs. While it is easy to understand how a passageway is necessary in this process, what possible function can be carried out by the hollow spaces?

The hollow spaces, known as the paranasal sinuses, are located in pairs behind the eyebrows, in each cheekbone, behind the nose, and between the eyes. Because they are filled only with air, they act as a sort of "echo chamber," giving resonance to your voice. They also lessen the weight of your skull, cushion it against shocks, and give you better balance. The most important function of your sinuses, however, is as a "conditioner" for inhaled air on its way to your lungs. Normally, the membranes lining the nose and sinuses produce between a pint and a quart of mucus and secretions a day. This discharge passes through the nose, sweeping and washing the membranes and picking up dust particles, bacteria, and other air pollutants along the way. The mucus is then swept backward into the throat by tiny undulating hairs called cilia. From there, it is swallowed into the stomach, where acids destroy dangerous bacteria. It's all in a day's work for the lining of the sinuses and the nasal cavity.

But when those nasal passages become irritated or inflamed by an allergy attack, air pollution, smoke, or a viral infection such as a cold or the flu, the nose and sinus membranes secrete more than the normal amount of mucus. They also swell, blocking the openings and preventing an easy flow of mucus and air and setting the stage for bacteria to flourish.

Sinus trouble comes in two versions: acute and chronic. The acute attack of sinusitis, which lasts

Know Thy Headache

"A big problem associated with 'sinusitis' is that many people think they have it when they really don't," says Joel R. Saper, M.D., director of the Michigan Headache and Neurological Institute in Ann Arbor. "Only one out of ten persons seeking help for 'sinus trouble' actually suffers from sinus disease."

Thinking their sinuses are the source of the problem, many people treat themselves with over-the-counter drugs designed to relieve "sinus headaches." They may never know they're not treating the real cause because, as Saper points out, these preparations may offer relief—at least in the short run. "Commercial preparations contain not only an analgesic component to counter the discomfort but a mild vasoconstrictor, as well. This narrows the swollen blood vessels that contribute to sinus pressure, congestion, and pain."

To determine the exact source of your discomfort, see an ear, nose, and throat specialist.

for a week to ten days, produces a headache that can range in intensity from minor to what feels like bone-shattering. Chronic sinusitis—which occurs when the sinus opening is blocked for an extended period—seldom causes head pain, although it does cause unpleasant discharge, chronic coughing, recurrent ear infections, and a roaring case of postnasal drip. But the lack of real pain is misleading; chronic sinusitis can be serious indeed,

♦♦ Avoid Rebound ♦♦

Advertisements touting relief from sinus pressure, congestion, and pain are everywhere. Do they deliver what they promise? "In the short run, nasal decongestants and nose drops may afford some relief," says Joel R. Saper, M.D. "But if your sinuses are the problem, use for a longer period of time puts you at risk for a chronic situation of diminishing returns." What happens is that each time the medication wears off, there is more swelling, more congestion, and more discomfort, not because of the original infection, but because of withdrawal from the constricting effect of the spray.

In addition, some people with asthma have aspirin intolerance, and if they use any of the medications containing aspirin, they may unwittingly intensify their problems, perhaps triggering a stuffy nose or even an asthma attack. These reactions often don't occur until three or four hours after taking aspirin, so many users don't make the cause-and-effect association.

If your symptoms don't improve within a few days of home treatment, see your doctor.

Take good care of yourself. "Sometimes, it is impossible to avoid catching a cold," says Daniel Kuriloff, M.D., associate director of the Department of Otolaryngology–Head and Neck Surgery at St. Luke's–Roosevelt Hospital Center in New York. "But you can probably maintain your resistance and thereby reduce the incidence of colds and flu and also lessen their severity if you are in good general health. That means eating a well-balanced diet, getting sufficient exercise, and, most of all, getting adequate rest."

Live the sanitary life. "Certainly you can't walk around with a surgical mask over your face to avoid contact with infectious organisms," notes John W. House, M.D., associate clinical professor in the Department of Otolaryngology, Head and Neck Surgery at the University of Southern California at Los Angeles. "But you don't have to stand right next to a person who is sneezing and coughing if you are in a public place. If a member of your family has a cold or flu, don't share eating utensils and other personal belongings."

Hydrate. "If you aren't drinking at least eight tall glasses of water a day, increase your intake," advises James Stankiewicz, M.D., professor and vice-chairman of the Department of Otolaryngology–Head and Neck Surgery at Loyola University Medical School in Maywood, Illinois. Fill a tall bottle with cool water and keep it at your desk so that you can take small sips throughout the day.

Clear the air. Avoid pollutants in the air, stay indoors if the air quality is poor, and above all, avoid cigarette smoke.

Control allergies. "If you know you are allergic to specific substances, take precautions to avoid them," says Kuriloff (see ALLERGIES). If that is not possible, see an allergist about desensitization treatments designed to help the body develop immunity to the offending substance. ♦

because bacteria can become so entrenched after repeated infections that no antibiotic can touch them. That's why it's wise to have your sinus problem checked out by a doctor, especially if your sinus drainage is greenish in color or if you have a fever.

If your sinuses make your life miserable, do you have to live with it? Not necessarily, say experts; there are many ways to head off the worst of the symptoms.

◆ SLEEPWALKING ◆

13 Ways to Handle It

Sleepwalking is not a sleep disorder, but a parasomnia—a disorder characterized by partial arousals. In normal sleepers, tiny disturbances throughout the night, say a noise or a jerky leg movement, cause a momentary awakening and a quick return to sleep. However, in people who are prone to sleepwalking, such disturbances can propel the sleeper into a state that is halfway between sleeping and waking. Unable to go back to sleep, the individual is partially conscious and struggles to comprehend his or her surroundings. The sleepwalker then becomes confused and tries to complete complex, although sometimes nonsensical, tasks.

"There is no magic switch between wakefulness and sleep," says Mark Mahowald, M.D., president of the American Sleep Disorders Association and director of the Minnesota Regional Sleep Disorders Center at Hennepin County Medical Center in Minneapolis. "People are awake enough to exhibit extremely complex motor behaviors but are not conscious of them and don't remember them in the morning. Most of us have answered the phone in the middle of the night, talked coherently, went back to sleep, and, in the morning, didn't remember it at all. So, there's a little bit of sleepwalking in all of us."

Sleepwalking is very common, occurring in up to 30 percent of healthy children, 5 percent of whom have frequent episodes. It also occurs in one to three percent of adults. The behaviors of sleepwalkers may range from walking into the kitchen to make a sandwich to walking outside barefoot in the snow or trying to drive a car. "The most important thing to remember is that these are normal phenomena and do not represent any serious psychological problems," says Mahowald.

When should sleepwalkers seek medical help? Probably when the episodes provoke fear or concern in those around them, or if the sleepwalkers are putting themselves in danger during their late-night excursions, experts agree. A good sleep specialist or family physician may be able to prescribe medications or other therapies that can decrease the frequency of sleepwalking or stop it altogether. If the sleepwalking is mild, however, read on. The following tips may help.

Maintain a regular sleep-wake schedule. "If you are very sleepy when you go to bed, your chances of sleepwalking may be greater," says Lee J. Brooks, M.D., assistant professor of pediatrics at Case Western Reserve University in Cleveland and director of the Sleep Disorders Center at Rainbow Babies and Children's Hospital, University Hospitals of Cleveland. "Regular bedtimes and regular awakenings could help." Overtired children are also notorious for sleepwalking.

Make sure the environment is safe. One important guideline is to make sure that there is nothing dangerous in a sleepwalker's path, says Brooks. "That means making sure that the person doesn't have the opportunity to jump out of windows," he says. "If it is a young child, you probably want to place a gate in front of the stairs and safety locks on the windows. You can buy products from the hardware store that allow you to open the window a small amount, but which will prevent somebody from jumping out. Make sure knives are not kept out. Don't let a sleepwalking child sleep on the top bunk of a bunk bed. Different people are more severe than others. You need to judge the individual as to what lengths to go to." Other safety tips include placing locks high on doors, keeping clutter off of floors and stairs to prevent the possibility of tripping, and moving tables, nightstands, and other furniture out of the path to the bedroom door.

Don't drink alcohol. Alcohol fragments sleep, making it less sound than normal, according to Mahowald. In adolescents and adults, this fragmentation can also trigger sleepwalking, he says.

Empty your bladder before retiring. Since sleepwalking is usually triggered by a partial arousal from sleep, try to eliminate all possible disturbances. At the top of the list is a full bladder. "Some people think that a full bladder can precipitate sleepwalking in a susceptible patient," Brooks says. It's also wise to limit nighttime fluid intake.

Treat a cough. Fever, coughs, and sneezing can all bring on sleepwalking by partially awakening the sleeper, according to Mahowald. Treating ailments with over-the-counter medications before bedtime may help to prevent a sleepwalking episode.

Check your medications. Certain medications, such as lithium and benzodiazepines or other hypnotics, can precipitate sleepwalking in people who are predisposed to nighttime rambling, according to Brooks. If you suspect that a drug is causing your problem, he suggests calling your doctor.

Learn self-hypnosis. "Hypnosis can be helpful for mild cases of sleepwalking," says Mahowald. "Not in-depth hypnotherapy, but self-hypnosis or relaxation that can be taught in one or two visits to an experienced medical hypnotherapist."

Guide the sleeper back to bed. If you notice someone in your household sleepily ambling around, take them by the elbow and gently guide them back to bed, says Brooks. At the same time, whisper reassuringly into the sleeper's ear. Chances are, they'll allow themselves to be easily led and will quickly return to sleep.

Don't touch the sleeper if he or she seems agitated. "If a sleepwalker seems agitated, don't attempt to

---

◆◆◆ Should You ◆◆◆ Wake a Sleepwalker?

Legend used to have it that it could be dangerous to awaken a sleepwalker. But is there any truth to this old wives' tale?

"First off, it may be very difficult, even impossible, to wake a sleepwalker," says Mark Mahowald M.D. "However, that old story came from a myth in primitive cultures, who thought that the soul left the body while it slept. If you awakened the sleepwalker, you would have a person without a soul."

The best advice is to simply lead the sleepwalker back to bed, he says.

---

touch him or try to lead him back to bed," says Richard Ferber, M.D., director of the Center for Pediatric Sleep Disorders at Children's Hospital, Boston, and assistant professor of neurology at Harvard Medical School in Boston. Touching an upset sleepwalker may cause him or her to flail out violently, putting you in danger.

Give the sleeper some space. If you are unable to lead a sleepwalker peaceably back to bed, back off and give them room to do their thing, says Ferber. If they appear to be in danger, move objects out of their path or redirect them, he advises. "If they are hot and bothered and are about to fall down stairs, do something about it," he suggests. "If they are feeling their way along the wall, talking in an upset way, you can also try to talk to them quietly and calm them down."

Keep it quiet. Any nighttime disturbances can propel a sleepwalker into a state halfway between

Anatomy of a Sleepwalker

Although almost everyone has had some type of a sleepwalking experience in his or her life, certain individuals are predisposed to having frequent episodes of sleepwalking. What makes an individual more likely to sleepwalk?

Sleep researchers think that family history may play a role. Many published studies show that children who sleepwalk are often members of families with other sleepwalkers. One study even showed that identical twins were more likely to exhibit the same sleepwalking tendencies than fraternal twins were, suggesting that certain genes may be responsible.

Sleep apnea, a serious sleep disorder that is linked with cardiovascular disease, has also been associated with a higher incidence of sleepwalking, at least in children. In sleep apnea, the individual has gaps in breathing that may cause an oxygen deficiency. The breathing difficulty may cause a partial arousal and, hence, a sleepwalking episode.

Children with migraine headaches also have a much higher frequency of sleepwalking than children without migraines, studies show. This may be because children with migraines have more disturbed sleep.

Sleepwalking is actually one side of the spectrum of arousal problems. It is a different manifestation of the same biological factors that cause mumbling in sleep, confused half-awakenings without walking, and night terrors, where the sleeper bolts out of bed, terrified and possibly screaming. It is, however, a different phenomenon than nightmares, which occur in the rapid-eye movement (REM) stage of sleep. While a sleeper will remember a nightmare in the morning, a sleepwalker almost never will remember walking in his or her sleep.

sleeping and waking, according to Brooks. Keep the household as quiet as possible, eliminating any unnecessary noise. If your home is extremely noisy, say due to proximity to an airport or railroad track, earplugs can offer welcome relief.

Put a bell on the bedroom door. It is probably dangerous to allow a young child to wander around the house unattended (especially if there are stairs), says Ferber. His advice is to put a bell on the bedroom door that will ring when the door is opened, to alert you that the sleepwalker is up and about.

Wait it out. "It's important to remember that sleepwalking, especially in children, improves with time and does not represent any serious psychological problems," says Brooks. He recommends seeing a doctor if the episodes provoke concern or pose the threat of an injury to the sleepwalker or other household member. ◆

◆ SLIVERS ◆

5 Ways to Remove Them Safely

I t's cold and you're hauling in firewood. But you forgot to wear gloves. Suddenly, you feel a sharp pain in your hand—yep, you've got a sliver.

Essentially, a sliver (or splinter) is a puncture wound with debris in it—in this example, a sliver of wood. You can, of course, also get slivers of glass, metal, or plastic, but wood slivers are by far the most common.

While a cut is a vertical slice and a scrape is the horizontal removal of the outer skin, a puncture wound is a stab deep into the tissue. In the case of a sliver, it's the foreign object— the sliver—that causes the puncture and stays in the tissue. Most slivers aren't serious and can be treated at home. Here's how:

Tweeze it. "If the sliver is sticking above the skin, it's pretty easy to remove it with tweezers. Sterilize the tweezers with alcohol, grasp the sliver as close to the skin as possible, and gently pull it out," says Louisa Silva, M.D., a general practitioner who sees plenty of slivers in her private practice in Salem, Oregon.

Needle it. When slivers don't stick out of the skin, sterilize a needle with alcohol and use it to push the sliver out from the bottom, says Paul Contorer, M.D., chief of dermatology for Kaiser Permanente and clinical professor of dermatology at Oregon Health Sciences University in Portland. "It's important to push the sliver out from the bottom," he says, "or it's likely to break up and leave parts of the sliver in the skin."

Slice it. Too often, slivers are deep and people poke and prod with tweezers and end up bruising the tissue all around the sliver site, according to Robert Matheson, M.D., a dermatologist in private practice in Portland, Oregon. "Use a new, clean razor blade," he advises, "and make an incision parallel to the sliver, right above it. Then gently spread the incision and pick out the sliver." While slicing into your skin may sound gruesome, Contorer says it shouldn't hurt. "The top layer of skin is dead tissue," he explains. "As long as you use a sharp razor or knife and don't cut too deeply, you won't even feel it." Be sure to sterilize the instrument with alcohol first.

Clean it. Once you've got the sliver out, clean the wound thoroughly with soap and water. "Clean it really well," advises Silva. "There's a much higher rate of infection with puncture wounds that are deep and dirty." After cleaning with soap and water, Contorer likes to use hydrogen peroxide to make sure all the debris has been cleaned out. "The hydrogen peroxide releases oxygen, kills bacteria, and speeds healing," he says.

Squeeze on the antibacterial ointment. If the wound hasn't immediately closed up or if you've used the slice technique to remove the sliver, apply an antibacterial ointment like Polysporin or Neosporin and cover with a bandage. Contorer says he prefers Polysporin because fewer people have allergic reactions to it. ◆

◆ SNORING ◆

9 Ways to Turn Down the Volume

Snoring is a problem that, it would seem, hardly needs an introduction. However, as a definition, snoring is "a harsh and noisy sound made by the nose and mouth during sleep," according to Philip R. Westbrook, M.D., F.C.C.P., director of the Sleep Disorders Center at Cedars–Sinai Medical Center in Los Angeles and past president of the American Sleep Disorders Association. It is a common affliction, affecting 20 percent of men and 5 percent of women between the ages of 30 and 35, and 60 percent of men and 40 percent of women at age 60. Despite its frequency, however, snoring is a sleep disorder that can have serious medical and social consequences. The tips that follow may help you sleep more peacefully. Pleasant dreams!

Sleep on your side. "Much of the reason for snoring is positional," says Westbrook. "It occurs when the individual is on his back, not on his side. 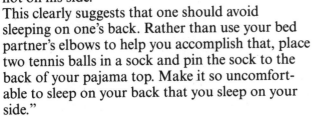 This clearly suggests that one should avoid sleeping on one's back. Rather than use your bed partner's elbows to help you accomplish that, place two tennis balls in a sock and pin the sock to the back of your pajama top. Make it so uncomfortable to sleep on your back that you sleep on your side."

Avoid alcohol and tranquilizers. Alcohol and sleeping pills can depress your central nervous system and relax the muscles of your throat and jaw, making snoring more likely, according to Karl Doghramji, M.D., director of the Sleep Disorders Center at Jefferson Medical College of Thomas Jefferson University in Philadelphia. These

substances are also known to cause sleep apnea, a dangerous condition that has been linked with cardiovascular disease, he says.

Lose weight. Excess body weight, especially around the neck, puts pressure on the airway, causing it to partially collapse, Westbrook says. "It becomes like trying to suck air through a wet [paper] straw. It limits the amount of air that comes in. Turbulence is created, and the soft tissues flap in the breeze, so to speak, creating the noise." He says that it usually takes a significant weight loss, about ten percent of your total body weight, to make an improvement.

Get your allergies treated. Chronic respiratory allergies may cause snoring by forcing sufferers to breathe through their mouths while they sleep, says Doghramji. A decongestant or antihistamine before bedtime may help, he says. Another help for a blocked nose is saline spray, which may be purchased at any drugstore, says German Nino-Murcia, M.D., founder and medical director of the Sleep Medicine and Neuroscience Institute in Palo Alto, California. (You can make your own saline solution by mixing a cup of water at body temperature, a half teaspoon of salt, and a pinch of baking soda. Then put the solution in a clean nasal spray bottle or nasal syringe and squirt it into your nose.) "An ultrasonic humidifier is also a good idea," he adds (see ALLERGIES).

Buy a mouth guard. Your dentist or doctor may be able to prescribe an antisnoring mouth guard, says Doghramji. "The guards fit into the mouth and make sure that the upper and lower teeth are held together," he says. "It prevents the lower jaw from sagging backwards."

Stop smoking. "Smoking can be very irritating to the lining of the upper airway, including the nose,"

What's Wrong with Snoring, Anyway?

We have come to think of snoring as a normal phenomenon in our society. Just ask any child to act out being asleep: He or she will lie down on the floor and feign snoring. However, there are serious problems associated with the annoying noise. Medically, the biggest danger is an association with sleep apnea, a disorder that has been linked with cardiovascular disease. Apnea should be suspected if snoring is excessively loud or if there are gaps in the sleeper's breathing, says German Nino-Murcia, M.D. Other symptoms are extreme daytime sleepiness (although most snorers, not just those with apnea, are sleepier than nonsnorers during the day) and uncontrollable weight gain, says Karl Doghramji, M.D. If any of these symptoms accompanies your snoring, you should see a doctor without delay.

There are also serious social consequences of snoring, which should not be trivialized, according to Philip R. Westbrook, M.D., F.C.C.P. "Although snoring has been an object of derision and humor, it certainly is not very funny for the person who has to listen to it," he says. "And a lot of wives have moved out of bedrooms and houses because of snoring. People may refuse to take trips because they snore. While some of the complaints are not always justified [they may serve as an excuse for other underlying problems], snoring can be loud enough to harm the hearing."

If snoring has not improved after a month of trying out the suggestions described here, your family doctor may be able to help.

says Westbrook. "Your snoring may improve if you quit."

Keep a regular schedule. "People who are sleep deprived will tend to snore," says Thomas Roth, Ph.D., chief of the Division of Sleep Disorders Medicine at Henry Ford Hospital in Detroit. "If you find that you are sleepy during the day, you may not be getting enough sleep." Sleep deprivation also increases the volume of the snoring, says Nino-Murcia, and may cause sleep apnea, although physicians aren't sure why. "Keeping a regular sleep-wake cycle is also helpful," Nino-Murcia says.

See a doctor if you are pregnant and snoring. Sometimes, women who are pregnant will begin to snore, according to William C. Dement, M.D., a professor of psychiatry and behavioral sciences in the School of Medicine at Stanford University and director of Stanford University's Sleep Disorders Center in California. The snoring may begin because of the increased body weight and because the hormonal changes of pregnancy cause muscles to relax. Whatever the cause, snoring during pregnancy may be a sign of sleep apnea, which can decrease the oxygen supply to the fetus, Dement says. "Snoring during pregnancy is a serious problem that people haven't paid much attention to," he says. "During pregnancy, sleep is already disturbed by the need to urinate and by discomfort, which may mask other problems."

Elevate your head. Sleeping with your head raised may take some of the pressure off of the airway, making breathing easier, according to Roth. "Sleep halfway sitting up," he says. "Prop yourself up with pillows." ◆

◆ SORE THROAT ◆

10 Steps for Quick Relief

A sore throat can be a minor, but annoying, ailment, or it can be a symptom of a serious illness. Causes range from a stuffy nose or a cold to strep throat, an infection caused by the streptococcus bacteria. Since untreated strep throat can lead to rheumatic fever and scarlet fever, it's important to get medical help as early as possible into the illness. Symptoms of strep throat include fever, body aches and pains, malaise, and severe sore throat. If you have these symptoms, or if you have a sore throat lasting more than two or three days, it makes good sense to see a doctor. For mild sore throats that accompany a cold or an allergy, the tips below may help ease your discomfort.

Gargle with warm salt water. "If you are a good gargler, do it with very warm, normal saline solution," says V. E. Mikkelson, M.D., a recently retired general practitioner in Hayward, California. "Use one-half teaspoon of salt to a cup of water. It is an extremely comforting fluid and won't do any harm."

Gargle with Listerine. Another good gargling fluid is the mouthwash Listerine, according to Robert S. Robinson, M.D., a general practitioner in Metter, Georgia. "Take it straight from the bottle [but don't share the bottle with anyone else] and do it frequently," he says.

Drink hot liquids. If you're not good at gargling, drink hot fluids, be they coffee, tea, or hot lemonade, Mikkelson says. "The act of swallowing will bathe most of the tissue involved with heat," he explains. "There is something almost mysterious about moist heat. I think microorganisms find it very noxious. I have seen so much benefit in applying hot packs to the skin to fight infection. The same principle holds for the inside of the throat. But since you can't put a hot pack down there, the next best thing is sloshing hot water on it frequently."

◆ Dr. Mikkelson's ◆ Sore-Throat Tonic

What do good, old-fashioned general practitioners prescribe for a sore throat? Besides the tips described here, mixed with a little tincture of time, some advise special brews guaranteed to soothe both body and soul. The following is a favorite of V.E. Mikkelson, M.D.; it was extracted from a book of home remedies published more than 130 years ago. He says he's tried it and swears that it is surprisingly palatable and works wonders.

> *1 tablespoon honey, any kind*
> *1 tablespoon vinegar, preferably apple-cider vinegar*
> *8 ounces hot water*

Mix all the ingredients together in a mug and sip slowly (but don't let it get cold). Use as often as desired.

Take an analgesic. Plain old aspirin, acetaminophen, or ibuprofen can do wonders for sore-throat pain, according to Stephen Kriebel, M.D., a family physician in Forks, Washington. However, aspirin should not be given to children under the age of 21 because of the risk of Reye's syndrome, a potentially fatal condition. Pregnant and nursing women should check with their doctor before taking any medication.

Rest and take it easy. Common sense dictates staying in bed and resting when a sore throat's got you down. Taking it easy leaves more energy to fight the infection, Mikkelson says.

Suck on hard candy. 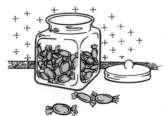 "Hard candy and lozenges help the pain get better," according to Kriebel. "The sugar itself helps as much as anything. It has a soothing effect. It also helps with tickly coughs. And you don't have to go with brand names."

Keep your nasal passages clear. Doctors agree that two of the most common causes of sore-throat pain are postnasal drip and a dry throat that results from sleeping with your mouth open when your nasal passages are blocked. Decongestants, especially those containing pseudoephedrine (read package labels), may be helpful in stopping the flow, according to Alvin J. Ciccone, M.D., F.A.A.F.P., a family physician and an associate professor in the Department of Family Medicine at Eastern Virginia Medical School in Norfolk. Kriebel recommends using a nasal saline spray and investing in a humidifier for use at night.

Spray it. Analgesic sprays, such as Chloraseptic, may be effective in temporarily relieving sore-throat pain, says Kriebel. The only problem is that the effect doesn't last long. You may have to spray several times an hour. However, the sprays won't harm you and may take the edge off of an extremely painful throat.

Steam it out. One old-fashioned remedy for a cold or sore throat is a steam tent—sitting with your face over a bowl of steaming hot water. Draping a towel over your head serves to keep the steam in. The effectiveness of this remedy is more than an old wives' tale, according to Kriebel. "There have been a couple of scientific studies done on steaming," he says. "They show that it may shorten the length of time it takes for the infection to go away."

Keep the fluids coming. Ciccone advises his patients to drink as much fluid as possible—at least eight to ten eight-ounce glasses per day. "Fluids lubricate the throat and prevent it from drying out," he says. They also soothe and help prevent irritation. They may even help to shorten the course of the illness." ◆

◆ STAINED TEETH ◆

8 Ways to Keep Them Whiter

Pearly whites gone dingy are one of the most common complaints dentists hear from their patients. And some folks simply go ahead and take matters into their own hands, risking damage to their teeth and gums in the process.

What causes stained teeth? Tobacco—whether it's smoked or chewed—is one of the worst offenders. Coffee, tea, and colas are culprits as well. Other possible causes include fruit juices (especially grape), red wine, fruits such as blueberries, soy sauce, and curry. "If it will stain your carpet permanently, it's not great for your teeth," says Christine Dumas, D.D.S., assistant professor of clinical dentistry at the University of Southern California in Los Angeles and a consumer advisor/spokesperson for the American Dental Association.

Aging also contributes to the yellowing of teeth. The enamel, which is the hard outer coating of your teeth, wears thin, allowing the underlying layer of yellowish dentin to show through.

And some stains are what's called intrinsic. That is, they actually occur on the inside of the tooth. For example, children who take the antibiotic tetracycline (or whose mothers took it during pregnancy) often have such stains. Silver-colored fillings can sometimes leach out and stain the surrounding tooth, says Cary Goldstein, D.M.D., special lecturer in esthetic dentistry at Emory University School of Dentistry in Atlanta.

So before you can take action, you have to understand what kind of stains are dulling your teeth. You also need to be realistic, too, in what you want: "Teeth are not naturally pure white," says Becky DeSpain, R.D.H., M.Ed., director of the Caruth School of Dental Hygiene at Baylor College of Dentistry in Dallas. "People have unreasonable expectations of what their smiles should look like."

Only your dentist can correct intrinsic stains through the use of such cosmetic procedures as composite resin bonding and porcelain laminate veneers. Stains from food and drink can often be removed with a professional dental cleaning. A more expensive and time-consuming option is in-office bleaching.

Once you've had the stains professionally removed, here's what you can do to keep them from occurring in the future:

Keep your teeth clean. That means brushing your teeth at least twice a day, especially after meals. An electric brush may be more effective if you don't do a thorough job manually, Goldstein says. "Don't make the mistake of scrubbing the teeth too hard," warns DeSpain. "You can wear grooves into the tooth at the roots."

Floss. Ever notice how stained teeth look worse around the edges? That's because the plaque (a thin, nearly invisible layer of bacteria and food debris) that accumulates between teeth and at the gum line attracts stains like a magnet. Keep that plaque down with thorough daily flossing and you'll help fight stains.

Quit smoking. Much easier said than done, but if you won't stop for your health, will you do it for a more-attractive smile?

Cut down on coffee. You know how coffee can stain a porcelain cup. It, along with tea and colas, does the same thing to your teeth. Don't sip on such drinks throughout the day. Try to brush after drinking them, too.

Use a straw. OK, sipping hot coffee through a plastic straw is hardly appealing, but it'll work for iced tea, cola, and fruit juices. "It helps minimize the contact with the teeth," says Dumas.

Use stain-removing toothpastes with caution. The smokers' toothpastes are abrasive, says Goldstein. "These shouldn't be used unless you've got a real problem with stains," warns Richard Simonsen, D.D.S., M.S., editor-in-chief of *Quintessence International,* an international dental journal, and a professor in the College of Dentistry at the University of Tennessee in Memphis. Goldstein says he tells patients to limit the use of such products to two or three times a week.

Get a "cosmetic cleaning." If your teeth stain easily, call your dentist for a cosmetic cleaning between checkups. "About ten percent of our patients come in once a month for this," says Goldstein. It takes about 20 minutes and costs about half the price of a regular cleaning (it is not, however, meant to take the place of regular checkups).

Don't get creative. "Patients can scratch composite resins and porcelain veneers [types of restorations] with baking soda," says Dumas. "And that makes these materials more prone to picking up stains." She's also seen people use a dental pick at home and "do more harm than good." Another dangerous home remedy: applications of chlorine bleach. ◆

◆◆◆ At-Home Products: ◆◆◆ Are They Safe?

Late-night commercials and glossy advertisements in some consumer magazines promise the brightest teeth ever with the use of certain home tooth-whitening products.

But before you reach into your wallet (pretty deeply for some of these products), be aware that both the American Dental Association (ADA) and the U.S. Food and Drug Administration (FDA) have expressed doubts concerning over-the-counter tooth whiteners.

In fact, the FDA has ruled that these products make claims that take them out of the cosmetics category and that they are actually new drugs. That means they need FDA approval of their safety and effectiveness before being marketed.

The ADA's Council on Dental Therapeutics has jumped into the fray, issuing a statement expressing concern over long-term safety. Published scientific studies have shown that the ingredients used (primarily carbamide peroxide, which converts to hydrogen peroxide in the mouth) may damage teeth and gums, delay healing of damaged tissue, and possibly cause cancer.

The ADA also pointed out that one toothpaste carries a seal of approval of the American Society of Dental Aesthetics (not affiliated with the ADA), whose president just happens to have invented that product.

Other over-the-counter tooth whiteners that don't rely on bleaching ingredients are nothing more than a cover-up. "You paint it on like a nail polish," says Cary Goldstein, D.M.D. "And it just doesn't look natural."

Then there's the cost of some products. "The consumer gets ripped off," says Richard Simonsen, D.D.S., M.S.

So rather than getting taken to the cleaners, take your stained teeth to a dentist to have them cleaned safely.

◆ STINGS ◆

14 Ways to Avoid and Treat Them

You hear the buzz, you see the bee, but before you know it—zap, you're stung. Almost all of us have had this experience at least once, and it's no fun. But if you know what to do, you can take the ouch out of being stung and perhaps prevent the attack from happening in the first place.

Bees, yellow jackets, hornets, wasps, and fire ants all have stingers that inject venom into their unfortunate victim. The normal reaction is redness, pain, itching, and perhaps some swelling around the sting area, which lasts for a few hours.

For the one to two million people who are highly allergic to the venom of stinging insects, the consequences can be much worse, according to the American Academy of Allergy and Immunology. "Some may have a local allergic swelling, which is usually larger than five inches and can encompass the entire arm or leg or face," says David Golden, M.D., assistant professor of medicine at Johns Hopkins University in Baltimore and chair of the Insect Committee at the American Academy of Allergy and Immunology. This swelling isn't immediate; it develops over a 12- to 24-hour period.

The most serious allergic reactions involve the whole body. Symptoms may include hives, wheezing, difficulty in breathing, dizziness, and nausea, after which shock and unconsciousness may occur. People suffering from these types of allergic reactions need emergency medical treatment. It's estimated that fifty people die every year from anaphylactic shock brought on by insect stings.

Thankfully, for most of us, a sting is little more than a minor nuisance. And it's a nuisance you can do something about.

EASING THE PAIN

Here are some simple suggestions for minimizing a sting's pain quickly and easily. Be sure to keep an eye out for signs of a more-severe reaction so that medical help can be sought immediately if necessary.

Apply unseasoned meat tenderizer. "Take a teaspoonful of meat tenderizer, mix it with a few drops of water, and put it right on the sting," says Jerome Z. Litt, M.D., assistant clinical professor of dermatology at Case Western Reserve University School of Medicine in Cleveland. "You can get almost instantaneous relief." This works thanks to an enzyme in the tenderizer called papain or bromelain, which dissolves the toxins the insect has just injected into you. Litt recommends carrying a bottle with you when you know you're going to be outdoors in areas where bees are likely to be present. That's probably a good idea, because if you don't put it on fairly soon after you've been stung, it won't work. "Once the venom proteins are really into the skin, then it's too late for the meat tenderizer to reach those proteins and degrade them," says Golden.

Try a baking-soda paste. Think of this as "plan B" if you don't happen to have any meat tenderizer available. "Baking soda will relieve some of the itching and swelling but won't neutralize the venom," says Litt.

Scrape the stinger out. Bees and some yellow jackets have barbed stingers that anchor in your skin after you're stung. (Other stinging insects have smooth stingers that remain intact on the bug.) You should get the stinger out as soon as possible, because it will continue to release venom into your skin for several minutes after the initial sting. Resist the urge to squeeze, grab, or press the stinger, however. Doing that will just make matters worse by pumping more venom into your skin. "Instead, lift the stinger up gently with a clean fingernail or knife blade," says Litt. "Then scrape gently and the stinger will come out."

Put it on ice. Rub ice over the sting site. This may help to reduce some of the inflammation and swelling, says Litt.

Take an antihistamine. If the itchiness from a sting is bugging you, you might try an over-the-counter antihistamine for relief, suggests Golden.

PREVENTING FUTURE STINGS

Even better than calming the discomfort of a sting is preventing one from happening in the first place. Here's what you can do to protect yourself.

Keep your cool. If a wasp, yellow jacket, or any stinging insect flies near you, stay calm. "You should move away very slowly and don't flap, wave, or swat," says Litt. Getting agitated like that may incite the insect to sting.

Unsweeten your sweat. Ever notice how certain people just seem to attract insects more than others? "What it is that attracts those insects is not clear," says Golden, but it may have to do with the smell of a person's sweat or his or her body odor. One theory, though so far unsubstantiated, is if you can change the smell of your sweat, insects may keep their distance. "I believe eating onions and garlic or taking high doses of vitamin B sometimes can prevent insect stings," says Litt. You may attract fewer insects, but you won't win any popularity contests. Don't take large doses of any vitamin without your doctor's OK.

◆◆◆ Killer-Bee Update ◆◆◆

Killer bees have finally arrived, and they're here to stay. On October 15, 1990, the first colony of killer bees in the United States was discovered near Hidalgo, Texas, after crossing the Mexican border. Since then, they've continued to spread in Texas. "We expect the first swarms to reach Louisiana sometime this year [1992], and they'll reach Arizona in the next two years certainly. They should be in California in the next three to five years," says Mark Winston, Ph.D., professor of biological sciences at Simon Fraser University in Burnaby, British Columbia, and author of Killer Bees: The Africanized Honey Bee in the Americas. *Just how far north they'll go in the United States is a hotly debated issue, but Winston believes they won't make it past the southern third of the country, no farther north than the Carolinas.*

What will stop their advance? Nothing high tech, just cold temperatures. That's one big difference between killer bees and the European bees we're used to. Africanized bees can't withstand long, cold winters. Another well-known difference is that "africanized bees can be extraordinarily aggressive with very little provocation. They're very, very quick on the trigger," says Winston. "There have already been some serious stinging incidents in Texas, and it's just a matter of time before there's a fatality."

So what should you know if you enter killer-bee country? Keep your eyes open, because killer bees nest in a much greater variety of places then European bees do. If you see a hive, don't disturb it, no matter what. Slowly and carefully walk away. If you start getting stung, you need to get out of there fast. Sting for sting, killer bees are no worse than other honeybees, but they sting in much greater numbers. Winston advises that you run as fast as you can or get into a car or building. "Even though Africanized bees will pursue you for quite a distance, it is possible to outrun them," Winston says. "If you dive to the ground and swat and panic you're going to get a lot more stings and it could be a very serious situation."

Don't wear bright, flowery clothes or rough fabrics. These seem to attract insects for some reason. Stick to smooth fabric and light-colored outfits in tones of white, tan, green, or khaki when you plan to spend time outdoors.

Go fragrance-free. Perfumes, colognes, after-shaves, hair sprays, and scented soaps will attract insects. You may feel a bit bland without your favorite fragrance, but it may be well worth it in terms of preventing painful stings.

Leave bright, shiny jewelry at home. "Insects find bright jewelry and other metal objects very alluring," says Litt. You may lack some pizazz, but in this case, making less of a fashion statement is in style.

Keep your shoes on. Walking barefoot outside may feel great, but when you're in grassy areas, it's not such a wise idea. "Bees love clover, and the yellow jackets live in the ground, so bare feet are very vulnerable to insect attacks," says Litt.

Keep food covered when outside. Picnics are a summer family favorite, but open food attracts stinging insects. Keep covers on food as much as possible and keep the lids on garbage cans as well. You're best off to steer clear of public trash cans that are partially open on top.

Watch what you drink from. If you're downing a cold drink outdoors, use caution. "Never drink from a soda can or anything that you can't see inside," says Golden. "There's nothing worse than getting stung on your tongue or throat."

Be aware of your surroundings. When doing yard work or gardening, be on the lookout for hives. Nests can be found in the eaves and attic of your home and in trees, vines, shrubs, wood piles, and other protected places. Disturbing a nest, even by accident, can irritate the insects. The American Academy of Allergy and Immunology suggests using extreme care when operating power lawn mowers, hedge clippers, or tractors. ◆

◆ STOMACH UPSET ◆

23 Ways to Tame Your Tummy

If your tummy is bothering you, play detective with your symptoms. It's alimentary, my dear Watson.

First question: How long has this been going on? Chronic, long-term stomach upset is something you should be discussing with your doctor. But if your temperamental tummy is something that hit you after a big meal or a party, it's likely that it's a temporary discomfort.

"We try to separate out the temporary 'I ate too much pizza' from the long-term," says Sherman Hess, B.S., R.Ph., a pharmacist in Portland, Oregon, who has guided many a gastronomically upset customer to the antacid shelf.

Temporary stomach upset may be due to indigestion or flu. Often, it's the result of something—or the quantity of something—you ate. Here are some tips that can help you.

Try some soda. Soda pop, particularly 7-Up and other noncaffeinated varieties, helps to settle stomachs, says Hess.

Take fruit juice for flu. If you have the flu, with diarrhea and/or vomiting, fruit juice will help resupply the potassium and other nutrients your body has lost.

Don't count on milk. Douglas C. Walta, M.D., a gastroenterologist in Portland, Oregon, says milk often hinders rather than helps stomachs because some people can't digest it easily. "Milk is probably the biggest contributor to gut upset that I see in the population over 30," he says.

Ease off on coffee. Coffee may irritate the stomach. "It's controversial whether it's the acid or the caffeine or both," says Walta.

Hold off on the booze. Alcohol also is an irritant to the stomach lining, Walta says.

Lighten up on pepper. Red and black pepper are frequently identified as gastrointestinal irritants,

says Kimra Warren, R.D., a registered dietitian at St. Vincent Hospital and Medical Center in Portland, Oregon. Try cutting back to see if your symptoms improve. If they don't, then pepper isn't your problem.

Don't smoke. Walta notes that smoking is often associated with ulcers. Cigarette smoke is a gastrointestinal irritant.

Watch your diet. Do your stomach a favor and eat foods that are easy to digest. David M. Taylor, M.D., a gastroenterologist and assistant professor of medicine at Emory University in Atlanta and the Medical College of Georgia in Augusta, says the stomach has a tough time with fatty, fried foods. "A high-carbohydrate, low-fat, high-bulk diet is the best thing," he says.

Increase fiber gradually. A high-fiber diet is good for your health, but don't go too high too fast. A gradual change of diet, with a slow but continual addition of fiber, will help to offset tolerance problems.

Choose veggies carefully. You may love broccoli, but if you have a problem with gas, perhaps you should cut back, suggests Warren. Too much of certain gassy vegetables, namely broccoli, cauliflower, and brussels sprouts, can be a problem.

Limit problematic fruits. Some people get tummy problems from eating apples and melon. Pay attention to whether your stomach upset followed eating one of these. If so, skip them.

Worry about the quantity, not quality. Walta says it's a myth that hot, spicy foods create stomach problems. So go ahead and eat spicy food. Just don't overload your stomach.

Cook gasless beans. Warren says if you throw out the water in which you've soaked the beans overnight, and cook them in fresh water, you'll significantly decrease their gas-causing potential.

Think about your diet. Problem foods can be very individualistic. Identify the foods that you are sensitive to, then avoid them.

Exercise your body. "Exercise is very helpful," says Taylor. Even a brief walk, particularly after meals, may aid in digestion and help you feel better.

Drink plenty of water. Nutritionists recommend six to eight glasses of water a day to help with digestion.

Avoid laxatives. If you have constipation, it's better to avoid laxatives, says Taylor. Instead, go the more natural route and take bran or a commercial bulking agent such as Metamucil.

Lay off the aspirin. Aspirin and nonsteroidal anti-inflammatory drugs, such as ibuprofen, can actually create ulcers. "What causes ulcers to bleed is aspirin," says Walta. If you have a sensitive stomach but you need pain relief, try aceta-minophen or enteric-coated aspirin.

Take an antacid. Antacids are very effective in soothing stomachs, but they can have side effects. For example, magnesium-based antacids can cause diarrhea, while calcium-based antacids can cause constipation. Antacids with aluminum hydroxide also can cause constipation.

Switch brands. Sometimes, a different brand of antacid may prove to be more effective.

Don't take an antacid too long. Side effects from antacid use usually don't appear unless a person has taken the medication for several days. But if the problem has persisted that long, it's time to call the doctor.

Try an antacid in tablet form. Hess suggests taking an antacid in tablet form because the dose is lower than in liquid preparations and therefore may not contribute to constipation or diarrhea.

◆ What's It to You? ◆

"What you consider indigestion and what I consider indigestion is very variable," says Douglas C. Walta, M.D.

The word can be tagged to a wide range of maladies, some of them simple, some of them serious. Walta says he tells patients to drop the word "indigestion" and to just describe to him their gut feelings. Also, it's helpful to him to know if patients feel better or worse after eating. They may be describing what could be a pre-ulcer disease or a gallbladder problem. In some cases, especially in older individuals, the symptoms may be tied to a cancerous condition.

That's why Walta is concerned about attaching the label "indigestion" to too many symptoms. The rule of thumb is, if the condition persists, see a doctor.

Relax. After disease is ruled out as the cause of stomach discomfort, the underlying culprit often turns out to be stress. Stress frequently translates into physical problems. Along the gastrointestinal tract, these problems can include indigestion, irritable bowel syndrome, constipation, and diarrhea.

The cure: Unwind. Relax. Enjoy yourself. Taylor says he recommends "hobbies, running or tennis or hiking or karate, or communing with nature, or sex, or whatever" to patients whose stomach troubles seem to be stress related. He says one of the most effective prescriptions is to take a trip. "They come back and say, 'Gee, doc, it's remarkable. I went away skiing and now I don't have any trouble.'" ◆

◆ STRESS ◆

14 Ways to Combat It

With the fast-paced, high-pressure life that many of us lead, full of hefty job and family responsibilities, it's no wonder that many of us feel stressed to the limit. We all have to live with stress, but if not reined in, it can profoundly affect both mind and body. Fortunately, you can curb stress.

We all know stress when we see it (or feel it), yet it's hard to define. One way of describing stress is "the individual's perception of losing control of his or her life," says Robert Eliot, M.D., director of the Institute of Stress Medicine and professor of cardiology at the University of Nebraska Medical Center in Omaha. "It's a mismatch between expectations and reality."

Stress doesn't just arise from unpleasant, aggravating events. Positive happenings like getting married, starting a new job, being pregnant, or winning an election can also tense us up.

Stress isn't all bad, either. In fact, it protects us in many instances by priming the body to react quickly to adverse situations. This fight-or-flight response helped keep human beings alive when their environment demanded quick physical reactions in response to threats.

The problem in modern times is that "we put the physiology of stress into overdrive even when there's not a life-threatening situation. This causes wear and tear on the body that can make a person feel miserable," says Raymond Flannery, Jr., Ph.D., clinical psychologist and assistant professor of psychology in the Department of Psychiatry of Harvard Medical School at Cambridge Hospital in Massachusetts.

How you'll be affected by stress depends on what the "weak plank in your body's platform of resistance is," says Eliot. Everything from headaches, upset stomach, skin rashes, hair loss, racing heartbeat, back pain, and muscle aches can be stress related. "Every organ in the system can be affected, from the skin to the gut to the heart," says Paul Rosch, M.D., president of The American Institute of Stress in Yonkers, New York.

Most importantly, the perception of stress is highly individualized. What jangles your friend's nerves may not phase you in the least, and vice versa. Rosch likens it to a roller-coaster ride, which has thrill-seekers who savor every dip and turn, others who sit white-knuckled praying for the ride to end, and the rest who fall somewhere in between. "It's not external events that are stressful but your perception of them. And you have the power to change that," says Rosch.

Just as the things that cause tension vary from person to person, so do the tools of stress management. "Some people find meditation dull, and others think it's great. You have to find out what works for you," says Rosch. He advises that you develop a "smorgasbord" of stress busters. Here is a menu of practical techniques you can choose from to help de-stress yourself:

Get a support system. You'll be able to cope with stress much better "if you have a sense of links, or caring attachments, to other people," says Flannery, whether those links are with friends, relatives, or both. For example, "for both sexes of all races and all age groups in all countries, married people have better health than single people," says Flannery.

Take reasonable control over your life. You can't control everything around you, but if you've got a good handle on your job and relationships, you'll be better able to deal with stress. "What we find is that anybody under control is apt to be cool," says Eliot. "Take them out of control, and they're apt not to be cool." In fact, having little autonomy on the job is one of the factors that's been shown to lead to stress at work (see "Stress on the Job").

Have a sense of purpose to your life. Waking up each morning with a good reason to get up and a sense of purpose is crucial to stress management. "You can smell the roses forever and jog until your heart gives up, but if you don't have a meaning in life, you're never going to have good physical and mental health and be able to cope with stress," says Flannery.

Laugh a little. "Humor's important because it helps us to keep things in perspective," says Flannery. He studied 1,200 stress-resistant people over the course of 12 years and found that among other attributes, they either had a good sense of humor or chummed around with people who did. Laughing itself also causes chemical changes in your body that elevate your sense of well-being. Eliot agrees that humor is vital and says, "Humor is the lotion on the sunburn of life."

Work out your troubles. Aerobic exercise can do a lot for your body and mind. Flannery says it can induce a sense of well-being and tone down the stress response. And you don't need to run a marathon, either; three 20-minute periods of exercise each week is enough. So take a break and get out there and walk, swim, bike, jog, or aerobicize. Check with your doctor first before starting any program if you're not a regular exerciser or if you have any significant health problems.

Opt for an unstimulating diet. Cut back on caffeine, a dietary stimulant that Flannery says can make you feel anxious even when you have no problems. Who needs the extra jitters? Nicotine can do the same, so reduce or give up the cigarette habit.

Change the self-talks in your head. We all have silent conversations with ourselves every day, and Eliot believes these "self-talks" can have great power over our stress levels. Negative, tension-

Stress on the Job

More work with fewer people to do it. That seems to be what an increasing number of folks are saying about their jobs. The outcome? Rising levels on the stress barometer.

"Perhaps the leading adult health problem in the country today is job stress," says Paul Rosch, M.D. Indeed, a 1991 study of 600 full-time workers nationwide by Northwestern National Life Insurance Company found that job stress is a major thorn in the side of many employees. Of the respondents, 46 percent said they find their jobs very or extremely stressful. Seventy-two percent said they frequently experience stress-related physical or mental conditions. The ailments they cited were: exhaustion, anger or anxiety, muscle pain, headache, inability to sleep, respiratory illness, ulcers or intestinal disorders, depression, and hypertension.

What's the solution? That's a tough question to answer, but the study offered five ways that employers can cut stress:

• Give employees control of their jobs.

• Offer supportive work and family policies.

• Improve communication between management and employees.

• Provide health insurance for mental illness and chemical dependency.

• Allow flexible scheduling of work hours.

causing thoughts—such as, What will the IRS do to me? Will I get that promotion?—aren't helpful. They paint us into a corner and offer us no choices. Rational, more-positive self-talks can "give us some choices and allow us to cool off," says Eliot. Irrational self-talks may be a long-standing habit with you, so Eliot suggests you slowly try to modify them, a little at a time.

Realize you can't control all stresses. Though we'd like to reduce stress to ground zero, there are some situations we can't do anything about. Hurricanes, death, and earthquakes, for instance, are beyond your control. "Some stresses you can't hope to control, and some you can do something about. The wisdom is in learning how to distinguish between the two so you don't waste your time and talent constantly being frustrated by trying to change things you can't influence," says Rosch.

Take time out to relax. Another common thread among Flannery's stress-resistant group was that they all set aside 10 or 15 minutes each day to do something relaxing. Some benefited from practicing relaxation exercises on a daily basis to calm themselves or to reduce their butterflies before certain stressful events, like giving a speech. Relaxation exercises that release muscle tension can help a lot. To do them, you tighten certain groups of muscles as you inhale and then relax them as you exhale. Start with your toes and slowly work your way up to your face. Or you may want to try visualization. With this, you pick a pleasant and relaxing place where you've been or maybe someplace you'd like to visit. Then imagine you are there and try to picture what it would look, smell, taste, and feel like. Breathe slowly throughout, and play the scene in your mind for about five minutes. Some people don't find these techniques relaxing, so they should try something else. Other options you might want to try include dance, crocheting, photography, art, or music, says Flannery.

Get your finances in order. Shaky financial situations can create great strain. A lot of folks get in over their heads using credit cards. "The single greatest source of stress for most people in our society is credit-card debt," says Flannery. "It's one of the leading causes of divorce." So if you avoid the temptation to throw your purchases on plastic and overspend, you'll probably ward off lots of problems and help control your stress levels.

Don't try to have it all. Society pushes us to attain wealth, power, and success along with a great personal and family life. "That's probably the biggest stressful dilemma in life. People are trying to pursue all of the material goods and all of the personal strivings," says Flannery. "The problem is that there aren't enough hours in the week for everybody to do everything." Decide what's most important to you and focus on that.

Get help if you have major stressful problems that you can't deal with. Seek good advice from the best source you can, suggests Eliot. "Often self-help will go so far, but when you have major problems with your job, marriage, spiritual beliefs, friends, or children, don't be afraid to ask for outside help." If you can get these basic areas under control, you'll reduce stress tremendously, and a lot of other things will slide into place.

Breathe deep and slow. Taking steady, slow abdominal breaths can help you cool off in a stressful situation so that you can think more clearly, says Eliot. Flannery teaches breathing techniques based on five-second intervals. For five seconds, you inhale. Hold that breath for five seconds. Exhale for five seconds. Hold it for five seconds, and repeat one more time. (Don't go much beyond that, however, because you could start hyperventilating.) Be patient. It may take some practice to get this down; smokers, in particular, may have trouble.

Don't take your frustrations out on the wrong person. "If you're angry at your boss, coming home and being crabby and irritable with your wife and kids won't solve the problem," says Flannery. Instead, you need to clearly identify the problem, figure out some strategies to solve it, and then put them into action. Otherwise, you'll simply be compounding the stress you feel. ◆

◆ STY ◆

6 Treatment and Prevention Tips

It's just a tiny red bump at the root of an eyelash, but a sty can be mighty uncomfortable—and mighty unsightly.

A sty occurs when a gland at the root of an eyelash becomes blocked due to an infection. The gland swells and turns red, causing pain and discomfort. It may eventually come to a head as it fills with pus.

Doctors—from family physicians to ophthalmologists—agree that you can take the first steps in treating a sty at home and keeping sties from coming back. Here's how:

Use warm compresses. Wring a *clean* washcloth out in warm water—as warm as you can tolerate, but be careful not to burn the skin. Place it on the eyelid for five minutes at a time. You may have to run the cloth through warm water several times to keep it hot enough. Do this at least two or three times a day. "The heat increases the circulation of the blood," explains Barbara J. Arnold, M.D., associate clinical professor at the University of California Davis. "That allows your own white blood cells—part of the body's defense system—to clean up the problem."

Do *not* squeeze, poke, push, or pick at the sty. You risk spreading the infection. Even if the sty has come to a head, let it drain on its own.

Skip eye makeup while the sty is present. Otherwise, you risk contaminating your makeup and applicators with bacteria.

Always practice good lid hygiene. To keep sties from returning, try washing the roots of your lashes each day with diluted baby shampoo or mild soap on a cotton ball or washcloth. Monica L. Monica, M.D., Ph.D., an ophthalmologist in private practice in New Orleans, recommends using over-the-counter Cetaphil, because it won't sting or excessively dry the skin.

◆◆ Hello, Doctor? ◆◆

Any time a child has a swollen eyelid for more than 24 hours, it's time to see the doctor, stresses Monica L. Monica, M.D., Ph.D. "Problems can progress more quickly in children," she says.

And if an adult fails to see any improvement with warm compresses in two or three days, it's time to get medical attention.

Monica also stresses that if you're suffering from recurring sties or you have any sort of bump on the lid that remains for weeks or months, you need to see your doctor. You may have a chalazion instead of a sty. A chalazion is also a blocked gland—but a different one than that at the root of an eyelash. Warm compresses are the first line of treatment for a chalazion. If it doesn't clear up eventually or is unsightly, a physician can drain it. Do not try to drain it on your own, however.

Remove eye makeup. Once you start wearing makeup again, be diligent about removing it daily. "Take your eye makeup off Friday night, not Saturday morning," says Arnold. Wash the lids again in the morning before re-applying makeup.

Don't share eye makeup or applicators. You could pass infection on to others, or vice versa. ◆

◆ SUNBURN PAIN ◆

12 Ways to Soothe the Sizzle

The sun. People have worshipped it for thousands of years. But only in the last century have people worshipped the sun by baking themselves in it to a golden tan—or, as may be more often the case, to an angry red burn. But the sun can do much more damage than simply give you a painful sunburn. Dermatologists say that prolonged exposure to sunlight causes brown spots; red, scaly spots; and drying and wrinkling. Worst of all, it can cause skin cancer.

Although few things can penetrate the skin's outer layer (stratum corneum), the sun's ultraviolet rays easily pass through this layer and damage the cells and structures beneath. Ultraviolet light comes in two varieties: ultraviolet A (UVA), the so-called "tanning rays," which do not cause sunburn (except at very high doses), and ultraviolet B (UVB), the "burning rays." UVA rays can pass through window glass in cars, houses, and offices, while UVB cannot. Both types penetrate the outer layer of the skin and cause damage.

Ultraviolet rays that pass through the stratum corneum cause pigment-producing cells called melanocytes to produce brown pigment (melanin). This is the skin's effort to protect itself from the invading rays and prevent further damage to skin structures. How much and how quickly the melano-cytes can produce pigment depends largely on genetics. Dark-skinned people more readily produce melanin, while light-skinned individuals, especially those of Northern European ancestry and Orientals, don't produce it well or produce it in blotches that appear as freckles. These people can't tan no matter how hard they try and tend to be "quick fryers," readily burning even with mild sun exposure.

If your skin doesn't produce the protective melanin pigment well, or if you're overexposed to the sun before the pigment can be manufactured and dispersed, the ultraviolet rays damage the epidermal cells. "The sun's rays actually cause the skin cells to die," says James Shaw, M.D., chief of the Division of Dermatology at Good Samaritan Hospital and Medical Center and associate clinical professor of medicine at Oregon Health Sciences University, both in Portland. "Even if you develop only a mild redness, you're killing the top layer of your skin just as you would with a thermal burn from touching something hot."

Damage to skin cells is more prevalent among fair-skinned people, and the immediate effect is a sunburn. Over time, the effects can be much more serious—blotchy brown spots and even skin cancer.

Ultraviolet light can even damage the dermis, the layer of skin that gives your skin its shape, texture, strength, and elasticity. Sunlight breaks down the thick, strong tissue structure of the dermis, rendering it weak, thin, and less elastic and making it appear wrinkled and saggy.

You'd probably never expose yourself to a sunburn again if you could see the dramatic damage to your skin under a microscope—cells are shriveled and dead; formerly thick, red bundles of connective tissue have been ground into a gray smudge; thin-walled, superficial blood vessels are dilated and may be leaking fluid; and DNA sequences, the "software" that tells the skin how to repair and replicate itself, are damaged, causing the skin to produce abnormal precancerous cells and, in some cases, cancerous cells.

Many of us ignore doom-and-gloom sun-exposure warnings. After all, that bronze tan looks wonderful. If you've overexposed your skin to the sun and end up with a sunburn, the home remedies that follow can make you feel better until Mother Nature can heal the burn. Keep in mind, though, that the remedies given here cannot reverse the damage caused by the sun's rays. "Once you've been overexposed to the sun," says Shaw, "the damage to the skin is already done. But you can make yourself more comfortable while you wait for it to get better."

Apply cool compresses to the skin. Shaw advises using cool compresses to help ease the pain of a sunburn. To do this, soak a washcloth in cool water and apply it directly to burned areas. Don't use ice on the sunburned skin. Rewet the compress often and reapply it several times a day. You can also add a soothing ingredient, such as baking soda or oatmeal, to the compress water. Simply shake a bit of baking soda into the water. Or wrap dry oatmeal in a cheesecloth or a piece of gauze and run water through it. Then toss out the oatmeal, soak the compress in the oatmeal water, and apply it to the skin.

Stay out of the sun. Skin that is sunburned is much more vulnerable to additional burning. "Stay indoors and out of the sun for several days after getting burned," says Margaret Robertson, M.D., a dermatologist in private practice in Lake Oswego, Oregon. Be aware that when you're outdoors during the day, even if you're in the shade, you're being exposed to ultraviolet light. While shade from a tree or an umbrella helps, much of the sunlight your skin is exposed to comes from light reflected off surfaces such as concrete, sand, and boat decks. Ultraviolet rays can also penetrate clothing. As much as 50 percent of the sun's damaging rays can get through clothing. So if you're already sunburned, indoors is the best place for you.

In addition to staying out of the sun while you have a sunburn, Robertson says it's important to stay cool. A burn causes the skin's blood vessels to dilate and literally radiate heat from your skin. You'll be more comfortable if you drop the room temperature down and keep it cool inside. So turn on the air conditioner or switch on a fan.

Cool off with a soak. A good way to cool the burn, says Shaw, especially if the burn is widespread, is to soak in a tub of cool water. Avoid using soap, which can irritate and dry the skin. If you feel you must use soap, use a mild one, such as Dove or

---

◆◆ Hello, Doctor? ◆◆

While most sunburns can be effectively treated at home with the remedies described here, you should call the doctor if:

- *You have extensive blistering.*

- *You have a total body burn.*

- *Your blisters break and become infected.*

- *You develop chills and a fever and feel shaky.*

- *You feel unwell, as if you have the flu.*

- *The pain and itching get worse after the first 24 hours.*

Aveeno Bar, and rinse it off well. Definitely skip the washcloth and bath sponge. Afterward, pat your skin gently with a soft towel.

Robertson says she prefers cool showers to baths for treating sunburns. "If you soak too long in a tub," she explains, "you can dry out the skin and increase peeling."

Toss in some oatmeal. Frank Parker, M.D., professor and chairman of the Department of Dermatology at Oregon Health Sciences University in Portland, likes the cool-soak idea, too, but he suggests adding skin soothers such as oatmeal or baking soda to the bath. Prepare the oatmeal like you would for an oatmeal compress—wrap the dry oatmeal in a cheesecloth or piece of gauze, run the water through it as it's coming out of the faucet, then throw out the oatmeal. Another way to do this is to buy Aveeno powder, an oatmeal powder, at your local pharmacy or health-food store; follow the package directions. If you use baking soda, sprinkle it liberally into the water. Keep the soak to 15 to 20 minutes in order to avoid overdrying the skin. When you get out, let the water dry naturally on your skin so that you don't wipe off the baking soda or oatmeal.

◆◆◆ Protect Yourself ◆◆◆

For years, we've heard doctors warn us about the drying, wrinkling, burning, and cancer-causing effects of the sun. Many of us ignore those warnings because a golden-brown tan looks great. But recently, scientists have found the danger may be even worse than they thought.

Scientists know that the earth's layer of ozone, a gas that absorbs ultraviolet light and protects us from much of the damaging effects of the sun, is being destroyed at an alarming rate. Originally, scientists believed that the ozone depletion was centered only over the unpopulated South Pole. Australia, near the South Pole, already has the highest rate of deadly skin cancer (melanoma) in the world. Now, new evidence from the National Aeronautics and Space Administration (NASA) seems to suggest that a hole in the ozone layer may form over the northernmost parts of the United States, Canada, Europe, and Russia within the next decade.

The Skin Cancer Foundation says one in three cancers diagnosed this year will be skin cancer. One in six Americans will develop skin cancer in his or her lifetime. And 1 in 105 people developed melanoma, the most deadly form of skin cancer, in 1991; that's more than twice as many as diagnosed in 1980.

Fortunately, there is plenty you can do to protect your skin from the damaging effects of the sun.

Cover up. The Skin Cancer Foundation says that hats and clothing made of dark, tightly woven materials absorb ultraviolet light better than cotton fabrics in lighter shades. Dry fabrics offer more protection than wet ones.

Spread on the sunscreen. Frank Parker, M.D., says people need a sunscreen with a sun protection factor (SPF) of at least 15. "Fair-skinned people should always wear a sunscreen with an SPF of 15 to 20," he says.

If you're fair-skinned, you might want to put an extra layer of sunscreen on the night before sun exposure, says Margaret Robertson, M.D. "If you put it on the night before, it absorbs into the stratum corneum."

Spread it on thick enough, too. Applying only a thin coating of a sunscreen with an SPF of 15 can reduce the effectiveness of the product by as much as 50 percent. Apply the sunscreen 15 to 30 minutes before exposure to allow the skin to absorb it. And reapply it every two hours—more often if you're sweating or getting wet.

Protect your ears. Too often, people forget to protect sensitive spots like the tops of the ears, the hairline, the "V" of the chest, the nose, and the hands. The Skin Cancer Foundation says 80 percent of skin cancers occur on the head, neck, and hands. The Foundation therefore recommends that you wear a hat made of a tightly woven fabric such as canvas rather than one of straw and that you wear a sunscreen with an SPF of 15 on your hands. Horizontal surfaces like the nose present special sun-protection problems. Lifeguards often wear zinc oxide paste on their nose, but it only provides an SPF of about seven. Instead, apply a sunscreen with an SPF of at least 15, let it soak in a few minutes, and, for maximum protection, then apply zinc oxide paste.

Protect yourself from reflected light. Keep in mind that even umbrellas or shade trees provide only moderate protection from ultraviolet light, and they don't protect you from rays reflected from sun, snow, concrete, or other surfaces. Ultraviolet light isn't reflected by water, but it can easily penetrate water, so being in the water doesn't protect you, either. Be careful to protect surfaces such as the under part of the chin that are especially vulnerable to reflected light.

Be careful between 10:00 A.M. and 3:00 P.M. The sun's rays are most intense during this time of the day, says Parker. Stay indoors during this time, or if you must be outdoors, cover up and wear sunscreen.

Take care on cool, cloudy days. Ultraviolet light can penetrate cloud cover. Take precautions even when the sun isn't shining brightly.

Don't let the snow fool you. *During the winter months, many winter recreationists, such as snow skiers, learn the hard way that high altitudes (which have little atmosphere to filter out the sun's rays), blustery wind, and white snow can be a painful combination. Cover up with appropriate clothing and a sunscreen with an SPF of at least 15. Don't forget to wear sunglasses, too, to avoid "sunburning" your eyes.*

Don't forget your lips. *"The lips are very vulnerable to sunlight," says James Shaw, M.D. "A lot of skin cancers occur on the lips." Use a lip balm with an SPF of at least eight and reapply often.*

Avoid sunbathing. *"Most Caucasians shouldn't try to get tan," says Parker. "Everyone should minimize attempts at tanning, but for fair-skinned people, it really makes no sense. In fact, many light-skinned people won't tan no matter how hard they try."*

If you feel you must sunbathe, take it slowly and let your skin gradually build up protective melanin. And don't use tanning oils. "They're like using Crisco on your skin," says Shaw. "They enhance the ultraviolet light and can make a burn even worse."

Watch for photosensitivity. *Some drugs, such as tetracycline and diuretics, can make your skin extra sensitive to sun exposure and increase the risk of sunburn. Talk with your doctor or pharmacist about this possibility if you are taking any medications.*

Stay out of tanning booths. *In search of "safe" tanning, many people resort to tanning booths or tanning beds. While tanning companies will tell you their light machines produce only UVA radiation, the nonburning type, they are far from safe. "UVA rays penetrate the skin even deeper than UVB rays do and can damage it," explains Shaw. "In the long run, they cause skin drying and wrinkling and increase the risk of skin cancer."*

Bring on the aloe vera. The thick, gel-like juice of the aloe vera plant can take the sting and redness out of a sunburn, says Shaw, especially if it's applied immediately to a new burn. "Aloe vera causes blood vessels to constrict and can take some of the redness and soreness out of your burn," he says. Aloe vera is available at nurseries in plant form. Simply slit open one of the broad leaves and apply the gel directly to the burn. Apply five to six times per day for several days.

Take an over-the-counter pain reliever. Nonprescription pain relievers such as aspirin and ibuprofen can relieve pain and cut the inflammation of a sunburn, says Robertson. Take the medication with food as directed on the bottle. If you find that aspirin or ibuprofen upsets your stomach, try taking an enteric-coated form of aspirin. 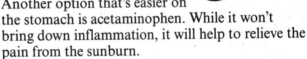 Another option that's easier on the stomach is acetaminophen. While it won't bring down inflammation, it will help to relieve the pain from the sunburn.

Drink up. You can easily become dehydrated when you've got a bad sunburn. Robertson says to drink plenty of fluids, especially water, like you would if you had a fever. "It's important to stay hydrated," she says. "Keep drinking until your urine is relatively clear. If your urine is cloudy, you may not be drinking enough."

Try a topical anesthetic. Topical anesthetics like Solarcaine may offer some temporary relief from pain and itching, says Robertson. She recommends that you look for products that contain lidocaine, which is less likely than some of the other anesthetics to cause an allergic reaction. Because some people do have allergic reactions to such products, she advises testing a small area of skin before using it all over.

Topical anesthetics come in both creams and sprays. The sprays are easier to apply to a sunburn. If you use one, avoid spraying it directly onto the face. Instead, spray some onto gauze and gently dab it on your face.

Get relief with hydrocortisone. Over-the-counter hydrocortisone creams or sprays can bring temporary relief from sunburn pain and itching, says Parker. Look for those containing 0.5 percent or 1 percent hydrocortisone.

Moisturize. The sun dries out the skin's surface moisture and causes cells and blood vessels to leak, drying the skin out even further. In addition, while cool baths and compresses can make you feel better, they can also dry your injured skin. To prevent drying, apply moisturizer immediately after your soak, says Shaw. For even cooler relief, chill the moisturizer in the refrigerator before using.

Watch the blisters. If a sunburn is bad enough, the skin blisters. Robertson warns, "A bad sunburn with extensive blistering can be life-threatening." If you have extensive blistering, see your doctor immediately.

If you have just a few blisters, watch that they don't become infected. Don't pop them and don't remove their protective skin covering, says Robertson.

Take a tincture of time. Ultimately, the one thing that will heal your sunburn is time, says Robertson. No product can speed the process. Even when your sunburn is healed, be careful in the sun, because it'll take several months for your damaged skin to return to normal. If you overdo it in the sun while your skin is still healing, your skin will burn faster and be more damaged than before. ◆

◆ SWIMMER'S EAR ◆

5 Ways to Sidestep It

The water, the sun, plenty of swimming and splashing around—to many people, these are the ingredients for a perfect summer day spent by the pool or at the beach. Add a painful ear infection to the picture, and the scenario quickly slides downhill. That's what can happen to you if swimmer's ear strikes, unless you know how to prevent the problem.

Swimmer's ear, an infection of the outer ear canal, sometimes can be caused by a fungus, but common bacteria is usually the culprit. "It got the name swimmer's ear because it's quite prone to happen in the summer, when people are in the water a lot and they have water lying in the ear for a long period of time," says Donald B. Kamerer, M.D., F.A.C.S., a professor in the Department of Otolaryngology at the University of Pittsburgh School of Medicine and staff physician at the Pittsburgh Eye and Ear Hospital. Those are just the right conditions for the development of swimmer's ear, because bacteria thrive in a warm, damp, moist environment. Also, exposure to large amounts of water tends to wash away the oily, waxy substance that normally lines and protects the ear canal. "Then the antibacterial protection is lost, bacteria begins to enter, and it can get out of hand," says Jay E. Caldwell, M.D., director of the Alaska Sports Medicine Clinic in Anchorage.

External ear infections don't just occur in swimmers or in the summertime. "We see them all year round," says Kamerer. Getting water in the ear from showers may cause them, but sometimes you don't need to be around water at all. "People who play inside their ear canals with bobby pins or all sorts of implements sometimes get infections started by scratching the very delicate skin in the ear canal," says Kamerer. Many people also use cotton swabs to clean their ears daily, which can actually hinder their efforts to keep their ears healthy. "The ear has a way of keeping itself clean," says Caldwell. "Q-tips or bobby pins or

> ## ◆◆ Hello, Doctor? ◆◆
>
> *Mild cases of swimmer's ear may improve if you keep your ears dry and use antiseptic eardrops for a few days. But Alexander Schleuning, M.D., suggests that if you have persistent pain in your ear that lasts more than an hour or if there's discharge from the ear, you should see a physician. The Academy of Otolaryngology-Head & Neck Surgery cautions that if you have ever had a perforated, punctured, ruptured, or otherwise injured eardrum or have had ear surgery, you should consult an ear doctor before you go swimming and before you use any type of eardrops.*

whatever you put in there just scrapes the surface and breaks down the fairly resilient barrier against bacteria."

Swimmer's ear usually starts with an itching or tingling in the ear. Resist the urge to scratch, though, which will only make the problem worse. After that, you may experience mild to severe pain. With more serious cases, discharge drains from the ear, and you may have some hearing loss from swelling of the ear canal. You should see your doctor right away if this occurs (see "Hello, Doctor?"). One way to help you determine if the infection is in the outer ear is to gently pull on your ear, wiggle it, and move it back and forth. If that hurts, it's likely to be an outer-ear infection such as swimmer's ear.

So that you won't have to suffer through this, here's what you can do to prevent swimmer's ear:

Watch where you swim. Avoid jumping into pools, ponds, lakes, oceans, or any other body of water in which the water may not be clean. Dirty water means more bacteria.

Get the water out. A key to preventing swimmer's ear is to not let water sit in the ear. You can usually feel water swish around in your ear if there's still some in there after a shower or swim. "Shake the water out of your ear if you've been swimming or diving," says Alexander Schleuning, M.D., professor and chairman of the Department of Otolaryngology/Head and Neck Surgery at Oregon Health Sciences University in Portland.

Add a few drops. Over-the-counter antiseptic eardrops, such as Aqua Ear, Ear Magic, or Swim Ear, used after swimming may help to prevent or ease the problem for those who swim a lot and are already familiar with the symptoms of swimmer's ear. According to the Academy of Otolaryngology–Head & Neck Surgery, you can also whip up an antiseptic mixture of your own using equal amounts of

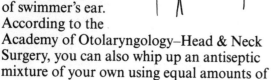

rubbing alcohol and white vinegar, as long as you have normal eardrums and your doctor says it's safe (see "Hello, Doctor?"). White vinegar kills bacteria and fungus. The alcohol absorbs water and may kill bacteria and fungus as well. You can buy a dropper bottle at a pharmacy. Along the same lines, Kamerer recommends that people who swim a lot put a couple of drops of rubbing alcohol in their ears following swimming or drop in a mixture of half white vinegar, half water.

Pull on a bathing cap. While this may not afford much protection for a competitive swimmer who's constantly in the water, says Caldwell, it may keep water out for the casual swimmer. "If it's a tight bathing cap that fits over the ears, across the forehead, and around the back of the neck, it may help," says Kamerer.

Don't poke around in your ears. "I always tell my patients not to put anything in their ear smaller than their elbow," says Caldwell. You can exacerbate a mild case of swimmer's ear or get an infection started by poking, swabbing, or scratching inside your ears. Wax produced in the ear puts up a barrier that is antibacterial and protects against moisture. "If you undo nature's system, you set yourself up for trouble," says Kamerer. ◆

◆ TARTAR AND PLAQUE ◆

16 Tips to Control Them

Advertising claims have added the terms "tartar" and "plaque" to the vocabulary of the average American, as products promise to rid our mouths of these pesky substances. How true are these claims? And what roles do tartar and plaque play in our oral health?

For starters, let's define the two players. Plaque, which is actually by far the most villainous, is a soft, sticky, nearly invisible deposit that accumulates on teeth and dental restorations (fillings, crowns, and dentures, for example) and on the gums and the tongue. "It's an organized mass of oral bacteria," explains Erwin Barrington, D.D.S., professor of periodontics at the University of Illinois in Chicago. Some of those bacteria cause tooth decay, and some are responsible for periodontal, or gum, disease.

Plaque is always with us. A newborn's mouth is sterile, but only for the first ten hours or so of life, according to Sebastian G. Ciancio, D.D.S., professor and chairman of the Department of Periodontology, clinical professor of pharmacology, and director of the Center for Clinical Dental Studies at the School of Dental Medicine at the State University of New York at Buffalo.

Tartar is a calcified material that often contains bacterial debris and sometimes plaque. It's a white, chalky substance. Although tartar (also called calculus) can make it easier for plaque to stick around, the stuff is generally considered to be primarily a cosmetic problem.

Plaque is the culprit in cavities and gum disease. "As plaque matures and gets older, it becomes even more dangerous because it changes," says Michael G. Newman, D.D.S., adjunct professor of periodontology at the University of California at Los Angeles School of Dentistry and president of the American Academy of Periodontology. As certain bacteria in plaque feed off fermentable carbohydrates (which include sugars, even those in fruit and milk, and starchy foods such as breads, pastas, and crackers), they produce an acid that eats away at tooth enamel, causing cavities. Other bacteria infect the gums, resulting in redness, inflammation, and bleeding. These are symptoms of gingivitis, the earliest stage of gum disease (see GINGIVITIS). If left untreated, gum disease may progress to the point that the infection literally destroys the bone that anchors the teeth roots. That's why gum disease is the major cause of tooth loss among adults over age 35.

Both plaque and tartar can form above and below the gum line. It takes a dentist or hygienist to remove tartar from anywhere in the mouth and to remove plaque from below the gum line. And regular professional cleanings—as often as your dentist recommends—will help make your home care more effective, points out Christine Dumas, D.D.S., a Los Angeles dentist who is a consumer advisor/spokesperson for the American Dental Association (ADA) and an assistant professor of clinical dentistry at the University of Southern California. It's also important to have the condition of your gums checked through a periodontal probing. "It should be as routine as getting your blood pressure checked," she says.

You can, however, try to keep plaque under control. "It takes physical contact," says Barrington. "You can't rinse it away."

Here's what you can do.

Brush. "It's not how often but how well you brush," says Barrington. "You can brush ten times a day, but if you do a sloppy job, you're getting no benefits."

The ADA recommends the following method:

1. Hold the brush at a 45-degree angle against the gum line. "Most of us, when we brush in the morning, are worried about getting the cornflakes out from between our teeth," explains Dumas. "But we completely miss the gum line." Point the brush upward, or toward your nose, when you're cleaning the upper teeth; downward, or toward your chin, when you're doing the lower teeth.

◆◆◆ The FDA and ◆◆◆ Plaque Fighters

The Food and Drug Administration (FDA) has stepped into the plaque-fighting arena. In the last few years, some 40 products, ranging from toothpastes to rinses, have claimed to reduce plaque and even treat gingivitis, the early stage of gum disease.

That has led to questions from the FDA, which convened a review panel in early 1992 to examine the safety and effectiveness of these products. An FDA spokesperson said there are no safety concerns in particular, but "there's not really a lot known about the safety and effectiveness of these products." The review should be completed in 1994 or 1995.

One reason for concern: Gingivitis, the early stage of gum disease, is not a condition that can be diagnosed by the consumer. And the use of some antibacterial products may disguise some of the obvious symptoms of gingivitis at the gum line while the disease continues to progress, says Michael G. Newman, D.D.S.

That can also result from the use of baking soda and peroxide, a mixture popularized in the early '80s as the Keyes Technique, which made dental headlines with the promise of no more periodontal surgery. Studies failed to back up those claims, but consumers still cling to the hope that they can treat their periodontal disease at home. By trying to do so, they may end up with worse problems.

"I've seen several cases where people stripped the surface of their gum tissue raw," says Newman. "They think a little's good so a lot's better."

2. Use a short (about the width of half a tooth) back-and-forth motion to clean the outer surfaces of your teeth. Focus on just one or two teeth at a time. And be gentle; you're not scrubbing the floor or the bathtub. "People try to use too much force, and that can injure the gums," says Marilyn C. Miller, D.D.S., F.A.G.D., codirector of the Princeton Dental Resource Center in New Jersey.

3. Use this same stroke on the inside surfaces of all the teeth, except the front ones. Remember to keep the brush angled (at 45 degrees) toward the gum line.

4. Scrub the chewing surfaces of your back teeth with the brush held flat in the same back-and-forth motion.

5. Tilt the brush vertically, and use the front part of the brush in short up-and-down strokes to clean the inside surfaces of the front teeth. "People tend to ignore the back sides of their front teeth," says Miller.

6. Don't forget to brush your tongue. It can harbor disease-causing plaque, too.

Use the right tools. The ADA recommends a soft nylon brush with end-rounded, polished bristles. Hard bristles can wear away the enamel that protects your teeth and can form grooves in the teeth. Using such bristles, which Dumas calls "the Brillo pad philosophy of cleaning," can damage tender gums, too, causing them to recede, or pull away, from teeth. Get a brush that's small enough to reach all of your teeth, especially those in the back. Some adults may actually prefer using a child-sized brush. Don't be stingy with toothbrushes, either—replace your brush every three months, or sooner, if the bristles become frayed, splayed, or worn.

Don't worry about going hi-tech. You can wield your old-fashioned manual toothbrush as effectively as any electric product. But if your manual dexterity's not up to par, or you're just plain lazy, one of the new electric brushes on the market may be for you. "They can be a great motivator," says Dumas.

Use a fluoridated toothpaste. Choose a product with the ADA's seal of acceptance. What's so wonderful about fluoride? It combines with the minerals in saliva to "remineralize," or strengthen, the teeth, preventing cavities in both children and adults. You may think you don't get cavities anymore, but as you get older, your gums recede, exposing the roots of teeth, which lack the protective coating of enamel and are prone to a type of decay known as root caries.

Try a tartar-control toothpaste. If you're one of the people who tend to develop a lot of tartar, using such a product can help. "It doesn't stop tartar from forming, but it slows down the formation rate," points out Barrington. Chemicals such as pyrophosphate in the toothpaste interfere with the deposits of calcium salt. Ciancio says studies show up to a 30 to 40 percent reduction in the amount of tartar deposits.

Floss. Too many people think of flossing simply as a way to get the roast beef or popcorn kernels out that are stuck between the teeth. "But it's really the best way to clean between the teeth and to clean under the gums," explains Miller.

Here's how to floss correctly:

1. Start with 18 to 24 inches of floss, and wind most of it around the middle or index finger on

◆◆◆ The Foods You Eat ◆◆◆

"Grazing" all day long can be cruel to your teeth. Every time you eat, you also feed the plaque in your mouth. Those bacteria like to feast on far more than the simple sugars we once learned cause cavities. They like all "fermentable carbohydrates"—that includes starches such as bread, crackers, and pasta. Natural sugars, such as honey and molasses, are tasty to the bacteria, too, as are the sugars found in fruits and even milk.

You can't stop eating these foods, but you can try to adopt some habits that are kinder and gentler to your teeth. Here's how, according to Carole Palmer, Ed.D., R.D., cochair of the Division of Nutrition and Preventive Dentistry at Tufts University School of Dental Medicine in Boston:

Limit how often you eat sugar-containing foods. *"Have your cake with your meal if you brush afterward," Palmer suggests. Don't suck on hard candies all day long. "It's really not the amount of sugar you eat but the patterns of usage."*

Don't sip. *"If you drink sweet drinks like soda or sugar-sweetened tea or coffee, drink it pronto— don't dillydally," she says. Using a straw may help limit the exposure to teeth.*

Chew sugarless gum. *The gum stimulates the flow of saliva, which helps cleanse the mouth and protect the teeth.*

Choose tooth-healthy snacks. *Munch on raw vegetables, crunchy fruits like apples (which, though they contain natural sugars, are low on the danger-to-teeth list), plain peanuts, and cheeses. The French have the right idea, apparently, with ending a meal by eating cheese (although some varieties are high in fat and sodium). Drink plain club soda or unsweetened or artificially sweetened tea, coffee, or soda instead of sugar-containing drinks.*

one hand (whichever finger is the most comfortable for you).

2. Wrap the rest of the floss around the same finger on the other hand. Think of this other finger as the take-up spool for the used floss. Don't scrimp. "Floss is cheap," says Miller. "And if you don't use enough, you're just re-introducing the bacteria to another spot when you don't use a clean section of floss for each tooth."

3. Hold the floss tightly with your thumbs and forefingers, leaving about an inch of floss between them. The floss should be taut.

4. Use a gentle "sawing" kind of motion as you pull the floss between the teeth. Be careful not to snap it into the tender gum tissue.

5. When you've reached the gum line, curve the floss into a "C" shape to fit snugly around the tooth, and slide it into the space between the gum and tooth gently.

6. Bring the floss out from the gum and scrape the side of the tooth. "Remember, you're following the shape of the tooth to remove the plaque from that side," says Virginia L. Woodward, R.D.H., past president of the American Dental Hygienists' Association. After you pull it out, use a clean section of floss to clean the tooth on the other side of that space.

7. Be sure to clean the back side of the last tooth on each side.

Relax about wax. Don't worry about choosing between waxed or unwaxed floss. Pick what's comfortable. Flavored flosses are fine, too, especially if you find yourself using them more frequently. If your fingers are too awkward, you suffer from arthritis, or you have a lot of bridgework, you may find floss threaders or floss holders helpful; they're available at drugstores. Ask your dentist or hygienist if you have questions about how to use these devices properly.

Know that there's no substitute for flossing. Flossing is your best bet. "Nothing can substitute for floss," says Woodward. "There's nothing available that can clean between the teeth as well."

But if you absolutely, positively refuse to floss, ask your dentist or hygienist about alternatives. Barrington recommends soft wooden interproximal cleaners, like Stim-u-Dents. Interproximal brushes, which look like tiny bottle brushes, work, too, but won't always fit in tight spaces between teeth. Oral irrigators "can be a terrific adjunct," says Newman, but again, are no substitute for flossing.

Dumas warns against using Stim-u-Dents, the rubber tips on some brushes, or oral irrigators until after you've brushed and flossed, because of the danger of pushing debris or plaque deeper into a pocket. "This is why it's important to know the state of your periodontal health," she stresses.

Establish a routine. For both brushing and flossing, start at the same spot in your mouth each time and work your way around. By getting into this habit, you may be less likely to miss cleaning any tooth surfaces.

Test yourself. Disclosing tablets or solution, available at drugstores, can reveal the plaque that's left after you've cleaned your mouth. "You may be aghast at what you see," warns Woodward. Don't get discouraged: "There's no way you can remove 100 percent of the plaque," says Barrington. But such tablets can show where you're not cleaning as thoroughly.

Wet your whistle. Saliva naturally cleanses the mouth and helps fight bacteria, says Irwin D. Mandel, D.D.S., professor emeritus of dentistry at Columbia University School of Dental and Oral Medicine in New York. But dry mouth is a side effect of some 300 to 400 different medications, including antidepressants, antihistamines, and drugs used to treat high blood pressure and Parkinson's disease. A disease called Sjogren's syndrome, which can accompany some rheumatoid conditions, also slows down the flow of saliva (and causes dry eyes, too). If you've had radiation therapy to the head and neck for cancer, your saliva glands may have been damaged.

You can fight dry mouth with sugarless gum or candy or with artificial saliva, available over the counter, suggests Mandel. Take frequent sips of water. Rinse with a mixture of one teaspoon of glycerine in a glass of water. Coat the lips, mouth, and tongue with mineral oil (then spit it out), especially at night when dry mouth tends to worsen.

Don't rely on "miracle" rinses. You can't rinse plaque and tartar away. The commercials on television look so appealing: A swig of this product, a few swishes in the mouth, and, like magic almost, all that nasty plaque is gone. If it were only that simple.

Only two products have the acceptance of the ADA's Council on Dental Therapeutics for reducing plaque: Peridex, available by prescription only, contains 0.12 percent chlorhexidine, a powerful germ-fighter, and over-the-counter Listerine, which relies on a combination of oils like menthol, eucalyptol, and thymol, along with alcohol. "These products are not substitutes for brushing and flossing," warns Barrington.

As for Plax, a prebrushing rinse, several studies have disputed its claims. And in 1989, the National Advertising Division of the Council of Better Business Bureaus asked the company to discontinue its ads citing it was 300 percent more effective in removing plaque than brushing alone.

Newman looks at it another way. "Do you really want to use more chemicals in your body than you need to?" he asks, when thorough brushing and flossing can keep plaque and tartar under control for most people. ◆

◆◆ Hello, Doctor? ◆◆

Careful dental hygiene at home, along with regular professional cleanings and checkups, can help control tartar and plaque and prevent gum disease. In addition, you should keep an eye on the state of your mouth so that any problem that may develop can be taken care of promptly. The American Dental Association recommends calling your dentist if:

• *You have persistent bad breath.*

• *There is pus between the teeth and gums.*

• *Your "bite," the way your teeth fit together, has changed.*

• *You have loose or separating teeth.*

• *Your gums consistently bleed.*

• *The gums at the gumline appear rolled instead of flat.*

• *Your partial dentures fit differently than they used to.*

◆ TEETHING ◆

9 Tips to Ease Baby's Discomfort

Drooling. Gum inflammation. Irritation. Fussiness. Any parent who has cared for a baby knows well the symptoms of teething, the process of the first (primary) 12 teeth erupting through the surface of the gums. The teeth, which form before the baby is born, usually begin surfacing around six or seven months of age with a single lower central incisor. Most children have all of their primary teeth by age three. But, like many things in nature, teeth don't come in on a set schedule. "Parents often have the wrong idea about when their baby's teeth should come in," says Ken Waddell, D.M.D., who sees many children in his private practice in Tigard, Oregon. "The first tooth usually comes in at 6 or 7 months, but it's also normal to come in at 2 months or 12 months of age."

Although there can be a wide range of timing among children, generally, the central incisors, the teeth right in the middle of the jaw on the top and bottom, come in at 6 to 12 months; lateral incisors at 9 to 13 months; canine (cuspids) at 16 to 22 months; the first molars at 13 to 19 months; and the second molars at 25 to 33 months of age.

The process of teething, or "cutting" all of these baby teeth, can be painful for both the baby and the parents. When a tooth pushes through the sensitive gum mucosa, it hurts, and the baby is likely to become cranky and fussy. But each baby is individual, emphasizes Susan Woodruff, B.S.N., childbirth and parenting education coordinator at Tuality Community Hospital in Hillsboro, Oregon. "Every baby responds differently to the process of teething," she says.

Some babies seem to sail through cutting new teeth without so much as a whimper, while others are enraged and restless the entire time. How long teething lasts varies widely, too. Jack W. Clinton, D.M.D., associate dean of Patient Services at the Oregon Health Sciences University School of Dentistry in Portland, says, "Some babies can pop a new tooth through in a matter of a few hours. For others, it may take as long as a couple of days."

Teething symptoms often include crankiness, drooling, chewing, crying, gum redness, decreased appetite, and difficulty sleeping. In addition, some babies spit up and have mild diarrhea due to gastrointestinal reactions to changes in the character and amount of their own saliva. Other babies develop a red and slightly swollen rash on the cheeks, chin, neck, and chest from the saliva's contact with the skin. Sometimes, teething causes babies to develop a mild fever, congestion, and ear pulling that often mimics middle-ear infection. Relax. All of these symptoms are normal.

With the helpful hints that follow, you can make your baby more comfortable during teething:

Massage those gums. "Pressure often helps relieve the pain," says Clinton. He suggests gently rubbing baby's gums with a clean finger.

Cool it. Woodruff says giving the baby something cold to chew on helps soothe inflamed gums and distracts the child. She recommends a cold washcloth, chilled pacifiers, a frozen banana, or cold carrot. "Anything cold that is safe is great," says Woodruff. "Babies especially enjoy things like bananas that taste good."

Clinton suggests giving the baby an ice cube wrapped in a clean washcloth to suck on. You'll have to hold the washcloth for a very young child. Don't let the child chew directly on ice, because this can harm the gums. And, of course, keep an eye on the child at all times to make sure that he or she doesn't choke.

Baby-bottle it. One of the tricks Woodruff teaches her new mothers is to fill a baby bottle with water or juice, tip it upside down so the liquid flows into the nipple, and freeze it. The baby then can happily chew on the bottle's frozen nipple.

Let 'em chew. "Anything the baby can chew on will help the tooth work through the gum," says Waddell. "Be imaginative and find things the baby will like." He suggests apple wedges, or for younger babies, apple wedges placed in a washcloth that the parent holds. Woodruff likes to let teething babies chew, too. She says commercial teething biscuits are good (though they can be messy), and slightly stale bagels make excellent baby chewies.

Distract them. Ronald Wismer, D.M.D., a general dentist in Beaverton, Oregon, says distracting teething babies may be the best solution. Try playing with them with a favorite toy or rocking or swinging them. Sometimes, a rousing game of peekaboo is all that's needed to distract baby from the discomfort.

Try pain relievers. Over-the-counter pain relievers like Children's Liquid Tylenol (not aspirin) can offer relief for up to four hours, says Woodruff. However, since you can't give children pain relievers around the clock, choose a time like bedtime when pain relief is most needed. Don't give more often than three times in 24 hours.

Numb those gums. Commercial oral anesthetic teething gels (for example, Orajel and Anbesol) give temporary relief (30 to 40 minutes worth) and can often get baby over a difficult time, Wismer says.

◆◆ Hello, Doctor? ◆◆

Sometimes, teething symptoms can mimic other, more serious health problems. Call the doctor if the baby develops:

• *A very severe rash that covers the back, arms, and legs. This may indicate a bacterial or viral infection.*

• *A sustained fever or pus in the eyes. The baby may have a respiratory infection.*

• *Fever, fussiness, vomiting/diarrhea, and pulling on or gesturing to the ear. The baby may have an ear infection.*

Try teething tablets. Pharmacies carry so-called herbal "teething tablets" that dissolve almost instantly in the mouth, are safe for the baby, and provide temporary relief, says Woodruff.

Keep a towel handy. Teething often causes plenty of drooling, and the saliva can cause skin irritation. Wismer advises carrying a soft towel to clean up baby often. If that isn't enough, protect the skin with petroleum jelly or zinc-oxide ointment. ◆

◆ TEMPOROMANDIBULAR ◆ JOINT SYNDROME (TMJ)

6 Strategies to Ease TMJ Discomfort

Is It TMJ Disorder?

The American Dental Association says that if you answer yes to any of the following questions, you may have a TMJ disorder and should seek help from a TMJ specialist:

- *Do you have frequent headaches, especially in the morning?*

- *Do you clench or grind your teeth?*

- *Have you noticed any teeth, especially the eye teeth, wearing down?*

- *Do your jaw muscles feel tender?*

- *Does your jaw make popping or clicking sounds when you open your mouth?*

- *Do you have difficulty opening your mouth?*

- *Do you have facial pain? Neck pain? Teeth pain? Shoulder pain?*

- *Is it painful to chew, yawn, or open your mouth widely?*

- *Does your jaw ever get stuck open or closed?*

- *Do you have pain in or around the ear?*

- *Do your ears feel stuffy or itchy?*

- *Do you suffer from earaches without ear infections?*

- *Do you have ringing, roaring, hissing, or buzzing in the ears?*

- *Do you often feel dizzy?*

If you experience headaches, bothersome clicking and popping in the jaw, or pain in the face, neck, or shoulders, the problem may literally be all in your head. You may suffer from a misalignment of the temporomandibular joint (TMJ), the joint that allows your mouth to open, close, and move sideways. The American Dental Association estimates that as many as ten million Americans may have TMJ syndrome or TMJ dysfunction. Unfortunately, it's a condition that often goes undiagnosed or misdiagnosed and untreated.

Five pairs of muscles and the temporomandibular joint that connects the upper and lower jaws allow you to open and close your mouth and control the forward, backward, and side-to-side movements of the lower jaw. Any problem that prevents this complex system of muscles, ligaments, bones, and joints from working together may result in the pain and other problems known as TMJ syndrome.

The jaw joint can become misaligned from a variety of causes—teeth that don't fit together properly due to genetics, orthodontia, or tooth grinding (bruxism); habits like cradling the phone between the ear and shoulder; or injuries like whiplash or a blow to the jaw. Stress plays a major role, too, and people often experience their first TMJ discomfort during stressful times.

According to Ronald Wismer, D.M.D., former president of the Washington County Dental Association in Oregon, nearly half the patients in his Beaverton, Oregon, practice have misaligned jaw joints, but only half of those experience any symptoms. In some cases, he says, conservative home care can alleviate the pain and discomfort. In others, professional help is important.

The following are some tips for coping with your TMJ disorder. If the conservative treatments described here don't give you relief, seek help from a dentist, preferably one who is a TMJ specialist.

Massage those jaws. Ken Waddell, D.M.D., a TMJ specialist in Tigard, Oregon, recommends conservative treatment first. "Muscle spasms cause pain," he says. "To relax the muscles, try massaging the jaw joint just in front of the ears."

Heat it up. Heat is an excellent muscle relaxant, says Wismer. Use a hot pad or hot-water bottle to ease aching jaw, neck, and shoulder muscles. Keep the heat low enough not to cause burns.

Cool it down. Ice packs are also excellent for relieving pain, says Waddell.

Take over-the-counter pain relievers. Wismer says that over-the-counter products like aspirin, acetaminophen, and ibuprofen can relieve pain in the muscles. Aspirin and ibuprofen can also help bring down inflammation.

Teach an old dog new tricks. Become aware of and eliminate habits—such as resting your head on your hand, cradling the phone between your shoulder and cheek, or clenching your teeth—that tend to stress the jaw joint.

Relax. "Stress is a major player in TMJ problems," says Waddell. Gregg R. Morris, D.C., a chiropractor in private practice in Beaverton, Oregon, who has worked with TMJ patients for more than ten years, agrees, "Stress can create a cycle of muscle tension and pain that needs to be broken." Both Waddell and Morris recommend relaxation techniques, such as progressive relaxation, in which you consciously relax muscles starting with the head and working down the body to the feet.

You might also try visualization exercises to let go of stress. Find a quiet, comfortable place where you won't be disturbed. Close your eyes and take a couple of deep breaths. Now, imagine yourself in one of your favorite places—a beach, a mountain meadow, a country lane. Let yourself feel the sights and sounds. Feel yourself relaxing in this special place. You have nothing you have to do, nowhere you have to go. After several minutes of enjoying this visualization, take a couple of deep breaths

---

◆ Find a TMJ Pro ◆

Your TMJ symptoms may require professional help. A TMJ dental specialist may need to create a special mouthpiece, or "splint," to help the muscles relax. The jaw may need to be permanently realigned through subtle tooth grinding (equilibration), moving teeth (orthodontics), or moving bony structures (orthopedics). In a few cases, surgery may be required.

Successful treatment may also require the services of an orthopedist; a neurologist; an ear, nose, and throat specialist; and a physical therapist or chiropractor. Stress reduction may require the help of a mental-health professional. Look for professionals with whom you feel comfortable and who will take the time to explain things to you. TMJ specialist Ken Waddell, D.M.D., advises, "Look for someone who is honest and who doesn't promise you the moon." Ask these questions:

• What is your experience in treating TMJ disorder?

• What special training have you received in treating TMJ?

• How many TMJ patients have you treated? What is your success rate?

• How long does treatment usually last? How much does it cost?

• How do you feel about a team treatment approach? What specialists do you typically use?

---

and slowly open your eyes. You may find that you feel amazingly relaxed and refreshed from this "mental vacation."

If neither of these works for you, find something that does help you relax when you feel tense. ◆

◆ TENDINITIS ◆
17 Ways to Take Care of Your Tendons

Sometimes, it's hard to tell what hurts more: The constant throbbing of the tendinitis itself or the fact that you can't do all the activities you were doing before you got sidelined by the pain. The tendons are sinewy connective tissue fibers that attach muscle to bone. Tendinitis, or inflammation of these tissues, is the price you pay for doing too much of what you thought was a good thing or working at too quick a pace—on a keyboard or at the track—without the proper training or warm-up.

As you're swearing that you'll take the right steps next time, here are tips to help you get through today's pain and get back in the game.

Ice the area. When a tendon flares up, cold can reduce the inflammation. Fill a bag with ice or try a reusable cold pack, a bag of frozen peas, or a sealed bag of frozen unpopped popcorn. "Place a wet towel between you and the ice to help prevent hives or an ice burn," says Joan Couch, M.S.A.T.C., assistant professor and athletic trainer at the University of Delaware in Newark.

"Apply the ice for five to ten minutes, three or four times a day until the symptoms subside," says Lawrence Magee, M.D., coordinator of the Sports Medicine Clinic at the University of Kansas in Lawrence.

Cup the pain. For a longer-lasting application of ice, try a cup instead. Fill paper cups with cold water and freeze them. When needed, "tear the lip and the top portion of the cup off to get to the ice," recommends Couch. Place a wet towel on the affected area, and rub the ice over that.

Get help from aspirin. Aspirin and ibuprofen are two over-the-counter anti-inflammatory medications that can help alleviate pain and stiffness. Acetaminophen can help reduce pain, but it does not reduce inflammation. Keep in mind, too, that these drugs "will not speed the healing process," says Magee.

Elevate the area. This will help control the swelling.

Tape the tendinitis. A fabric bandage wrapped around the knee or ankle may help support the joint and keep swelling to a minimum. However, the bandage will be of no use if it is not wrapped properly and securely (but never too tightly). Read package instructions or consult a health-care practitioner.

Splint it. Some experts recommend a splint instead of tape because it's stiffer and will keep the affected area in a certain position, says Sandra H. Phipps, P.T., a physical therapist at Slippery Rock University in Pennsylvania.

Consider cross-training. Since tendinitis is often brought on by constant and repetitive activities, you may want to alternate your favorite exercise with other ones. This way, one set of muscles won't be overworked and, as a result, be prone to tendinitis. For instance, swimming doesn't pound the legs like running can. Cross-training also "creates a balance of all muscle groups, making you more fit all over," says Phipps.

Build up your body. Before undertaking an exercise routine, such as running or swimming, condition the muscles you'll be depending on. Weight training is the best way to firm up specific muscle groups. Do arm or leg curls, for instance, with free weights or on a weight-training machine.

Warm up before you warm up. For the physically active, stretching is synonymous with warming up. But there's more to it than a few tugs and pulls. Before doing any stretches, you should do some form of mild, body-warming aerobic exercise for a few minutes, since stretching cold muscles can lead to tendinitis. A few pre-warm-up warm-ups: Running in place, jumping rope, stationary bicycling, walking.

Don't stretch to the point of pain. "Some people don't realize that you shouldn't stretch until you feel pain, but only to feel a slight pull," says Couch. This should be done gently and slowly, with no bouncing or jerky movements.

Take it slow. If you're starting a new exercise activity or getting back into an old one after a bout of tendinitis, start off with an abbreviated, not-too-taxing routine. Run a few miles, not ten; bicycle flat terrain, not a hilly course. Before setting out, do some range-of-motion exercises.

Wear the right shoes. Athletic footwear is specially designed for virtually every type of activity, so you shouldn't expect a tennis shoe to be good to you when you're running. When buying a new pair of shoes for a sport with lots of pounding or jumping, look for the kind with air chambers in them, recommends Phipps. These will have the extra cushioning you need to absorb some of the shock that would otherwise travel up your leg and into your ankles and knees. How you wear your shoe can make a difference, too (see "Check Your Shoes' Warning Signs").

Vary your terrain. Runners often use the same route on the same surface day after day. This repetitive routine can lead to tendinitis, says Phipps. Instead, try new routes on different types of surfaces, whether asphalt, grass, or clay. You should also change the direction of the route, says Phipps. This is because the camber, curves, dips, and bumps of a surface can cause your feet to do the same moves over and over. Instead, run a trail on the opposite side or begin at the opposite end. (On roads, however, always run with the traffic.) No matter what the surface, "it should never be too hard or too soft," says Magee.

Bag the sand. Sand is not a good surface for a workout, says Magee. Sand, as well as snow, can

Check Your Shoes' Warning Signs

Wearing the right shoe when working out is important, but so is wearing the correct shoe correctly, says Sandra H. Phipps, P.T. Once laced up, your foot should be able to wiggle a bit but not slip around. If your shoe is too loose, your body must work harder to keep your foot in the proper position. And if your shoe is too tight, you won't be giving your feet and legs the natural maneuverability they need to perform properly. In addition, look at the sole below the heel. Has the sole worn unevenly?

Besides needing a new pair of shoes, you may also need orthotics, says Lawrence Magee, M.D. These specially made shoe inserts help correct structural discrepancies, such as pronation (your feet tend to go inward) or supination (your feet rotate outward). By setting the foot right, your whole body will work right when you're active, and it's less likely tendinitis will stop you.

cause your legs to twist and slip, leading to strains, sprains, and tendinitis.

Cool down. Gently stretch after a workout, and if you're prone to tendinitis, ice the area to help prevent a flare-up, says Magee.

Use caution with cleats. A tendon is more likely to take the full force of a hit when you're wearing this type of shoe, which anchors the foot.

Wear knee pads. These protect your knees by cushioning the blow from direct hits in such sports as volleyball, baseball, softball, and football. ◆

◆ THUMB SUCKING ◆

10 Ways to Help Your Child Kick the Habit

It was cute when she was a baby, but now that your daughter has reached kindergarten age, you're starting to worry about her having her thumb in her mouth all the time. You feel embarrassed when you're out in public with her and are concerned about what her peers will say in school.

You're not alone: Pediatricians estimate that about 18 percent of children between the ages of two and six suck their thumbs. Why do they start? "The infant's repertoire is very limited," says Patrick C. Friman, Ph.D., a clinical psychologist at Father Flanagan's Boys Home in Boys Town, Nebraska; an associate professor of pediatrics at the University of Nebraska Medical School; and an associate professor of human communication and otolaryngology at Creighton University Medical School in Omaha. "Their most highly developed behavior is sucking." Thumb sucking is one of the few self-comforting methods available to a young child.

Most experts recommend that parents not try to stop a child's thumb sucking until the child demonstrates that he or she is ready to stop. If your child has reached that point, read on.

Let the child decide it's a problem. If there's one message that pediatricians have about thumb sucking, it's this: The best way to get a child to continue thumb sucking is to tell him or her to stop. "The time to take action is when the child comes home saying that they've been teased about their thumb sucking and they don't know how to stop," says Daniel P. Kohen, M.D., director of the Behavioral Pediatrics Education Program at Minneapolis Children's Medical Center. In other words, if the child is not motivated, you're unlikely to be able to help him or her kick the habit.

Use a reward system. Kohen endorses a game-playing, reward-based system for helping kids stop thumb sucking. He suggests buying a calendar and placing it on the refrigerator. For each day you don't see the child sucking his or her thumb, you can put a smiley-face sticker on the day. At the end of a set period of time, say a month, you can offer a modest reward, such as a toy or dinner at the child's favorite restaurant.

Don't force the child to quit outright. "When a child sees me about thumb sucking in my clinic, I never bring the subject up," says Friman. "I pretend that I don't know that that's why they're here. Finally, they bring it up. We talk about it, and then I bring up the game with them [he plays a reward game similar to Kohen's]. It's a much more powerful approach than to take it head-on and force the child to quit."

Try ordeal therapy. Kohen tries a crafty trick. "I ask them why they suck only their thumbs," he says. "I say 'Is that fair?' Then I give them a timer to take home and tell them to make sure they suck all their fingers equally. They usually get so tired of the whole process that they give it up. It also shifts the thumb-sucking 'program' in their brains." The only problem with this sort of "reverse psychology" approach is that kids are likely to see through it when it comes from a parent. If you suspect this will be the case, a pediatrician or close friend of the family may be able to help.

Offer the option of thumb sucking in private. Friman's definition of success focuses on not having any adults see the child thumb sucking. "It is not possible for them to suck their thumb enough in private to cause other problems," he says. "All of my systems are based on not having any adults see them thumb sucking."

Never use negative reinforcement. If the child has a slip, it may be destructive to use a negative reward, such as a sad-faced sticker, says Kohen. Failure has a nasty way of perpetuating itself.

Try "reminder fluid." Although some doctors see it as cruel, Friman endorses the use of bad-tasting fluids that are put on the thumb to keep the child from sucking. However, he stresses that the method should not be used as a punishment. Rather, he tells the child that it will help them succeed by reminding them of their goal. Another option is to place a glove or mitten on the child's hand as a reminder to keep the thumb out of the mouth.

Start with the easy stuff. One strategy is to try to help your child stop sucking his or her thumb at the times that your child does it the least, say in public, and then move on to the times when the habit is most ingrained, such as bedtime, says Jeffrey L. Brown, M.D., a clinical associate professor of pediatrics in the Department of Pediatrics and the Department of Psychiatry at The New York Hospital–Cornell Medical College in New York. "Start during the periods where kids can easily comply," says Brown. "Save the most difficult times for last. You can even give a double reward for days when the child doesn't suck his thumb during the most difficult times."

Don't yell. Although you may feel frustrated when your child slides back into his or her thumb-sucking behavior, save it for the tennis court, says Brown. Whatever you do, don't punish or yell at the child. "Yelling makes them nervous," says Brown. "And nervousness makes them suck their thumbs even more."

Wait it out. You know what happens to most kids who suck their thumbs at four, five, or even six years of age? They stop, says Kohen. "The parents will tell you that this year, their child does it less than last year, or that the child only does it when he's tired or watching television. Most of the time, by age six or seven, a child will stop, because their peers comment on it. They will be shamed out of it. If the thumb sucking is a symptom of something else, like sadness or anxiety, then it behooves the family or someone close to the family to figure that out. In that case, thumb sucking is no different than any other symbol of anxiety. Children suck their thumbs as a matter of self-comforting. The quickest way *not* to undo the behavior is to insist that it be changed." ◆

◆◆ How Important Is It? ◆◆

The old school of thought about thumb sucking was that it was a nasty habit that might cause dental problems and should be curtailed. However, times have changed.

"At age four or five, parents typically get worried about thumb sucking," says Daniel P. Kohen, M.D. "They often worry about the habit's reflection on them. It's normal for parents to worry about stuff like that, but it's not OK to put that worry onto the kid. What's important is that parents recognize the stage that the child's in, and not to overinvest themselves in it or do the wrong thing to help."

Patrick C. Friman, Ph.D., says that he will only take a child in his clinic for thumb sucking if the child is over five years old and has a chronic habit that appears to be causing a real problem, such as an infection of the thumbnail, malformation of the thumb itself, teasing at school, or the possibility of poisoning (from touching dangerous substances and then putting the thumb in the mouth).

And what about dental problems? Do thumb suckers end up in braces? "In truth, not nearly as many kids have thumb sucking contributing to their teeth problems as people would have us believe," says Kohen. "Some dentist friends of mine have told me that in many cases, kids who suck their thumbs are kids whose tooth alignment would have been a problem anyway." There are a variety of dental devices that can be used to help a child stop thumb sucking, Kohen says, but he only recommends their use if the child doesn't mind them. "Forcible or insistent use is probably bad for the kid's psyche," he says, "and the psyche is probably more important than the teeth."

◆ TOOTHACHE ◆

9 Ways to Ease the Pain

◆ Toothache Myths ◆

Don't fall for these myths—you could end up causing more damage by believing in them.

Put an aspirin on the tooth. *If you want to use aspirin to help relieve the pain of a toothache, swallow it with a glass of water. Do* not *place it on the tooth or surrounding gum. "That's a fallacy," says Joseph Tenca, D.D.S., M.A. "Aspirin does not work locally." What's worse, you may end up with a severe burn from the aspirin on your gum or cheek that can take four to five days to heal. "You're only adding to your problems," he says.*

A toothache means you'll lose the tooth. *Not so anymore. "Just because you have a bad toothache doesn't mean the tooth will have to be extracted," reassures Tenca. Root-canal therapy can save an abscessed tooth or one with damaged pulp. Root-canal therapy involves making a small opening in the tooth, removing the pulp in the root canal (that's where the name of the procedure comes from), filling the canal with a material called gutta percha, and then, usually, crowning the tooth. Sometimes, tiny metal posts are placed in the canal to help strengthen the tooth.*

If the pain disappears, the problem's gone. *"You don't have that kind of pain for no reason," says Alan H. Gluskin, D.D.S. He points out that coronary problems can cause pain in the lower jaw, while mouth pain can be referred to the ears, neck, or even shoulder. "Don't ever ignore pain in the head and neck."*

"For there was never yet philosopher that could endure the toothache patiently." Shakespeare was right. The toothache isn't easy to endure. The good news: With improved dental care and regular checkups, the excruciating pain of a toothache is not as common as it once was. But when pain does occur in the mouth, it's an important signal that you should not ignore—even if it goes away on its own.

Tooth pain is varied. Perhaps most common is the minor pain caused by sensitive teeth. You eat or drink something hot, cold, or sweet and feel a momentary twinge. (See SENSITIVE TEETH for advice.) Some people suffer achy teeth because of sinus problems; that's probably the case if you notice that the pain is limited to your upper teeth and that several teeth are affected at one time. Recent dental work can cause a tooth to be sensitive to temperature changes for a few weeks.

But some types of pain deserve immediate attention from your dentist. If you feel a sharp pain when you bite down, for instance, you may have a cavity, a loose filling, a cracked tooth, or damaged pulp (that's the inner core of the tooth that contains the blood vessels and nerves). Pain that sticks around for more than 30 minutes after eating hot or cold foods can also indicate pulp damage, either from a deep cavity or a blow to the tooth. And the stereotypical toothache with constant and severe pain, swelling, and sensitivity is definitely a sign of trouble. "If the pain wakes you up at night, it's serious," says Joseph Tenca, D.D.S., M.A., past president of the American Association of Endodontists and professor and chairman of the Department of Endodontics at Tufts University School of Dental Medicine in Boston. You could have an abscessed tooth; that means the pulp of the tooth has died, resulting in an infection that can spread to the gum and even to the bone.

Pain associated with the pulp of the tooth is kind of tricky. It can let you know that damage has occurred. "But the degeneration of the nerves (in the pulp) can be very rapid," points out Alan H. Gluskin, D.D.S., associate professor and chairperson of the Department of Endodontics at the University of the Pacific School of Dentistry in San Francisco. "They can die within a 12-hour period." So the pain disappears. But then the tooth hurts again as the dead tissue becomes infected, or abscessed.

That's why putting off dental attention for a toothache can mean bad news. But if it's 3:00 in the morning or the middle of Sunday afternoon, you can take some temporary measures to deal with the pain until you can get into the dental office:

Take two aspirin . . . or acetaminophen or ibuprofen, "whatever over-the-counter analgesic you use to relieve your headaches," says Tenca. Roland C. Duell, D.D.S., M.S., professor of endodontics with the Department of Oral Health Practice at the University of Kentucky College of Dentistry in Lexington, points out that ibuprofen is best at relieving inflammation, which may accompany a toothache.

Apply oil of cloves. You can pick this up at the pharmacy. Follow the directions for use, and be sure to put it only on the tooth and NOT on the gum. Otherwise, your burning gums may distract you from your toothache. And remember, oil of cloves won't cure the toothache; it just numbs the nerve.

Cool the swelling. Put a cold compress on the outside of your cheek if you've got swelling from the toothache.

Chill the pain. Holding an ice cube or cold water in the mouth may relieve the pain, says Tenca. But if you find that it simply aggravates your sensitive tooth, skip it.

When Pulp Goes Bad

Most of us don't think of our teeth as being alive, but they are. Each tooth contains what's called the pulp, composed of nourishing blood vessels and nerves.

If that pulp is damaged or exposed, the nerves can die, and the tooth can become infected, or abscessed. What can cause this? A deep cavity, a cracked tooth, or a hard blow to the tooth (from biting down on a popcorn kernel, for example).

"Once the pulp has been damaged or exposed, it can't repair itself," says Roland C. Duell, D.D.S., M.S. "It will need treatment." That's why you need to pay attention to any pain you experience from your teeth.

Keep your head up. Elevating your head can decrease the pressure in the area, says Duell.

Rinse. You can't really rinse away the pain, but you can rinse with warm water to remove any food debris. Tenca suggests using one teaspoon of salt in a glass of warm water.

Floss. No, it's not a cure, but flossing is another way to remove any food debris that could be trapped. The rubber tip on your toothbrush or a toothpick (if used with caution) can help dislodge any stuck food. "Sometimes, food can get lodged in the gum, and the pain mimics that caused by pulpal problems," says Tenca.

Be careful with the hot, the cold, and the sweet. These foods and beverages may aggravate an already sore and sensitive situation.

Plug it. If the tooth feels sensitive to air, cover it with gauze or even sugarless chewing gum until you can get to the dentist. ◆

◆ TRAVELER'S DIARRHEA ◆

20 Ways to Battle It

Montezuma's revenge, Delhi belly, Turkey trot, and Casablanca crud. Such colorful names give you a good idea of the misery to expect from traveler's diarrhea, a disease that can spoil an expensive and eagerly anticipated vacation.

It was once believed to be caused by a change in water, indulgence in spicy foods, or too much sun. Not so anymore. Researchers have found specific bacteria to blame. These bugs take up residence in the upper intestine and produce toxins that cause fluids and electrolytes (minerals like sodium and potassium that help regulate many body functions) to be secreted in a watery stool.

If you visit nearly any developing country in Latin America, Africa, or Asia, you've got a 30 to 50 percent chance of spending a few days in close contact with your bathroom. Less risky are countries such as southern Spain and Italy, Greece, Turkey, and Israel, where some 10 to 20 percent of tourists come down with traveler's diarrhea. Posing the lowest risk are Canada and northern Europe.

Your actions, however, can help influence that risk. If you really want to try food from the local street vendor or insist on drinking tap water, you're increasing your chances of coming down with traveler's diarrhea.

If you do get sick, it will probably last for two to four days, although some ten percent of cases can last for more than a week. And you may also experience—as if the diarrhea weren't enough—abdominal pain, cramps, gas, nausea, fatigue, loss of appetite, headache, vomiting, fever, and bloody stools.

Most common is watery diarrhea, sometimes accompanied by vomiting and a fever under 101 degrees Fahrenheit. If you actually get bacillary dysentery (caused by the Shigella bacteria), you'll have a fever over 101 degrees Fahrenheit, much more abdominal pain and cramping, and, often, blood in your stools, says David A. Sack, M.D., associate professor in the School of Public Health and director of the International Travel Clinic at Johns Hopkins University in Baltimore.

◆◆ What If There ◆◆ Is No Bottled Water?

If you're roughing it in the wilds of some underdeveloped nation, bottled or even boiled water may not be a practical option. You've got two alternatives, says David A. Sack, M.D.:

• Purify the water by adding iodine drops or chlorine tablets, which can be purchased at a camping-supply store in the United States before your departure.

• Pack a water purifier. The type with both a filter and iodine resin has been tested and shown to remove bacteria, viruses, and parasites.

The following are prevention and treatment options that can help save your vacation or business trip.

PREVENTION STRATEGIES

Here's what you can do to try to prevent a case of traveler's diarrhea from spoiling your trip. "A lot of it involves using your head about your eating or drinking," says Sack.

Give up ice cubes for the duration. They're made with tap water, and despite some people's beliefs, freezing will not kill the bacteria. Neither will floating those cubes in an alcoholic drink; the alcohol isn't strong enough to kill the bugs.

Drink bottled water. Don't drink water delivered to your table in a glass and don't drink water straight from a tap. And if you don't like the looks of the water in the bottle, "if it looks scummy," don't drink it, advises Peter A. Banks, M.D., director of the Clinical Gastroenterology Service at Brigham and Women's Hospital in Boston.

Open your own bottles. Whether it's water, a soft drink, or beer, open the bottle yourself. Otherwise, says Banks, "you don't know whether someone took an empty bottle and filled it up at the back sink." What's more, Banks adds, "Some people are not terribly clean and may rub their grimy hand or a dishtowel over the top of a bottle that's been opened to theoretically clean it."

Use caution with other beverages. Fresh lemonade may sound appealing, but you don't know the source of the water. Boiled beverages are OK— that means tea and coffee can be safe.

Know your dairy products. Don't drink unpasteurized milk and dairy products.

Stick to cooked foods. This is not the time to indulge in raw oysters. You'll have to pass on that green salad, too. Avoiding raw vegetables is one of the most important things you can do, stresses Sack.

Eat your cooked foods while they're hot. If they have time to sit around and cool off, bacteria-carrying flies have time to visit your food before you eat it.

Eat only fruits you peel yourself. "Pass up that pretty grapefruit salad and get a grapefruit you can peel yourself," says Banks. The same advice goes for hard-boiled eggs. Sack points out that the bacteria isn't *in* the food, it's *on* the food.

Take your own care package. "Bring along some granola bars, tea bags, packets of instant cocoa," says Banks. You can make your own tea, for example, if you boil the water *thoroughly.*

◆ Take a Suitcase ◆ of Pepto-Bismol

Researchers have found that taking Pepto-Bismol can prevent traveler's diarrhea. In fact, they managed to reduce the frequency anywhere from 23 to 61 percent.

The only problem: You've got to take a bottle of the stuff a day (that's two ounces, four times daily). And there's no guarantee you still won't be in the percentage that gets sick, points out David A. Sack, M.D.

"You can ruin a vacation with one bad meal," Banks says. "You're entitled to be careful."

COPING TIPS

If, despite all your precautions, you still get sick, don't despair. Simply follow the same instructions for diarrhea that you would at home:

Beware of becoming dehydrated. The danger in diarrhea is in losing both fluids and electrolytes, minerals like sodium and potassium that regulate many different functions in the body.

Try oral rehydration therapy (ORT). "You can usually buy a packet of oral rehydration solution to mix with water in a drugstore in any country except the United States," says Sack. "Mix it with the best water available, but don't worry if you have to mix it with tap water. It's important to get fluids, and besides, the horse is already out of the barn at this stage."

Make your own ORT. If you can't get to a drugstore, you can use common kitchen ingredients to make your own oral rehydration therapy solution. Mix four tablespoons of sugar, one-half teaspoon of salt, and one-half teaspoon

Preventive Antibiotics

One possibility: Take antibiotics along to take every day as a preventive measure. That's usually not recommended for most people, although there are exceptions:

• If you're over 65 or have a history of heart disease or stroke so that diarrhea could compromise your health.

• If you're a businessman on a tight schedule.

• If you're on your honeymoon. "It's just not nice to have diarrhea on your honeymoon," says David A. Sack, M.D.

of baking soda in one liter of water. "Be sure to eat lots of oranges and bananas for potassium with this," points out Sack. "There's no common kitchen ingredient with potassium to include."

Drink a combination of fluids. Remember, the biggest danger in diarrhea is becoming dehydrated. You're also losing electrolytes, so drink a combination of liquids besides water, such as weak tea with sugar, broth, moderate amounts of fruit juices (be careful—some have a laxative effect), defizzed nondiet and noncaffeinated soda pop, or Gatorade.

Sip, don't guzzle. Try to take frequent small drinks; it's less irritating to your gut that way.

Eat a bland diet. Forget the enchiladas and salsa. This is the time for toast, rice, noodles, bananas, gelatin, soups, boiled potatoes, cooked carrots, and soda crackers.

Pack the pink stuff. Pepto-Bismol is definitely the first choice when it comes to treating traveler's diarrhea. "It actually has a mild antibacterial

effect, so it's especially useful in traveler's diarrhea," says Rosemarie L. Fisher, M.D., professor of medicine in the Division of Digestive Diseases at Yale University School of Medicine in New Haven, Connecticut.

Don't rely on over-the-counter medicines that decrease motility. In plain English, avoid Imodium and Kaopectate; they slow down the movement of the bowel. "That can have serious consequences, especially if you've got dysentery [signified by bloody diarrhea]," says Fisher.

Bring along an antibiotic—just in case. Visit your doctor *before* you leave on vacation and get a prescription antibiotic such as doxycycline, sulfamethoxazole, or quinolones (Sack's first choice). "If you start taking it early in the disease, you'll shorten the duration [the average duration is four to five days] to one to two days," says Sack. He stresses the need to visit your doctor or a travel clinic before leaving. "I've heard too many horror stories about tourists calling the hotel doctor and what kind of remedies he's given them. It's worth the expense to see a doctor ahead of time when you've invested so much in a trip."

Don't be alarmed if your diarrhea waits until you get home to show up. If you've picked up a parasite like giardia, its appearance may be delayed. And some travelers relax their restrictions on the plane home—forgetting the food was prepared in the country they just left. ◆

◆ ULCER ◆

7 Care Tactics

Everyone has a favorite image of a person who has ulcers: He's middle-aged, compulsive, anxious, angry, and hostile, and he seems resigned (even proud) that this condition is a price he's paying for his position in life.

Well, here's a surprise: "He" is very likely to be a "she" these days. Thirty years ago, the ratio of male-to-female ulcer sufferers was twenty to one; today it's probably one to one. What's more, while certain personality characteristics and life stresses may hasten the development of an ulcer, they are not the sole cause. And nobody, given a choice, would opt for the kind of success that means having a hole in the gastrointestinal tract.

Actually, the erosion can appear in the stomach or in the duodenum (the first part of the small intestine). In the course of a day, as food travels through the digestive system, two substances—pepsin and hydrochloric acid—go into action to break down the food. Once the food is broken down, the digestive fluid rests in wait for the next meal. Sometimes, however, the system works too well, activating digestive juices even when there is no food to work on, which means that the juices have no recourse but to try to consume the digestive tract itself.

Why do some people develop ulcers while their neighbors don't? Various theories have come and either gone or stayed around, including the assumption that ulcer sufferers generate an excess of hydrochloric acid (in fact, some individuals with ulcers generate *less* acid) and that ulcers are an aftermath of a bacterial infection of the stomach (not everyone is convinced that it is so simple).

Treatment is not so simple, either. Many of the methods that have been used in the past have been found to be less than satisfactory. Unfortunately, some ulcer sufferers may be following regimens that are, at best, ineffective and, at worst, harmful. If you have—or suspect you may have—an ulcer, you should be under the care of a doctor. However, there are also some steps you should be taking at home to care for your digestive tract. Here are the most recent recommendations for those who have been diagnosed with a peptic ulcer:

Go by gut reactions. Highly spiced and fried foods, long thought to be prime culprits in instigating ulcers, are now considered to have little bearing on either the development or course of an ulcer. "You don't have to relegate yourself to a bland and boring diet of soft, unseasoned foods," says Norton Rosensweig, M.D., associate clinical professor of medicine at Columbia University College of Physicians and Surgeons in New York. Nevertheless, individual tolerances vary. If you find that spicy meals, for example, are always followed by a severe gnawing pain, assume that there may be a cause and effect. The same goes for any other food that seems to cause you discomfort.

Eat wisely. The real key to keeping gastric juices from attacking the lining of the digestive tract is to keep some food present as much of the time as possible. Try eating smaller meals more frequently. "That doesn't mean overeating," says Lawrence S. Friedman, M.D., associate professor of medicine at Jefferson Medical College of Thomas Jefferson University in Philadelphia. Too much food causes formation of more gastric juices—as well as weight gain.

Skip the milk solution. One of the earliest treatments for ulcer flare-ups was milk, which was believed to neutralize stomach acid. "Foods high in calcium stimulate stomach acid," says Friedman. So while the protein part of the milk may soothe, the calcium may make matters worse.

Rechannel stress. The idea that one has to eliminate stress is unrealistic, since stress is very much a part of everyday life. "Trying to avoid stress may be a futile endeavor," says Gayle Randall, M.D., assistant professor of medicine in the Department of Medicine at the University of California at Los Angeles School of Medicine. It's

◆◆ How to Reach ◆◆ for Relief

The good news about antacids is that, when taken as directed, they are effective in relieving the discomfort of a peptic ulcer attack. Even better news is that by neutralizing the acid in the digestive fluids, they may help the ulcer to heal. On the downside, these products come with risks and precautions:

• Aluminum-based antacids frequently cause constipation and may also interfere with absorption of phosphorus from the diet, resulting in weakness and bone damage over a long period.

• Magnesium-based antacids can cause diarrhea. And in individuals with impaired kidney function, blood levels of magnesium may increase, causing weakness and fatigue.

• Prolonged use and then sudden stoppage of these medications can lead to an increase in stomach acid.

• All such products interfere with absorption and metabolism of other drugs. Check with your pharmacist about possible interactions with your prescription medications.

• Consistent use of antacids can possibly mask the symptoms of a more serious disorder.

• Consult with your doctor before taking antacids over a long period of time. If you find yourself needing to take more and more of an antacid for relief, contact your doctor.

not stress but the inability to cope with it satisfactorily that can be harmful to an ulcer-prone individual." The same faulty coping process can aggravate heart disease in one person and migraine headaches in another. Work on ways to help cope with stress more effectively. Take a stress-management class, take up a hobby, learn to meditate, start an aerobic exercise program, or do whatever helps you to blow off some steam and manage stress more effectively.

Avoid the smoke screen. One point that hasn't changed over the years: Smoking cigarettes is courting trouble. Smoking inhibits the secretion of natural body substances called prostaglandins, which might normally act in defense of an attack by hydrochloric acid and pepsin. "The gut is left vulnerable," says Rosensweig. Aspirin and other drugs in the family of nonsteroidal anti-inflammatory drugs also inhibit prostaglandins and, thereby, reduce the digestive system's defenses.

Drink lightly. The question of alcohol's impact on ulcer formation remains unanswered. Many medical experts believe that individuals who drink heavily are at higher risk of developing ulcers than those who drink lightly or not at all. "Until a verdict is in, there is good reason to recommend that ulcer patients minimize their intake of alcoholic beverages," says Randall.

Self-medicate with care. Ulcer sufferers are never far away from their antacids. But if you use these medications, do so with care. "People may take more and more of the drugs," says Friedman. "They may end up overmedicating." Not to mention overspending—you may end up paying as much as you would for prescription drugs (see "How to Reach for Relief"). ◆

◆ VARICOSE VEINS ◆

16 Coping Techniques

The circulatory system could be compared to a big city's freeways, where the bumper-to-bumper cars, in this case the frenetic blood cells, are delivering oxygen and nutrients to every part of the body. The pumping heart maintains the pulse of the "traffic" by pushing the blood cells on their way through the arteries.

On the cells' return trip to the heart and lungs, the veins have a harder time of it. For one thing, the pressure caused by the pumping heart is decreased. For another, the veins below the heart, in the legs and torso, must work against gravity, as the blood makes its way up from the feet. So these vessels depend more on the leg muscles to help pump the blood back to the heart. The veins also contain valves to help keep the blood moving along. The valves work like locks in a canal. As blood flows through a valve, its "doors" slam shut so the blood can't go backward.

When any one of these valves fail, blood can seep back and begin to pool, often in the lower legs. The extra pressure of the increased volume of pooling blood can, over time, cause subsequent valves to fail. Then the vein's walls begin to bulge and become misshapen. At this point, the vein may show through the skin surface, looking knotty and gnarled, blue and bumpy.

It's estimated that 25 percent of all women and 10 percent of all men are affected by varicose veins. Fortunately, there are ways to prevent or, at the very least, postpone, their development and decrease their severity. Here's how:

Check your family tree. "The tendency to develop varicose veins can run in families," says Hugh Gelabert, M.D., assistant professor of surgery in the Section of Vascular Surgery at the University of California at Los Angeles School of Medicine. The reason for this is unknown. Some experts believe there is a weakness in the gene that governs the development of the veins. This may lead to defects in the structure of valves and veins or, in some people, a decrease in the number of valves in the veins, causing the few that are there to get

> ## ◆◆◆ Spider Veins: ◆◆◆ "Cousin" to Varicose Veins
>
> *Eighty percent of varicose-vein sufferers will also develop spider veins, says Luis Navarro, M.D. And half of all spider-vein sufferers also have varicose veins. But unlike knotty varicose veins, spider veins are thin and weblike in appearance (thus the name) and most often show up on the legs, neck, and face. These veins are actually dilated blood vessels that appear no thicker than a thread or hair. Except for their link to pregnancy and hormones (see "Advice for Moms-to-Be"), no one knows for sure why they crop up. Because the cause hasn't been pinpointed, the veins can't be prevented. But on the plus side, they rarely cause problems—perhaps only a little itching now and again.*

overloaded in their duties. If you do find a history of varicose veins in your family, the sooner you follow preventative measures the better.

Get moving. "Exercise works by keeping the veins empty of pooling blood," says Gelabert. "Every time a muscle contracts in the buttocks, thighs, or lower legs, blood is helped on its way back to the heart." However, it's hard to say if exercise will only postpone, or if it can prevent, varicose veins. "If there's a strong family history of the condition present, then exercise will probably only postpone the condition," says Gelabert. To get your legs moving, almost any exercise that involves the legs will do, from aerobics to strengthening to spot-

Clots: Be Careful!

Though thankfully rare, clots can form in varicose veins. Thrombo-phlebitis, the inflammation of a vein caused by a clot, can be potentially dangerous if the clot begins to travel through the veins. The traveling clot, then called an embolism, can end up blocking part of the blood flow in the heart or lungs, possibly resulting in a pulmonary (lung) embolism or heart failure.

If the clot forms in what's called the superficial venous system, "you may see localized redness at the site, as well as tenderness and pain," says Alan M. Dietzek, M.D. If the clot forms in what's known as the deep venous system, you won't be able to see the clot, but you may have swelling and tender-ness in all or part of either leg, he says. If you experience any of these symptoms, see your doctor.

Some of the best measures to help prevent clotting: Keep active; maintain a desirable weight; and take breaks from sitting, especially on long car and plane rides and during long hours of sitting at work.

Lose weight. Obesity "puts a strain on every part of the body," explains Luis Navarro, M.D., founder and director of the Vein Treatment Center in New York and author of *No More Varicose Veins*. "Furthermore, people who are overweight tend to be more immobile and get less exercise." As a result, overweight people usually have muscles that can't as efficiently help the veins pump their blood back to the heart. In addition, an overweight person's blood vessels carry more blood than a thinner person's, so the strain is greater on the vessels themselves.

Eat a balanced diet. Besides helping you to maintain proper weight, a balanced diet can give you nutrients that may actually help prevent varicose veins. Protein and vitamin C are both components of collagen, part of the tissue in the veins and valves. If the collagen is in good shape, the tissues may not fall apart as readily. However, "diet will not reverse a case of varicose veins," says Frank J. Veith, M.D., professor of surgery and chief of Vascular Surgical Services at Montefiore Medical Center–Albert Einstein College of Medicine in New York.

Take a break from standing. "When you're upright, the feet are the furthest possible distance away from the heart, so the blood has far to go, against gravity no less, to get back to the heart," says Gelabert. As a result, the blood can have a tendency to pool in the lower legs, leading to the development of varicose veins.

But don't sit too long, either. Some experts theorize that even sitting can contribute to varicose veins. "They believe since the knees and groin are bent while sitting, the blood flow has a difficult course back to the heart," says Navarro. So it's very important on a long car or plane ride or during a day of sitting at the office that you get up and stretch your legs once in a while. Navarro suggests this rejuvenator: Stand on your toes and flex the heel up and down ten times.

toning activities, say the experts. Ride a bike, take an aerobics class, go for a walk or a run, use the stair machine in the gym—these are all good exercises for the legs. Spot-toning exercises, such as leg raises, that specifically build up the muscles in the buttocks, thighs, and lower legs are also recommended.

Get support from your stockings. Support panty hose are better than regular hosiery for helping to control the development of varicose veins. Better yet are the support stockings available by prescription. These 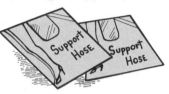 stockings help by keeping the veins in the legs from bulging, and as a result, keeping fluids from collecting in the legs. How do they work? They apply more pressure to the lower legs than to the thigh area. Since more pressure is exerted on the lower legs, blood is more readily pushed up toward the heart. The stockings' compression on the legs is measured in millimeters of mercury, called mm Hg, and ranges from 20 mm Hg for milder cases to 60 mm Hg for severe varicosity. (In comparison, support panty hose from a department store have a strength of 14 mm Hg to 17 mm Hg.) The prescription stockings also come in a variety of lengths: below the knee, midthigh, full thigh, and waist high. The lower-strength stockings are sometimes recommended for pregnant women (see "Advice for Moms-to-Be"). Since the stockings are only available in a few colors, some women prefer to wear them under pants. The downside: The stockings have a tendency to feel hot.

Slip into spandex pants. Like store-bought support panty hose, this type of stretch pant applies pressure to the legs, says Gelabert.

Cover up the blues. If you've stopped wearing shorts or going to the beach because you're embarrassed about your varicose veins, make them "disappear." There are products specially made to cover the blue vein lines that are causing you to take cover. Available in a variety of shades to match your skin, the cream is applied by hand and blended. Leg Magic by Covermark Cosmetics is waterproof and even has a sun protection factor (SPF) of 16 to protect your legs from the sun's

◆◆◆ Advice for ◆◆◆ Moms-to-Be

Pregnancy can also lead to the development of varicose veins and spider veins. Surging hormones weaken collagen and connective tissues in the pelvis in preparation for giving birth. Unfortunately, as a side effect, the hormones may also weaken the collagen found in the veins and valves of the body. These weakened tissues have a more difficult time standing up to the increased blood volume that comes with carrying a baby. In addition, the weight of the fetus itself may play a role in the development of varicose veins and spider veins in the legs, says Hugh Gelabert, M.D. Elevating the legs whenever possible can be helpful, and compression stockings in the 20 mm Hg to 30 mm Hg range may be prescribed. The good news is that for many women, the swollen veins subside after the baby is born.

harmful rays. Wearing stockings over the cover-up won't make it fade or rub off, and you can even go for a swim, says Richard Ottaviano, president of Covermark Cosmetics in Moonachie, New Jersey. While these types of products obviously won't fix the veins, they may make you feel better about yourself.

Consider the effects of estrogen. The hormone is generally believed to have a detrimental effect on the collagen and connective tissue of the veins. And "while the Pill probably does not have a direct correlation to varicose veins, it may have an indirect one," says Gelabert. "The Pill may lead to the development of embolisms, or clots in the blood, which can interfere with blood flow" (see "Clots: Be Careful!").

Prop up your legs. Elevating the legs is good, but raising them above your heart is even better. By doing this, you're working with gravity to help get the blood out of the ankles and back to the heart. "This is the oldest and most successful way to alleviate discomfort and facilitate drainage and reduce swelling," says Gelabert. As a matter of fact, Hippocrates in ancient Greece wrote of its benefits, he notes. Lie down on a couch and put your feet on the back of it. "If you can, elevate the legs for ten minutes every hour," recommends Alan M. Dietzek, M.D., vascular surgeon at North Shore University Hospital in Manhasset, New York, and assistant professor of surgery at Cornell Medical College in New York.

Flex your feet. "Flexing might help by making the muscles contract, which in turn helps squeeze the blood out of the veins," explains Gelabert. While your legs are elevated, try these three exercises to keep the blood pumping out of your feet and back to your heart:

• **The Ankle Pump:** Flex your foot up and down as you would when you pump a piano pedal or gas pedal.

• **Ankle Circles:** Rotate your feet clockwise and counterclockwise.

• **Heel Slips:** With your knees bent, slide your heels back and forth.

Sleep with elevated feet. For those with chronic swelling in the lower legs, it may help to put a few pillows under your feet while sleeping, says Gelabert.

Wear tennis shoes. If your feet habitually swell, it may be worthwhile to wear tennis shoes or other lace-up shoes that can be opened up or loosened to alleviate the pressure. ◆

◆ WARTS ◆

11 Ways to Wipe Them Out

Most of us have had one of these ghastly bumps at one point or another. Warts are caused by the human papilloma virus (HPV). Because they're brought on by a virus, they are contagious. That's why an initial wart can create a host of other ones. Common warts are the rough-looking lesions most often found on the hands and fingers. The much smaller, smoother flat wart can also be found on the hand but may show up on the face, too. Warts that occur on the soles of the feet are called plantar warts and can sometimes be as large as a quarter. Genital warts, which have become a growing problem, develop in the genital and anal area (see "Caution: Genital Warts"). If you suspect that you have a genital wart, see your doctor; do not try the remedies suggested here.

No one knows why warts occur and disappear and later recur in what appears to be a sponta-neous fashion. Andrew Lazar, M.D., assistant professor of clinical dermatology at Northwestern University School of Medicine in Chicago, tells a story to typify how warts remain a medical mystery. A woman came to him about the warts on her feet. As common practice, he asked her if she was on any medications or pregnant. She said she and her husband were trying to have a baby. Soon after, the woman found out she was pregnant. After she had the baby, the warts disappeared. About two years later, the woman came back to Lazar again with warts on her feet. Later she got the news she was pregnant for the second time. A few years after that, the woman called one day and told the doctor she had warts on her feet for the third time. "Doctor," she asked, "do you think I'm pregnant?" Sure enough, she was. (Of course, not all pregnant women get warts, nor are pregnant women the only people plagued by warts.)

A medical mystery also surrounds the fact that researchers have yet to find a way to get rid of warts for good. The solution may lie in developing a wart vaccine, but an approved, safe vaccine has yet to be developed. That leaves the wart sufferer

The Folklore Cures

While there is no scientific evidence that any of these age-old remedies works, if nothing else has worked for you, these might be worth a tongue-in-cheek try.

• *Tie a knot in a string for each wart that you have, then drop the string over your shoulder in the light of a full moon.*

• *For another take on the moonshine methods: Rub the wart with a chicken gizzard when the moon is waning; then bury the gizzard in the center of a dirt road.*

• *Touch the warts with a dishrag, then bury the rag.*

• *Rub a raw potato on the wart. Then, bury the potato in your backyard. A variation of this: Bury the potato in clay. Then repeat with another potato the next day.*

• *Have a relative "buy" your wart for a penny.*

• *Rub milkweed or dandelion juice on the wart.*

• *Tape the inside of a banana peel to the wart.*

with two options: Having a dermatologist or podiatrist treat the warts or trying a few methods on their own. As for home remedies, some people swear by certain tactics, while others will never have any success with them. This has led Jerome Z. Litt, M.D., a dermatologist in private practice in Beachwood, Ohio, and an assistant clinical

professor of dermatology at Case Western Reserve University School of Medicine in Cleveland, to observe: "Everything works and nothing works." And it seems that in some cases, prevention may be the best medicine. Here are some tips to help you be wart-free.

Make sure it's a wart. First and foremost, before you try any type of treatment, know whether your skin eruption is a wart or another condition. Warts (except the small, smooth flat wart) commonly have a broken surface filled with tiny red dots. (Some people mistakenly call these dots seeds, when in reality they are the blood vessels that are supplying the wart.) Moles, on the other hand, are usually smooth, regularly shaped bumps that are not flesh-colored (as flat warts can be). Rough and tough patches with the lines of the skin running through them may be a corn or a callus. There is also a chance that the lesion could be skin cancer. You may be able to recognize skin cancer by its irregular borders and colors. When in doubt, see your doctor. In addition, if you are diabetic, do not try any home therapy for wart removal; see your doctor.

Don't touch. The wart virus can spread from you to others, and you can also keep reinfecting yourself. The virus develops into a wart by first finding its way into a scratch in the skin's surface—a cut or a hangnail or a wound, for instance. Even the everyday task of shaving can spread the flat warts on a man's face. Inadvertently cutting a wart as you trim your cuticles can cause an infection. So keep the virus's travels to a minimum by not touching your warts at all, if possible. If you do come in contact with the lesions, wash your hands thoroughly in hot water. Children should also be told that picking or chewing their warts can cause them to spread.

Stick to it. Adhesive tape has shown to be especially successful on finger warts. Litt has been using this method with success since the 1950s. Here's how he does it: Wrap the wart completely with four layers of adhesive tape. The first piece goes over the top of the finger; the second around

the finger. Repeat these two steps with two more pieces of tape. Wrap the wart snugly but never too tightly. Leave the tape on for six and a half days. Then remove the tape for half a day. You may need to repeat the procedure for about three to four weeks before the wart disappears. You can try the procedure on a plantar wart, notes Litt, but use strips of tape that are long enough to properly secure the adhesive. "What's so good about this approach is that it's inexpensive and leaves no scar," says Litt.

◆◆◆ Caution: ◆◆◆ Genital Warts

The number of cases of genital warts is growing at a phenomenal rate, says the American Academy of Dermatology. The reason: Genital warts are extremely contagious. The usual mode of transmission is through sexual contact. It's also possible for an infected woman to pass on the virus to her fetus during pregnancy or birth.

The use of condoms can help protect against sexually transmitted diseases, including genital warts, says Joseph P. Bark, M.D. Yet, he says, many people still choose not to protect themselves. He points to "the immediacy-of-death rule" as the reason. "For instance, if someone was told that the next time they go out in the sun they would get skin cancer, they would be very careful about their exposure. The same goes for sexually transmitted diseases. Many people still believe it can't happen to them." One incentive for using protection may lie in the fact that certain strains of HPV have now been linked to cancer.

Try castor oil. The acid in castor oil probably does the trick by irritating the wart. The oil treatment works best on small, flat warts on the face and on the back of the hands, says Litt. He recommends applying the castor oil to the wart with a cotton swab twice a day.

"C" what you can do. Vitamin C is mildly acidic, so it may irritate the wart enough to make it go away, says Litt. Apply a paste made of crushed vitamin C tablets and water. Apply the paste only to the wart, not to the surrounding skin. Then cover the paste with gauze and tape.

Heat it up. One study found that having patients soak their plantar warts in very hot water was helpful because it softens the wart and may kill the virus. Make sure the water is not too hot, cautions Litt, or you may burn yourself.

Take precautions with over-the-counter preparations. The Food and Drug Administration (FDA) recently approved wart-removal medications made with 26 percent salicylic acid, reports Litt. Typically, remedies have contained about 16 percent. While the stronger formulas may work well for adults (except for those who have sensitive skin), Litt does not suggest using them on children. Salicylic acid works because it's an irritant, so no matter which strength of solution you use, try to keep it from irritating the surrounding skin. If you're using a liquid medication, do this by smearing a ring of petroleum jelly around the wart before using the medication. If you're applying a medicated wart pad or patch, cut it to only the size of the wart. Litt suggests applying over-the-counter medications at night and then leaving the area uncovered.

◆◆◆ Can You Wish ◆◆◆ Your Warts Away?

Some dermatologists agree that the power of suggestion, especially when used on children, can be very effective in making warts disappear. It may be that the warts were about to vanish anyway (children's warts usually disappear more quickly than warts in adults), or perhaps positive thoughts boost the immune system. No one knows for sure.

Taking the power of suggestion one step further, there have been studies of the use of hypnosis in the treatment of warts. At the mention of the word hypnosis, many people conjure up images of a Houdini-type magician gently swaying a crystal bauble in the face of an unwilling suspect who, unbeknownst to him, is about to reveal the truth—or cluck like a chicken. Unlike popular myth, hypnosis can't make you do something you don't want to do. Today, it's an acceptable way to quit smoking and can be used as an adjunct to losing weight.

Owen S. Surman, M.D., C.M., F.A.P.A., associate professor of psychiatry at Massachusetts General Hospital in Boston, used hypnosis to see if it would make warts go away. His study was done on 17 people who were treated with hypnosis once a week for five weeks. Seven other patients were not treated with hypnosis. Both groups were asked to abstain from any wart treatment, including home remedies. The patients who underwent hypnosis were told that they would experience a tingling sensation in the warts on one side of their body and only those warts would disappear. Nine patients lost more than three-quarters of all their warts, and four of them lost all the warts on both sides of their body. Meanwhile, the untreated group showed no improvement. Surman can only speculate on why the hypnosis may have worked. "Perhaps, a belief in the power of suggestion enhanced the activity of the body's T-cells, which combat viruses."

Chalk it up to the power of suggestion. Some physicians use this technique on children, who are still impressionable. The doctor tells the child that if the doctor rubs chalk on the child's warts, they will disappear. There are variations on this, including: Coloring the warts with crayon or drawing a picture of a child's hand with the warts crossed out and throwing the picture in the garbage (see "Can You Wish Your Warts Away?").

Don't go barefoot. "Millions of virus particles leak out of a wart," says Joseph P. Bark, M.D., chairman of dermatology at St. Joseph Hospital in Lexington, Kentucky. That fact puts people in public places at high risk for plantar, or foot, warts. The best protection: footwear. Locker rooms, pools, showers in fitness centers, even the carpets in hotel rooms harbor a host of viruses—not just wart viruses. You can catch any of a number of infections, from scabies to herpes simplex, says Bark. Never go barefoot, and at the very least, wear a pair of flip-flops, or thongs.

Keep dry. Warts tend to flourish more readily in an environment that's damp, especially in the case of plantar warts. That's why people who walk or exercise extensively may be more prone to foot warts, says the American Academy of Dermatology in Schaumburg, Illinois. So change your socks any time your feet get sweaty, and use a medicated foot powder.

Cover your cuts and scrapes. The wart virus loves finding a good scratch so it can make its way under your skin. By keeping your cuts and scrapes covered, you'll be helping to keep out the wart virus. ◆

◆ WEIGHT GAIN ◆

37 Ways to Fight the Battle of the Bulge

At any given moment, 33 to 40 percent of American women and 20 to 24 percent of American men are trying to lose weight. Yet an estimated one-fourth to one-third of Americans are still overweight, which increases their risk for heart disease, high blood pressure, and Type II (noninsulin-dependent) diabetes as well as for gallbladder disease, gout, some types of cancer, and osteoarthritis.

Traditional knowledge says that 3,500 calories equal one pound of weight. Cut the calories or burn more of them than you consume, and you'll drop pounds. That's been the approach for years—but it isn't working. Short-term calorie-restricted diets can help you lose, but as much as two-thirds of that weight is generally regained within a year and almost all of it within five years.

Weight loss is more complicated than a simple equation. That was part of the conclusion drawn from a conference sponsored by the National Institutes of Health in the spring of 1992. "Overweight is not a simple disorder of willpower, as sometimes implied, but is a complex disorder of energy metabolism," stated the conference report.

Many diets just don't work for the long haul. If you really want to keep the weight off for the rest of your life, you have to change your lifestyle. "Someday, I hope we'll look back on semistarvation diets the way we currently view such archaic practices as bleeding and purging," says C. Wayne Callaway, M.D., associate clinical professor of medicine at George Washington University in Washington, D.C., and a member of the 1989–1990 Dietary Guidelines Advisory Committee to the U.S. Department of Agriculture. "You have to look at weight loss as a lifetime management issue," says Callaway. "A weight problem is not like having pneumonia where you can take a course of antibiotics and cure it. You have to keep working on your weight."

Dieting becomes a way of life for some people, particularly women, who lose and gain over and over again in a syndrome of "yo-yo" dieting. A 1991 study published in *The New England Journal of Medicine* indicates that you may be shortening your life span if you engage in such practices. And most research has shown that such weight cycling probably makes it easier to regain the weight by messing with your metabolism (the rate at which your body burns calories). "You lose eight pounds of fat and two pounds of muscle the first time," explains Gabe Mirkin, M.D., associate professor at Georgetown University Medical School in Washington, D.C., and author of *The Mirkin Report,* a monthly newsletter on health, fitness, and nutrition. "Then you gain back ten pounds—all of it fat. So you've increased your amount of fat by two pounds," says Mirkin. Ironically, adds Callaway, you've lost muscle mass, and muscle actually helps burn more calories.

How do you lose fat wisely and increase your chances of keeping it off? The experts suggest:

Decide first if you truly need to lose weight. Look at your shape, height, weight, and history of obesity-linked diseases and the history of those factors in your family, suggests Callaway. Then consider when your weight problems began: Have you gained weight recently as the result of a marital separation or is this a gradual pattern since your teens? (See "Do You Need to Lose Weight?")

Analyze your eating and activity patterns. "If you're starving and bingeing, you first have to learn how to eat normally," says Callaway. He's seen numerous patients on low-calorie diets who persist in gaining weight, despite how much they cut down on what they eat. He blames constant dieting and erratic eating habits for reducing their metabolic rates, forcing their bodies into a starvation mode that hoards fat.

Keep a food diary for two weeks. Write down everything you eat, when you eat it, and how you're feeling at the time—bored, angry, or hungry, for example. "A food diary can be illuminating to a lot of people," points out Barbara Deskins, Ph.D., R.D., associate professor of clinical dietetics and nutrition at the University of Pittsburgh. "They don't realize they eat automatically." If you decide to visit a registered dietitian for assistance, take your food diary along.

Make a plan. Once you decide you're ready to change your lifestyle to reach a desirable weight, you'll have to figure out how to do that. Most experts recommend learning to make nutritionally sound food choices, eating an adequate amount of food each day, and increasing your physical activity. You may find the advice of your family physician, a registered dietitian, or an exercise physiologist helpful. (Callaway cautions, however, that you should make sure that the dietitian sticks to nutritional counseling and the exercise physiologist to exercise.) Some university medical centers and hospitals are adopting a multidiscipli-

nary team to handle weight loss; a registered dietitian, a physician, an exercise physiologist, and a behavioral psychologist join forces.

If you decide to go it alone, however, the tips that follow can help.

Don't plan to lose too much too soon. Rapid weight loss generally means a rapid weight gain down the road, says Callaway. Don't try to lose more than half a pound a week.

Pick a good time. "Don't decide to start this the week before your wedding or right after you lose your job," says Deskins. "You don't want to choose a period of high stress only to add additional stress."

Don't try to change everything at once. "It's unrealistic to think that tomorrow you'll completely redo your food habits in some 180-degree shift," says Deskins. Make changes gradually.

◆◆◆ Do You Need ◆◆◆ to Lose Weight?

Many of us, particularly women, don't care what the various charts say about our height-weight ratios. We're striving for a certain look, and unfortunately, that body image may be impossible for some of us to attain.

How do you know if you need to lose weight? You can check the Metropolitan Life Insurance Company Height and Weight Tables, which were revised in 1983. To determine your risk for weight-related health problems, however, consider the following:

• Are you at risk for high blood pressure, Type II diabetes, or heart disease? Your physician can help you with those answers by examining your medical

and family history, along with performing certain diagnostic tests.

• Where's your fat located? If it's concentrated around your belly, you need to lose. If it's around your hips and thighs but your belly's flat, you can relax a bit. That's because abdominal fat is linked with a higher risk for medical conditions than is fat on the hips and thighs. Divide your waist measurement by your hip measurement to get your waist/hip ratio: .70 to .75 is considered healthy for women and .80 to .90 is considered healthy for men. If you're above that, you need to lose.

• Calculate your body mass index (BMI). Divide your weight in pounds by 2.2 to get kilograms and your height in inches by 39.37 to get meters. Your BMI equals weight in kilograms divided by height in meters squared. Normal BMI is considered to be between 19 and 27.

Start with damage control. If you're the family food shopper, you can handle this one yourself. Or discuss it with the person who does the grocery shopping. It's pretty simple advice: If you don't have potato chips or chocolate around, you're not as likely to indulge in these high-calorie snacks. Instead, keep low-calorie snacks and foods on hand—raw vegetables or rice cakes, whatever works. The same thing goes in terms of the food that gets cooked for meals. Overweight tends to run in families, and part of that is due to shared eating habits, says John H. Renner, M.D., president of the Consumer Health Information Research Institute in Kansas City, Missouri, and member of the Board of Directors of the National Council Against Health Fraud.

Measure your foods. Doing this tedious chore for a few days can help train your eye to recognize portion sizes, says Johanna Dwyer, D.Sc., R.D., professor at Tufts University School of Nutrition and Tufts University Medical School and director of the Frances Stern Nutrition Center at New England Medical Center Hospitals, all in Boston.

Don't count calories. Opinions differ on this one, but most experts suggest changing the way you eat, rather than allotting yourself only so many calories a day.

Cut out the alcohol. You could say a martini is "empty calories"—it has no nutritional benefits. Callaway points out that alcohol may encourage fat distribution around the waist. The average American gets ten percent of calories from alcohol, says Deskins, so abstinence for some could mean a substantial drop in calories. "Some people can lose weight just by giving up beer," says Renner.

Eat breakfast. And lunch. And dinner. Callaway explains that skipping meals leads to binge eating. It's the body's attempt to make up for lack of food intake as it goes into starvation mode. He says if you get one-fourth of your calories at each meal, you'll lose the urge to snack as well.

Dieting and Pregnancy Don't Mix

One time not *to diet, say the experts: At the beginning of your pregnancy, even if you are overweight. "If you weigh 400 pounds, you still need to gain 20 pounds during pregnancy," says Gabe Mirkin, M.D. "It's important to eat regularly and not to skip meals," adds Barbara Deskins, Ph.D., R.D. Skipping meals can cause the body to break down its fat reserves, which create certain by-products known as ketones that may harm the fetus.*

Make sure you eat enough. That's music to any dieter's ears, but Callaway is concerned that starvation diets lead to bingeing and lowered metabolism.

Don't make a lapse a collapse. Just because you fail one day and pig out on the wrong foods doesn't mean you should give up for good, says Dwyer. Pick yourself up, dust yourself off, and start over again the next day.

Get your nutrients. You need two servings a day of meat, fish, poultry, or meat substitutes like eggs, legumes, or nuts; two servings of dairy products (three for children and four for teenagers); four servings of fruits and vegetables; and four servings of breads, cereals, pastas, and other grains.

Cut the fat. Fat is where it's at if you want to target one enemy of your waistline. And cutting out high-fat foods can benefit much more than your figure—you'll lower your risk for heart disease and some cancers. Fat is nature's way of crowding a lot of calories—or energy—into food. A gram of fat (one-fourth of a teaspoon) contains nine calories, while a gram of protein or carbohydrate has four.

How much fat is too much? The average American is consuming about 37 percent of calories from fat these days, down from 40 percent a few years ago, says Deskins. The American Heart Association recommends that no more than 30 percent of your calories come from fat, while Mirkin says if you also want to really reduce cholesterol, you'll have to go much lower than that.

High-fat foods can fool you, too. "They're small in amount but high in calories," says Dwyer. Follow these pointers to cut the fat:

• Switch to reduced-fat or nonfat salad dressing.
• Buy nonstick pans and use a tiny amount of oil or nonstick spray.
• Eat less meat and cheese; both can be high in fat.
• Buy lean cuts of meat and trim the fat before cooking. Remove the skin from poultry.
• Don't fry. Instead, roast, bake, broil, or simmer meat, poultry, and fish.

• Choose low-fat dairy products, such as skim milk.
• Fill up your plate with vegetables, fruits, and grains, and don't drown them in butter.
• Experiment with spices; use them to add flavor to your foods.
• Avoid nondairy creamers and toppings, which often contain high amounts of saturated fats from palm or coconut oils.

Exercise. Even nutritionists agree: Exercise appears to be the key in losing weight. "The leanest people in this country eat the most food, but they're the most active," says Callaway.

Obviously, exercise burns calories. But according to some researchers, it may also increase your metabolism, possibly for as long as 18 hours after you've worked out, says Mirkin. So you end up burning more calories, even after your workout.

◆◆◆ Fat Kids ◆◆◆

It's very likely that television has contributed to the creation of a generation of fat kids. Obesity is on the increase among children.

Although following the weight-control guidelines for adults can certainly help, you may want some advice specifically targeted to kids:

Teach them how to select foods. *"If you can't change where they eat, then teach them to make more healthy choices," says Ted Williams, M.D., a pediatrician in private practice in Dothan, Alabama, and a media spokesperson for the American Academy of Pediatrics. Encourage them to choose pizza with vegetable toppings instead of meat toppings, get a cheeseburger made with ground turkey, use low-fat cheese, pick a whole-grain bun over white bread, get pasta instead of french fries, and so on.*

Set a good example. *Don't just tell them what to do, show them by adopting the same healthy habits.*

Give them low-fat milk. *Once your children are over the age of two years, encourage them to drink low-fat milk. Williams says that children who consume one to one-and-a-half quarts of whole milk a day are getting a large amount of saturated fat in their diet.*

Kick kids out of the house. *Get them to exercise— it doesn't have to be a structured program. Encourage them to play; they'll burn off calories and excess weight that way, whether they're biking or at the playground.*

Take the children with you while you exercise. *Make sure you're getting some exercise on a regular basis. Walking's one way. "Take the kids with you," Williams suggests.*

Don't become overzealous. *Some parents attempt to put their children on a low-fat diet too early in life. Children under the age of two years actually need a certain amount of fat in their diet for the proper development of the nervous system, Williams points out.*

The effects of adding exercise to your life will vary depending on how active you already are. If you're a couch potato, the benefits you'll get from brisk walking may surprise you. If you're already exercising occasionally, you may need more aggressive exercise like running or cycling.

Callaway stresses the need to first change your eating patterns before working on adding physical activity to your life. Once you feel comfortable with those changes, concentrate on the physical. Get help from your local YMCA or hire a personal trainer if you need advice.

Use these tricks to get your body moving:
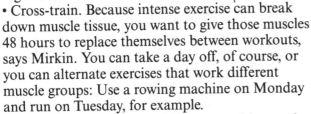
• Take the stairs instead of the elevator.
• Park farther away.
• Walk instead of riding or driving.
• Take several short walks if you can't fit one 30-minute workout into your schedule.

If you need more vigorous exercise:
• Cross-train. Because intense exercise can break down muscle tissue, you want to give those muscles 48 hours to replace themselves between workouts, says Mirkin. You can take a day off, of course, or you can alternate exercises that work different muscle groups: Use a rowing machine on Monday and run on Tuesday, for example.
• Alternate hard and easy. You can try this practice to avoid injury as well. Work out hard one day, easy the next: Run, then walk, for example. "Sixty-five percent of the people who take up running or aerobics quit within six weeks because of injury," Mirkin says. Alternating activities and intensity can help keep you from dropping out of exercise.
• Try strength training as well. "Lean body mass, or muscle, burns more calories," says Callaway. Aerobic exercise isn't the only way to lose weight. By including some resistance training in your program, you'll create more muscle mass. ◆

◆ Empty Promises ◆

Weight loss is big business in this country, with Americans spending more than $30 billion a year on various products and programs. It's an area ripe for quacks and frauds, who promise more than they can possibly deliver. In fact, the Federal Trade Commission has investigated the advertising and marketing claims of a number of diet products and programs over the last two years. Here's what John H. Renner, M.D., says to watch out for:

• *Words like "melt away," "no effort," "painless," "no exercise"*

• *Plans that promise excessive weight loss, such as a pound a day*

• *Programs that depend on artificial food or pills*

• *Claims that a food, such as grapefruit, possesses magical properties to get rid of excess weight*

• *Diets or gadgets that claim to cause weight loss from just one part of the body, such as the buttocks or chin*

• *Multilevel marketing plans that involve purchasing and selling products to people you know ("You shouldn't be buying your weight-loss products from your Sunday-school teacher," Renner points out.)*

• WRINKLES •

5 Ways to Fight Them

Wrinkles. Many of us dread the arrival of those lines, crinkles, and creases, but we know they'll etch their way into our faces sooner or later. You can't avoid aging, obviously, but it turns out that you don't have to end up with a prunelike complexion. If you follow some common-sense measures, you can prevent some wrinkling and continue to put your best face forward.

First, it's important to understand how skin ages and why we end up with wrinkles. One cause of skin aging occurs as the skin begins to wear out. "The skin thins out, the underlying fat disappears, and the skull actually begins to get thinner," says Melvin Elson, M.D., medical director of The Dermatology Center, Inc., in Nashville. "But that doesn't happen until very late in life, the seventh or eighth decade."

Most people think this intrinsic aging is the main cause of wrinkles, but it actually has a very small role. The big gun as far as wrinkle producers go is the sun. Getting a "healthy-looking" tan is anything but healthy for your skin. Another factor which comes into play over the years, moving everything downward, is gravity. "The corners of the lip are the first thing to come down, the eyelids fall, the jowl forms, the upper lip begins to disappear into the mouth, the tip of the nose begins to point down, and the ears get longer," says Elson. Sleep lines can add to your facial etchings, as can the facial expressions you've worn through the years. "Those lines occur simply from muscles pulling on the skin, when you laugh, cry, wink, blink, kiss, etc.," says Elson.

The following tips can help you minimize the effect of the wrinkle makers.

Wear a sunscreen every day. By doing this and shunning the sun from 10:00 A.M. to 2:00 P.M., "number one, you'll slow down the visible signs of aging and number two, you'll protect yourself from skin cancer," says Gary Rogers, M.D., associate professor of dermatology and surgery at the Boston University School of Medicine. Basking in the warm sun may feel wonderful, but the damage the sun's ultraviolet radiation

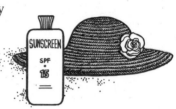

does to your skin is not. The sun does its dirty work by "injuring the scaffolding of the skin," says David J. Leffell, M.D., assistant professor of dermatology and chief of Mohs Surgery at Yale University School of Medicine in New Haven, Connecticut. The sun destroys both collagen (a fibrous protein) and elastin, found in the lower layer of skin. "The elastin fibers are blown away [by the sun]; they're fragmented into little snippets," says Leffell. This causes the skin to lose elasticity and form wrinkles.

How susceptible you are to sun damage depends on the kind of skin you inherited from your parents. Fair-skinned individuals burn more easily, while darker-skinned individuals have more of the pigment that protects against the sun's ultraviolet rays.

No matter what type of skin you have, however, your skin will thank you if you apply sunscreen every morning as part of your daily routine. And the sooner you start this habit, the better. "I have patients who have been especially protective of their skin or have avoided the sun, and their skin is relatively ageproof," says Leffell. Even more encouraging is a study of older people with sun-damaged skin who moved to a nursing home and stayed out of the sun. Researchers found that some of their wrinkles and blotchiness actually lessened, says Rogers. "If you protect yourself very conscientiously from the sun, you may actually be able to reverse some of the damage that you've already established."

Sleep on your back. Years and years of sleeping with your face pressed against the pillow can cause wrinkles. "It's like putting a napkin in a drawer.

When you take it out, you've got a crease in it," says Elson. Men tend to get sleep creases on the side of the forehead [on whichever side they snooze on], and women tend to get them on the cheeks, though they can appear anywhere, according to Elson. It may be a hard habit to break, but if you can train yourself to sleep on your back, you may end up with fewer facial lines.

Don't smoke. Not only can smoking cause cancer, but it can give you wrinkles. Donald Kadunce, M.D., and colleagues from the University of Utah Health Sciences Center in Salt Lake City studied smokers and nonsmokers. They found that premature wrinkling increased with cigarette consumption and the length of time the individual had been smoking. Heavy smokers were almost five times more likely to show excessive skin wrinkling than nonsmokers. The researchers speculate that smoking speeds wrinkling by damaging collagen. Squinting from smoke irritation can also cause or worsen crow's feet, and pursing the lips to puff on a cigarette can contribute to vertical lines around the mouth.

Moisturize. Using a moisturizer can temporarily improve the appearance of wrinkles by plumping up your skin, but it won't have a long-lasting effect. Moisturizers work by locking in moisture on the surface of the skin. Leffell says the optimal way to use a moisturizer is to apply it to wet skin and then pat your skin dry. (More and more moisturizers also contain sunscreen, so you get a double benefit).

Fine-tune your facial expressions. Some people often knot their eyebrows, frown, or crease their brow, and they've got the wrinkles to show for it. Often, we're not even aware of the expressions we make. If you watch yourself in the mirror and notice how you use your muscles to form expressions, you may be able to modify some of them, suggests Rogers. ◆

◆ Wrinkle-Fighting ◆ Myths

You may have heard one or more of the following suggestions for preventing or removing wrinkles. Unfortunately, they're simply wishful thinking.

Drink at least eight glasses of water a day. *The thought was that drinking that much water would plump up skin, so wrinkles wouldn't show as much. Absolutely bogus, says David J. Leffell, M.D. "The kidney closely regulates water intake. All that will happen if you drink eight glasses of water is that you'll go to the bathroom more."*

Skin massage can smooth away your wrinkles. *It's just not so. "Massaging the skin is no more effective at getting rid of wrinkles than massaging the scalp is at causing hair to grow," says Leffell.*

Hard scrubbing can rub away wrinkles. *The idea of using an abrasive cleanser or a "buff puff as an orbital sander to get rid of wrinkles is a mistake," says Leffell. "We've seen patients with very bad skin problems who have done that." Wrinkles are caused by damage below the skin surface, not on the top.*

◆ YEAST INFECTIONS ◆

12 Strategies to Beat Them

Most women are bothered at one time or another by the itching, burning, pain, and discharge that comes with a vaginal infection. Yeast infections can be caused by a number of organisms, many of which inhabit the healthy vagina. One of the most common causes of vaginitis is the fungus *Candida albicans.*

"Yeast infections are characterized by itching, caked discharge that smells like baking bread, and reddening of the labia and sometimes upper thighs," says Felicia Stewart, M.D., a gynecologist in Sacramento, California.

Yeast infections, especially recurrent ones, are a signal that your body is out of balance. *Candida* normally grows in a healthy vagina, but the slightly acid pH environment keeps *Candida* and other microorganisms from multiplying rapidly enough to cause infection. However, a variety of factors can make the body go "tilt" and alter the vaginal pH enough to allow one or more microorganisms to grow unchecked. The itching, burning, pain, and discharge are caused by the waste products of rapidly multiplying *Candida* (or other) organisms.

There are plenty of things that can throw your body out of balance. Many women find they are more vulnerable to yeast infection under these conditions:

• **Pregnancy.** The hormonal changes associated with pregnancy alter the vaginal pH and increase carbohydrate (glycogen) production, which provides food for infectious organisms.

• **Menstruation.** Some women report more yeast flare-ups just before or just after their menstrual period.

• **Antibiotics.** *Candida* live in the healthy vagina in balance with other microorganisms, especially lactobacilli. Tetracycline, ampicillin, and other antibiotics kill the vagina's lactobacilli and allow *Candida* to multiply, says Sadja Greenwood, M.D., assistant clinical professor in the Department of Obstetrics, Gynecology, and Reproductive Sciences at the University of California at San Francisco.

◆◆ Hello, Doctor? ◆◆

While mild cases of yeast infection can be effectively treated at home, Sadja Greenwood, M.D., says it's important to see a physician if:

• *You have abdominal pain.*

• *You have recurrent or significant amounts of bloody discharge between periods.*

• *The discharge gets worse or persists for two weeks or more despite treatment.*

• *You may have been exposed to a sexually transmitted disease.*

• *You have recurrent yeast infections. You may have diabetes or a prediabetic condition that is contributing to your yeast infections.*

• *Your discharge is thin, foamy, and grey or yellowish green in color.*

Some antibiotics, especially tetracycline, also appear to stimulate the growth of yeast organisms.

• **Diabetes or a high-sugar diet.** High blood sugar caused by diabetes or by a high-sugar diet can change vaginal pH and contribute to yeast infections. "Some women," says Stewart, "drink lots of fruit juice to prevent bladder infections. But fruit juice contains so much sugar, it may promote yeast infections."

• **Stressful times.** Doctors don't fully understand the stress/yeast connection, but many women report an increase in yeast infections during times of high stress.

While yeast infections can often be treated successfully at home, be sure yeast is the culprit. Other organisms, which require medical treatment, may be causing your symptoms. If the discharge is foul-smelling, yellowish, and frothy, you may be infected by one-celled protozoans called trichomonas or "trick." If you have a heavy discharge without much irritation and notice a fishy odor, particularly after intercourse, your symptoms may be caused by a bacterial infection doctors call "bacterial vaginosis." Bacterial infections are the most common cause of vaginitis. Both of these infections require treatment with prescription medication. In addition, symptoms similar to those of vaginitis may be caused by sexually transmitted diseases such as gonorrhea or chlamydia. *It's important to have your vaginal symptoms evaluated by a physician to ensure proper treatment.*

Many women who suffer from recurrent yeast infections have had their symptoms diagnosed by a doctor and know all too well the signs and symptoms of a yeast flare-up. If you're sure your vaginitis is caused by a yeast infection, try these home remedies:

Use a vinegar douche. At the first sign of infection, try douching with a mild vinegar or yogurt douche, suggests Stewart. For a vinegar douche, use one to three tablespoons of white vinegar to one quart of warm water; for a yogurt douche, make a dilute mixture of plain yogurt and warm water (see "Self-Care Douche").

Bring on the boric. Several studies have shown boric acid to be a safe, inexpensive, and effective yeast remedy. Amanda Clark, M.D., assistant professor of obstetrics and gynecology at Oregon Health Sciences University in Portland, suggests using boric-acid capsules as a suppository. "You can't buy the capsules already made up," she says. "Buy size 'O' gelatin capsules and fill them with boric acid. Then insert one per day vaginally for seven days." (Check with your pharmacist for the gelatin capsules and boric acid.)

Self-Care Douche

Routine douching isn't a good idea if you don't have vaginal symptoms. However, for women with yeast-infection symptoms, a mild vinegar douche can help restore the vagina's normal pH (which is about 4.5). Douching with yogurt that contains live lactobacillus or acidophilus bacteria may help restore the friendly microorganisms lost during infection or because of antibiotic use. For the best douche results, follow these easy steps:

1. Prepare the douche solution as outlined in the first remedy.

2. Make sure the container, tube, and irrigation nozzle are very clean. If not, clean them with a good antiseptic solution.

3. Lie in the tub with a folded towel under your buttocks and with your legs parted.

4. Suspend the container 12 to 18 inches above the hips.

5. Insert the nozzle into the vagina with a gentle rotating motion until it encounters resistance (two to four inches).

6. Allow the solution to flow in slowly. *Use your fingers to close the vaginal lips until a little pressure builds up inside. This allows the solution to reach the entire internal surface. An effective douche should take ten minutes or so.*

Boric acid hasn't been studied among pregnant women. If you're pregnant, Clark says to skip the boric acid. Instead, talk with your physician about other treatment options.

Use an over-the-counter fungal cream. Stewart says both miconazole (Monistat) and clotrimazole (Gyne-Lotrimin) are effective in treating yeast infections. They've recently become available in pharmacies without prescription. Use the suppositories nightly for three days or the cream once daily for one week. Don't stop using the medication when your symptoms subside. Use it for the full course. If recurrent yeast infections are a problem, try using one of these antifungal creams a few days before and/or after your menstrual period.

Try yogurt tabs. "Some women find relief using Lactinex (lactobacillus) tablets vaginally once or twice a day and douching with vinegar twice a day for two days," says Greenwood.

Wash out the secretions. The organisms that cause yeast infection produce secretions that are irritating to the genital tissues, says Clark. The nerve endings that sense the presence of the yeast are located at the vaginal opening. Although you may have an infection inside the vagina, you can often get symptomatic relief, she says, by simply washing away the secretions with water or with a douche.

Stay dry and loose. Yeast organisms like warm, moist conditions, with little or no oxygen. In order to deny them the perfect growing medium, be careful to dry your vaginal area thoroughly after bathing or showering. Avoid wearing tight, restrictive clothing that can hold in heat and moisture, and avoid lounging around in a wet

---

◆◆ Douche Danger ◆◆

The ads for douches admonish women to "feel fresh." And some women erroneously believe that douching after intercourse will prevent pregnancy (it doesn't). But new evidence shows that routine douching may be too much of a good thing and may actually do more harm than good.

Routine douching has been associated with an increased risk of pelvic inflammatory disease," says Felicia Stewart, M.D. "I don't recommend it."

Pelvic inflammatory disease, or PID, is an infection of the uterus, fallopian tubes, or ovaries. It can cause scarring of the fallopian tubes and result in infertility. If the infection spreads to the circulatory system, it can cause death.

According to a 1990 study in The Journal of the American Medical Association, *women who douched three or more times per month were three-and-a-half times more likely to have PID than women who douched less than once a month.*

The symptoms of PID include fever, chills, lower abdominal pain or tenderness, back pain, spotting, pain during or after intercourse, and puslike vaginal discharge. In most cases, a woman does not show all of the symptoms listed. If you have any PID symptoms, consult a physician immediately.

Not only has routine douching been associated with an increased risk of PID, some researchers believe it may increase a woman's risk of developing cervical cancer. A study that appeared in The American Journal of Epidemiology *showed that women who douched more than once a week were nearly five times as likely to develop cervical cancer as women who douched less often. The researchers suspect that vaginal secretions and normal vaginal bacteria may somehow protect the pelvic area and that routine douching may invite microbes that trigger cancer.*

The message is clear: While an occasional douche during an infection might be a good idea, don't make a habit of douching.

bathing suit for long periods of time. Opt for loose clothing and "breathable" cotton underwear and, if you must wear nylons, wear the type that has a cotton-lined panty or crotch.

Avoid harsh soaps, "feminine hygiene" sprays, and perfumed products. "Harsh soaps and hygiene sprays irritate the vagina and throw off its natural balance," says Susan Woodruff, B.S.N., childbirth and parenting education coordinator for Tuality Community Hospital in Hillsboro, Oregon. "Perfumed products contain alcohol that is drying to the tissues and hundreds of other chemicals that can cause irritation."

Rethink your contraception. Women who take birth control pills or use contraceptive sponges appear to be at greater risk for developing yeast infections. While researchers haven't established a cause-and-effect relationship between the Pill and yeast, some studies have shown that oral contraceptives increase the glycogen in the vagina (which provides more food for yeast reproduction).

Contraceptive sponges seem to be a yeast culprit, too. "We don't know exactly why contraceptive sponges increase yeast infections," says Stewart, "but we know they alter the vagina's normal ecology." If recurrent yeast infections are a problem for you, Stewart suggests considering an alternative birth control method like condoms, a diaphragm, a cervical cap, or an intrauterine device (IUD).

Have both partners treated. Sexual partners can play "Ping-Pong" with yeast infections by passing the infection back and forth unless both partners are treated. Often, men harbor yeast organisms, especially in the foreskin of an uncircumcised penis, but show no symptoms. When one partner is treated, the other should be treated to avoid reinfection, advises Woodruff.

Wash up and use condoms. Women with yeast infections should ask their lovers to wash up extra carefully before lovemaking. Couples who make love before the infection is completely cured should use condoms during intercourse.

Avoid routine douching. "The American culture is into cleansing," says Woodruff. "But the vagina doesn't need to be cleaned. It does that naturally. Routine douching upsets the vaginal pH and can actually cause yeast infections" (see "Douche Danger").

Practice good hygiene. While yeast is usually passed between sexual partners, Woodruff says it can also be passed to others like children through activities such as shared baths. To ensure you're not passing yeast, she recommends not bathing or sharing towels with your children, washing your hands frequently with soap and water, and washing your clothing in hot water. "The hot water in your washing machine should kill the yeast organisms present in your clothes," says Woodruff. "But if you're really worried about it, toss a cup of white vinegar into your rinse water." ◆

◆ INDEX ◆

A

Academy of General Dentistry, 40

Acetaminophen. *See also* Analgesics.
  and asthma, 30
  for back pain, 37
  for bladder infection, 50
  for breast discomfort, 57
  during breast infection, 62
  and bronchitis, 64
  and bruises, 66
  and bursitis, 71
  for canker sores, 72
  and colds, 89
  for denture discomfort, 109
  for ear infection, 135
  for fever, 148
  for flu, 158
  and fluid retention, 161
  for genital herpes, 176
  for hangover, 187
  and heartburn, 196
  and knee pain, 250
  and menstrual cramps, 261
  and neck pain, 272
  for shingles, 313
  for shinsplints, 316
  for sore throat, 327
  and stomach upset, 335
  for sunburn pain, 343
  for teething, 353
  for temporomandibular joint syndrome, 355
  for tendinitis, 356
  for toothache, 361

Acetic acid, 102

Acne, 12–15
  in adolescents, 12
  in adults, 12
  cystic, 15
  and diet, 15

Acne *(continued)*
  premenstrual, 12
  rosacea, 13
  treatments, 12–15
  vulgaris, 13

Acoustic neuroma, 301

Acupuncture, 85

Acyclovir, 91, 175, 312

Adenoids, 134

Adrenaline, 43, 217, 220

Aerophagia, 42

AIDS
  shingles in, 312
  virus, 111

Air conditioning
  in allergies, 18, 19
  for asthma, 27
  for heat exhaustion, 201

Air purifiers, 18, 27

Alcohol
  in asthma, 29
  in bladder infection, 49
  in bruising, 66
  and canker sores, 73
  and dry skin, 131
  and fever, 148
  in frostbite, 172
  in gout, 182
  and hangovers, 187–188
  and headaches, 192
  in heartburn, 196
  in heat exhaustion, 202
  and hypertension, 216
  and impotence, 222, 223
  and incontinence, 227
  and infertility, 233
  and insomnia, 238
  in irritable bowel syndrome, 243
  in laryngitis, 255
  in menopause, 256
  and motion sickness, 265
  and night terrors, 274
  and perspiration, 140

Alcohol *(continued)*
  in premenstrual syndrome, 292–293
  and snoring, 325
  in stomach upset, 334
  and ulcers, 366

Allantoin, 102

Allergies, 16–20
  black eyes in, 47
  and conjunctivitis, 96
  to cosmetics, 112, 113
  food, 17, 29, 218
  formaldehyde, 112
  latex, 111
  medication, 205
  PABA, 112
  patch testing for, 81
  pet, 19–20
  poison ivy, 286–288
  pollen, 18
  postnasal drip in, 289–291
  and snoring, 325
  symptoms, 16, 20
  treatment, 16–20

Amenorrhea, 282

American Academy of Dermatology, 372

American Academy of Otolaryngology, 133

American Academy of Periodontology, 178

American Council for Headache Education, 189

American Dental Association, 40, 330, 347, 348, 349, 351, 354

American Diabetes Association, 116

American Heart Association, 209, 210, 211, 212, 214, 217

American Podiatric Medical Association, 101

Amoebae, 123

Amphetamines, 197

Amputation, 118
in diabetes, 115
Analgesics. *See also*
Acetaminophen; Aspirin;
Ibuprofen.
for back pain, 37
in genital herpes, 176
for grinding teeth, 184
for headaches, 189
and infertility, 233
in shinsplints, 316
in sore throat, 327
in toothache, 361
Anaphylactic shock, 331
Anaphylaxis, 43
Androgens, 138
Anemia, 83, 151, 221
and hair loss, 185
iron deficiency, 73, 199
pernicious, 73
Anesthetic, topical, 313, 353
allergies to, 112
in cold sores, 91
for sunburn pain, 343
Angina pectoris, 317
Angiofibromas, 278
Antacids, 99, 194, 285
diarrhea-causing, 123, 194
for hiccups, 208
kidney stones and, 244
in stomach upset, 335
for ulcers, 366
Antibiotics, 30, 55, 80, 89, 90,
96, 135, 157, 285, 302, 364,
382. *See also* Medication.
in acne, 15
oral, 15
topical, 15, 235
Anticoagulants, 66
Antidepressants, 99
Antihistamines, 64, 89, 99, 135,
142, 238, 255, 291, 325
for allergies, 16, 20
for bites, 43
in dermatitis, 111
for hives, 218
for motion sickness, 265
for psoriasis, 296

Antihistamines *(continued)*
in restless legs syndrome, 299
topical, 111
Antiperspirants, 53, 78, 140,
169
Aphrodisiacs, 225
Arginine, 176
Arteriosclerosis, 278
Arthritis, 21–26
osteoarthritis, 21, 24, 183
rheumatoid, 21, 24, 74, 161
symptoms, 21
treatments, 21–26
Arthritis Foundation, 21, 22,
24, 26
Ascorbic acid, 102
Aspirin. *See also* Analgesics.
and asthma, 30
for back pain, 36
for bladder infection, 50
for breast discomfort, 57
for bronchitis, 64
and bruises, 65–66
for bursitis, 71
for canker sores, 72
for carpal tunnel syndrome,
76
and colds, 89
for cold sores, 91
for denture discomfort,
109
for fever, 148
for flu, 158
for fluid retention, 161
and food poisoning, 165
for genital herpes, 176
and gout, 182
and hangover, 187
and heartburn, 196
and hives, 218
and hyperventilation, 221
and knee pain, 250
and menstrual cramps, 261
and muscle pain, 268
and neck pain, 272
and nosebleeds, 277
for restless legs syndrome,
298

Aspirin *(continued)*
and Reye's syndrome, 135,
148, 158
and ringing in the ears, 301
for shingles, 313
for shinsplints, 316
for sore throat, 327
and stomach upset, 335
for sunburn pain, 343
and teething, 353
for temporomandibular joint
syndrome, 355
for tendinitis, 356
for toothache, 361
during weaning, 60
Asthma, 27–31, 32
allergic, 16
atopic, 27
and exercise, 30
medication, 197
and pets, 28–29
triggers, 27, 29, 31
Asthma and Allergy
Foundation of America, 19,
28
Astigmatism, 143
Atherosclerosis, 209, 213
Athlete's foot, 32–35, 150
medication, 33–34
symptoms, 32
treatment, 32–35

B

Back pain, 36–39, 336
prevention, 37–38
treatment, 36–37
Bacteria
in diarrhea, 123
oral, 108
pneumococcus, 96
staphylococcus, 54, 96
streptococcus, 96
Bad breath, 40–41, 179
Baker's Cyst. *See* Bursitis.

Balding, 185–186
  pattern, 185, 186
  treatments, 185–186
Barbiturates, 94
Bates Method, 143
Beau's lines, 151
Bed rest, 49, 63–64
  for back pain, 36
  in common cold, 88
Belching, 42, 156
Belladonna, 102
Benzocaine, 91
Benzoyl peroxide, 13, 15
Beta-blockers, 99
Bikini bottom, 234
Biofeedback, 293
Birth control.
    See Contraception.
Birth defects, 15
Bites, 43–45
  allergic reactions from, 43
  insect, 331–333
  snake, 44
Black eye, 46–47
Bladder control, 226–229
Bladder infection, 48–50
Bleeding
  as a cancer warning sign, 204
  in hemorrhoids, 203
  stopping, 44–45, 104, 105
Blindness
  in diabetes, 115, 119
  and hypertension, 214
  snow, 142
Blisters, 51–52, 80
  from burn, 68, 69
  fever, 72
  from frostbite, 172
  from genital herpes, 174
  in shingles, 312
  in sunburn, 341
Blood
  clotting, 66
  disease, 141
  disorders, 66
  pressure, 17, 50, 89, 99, 115,
    118, 125, 133, 181
  tests, 175

Body odor, 53
Boils, 54–55
Bone spurs, 21
Boric acid, 205, 383–384
Bowel
  irritable, 100, 124, 241–243,
    253, 335
  pattern, change in, 100
Breast
  cancer, 57, 258
  discomfort, 56–57
  engorgement, 56, 58, 59, 60
  fibrocystic, 56, 57
  infection, 59
  lumps, 57
  pump, 61
Breast-feeding discomfort,
    58–62
Breathing
  belly, 272, 317–318
  difficulty, 43
  exercises, 338
  hyperventilation, 220–221
  and stress, 338
Bromhidrosis. *See* Foot odor.
Bronchitis, 16, 63–64
  symptoms, 63
Bronchodilators, 30
Bruises, 65–67
Bruxism. *See* Grinding teeth.
Bun huggers, 78
Bunions, 168
Burns, 68–69
  prevention of, 69
  from the sun, 340–344
  treatment of, 68–69
Burping, 93. *See also* Belching.
Bursitis, 70–71

C

Caffeine
  in bladder infection, 50
  and breast pain, 57
  and constipation, 98

Caffeine *(continued)*
  in diarrhea, 124, 126
  diuretic effect of, 159
  and headaches, 192
  in heartburn, 196
  and heart palpitations, 198
  in incontinence, 227
  and insomnia, 238
  intolerance, 253
  in irritable bowel syndrome,
    243
  in menopause, 256
  and osteoporosis, 284
  and perspiration, 140
  in premenstrual syndrome,
    293
  in restless legs syndrome, 298
  in seasonal affective disorder,
    306
  in stomach upset, 334
  and stress, 337
Calamine lotion, 43, 110, 219,
    288
Calcium-channel blockers, 93,
    99
Calculus, 347
Calluses, 101–103, 168
  removal of, 102
Cancer, 100, 335
  bowel, 124
  breast, 57, 258
  cervical, 384
  colorectal, 204
  larynx, 255
  leukemia, 66
  lung, 64, 208, 217
  melanoma, 130, 151
  mouth, 309
  oral, 73
  skin, 82, 105, 130, 151, 295,
    342, 372
  uterine, 258
  warning signals, 124
Candida albicans, 382–385
Canker sores, 72–73
Carbohydrates
  and cholesterol, 211
  in diabetes, 115, 116–117

Carbohydrates *(continued)*
  fermentable, 347, 349
  in heartburn, 196
  and plaque, 347, 349
Carpal tunnel syndrome, 74–76
Casablanca crud. *See* Traveler's
  diarrhea.
Cellulitis, 34
Centers for Disease Control, 84
CFS. *See* Chronic fatigue
  syndrome.
Chafing, 77–78
Chalazion, 339
Chapped hands, 79–81
Chapped lips, 82
Charcoal, 156
Chicken pox, 148, 312
Chlamydia, 48, 383
Chlorhexidine, 53
Chlorine
  and conjunctivitis, 96
  and eye irritation, 142
  and skin chafing, 78
Chlorobutanol, 102
Chlorpheniramine maleate, 20
Cholesterol, 117, 118, 209–213
  and fiber, 212–213
  and heart disease, 209
  intake, 210
  levels, 212
Chondromalacia, 246
Chronic fatigue syndrome,
  83–86
  coping strategies, 83–86
  diagnosis, 83, 84
  symptoms, 83, 84
Clergyman's Knee. *See* Bursitis.
Climacteric. *See* Menopause.
Clotrimazole, 150, 384
Cold, common, 87–90
  medication, 89
  symptoms, 87
Cold sores, 72, 82, 91
  triggers, 91
Cold treatment
  in arthritis, 24
  for back pain, 36
  in black eyes, 46

Cold treatment *(continued)*
  in breast pain, 57
  in bruising, 65
  in burns, 68
  in bursitis, 71
  in carpal tunnel syndrome,
    76
  in conjunctivitis, 97
  for corns, 102
  in fluid retention, 160
  in foot pain, 167
  in headaches, 190
  in muscle cramping, 267–268
  for neck pain, 271
  for nosebleeds, 276–277
  in shingles, 312–313
  in shinsplints, 315
  in tendinitis, 356
Colic, 92–95
  medication, 94
Colitis, ulcerative, 124
Collagen, 66
  in arthritis, 21
  in scarring, 302
Colon, spastic, 241
Comedo, 14
Computers. *See also* Carpal
    tunnel syndrome.
  and eye irritation, 145
  and headaches, 189
Conception, 230
Condom dermatitis, 111
Conjunctivitis, 96–97, 141
  allergic, 96, 97
Constipation, 98–100, 125, 335
  and hemorrhoids, 203
  in irritable bowel syndrome,
    243
  treatments, 98–100
Contact dermatitis, 80
Contact lenses, 141, 143
Contraception, 161, 214, 261
  and bladder infection, 48,
    50
  condom dermatitis, 111
  oral, 12
  and yeast infection, 385
Contusions. *See* Bruises.

Corns, 101–103, 168
  hard, 101
  padding, 102
  removal, 102
  soft, 101, 102
Corticosteroids, 303
  nasal, 16
Cortisone, 141, 295–296
  for hives, 219
Cosmetics
  allergies to, 112, 113
  for dry skin, 131
  effect on acne, 12
  and fingernail problems, 152
  scar-covering, 303
  steroidal effects of, 57
  water-based, 281
Cough
  in bronchitis, 63
  in common cold, 87, 88
  drops, 64
  dry, 157
  productive, 159
  syrups, 64, 89
Crohn's disease, 73, 124
Cross-training, 250, 316, 379
Crying, in infants, 92–95
CTS. *See* Carpal tunnel
    syndrome.
Cumulative trauma disorders,
    74
Cushing's disease, 138
Cuticles, 151
Cuts, 104–105
Cystitis, 48
Cysts, 230
  ovarian, 230
Cytokines, 88
Cytotoxicity testing, 28, 29

D

Dairy products
  and cholesterol, 210
  in colic, 93

Dairy products *(continued)*
  in diarrhea, 126, 363
  in flatulence, 155
  in food poisoning, 165
  in heartburn, 195
  in hyperventilation, 221
  intolerance, 317
  in irritable bowel syndrome, 242
  in menopause, 258–259
  in stomach upset, 334
  and ulcers, 365
Dandruff, 106–107
Decongestants, 64, 87, 133, 135, 197, 221, 291, 325, 328
  nasal, 20
Deficiencies
  folic acid, 73
  iron, 73, 199, 299
  lactase, 155
  light, 304
  vitamin B_{12}, 73
Dehumidifying, 19
  for asthma, 27
Dehydration, 87
  in diabetes, 119
  in diarrhea, 123, 125, 363
  and fever, 148
  in flu, 159
  in food poisoning, 164
  in frostbite, 172
  and gout, 181
  in hangover, 187
  in heat exhaustion, 200, 202
  in incontinence, 227
  in laryngitis, 255
  in muscle cramping, 268
  in sunburn, 343
Delhi belly. *See* Traveler's diarrhea.
Denture
  adhesives, 108, 109
  care in diabetes, 120
  discomfort, 108–109
Deodorants, 53, 78, 169
Depilatories, 138
Depression, 83, 156, 256, 257, 292, 298, 304

Depression *(continued)*
  in chronic fatigue syndrome, 84
  stress-related, 337
Dermatitis, 110–114, 204
  allergic, 110, 112–113
  atopic, 113–114
  chronic, 129
  condom, 111
  contact, 80
  irritant, 110, 113
  seborrheic, 107
  treatment, 110–111, 114
Dextromethorphan, 64, 89, 159
Dextrose, 117
Diabetes, 115–120, 124, 169
  bad breath in, 41
  in children, 116
  and corns/calluses, 102
  foot care in, 119
  gingivitis in, 178
  and hair loss, 185
  and impotence, 223
  and ingrown toenails, 235, 236
  symptoms, 115
  treatment, 116–120
  Type I, 115, 116, 118
  Type II, 115, 116, 117, 118
  untreated, 115
  and warts, 372
Diamox, 238
Diaper rash, 121–122
Diaphragm. *See* Contraception.
Diarrhea, 123–126
  exercise and, 242
  in food poisoning, 164
  in infants, 125
  in irritable bowel syndrome, 241
  in lactose intolerance, 251
  medication for, 126
  from medication, 123
  in menstrual cramps, 260
  prevention, 362–363
  at-risk populations, 123, 125
  in stomach upset, 335
  traveler's, 123, 126, 362–364

Diarrhea *(continued)*
  treatment, 123–126, 363–364
  and vitamin C, 90
  watery, 362
Didronel, 284
Diet
  and acne, 15
  American Heart Association, 210
  antiheadache, 190–191
  and canker sores, 73
  and cholesterol, 209–211
  in chronic fatigue syndrome, 84
  and dandruff, 107
  in dermatitis, 114
  in diabetes, 116–117
  fasting, 85
  in irritable bowel syndrome, 242
  low-fat, 75, 118, 259
  low-purine, 182
  low-tyramine, 190
  in premenstrual syndrome, 292
  programs, 379
  in scarring, 303
  vegetarian, 211
  for weight loss, 375–379
Dilantin
  effect on acne, 12
  and gingivitis, 178
Diperodon hydrochloride, 102
Disease
  blood, 141
  cardiovascular, 22, 326
  celiac, 73, 124
  coronary-artery, 209
  Crohn's, 73, 124
  Cushing's, 138
  gum, 40, 178–180
  heart, 64, 115, 133, 259
  kidney, 115
  liver, 208
  Lyme, 43
  Meniere's, 300, 301
  Paget's, 284
  pelvic inflammatory, 384

Disease *(continued)*
  periodontal, 178–180, 183, 347
  pre-ulcer, 335
  rheumatic, 21–26
  sexually transmitted, 49, 50, 174–177, 230, 372, 383
  thyroid, 133, 141, 185
Diuretics, 98, 227, 255
  in gout, 182
  and hair loss, 185
  photosensitivity in, 343
Donnatal, 94
Douching, 383, 384, 385
Dramamine, 94, 265
Dreams, 238
Drugs. *See* Medication.
Dry hair, 127–128
Dry skin, 129–131
Dust mites, 18, 19, 27

E

Earache, 132–133
Ears
  cleaning, 345
  discharge from, 345
  and hearing loss, 132
  infection in, 64, 134–135
  pain in, 132–133
  perforated eardrum, 133, 300, 345
  piercing, 112
  ringing in, 300–301
  swimmer's, 134, 345–346
  wax in, 136, 300, 345
Eczema, 32, 34, 110–114, 153
Edema, 163
Electrocardiograms, 221
Electrolysis, 138
Embolism, 368
Emphysema, 64
Endogenous pyrogen, 146
Endometriosis, 230, 260
Endorphins, 192, 221, 293

Enzymes
  bromelain, 331
  lactase, 155, 251, 252
  papain, 331
Epilepsy, 223
Epsom salts
  for corns and calluses, 101
  for foot aches, 166
  for ingrown toenails, 235
Ergonomics, 76
Escherichia coli, 48
Esophagitis, 194
Estrogen, 56, 226, 256, 278, 282, 292, 293, 369–370
  replacement therapy, 258
Ethnicity
  and lactose intolerance, 251
  and scarring, 303
Excessive hair growth, 137–138
Excessive perspiration, 139–140
Exercise
  aerobic, 30, 215, 257, 261, 293, 306–307, 337
  after eating, 317, 318
  in arthritis, 21–22
  in asthma, 30
  for back pain, 38–39
  behavioral, 222
  breathing, 22, 36, 222, 338
  and bruxism, 184
  for carpal tunnel syndrome, 75
  and cholesterol, 213
  in chronic fatigue syndrome, 84
  and constipation, 98
  in diabetes, 116, 118–120
  eye, 143
  for feet, 167
  and headaches, 192
  for heartburn, 196
  and hemorrhoids, 205
  and hypertension, 215
  in hyperventilation, 221
  and incontinence, 228
  in infants, 95
  in irritable bowel syndrome, 242

Exercise *(continued)*
  isometric, 22, 273
  and kidney stones, 245
  for knee problems, 248–249
  in menopause, 257
  during menstruation, 260, 261
  neck, 272–273
  in premenstrual syndrome, 293
  range-of-motion, 21, 71
  relaxation, 193, 222, 338
  resistive, 229
  and stress, 337
  stretching, 22
  tests, 119
  and varicose veins, 367–368
  weight-bearing, 22
  and weight loss, 378–379
Extrasystole, 197
Eye
  astigmatism, 143
  black, 46–47
  blurred vision, 115, 141
  conjunctivitis, 96–97
  in diabetes, 115, 119
  drops for, 141, 142, 144
  dry, 96
  medication for, 97
  redness in, 141–142
Eyestrain, 143–145

F

Fatigue
  chronic, 83–86
  in diabetes, 115
  in flu, 158
  in premenstrual syndrome, 292
  stress-related, 337
Fats
  monounsaturated, 211
  polyunsaturated, 211, 217
  saturated, 210, 211

Feet
  aching, 166–168
  calluses, 101–103
  care in diabetes, 119
  corns, 101–103
  flat, 167
  odor from, 169–170
  overpronation, 247
  soaking, 101–102, 103
Fever, 146–148
  blisters, 72
  in children, 90, 146
  in common cold, 89
  in ear infections, 135
  in flu, 158
  and food, 148
  reading, 147
  rheumatic, 327
  scarlet, 327
  in sunburn, 341
  in teething, 353
  untreated, 146–147, 158
Fiber
  for colic, 93–94
  for constipation, 99, 100
  in diabetes, 117
  in flatulence, 155
  and hemorrhoids, 203
  in irritable bowel syndrome,
    243
  in stomach upset, 334
Fibroids, 230, 260
Fingernails, 149–152
  biting, 149
  clubbed, 151
  growth of, 150
  hangnail, 152
  infection, 150
  pitted, 151
  spooned, 151
Fissures, 153–154
  prevention, 154
  treatment, 153–154
Flatulence, 155–156
Fleas, 45
Flu, 157–159, 334
  analgesic use during, 148
  intestinal, 123

Flu (continued)
  myths, 158
  at-risk populations, 157–159
  shots, 157, 159
  symptoms, 157
  treatment, 158–159
Fluids
  balance of, 124
  in bladder infection, 49
  in bronchitis, 63
  in common cold, 87
  and constipation, 98
  in hangover, 187
  and hemorrhoids, 204
  intake in colds, 90
  in laryngitis, 254
  loss of, 148
  in postnasal drip, 291
  retention of, 57, 160–163, 293
  in stomach upset, 335
  for sunburn, 343
Fluoride, 284, 309, 349
Flushes, 256
Folic acid deficiency, 73
Folliculitis, 107
Food
  allergies, 16, 17, 29, 218
  asthma triggers, 29
  avoidance of irritating, 91
  bland, 126, 164, 364
  and body odor, 53
  and fever, 148
  in foot odor, 170
  and headaches, 190–191
  and heartburn, 195
  and hemorrhoids, 206
  as herpes trigger, 174
  in incontinence, 227
  intolerance, 16, 17
  in irritable bowel syndrome,
    242
  and motion sickness, 265
  and perspiration, 140
  and plaque, 349
  poisoning, 123, 164–165
Food and Drug
  Administration, 102, 186,
    205, 284, 330, 348, 373

Foot aches, 166–168
Foot odor, 169–170
Forefoot shock, 168
Formaldehyde, 112
Fragrances
  allergy to, 81
  insect-attracting, 333
Framingham Heart Study, 209,
    214
Frostbite, 171–173
  prevention, 172–173
  symptoms, 171
  treatments, 171–172
Fructose, 117
Fungus
  in asthma, 27–28
  trichophyton, 32

G

Gallbladder, 335
Gangrene, 118, 119, 171, 172
Gargling
  in bronchitis, 63
  in common cold, 88
Gas. See Flatulence.
Gastroenteritis, 123
Genes. See Heredity.
Genital herpes, 174–177
Giardia, 123, 364
Gingivitis, 178–180, 347, 348
Ginseng, 57, 85
Glands
  adrenal, 138, 185
  apocrine, 53, 139
  eccrine, 53, 139
  lymph, 55, 153
  mammary, 56
  oil, 12
  prostate, 48, 49, 50, 226
  sebaceous, 129
  sweat, 53, 129, 136, 139, 147,
    169
Glaucoma, 141, 143
Glucose, 115, 117

Glyceryl guaiacolate, 89
Glycogen, 266
Gonorrhea, 383
Gout, 21, 141, 181–182
    symptoms, 21
    treatment, 181–182
Grinding teeth, 183–184, 354
Griseofulvin, 34
Guaifenesin, 64

H

Hair
    analysis, 85
    brushing, 128
    dry, 127–128
    excessive growth of, 137–138
    ingrown, 234, 311
    loss of, 185–186, 336
    oily, 279
    thinning, 256
    vellus, 137
Halitosis. See Bad breath.
Hangnails, 152
Hangovers, 187–188
    prevention, 188
Hay fever. See Allergies.
HDL cholesterol, 118, 213
Headaches, 189–193
    cluster, 192
    diet in treatment of, 190–191
    migraine, 189, 192
    relaxation exercises for, 193
    stress-related, 336, 337
Hearing loss, 132, 135, 136
Heart
    arrhythmia, 146
    attacks, 209
    beat, 336
    conduction abnormality, 198
    disease, 64, 133
    disorders, 298
    failure, 214, 368
    palpitations, 197–199
    rhythm, 133

Heartburn, 194–196, 290
    in irritable bowel syndrome, 243
    symptoms, 194
Heat, and dry skin, 129–130
Heat exhaustion, 200–202
    in children, 202
    and medication, 202
    symptoms, 200, 201
Heatstroke, 201
Heat treatment
    in arthritis, 24
    for back pain, 36
    in bladder infection, 49
    for boils, 54
    in breast pain, 57
    in bruising, 65
    in bruxism, 184
    in frostbite, 171
    in headaches, 190
    for neck pain, 271
Heimlich maneuver, 195
Help for Incontinent People (HIP), 226
Hemorrhoids, 203–206
    external, 203
    internal, 203
    in pregnancy, 203
    prolapsed, 203
    treatment, 203–206
Herbal remedies, 28, 85, 87
Heredity
    in acne, 12
    in asthma, 27
    in athlete's foot, 32, 33
    and bruxism, 183
    and cholesterol, 209
    in chronic fatigue syndrome, 83
    and dry skin, 129
    in hair loss, 185
    and hemorrhoids, 203
    and hirsutism, 137
    and hypertension, 214
    kidney stones and, 244
    in menstrual cramps, 260
    in motion sickness, 264
    and psoriasis, 294

Heredity (continued)
    and sleepwalking, 323
    and sunburn, 340
    and varicose veins, 367
Hernia, hiatal, 194
Herpes virus
    and cold sores, 91
    genital, 174–177
    in pregnancy, 176
    in shingles, 312
    symptoms, 174
    triggers, 174
Hiccups, 207–208
    in infants, 207
    treatment, 207–208
High blood cholesterol, 209–213
High blood pressure, 214–217, 337
    and alcohol, 216
    and blindness, 214
    and heart disease, 209, 214
    and kidney failure, 214
    medication for, 215
    and nosebleed, 278
    in pregnancy, 214, 216
    treatment, 214–217
High-density lipoprotein. See HDL cholesterol.
Hirsutism, 137–138
Histamine, 87, 218
Hives, 218–219
    in allergies, 17
    in bites, 43
Hormones
    in acne, 12
    androgens, 138
    changing, 56
    estrogen, 56, 226, 256, 258, 278, 282, 292, 293, 369–370
    in gingivitis, 178
    imbalance, 178, 223
    insulin, 115
    melatonin, 304
    in menopause, 226, 256
    and oily skin, 280
    in pregnancy, 262
    progesterone, 292

Hormones *(continued)*
  progestin, 258
  regulating drugs, 161
  therapy, 56, 259
Hot flashes, 56, 256, 258
Housemaid's Knee. *See* Bursitis.
Human chorionic gonadotropin, 262
Humectants, 151
Humidifying, 81, 154, 159, 255, 277, 291, 297
  for asthma, 28
  in bronchitis, 63
  for dry skin, 130–131
Hydrocortisone, 43, 78, 105, 110, 205, 288, 344
Hydrogen peroxide, 104, 109, 330
Hypertension. *See* High blood pressure.
Hyperthermia, 85
Hyperthyroidism, 124
Hypertrichosis, 138
Hyperventilation, 220–221, 338
  in motion sickness, 264
  voluntary, 220
Hypoglycemia, 118, 292
Hypothalamus, 146, 147, 200, 201
Hypothermia, 173
Hysterectomy, 226

I

IBS. *See* Irritable bowel syndrome.
Ibuprofen. *See* Analgesics.
  and asthma, 30
  for back pain, 36
  for bladder infection, 50
  for breast discomfort, 57
  for bronchitis, 64
  for bruises, 66
  for bursitis, 71

Ibuprofen *(continued)*
  for canker sores, 72
  for carpal tunnel syndrome, 76
  for cold sores, 91
  for denture discomfort, 109
  for flu, 158
  for fluid retention, 161
  and food poisoning, 165
  for genital herpes, 176
  for gout, 182
  for grinding teeth, 184
  and heartburn, 196
  and knee pain, 250
  and menstrual cramps, 261
  and muscle pain, 268
  and neck pain, 272
  for shingles, 313
  for shinsplints, 316
  for sore throat, 327
  and stomach upset, 335
  for sunburn pain, 343
  for temporomandibular joint syndrome, 355
  for tendinitis, 356
  for toothache, 361
Ichthammol, 102
Imagery, 184, 242, 314
Immune system, 29
  in chronic fatigue syndrome, 83
  in common cold, 87
  infections and, 63
  in lupus, 21
  and smoking, 90
  vitamin C and, 89
Impotence, 222–225
Incontinence, 49, 226–229
  causes, 226
  overflow, 226
  reflex, 226
  stress, 226
  urge, 226
Indigestion, 334
Infection
  bacterial, 34, 48, 50, 63, 80, 82, 96, 97, 110, 254, 345, 353, 383

Infection *(continued)*
  in bites, 45
  bladder, 48–50
  from boils, 55
  breast, 59
  Candida albicans, 122
  in cuts and scrapes, 105
  in diaper rash, 122
  ear, 64, 132, 134–135, 345–346
  fever in, 146
  fingernail, 149, 150
  fungal, 32–35, 78, 149, 150, 154, 345
  inner-ear, 300
  middle-ear, 133, 134, 300
  parasitic, 124, 204, 364
  pelvic, 260
  secondary, 111
  sinus, 41, 64, 90, 289, 291, 319–320
  skin, 121
  strep, 297
  systemic, 297
  toenails, 150
  upper respiratory, 29, 30, 87, 157, 254
  urinary tract, 48–50, 245
  uterine, 384
  vaginal, 230
  viral, 123, 353
  yeast, 59, 122, 382–385
Infertility, 230–233, 384
  treatment, 230–233
Influenza, 148, 157–159. *See also* Flu.
Ingrown hair, 234
Ingrown toenails, 235–236
Inhalers, 16
Insomnia, 237–240
  stress-related, 337
  treatment, 237–240
Insulin, 115, 116, 117, 118
Interferon, 87
Iodine, 102
  effect on acne, 15
Iritis, 141
Irregularity. *See* Constipation.

Irritable bowel syndrome, 100, 124, 241–242, 253, 335
Isotretinoin, 15

J

Jock itch, 32, 78
Jogger's nipple, 77
Joints
 arthritis in, 21–26
 in bursitis, 70
 cartilage loss, 21
 and exercise, 21–22
 foot, 166
 immobilization, 182
 pain in gout, 181
 protecting, 24–26
 reducing strain on, 23
 temporomandibular, 132, 183

K

Ketoconazole, 34
Kidney
 disorders, 298
 failure, 208
 stones, 244–245
Knee pain, 246–250

L

Lactase deficiency, 155, 251
Lactation, 56
Lactobacillus, 126, 384
Lactose intolerance, 124, 155, 251–253, 283
La Leche League, 61
Lanolin, 81, 154
Laryngitis, 254–255

Laxatives, 99, 125, 243
 and hemorrhoids, 203, 204
LDL cholesterol, 213, 259
Leukemia, 66
Light
 deficiencies, 304
 in eyestrain, 143–144
 and seasonal affective
  disorder, 304–307
 sensitivity, 96, 97
 therapy, 304, 305
 ultraviolet, 34, 80, 82, 96,
  105, 295, 340, 342
Lips, chapped, 82
Lithotripsy, 244
Liver disease, 208
Low-density lipoprotein. *See*
  LDL cholesterol.
Lung
 in asthma, 27
 disorders, 298
Lupus, 21, 83
 and hair loss, 185
Lyme disease, 43
Lymphocytes, 87, 88
Lymphokines, 88

M

Malocclusion, 183
Massage, 22, 28
 for back pain, 37
 foot, 167
 in muscle cramping, 268–269
 in neck pain, 272
 scalp, 128
 in side stitch, 318
 in teething, 352
 in temporomandibular joint
  syndrome, 355
Mastitis, 56, 59
Measles, 185
Medication
 acyclovir, 91, 312
 allergy, 16, 20, 204

Medication *(continued)*
 antibacterial, 104
 antibiotic, 30, 55, 80, 89, 90,
  96, 135, 157, 235, 285, 302,
  364, 382
 antidepressant, 197, 223, 305,
  313, 314
 antifungal, 33–35, 78, 150,
  154
 anti-inflammatory, 36, 50,
  57, 62, 71, 76, 91, 135, 161,
  182, 250, 268, 272, 313, 356
 antiviral, 96, 175, 312
 asthma, 30, 197
 athlete's foot, 33–34
 attention deficit disorder,
  197
 for bites, 43
 for blisters, 51
 for boils, 55
 and bruising, 66
 canker sore, 72
 chemotherapeutic, 185
 for cold sores, 91
 colic, 94
 common cold, 89
 for constipation, 99
 constipation-causing, 99
 diaper rash, 121–122
 for diarrhea, 126
 diarrhea-causing, 125
 Dilantin, 12
 Donnatal, 94
 Dramamine, 94, 265
 and dry mouth, 350
 effect on acne, 12, 13
 hair loss, 185, 186
 heat exhaustion, 202
 hemorrhoidal, 204, 205
 hypertension, 215, 285, 290
 narcolepsy, 197
 for night terrors, 275
 phenobarbital, 94
 photosensitivity in, 343
 and psoriasis, 297
 sleep, 238
 thyroid, 197
 and yeast infection, 382

Meditation, 314, 336
Melanin, 340
Melanocytes, 340
Melanoma, 130, 151, 342
Melatonin, 304
Meniere's disease, 300, 301
Meningitis, 90
Menopause, 256–259
    and heart disease, 209
    hormones in, 56, 138, 226,
        256
    and osteoporosis, 282
Menstrual cramps,
    260–261
Menstruation
    acne in, 12
    canker sores and, 72
    cessation, 256
    changes, 256
    cramps, 260–261
    fluid retention, 57
    as herpes trigger, 174
    hormones in, 56
    irregular, 231
    and oily hair, 279
    and yeast infection, 382
Methylbenzethonium chloride,
    102
Methyl salicylate, 102
Miconazole, 33, 150, 384
Mildew, 28
Mink oil, 81
Minoxidil, 186
Moisturizers, 81, 114, 151, 281,
    344, 381
Mold, 19, 28
Moles, 372
Monoamine oxidase inhibitors,
    190, 197
Monocytes, 87
Mononucleosis, 83
Montezuma's revenge. See
    Traveler's diarrhea.
Morning sickness, 262–263
Motion sickness, 264–265
Mouthwashes, 40, 180
Multiple sclerosis, 83, 223
Muscle pain, 266–269

N

Narcolepsy, 197
Narcotics, 99
Nasal
    corticosteroids, 16
    decongestants, 20, 197, 277
    infection, 319–320
    mucus production, 87, 89
    polyps, 30, 289, 291
    sprays, 133
National Chronic Fatigue
    Syndrome Association, 83,
    85
National Headache
    Foundation, 189
National Institute of Diabetes
    & Digestive & Kidney
    Diseases, 251
National Institutes of Health,
    241
National Organization for
    Seasonal Affective
    Disorder, 305
National Psoriasis Foundation,
    294
Nausea, 270
Nebulizers, 277
Neck pain, 271–273
Nerves
    auditory, 300
    block, 313
    colon, 99
    compression, 75
    damage to, 74, 115, 118, 119
    phrenic, 207
    vagus, 207
Neuralgia, postherpetic, 312
Neuropathy, 118, 119
Nicotine. See Smoking.
Nifedipine, 161
Night terrors, 274–275, 323
Nodules, 15
    on vocal fold, 255
Nosebleeds, 276–278
Nursing. See Breast-feeding
    discomfort.

O

Oily hair, 279
Oily skin, 280–281
Onycholysis, 150
Orthotics, 247, 357
Osteoporosis, 56, 257, 258,
    282–285
Otitis media, 134
Ovaries
    cysts, 230
    infection of, 384
    polycystic, 138, 185
Overpronation, foot, 247
Ovulation, 230, 260
    prediction, 232
    suppression, 261

P

PABA, 112
Pacifiers, 95
Pain relievers. See Analgesics.
Pancreas, 115
Panthenol, 102
Parasomnia, 321–323
Penicillin, 89
Periodontitis, 178
Peristalsis motility, 242
Perspiration, excessive, 139–140
Petrolatum, 79, 80, 82, 91, 102,
    105, 127, 153, 154, 176, 205,
    277, 294
Petroleum jelly. See Petrolatum.
Phenobarbital, 94
Phenylpropanolamine, 118, 199
Phenyl salicylate, 102
Phlegm, 63
Photosensitivity, 343
Phototherapy, 295
Placebo effect, 85
Plaque, 41, 108, 180, 309,
    347–351
    in halitosis, 40

PMS. *See* Premenstrual syndrome.
Pneumococcus, 96
Pneumonia, 90, 157
  and bronchitis, 64
  and hair loss, 185
Poison ivy, 80, 286–288
  dermatitis in, 112
  myths, 288
  treatment, 287–288
Poison oak, 286–288
Poison sumac, 286–288
Pollen
  allergies, 18
  in asthma, 28
Pollution
  and conjunctivitis, 96
  effect on allergies, 17
  and eye problems, 141
  in sinusitis, 320
Polycystic ovary syndrome, 138
  and hair loss, 185
Polyps
  nasal, 30, 289, 291
  vocal fold, 255
Postnasal drip, 16, 42, 289–291, 319, 328
Potassium
  in muscle cramping, 267
  replacement, 165, 187, 201, 216, 334, 363, 364
  supplements, 85
PPA, 118, 199
Pregnancy, 230–233
  acne in, 12
  antibiotic use in, 15
  and bladder infection, 48
  and carpal tunnel syndrome, 74
  and dieting, 377
  and heartburn, 195
  and hemorrhoids, 203
  herpes virus in, 176
  hormones in, 56, 138
  hot baths during, 36
  and hypertension, 214, 216
  medication use in, 15
  morning sickness, 262–263

Pregnancy *(continued)*
  and oily skin, 280
  postnasal drip in, 289
  and snoring, 326
  and varicose veins, 367, 369
  and yeast infection, 382
Premenstrual syndrome, 292–293
Presbyopia, 143
Preservatives
  allergies to, 112
  in eye drops, 141
Progesterone, 262, 292
Progestin, 258
Prolactin, 233
Propranolol, 202
Prostaglandins, 87, 260
Prostatectomy, 226
Prostate gland, 48, 49, 50
Prostatitis, 48, 49, 50
Pseudoephedrine, 20, 89, 328
Psoriasis, 34, 107, 150, 151, 204, 294–297
  plaques, 294
  treatment, 294–297
Purines, 21
Pustules, 15

R

Rabies, 45
Radiation, 255, 350
Rectum, 154
Reflux, 194–196, 290
  in laryngitis, 254
Relaxation
  in asthma, 31
  in back pain, 37
  exercise, 222, 338
  and hypertension, 217
  progressive, 177, 184, 222, 241, 272, 355
  techniques, 193, 272, 355
Reserpine, 161
Resorcinol, 13

Restless legs syndrome, 298–299
Retin-A, 15
Retinoids, 15
Reye's syndrome, 135, 148, 158
Rheumatic fever, 327
Ringing in the ears, 300–301
Ringworm, 32
Rogaine, 186
Roughage. *See* Fiber.

S

SAD. *See* Seasonal affective disorder.
Salt. *See* Sodium.
Scabs, 104, 105
Scarlet fever, 327
Scarring, 302–303
  in acne, 15
Scleroderma, 124
Scopolamine, 265
Scrapes, 104–105
Seasonal affective disorder, 304–307
Seborrheic dermatitis, 107
Sebum, 12, 279
Sedatives, 94
Selenium, 186
Self-hypnosis, 313, 314, 322
Senile purpura, 66
Sensitive teeth, 308–309
Septicemia, 50
Serotonin, 306, 314
Sexual dysfunction
  erectile difficulties, 115
  impotence, 222–225
  infertility, 230–233
Sexual intercourse
  and bladder infection, 48
  and chronic fatigue syndrome, 86
  painful, 257, 384
  safe, 177
  urination following, 50

Sexually transmitted disease, 49, 50, 174–177, 230, 372, 382
Shaving discomfort, 310–311
Shingles, 312–314
Shinsplints, 315–316
Side stitch, 317–318
Simethicone, 156
Sinuses
   infection, 41, 64, 90, 289, 291, 319–320
   treatment in allergies, 17
Sinusitis, 133, 319–320
Skin
   aging, 380–381
   cancer, 82, 105, 130, 151, 295, 342, 372
   chafing, 77–78
   chapped, 79–81
   cracking, 78, 79, 153–154
   dermis, 340
   dry, 129–131
   in frostbite, 171–172
   itching, 80
   oily, 106, 280–281
   oozing, 78, 80
   plaques, 294, 295
   stratum corneum, 79, 129, 340
   in sunburn, 340–344
   swollen, 80
   wrinkles, 380–381
Skin Cancer Foundation, 342
Sleep
   apnea, 238, 323, 326
   deprivation, 298, 326
   disorders, 83, 237–240, 256, 274–275, 298–299, 321–323, 325–326
   REM, 238
   snoring, 325–326
Sleepwalking, 321–323
   in children, 323
Slivers, 324
Smoking
   in allergies, 17
   and asthma, 29
   and belching, 42

Smoking (continued)
   and bronchitis, 64
   and canker sores, 73
   and cholesterol, 213
   and colds, 90
   and ear infection, 134–135
   and eye irritation, 144
   and headaches, 192
   in heartburn, 196
   and heart disease, 209
   and heart palpitations, 198
   and hypertension, 217
   in incontinence, 227–228
   and infertility, 232–233
   in irritable bowel syndrome, 243
   in laryngitis, 254, 255
   and nosebleed, 278
   and osteoporosis, 285
   in scarring, 303
   and snoring, 325–326
   and stained teeth, 329
   and stress, 337
   and ulcers, 366
   and wrinkles, 381
Snoring, 238, 325–326
Society for Light Treatment and Biological Rhythms, 305
Sodium
   in breast pain, 57
   in fluid retention, 163
   in hypertension, 215–216
   intake, 210
   and kidney stones, 245
   in premenstrual syndrome, 293
   replacement, 363
Sore throat, 327–328
Sperm, 231
SPF. See Sun protection factor.
Spider veins, 367
Splinters, 324
Splints
   in temporomandibular joint syndrome, 355
   in tendinitis, 356
   wrist, 76

Sputum
   bloody, 63, 64
   loosening, 89
Stained teeth, 329–330
Staphylococcus, 54, 96
Steroids, 43
Stings, 331–333
   treatment, 331–333
Stomach upset, 334–335
   stress-related, 336
Streptococcus, 96
Stress, 336–338
   and acne, 12
   in asthma, 31
   and canker sores, 73
   in chronic fatigue syndrome, 83
   and dandruff, 107
   and excessive perspiration, 139
   and eyestrain, 143
   in flatulence, 156
   in foot odor, 170
   in gingivitis, 178
   in grinding teeth, 183, 184
   and hair loss, 186
   in headaches, 190
   in heartburn, 196
   in herpes, 174, 177
   in hyperventilation, 221
   and impotence, 222
   in infertility, 231
   in irritable bowel syndrome, 241
   job-related, 337
   management, 272, 293, 336–338, 366
   and night terrors, 275
   perceptions, 336
   positive aspects, 336
   and psoriasis, 297
   reduction techniques, 177
   in stomach upset, 335
   in temporomandibular joint syndrome, 355
   and ulcers, 365–366
   in yeast infection, 382

Stroke, 125, 214, 301
  and diabetes, 115
  and diet, 210
  symptoms, 217
Sty, 339
Sucrose, 117
Sulfites, 29
Sulfur, 13
Sun
  and acne, 13
  and dry skin, 130
  and psoriasis, 295
  and seasonal affective
    disorder, 307
Sunburn, 340–344
  from snow, 343
  treatment, 341–344
Sun protection factor, 15, 80,
  91, 105, 114, 130, 342
Sunscreens, 15, 80, 82, 91, 105,
  114, 130, 342, 380
Support groups
  in chronic fatigue syndrome,
    84
  herpes, 177
  irritable bowel syndrome, 243
  menopause, 258
Sweating. See Perspiration.
Swelling
  in fluid retention, 160, 162
  in frostbite, 171
  treatment, 65
Swimmer's ear, 345–346
Syphilis, 185

T

Tachycardia, 198
Tannic acid, 34, 62, 175
Tartar, 179, 347–351
Teeth
  abscessed, 360, 361
  aching, 360–361
  brushing, 41, 178–179, 180,
    329, 347–350

Teeth (continued)
  care in diabetes, 120
  clenching, 183–184
  dentin, 308–309
  dentures, 108–109
  disclosing tablets, 350
  enamel, 309, 329
  extraction, 108
  first, 352–353
  flossing, 41, 179, 329,
    349–350, 361
  grinding, 183–184, 354
  in infants, 352–353
  interproximal cleaners, 350
  loose, 179
  loss, 178
  oral irrigators, 350
  plaque, 40, 41, 108, 178, 180,
    309, 347–351
  porcelain laminate veneers,
    329
  pulp, 360, 361
  resin bonding, 329
  root–canal therapy, 360
  sensitive, 308–309, 360
  stained, 329–330
  tartar, 179, 347–351
  whiteners, 330
Teething, 352–353
Temporomandibular joint
  syndrome, 132, 143, 183,
    354–355
  symptoms, 354
  treatment, 355
Tendinitis, 356–357
TENS, 314
Testicles, 231
Tests
  blood, 175
  cardiovascular screening, 119
  cytotoxicity, 28, 29
  exercise, 119
  patch, 81
  Tzanck, 175
Tetanus shots, 45, 105
Therapy
  alternative, 85
  contrast, 268

Therapy (continued)
  dawn-simulator, 305, 307
  estrogen replacement, 258
  hormone, 56, 259
  light, 304, 305
  oral rehydration, 363
  ordeal, 358
  radiation, 350
  root-canal, 360
  sex, 222
Thermometers, 147
Thirst
  in diabetes, 115
  increased, 123
Throat, 132
  and laryngitis, 254–255
  sore, 88, 90, 289, 327–328
  strep, 90, 297, 327
Thrombophlebitis, 368
Thumb sucking, 358–359
Thyroid
  disease, 133, 141, 185
  disorders, 83
  medication, 197
  underactive, 100
Ticks, 44
  Lyme-carrying, 43–44
Tinea pedis, 32
Tinnitus, 300–301
TMJ. See Temporomandibular
  joint syndrome.
Toenails, 32, 34
  growth, 150
  infection, 150
  ingrown, 235–236
  trimming, 101, 167
Tolnaftate, 33
Tonsils, 132, 134
Toothache, 360–361
Tooth grinding. See Grinding
  teeth.
Tourniquets, 104
Transient ischemic attack
  (TIA), 217
Traveler's diarrhea, 123, 126,
  362–364
Tretinoin, 15
Trichomonas, 383

Triglycerides, 213, 301
Tryptophan, 306
Tumors
  angiofibromas, 278
  ear nerve, 301
  eye, 141
  fibroid, 230, 260
  ovarian, 138
  pituitary, 138
Turkey trot. *See* Traveler's
  diarrhea.
Tyramine, 188, 190, 192
Tzanck test, 175

U

Ulcers, 365–366
  duodenal, 194
  mouth, 73
  stomach, 194
  stress-related, 337
  treatment, 365–366
Ultraviolet
  light, 34, 80, 82, 96, 105, 295,
    340, 342
  polarized filters, 144
Undecylenic acid, 33
Urethral plugs, 228
Uric acid, 181, 245
  in gout, 21
Urticaria, 218–219
Urushiol, 286
Uterus, retroverted, 261

V

Vaginal
  burning, 111
  discharge, 382, 383, 384
  dryness, 256, 257
  infection, 230
  soreness, 258

Vaginitis, 115
Vaginosis, 383
Vaporizers, 28, 90, 131, 277
Varicose veins, 367–370
  pelvic, 260
  testicular, 231
Vaseline. *See* Petrolatum.
Viruses, 63
  AIDS, 111
  in chronic fatigue syndrome,
    83
  common cold, 87, 88
  contact, 174
  flu, 157
  herpes, 72, 91, 174–177,
    312
  human papilloma, 371–374
Vision
  blurred, 115, 141, 189
  changes in, 46, 141, 189
  in conjunctivitis, 96
  loss of, 217
Vitamin A, 81, 99, 102, 185,
  245
Vitamin B, 332
Vitamin B_6, 245, 263
Vitamin B_{12}, 73, 85
Vitamin C, 81, 87, 89, 90, 245,
  277, 373
Vitamin D, 99, 185, 283
Vitamin E, 81, 99
Vitamin K, 66, 99
Vomiting, 270

W

Warts, 371–374
  genital, 371, 372
  perianal, 204
  plantar, 371, 372, 373, 374
  treatment, 372–374
Weaning, 60
Weight
  in arthritis, 23
  in asthma, 31

Weight *(continued)*
  in carpal tunnel syndrome,
    74, 75
  in diabetes, 116, 117
  in fluid retention, 163
  in foot strain, 167
  gain, 375–379
  in gout, 181, 182
  in heat exhaustion, 202
  and hemorrhoids, 203, 206
  and hypertension, 215
  in incontinence, 227
  and knee problems, 247
  loss in diabetes, 115
  in neck pain, 272
  and osteoporosis, 282–283
  and perspiration, 140
  and psoriasis, 297
  and skin chafing, 77
  and snoring, 325
  and varicose veins, 368
Whirlpools, 23, 24, 231
Wipes, baby, 121
Wounds, puncture, 45
Wrinkles, 380–381

Y

Yeast infections, 382–385

Z

Zostrix, 314